Michael Stolberg
Learned Physicians and Everyday Medical Practice in the Renaissance

Michael Stolberg

Learned Physicians and Everyday Medical Practice in the Renaissance

Translated by
Logan Kennedy and Leonhard Unglaub

DE GRUYTER
OLDENBOURG

Revised version of „Gelehrte Medizin und ärztlicher Alltag in der Renaissance", De Gruyter: Berlin/Boston 2021, translated by Logan Kennedy and Leonhard Unglaub.

ISBN 978-3-11-127079-1
e-ISBN (PDF) 978-3-11-073354-9
e-ISBN (EPUB) 978-3-11-073362-4
DOI https://doi.org/10.1515/9783110733549

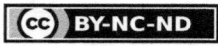

This work is licensed under the Creative Commons Attribution-NonCommercial-NoDerivatives 4.0 International License. For details go to http://creativecommons.org/licenses/by-nc-nd/4.0/.

Library of Congress Control Number: 2021943168

Bibliografische Information der Deutschen Nationalbibliothek
Die Deutsche Nationalbibliothek verzeichnet diese Publikation in der Deutschen Nationalbibliografie; detaillierte bibliografische Daten sind im Internet über http://dnb.dnb.de abrufbar.

© 2023 Michael Stolberg, published by Walter de Gruyter GmbH, Berlin/Boston
This volume is text- and page-identical with the hardback published in 2022.
The book is published open access at www.degruyter.com.

Cover image: Egbert van Panderen (1581-1637?), Physician (from: "The medical practitioner as Christ, angel, man and devil"), Wellcome Collection, London
Typesetting: Integra Software Services Pvt. Ltd.
Printing and binding: CPI books GmbH, Leck

www.degruyter.com

Contents

Introduction —— IX

Part I: Entering the World of Learned Medicine

Prologue: The "Learned" Physician. On the History of an Ideal —— 3

Choosing a Profession —— 11

The Study of Medicine —— 24
    Theoretical Medicine —— 32
    Practical Medicine —— 37
    Bedside Teaching —— 42
    Anatomy —— 60
    Pharmacy and Botany —— 67
    Surgery —— 73

Learned Habitus —— 82
    Poetry —— 84
    The *album amicorum* —— 89
    Letter Writing —— 92
    Historiography and Ethnography —— 99
    Loci Communes —— 104
    Scholarly Self-Fashioning —— 110

Part II: Learned Medical Practice

From theory to practice —— 117

Pathology —— 121
    Morbid Matter, Fluxes, and Obstructions —— 122
    Preternatural Heat —— 132
    Infection —— 135
    Obstructed Excretions —— 138
    The Myth of Humoral Imbalance —— 140

External Causes of Illness —— 146
    Environment and Lifestyle —— 146

The Moon, Stars, and Seasons —— 150

Diagnosis —— 155
    The Patient's Narrative —— 155
    Uroscopy —— 158
    Coproscopy —— 167
    Sputum and other Excretions —— 169
    Hematoscopy —— 170
    Pulse Diagnosis —— 173
    Physical Examination —— 176

Therapeutic Practice —— 181
    Cleansing and Purgative Remedies —— 183
    Bloodletting and Cupping —— 189
    Cauterization —— 200
    Sweating —— 201
    Thermal Springs and Healing Waters —— 202
    Dietetics: Eating, Way of Life, Emotions, and Sexuality —— 204
    Surgery —— 214

Diseases —— 221
    Fevers —— 226
    Consumption —— 241
    Gout and Podagra —— 247
    Stone Disease —— 255
    Cancer —— 265
    Dropsy —— 268
    Falling Sickness —— 273
    Apoplexy and Paralysis —— 278
    Melancholy and Madness —— 282
    The French Disease —— 289
    Toothaches —— 307

Pediatrics —— 316

Diseases of Women —— 323
    Disordered Menstruation —— 327
    Suffocation of the Womb —— 334
    Conception and Pregnancy —— 345

Birth and Childbed —— 351

Knowledge from Experience: The Rise of Empiricism —— 357
    Empirica, Experimenta, and Secret Remedies —— 360
    Paracelsianism and Chymical Medicines —— 363
    Experimental Drug Trials —— 377
    Case Histories: Observation at the Bedside —— 386
    Self-Observation: The Physician's Body as a Source of Knowledge —— 390
    Post-mortems —— 392
    Facticity —— 401
    Medicine and the "Scientific Revolution" of the Seventeenth Century —— 404

Part III: Physicians, Patients, and Lay Medical Culture

The rise of the learned medical profession —— 409

Private Practice —— 410

Municipal Physicians —— 414

Court Physicians —— 423

Everyday Practice —— 438
    The Physicians' Clientele —— 438
    Routines and Practices —— 442
    Epistolary Medical Practice —— 444

The Physician-Patient Relationship —— 447
    Interactions —— 448
    Authority in Jeopardy —— 455
    Diagnostic and Prognostic Uncertainty —— 457
    Money —— 463
    Self-Confident Patients —— 469
    Bitter Pills —— 475
    Strong-Willed Patients —— 477
    Undesirable Effects —— 482
    The Sense of Shame —— 485
    "Bystanders" and Caregivers —— 489

The Incurably Ill and the "Cura Palliativa" —— **495**
At the Deathbed —— **503**

Alternatives to Medical Treatment by Physicians —— **507**
Self-Treatment and Domestic Medicine —— **507**
Barbers and Barber-Surgeons —— **513**
Lay Healers —— **518**

Learned Physicians and Lay Medical Culture —— **524**
Learning from Laypeople —— **524**
A Shared World? —— **528**
Witchcraft and Magic —— **535**

Conclusion —— **544**

Sources

Visual sources – List of illustrations —— **553**

Manuscript Sources —— **555**

Printed Works —— **559**

Index —— **603**

Introduction

This book has a protagonist most readers will likely never have heard of. His name is Georg Handsch. He was born in 1529 in Leipa, today's Česka Lipa, a small prosperous town approximately eighty kilometers north of Prague.[1] He would return to this town shortly before his death in February of 1578. On his life's journey, which led him from Leipa to Goldberg, Prague, Padua, and finally Innsbruck, he collected a number of achievements. He studied medicine in Padua and earned his doctoral degree in Ferrara. Though not as their equal, he was in the company of some of the famous scholars and physicians of his time, including Matthaeus Collinus, the figure-head of the Bohemian humanism, and the well-known physician and botanist Pietro Andrea Mattioli. In the end, probably thanks to the advocacy of Mattioli, he gained the position of court physician for the Habsburg Archduke Ferdinand II.

Handsch remains a largely unknown figure, even among medical historians.[2] Apart from his German translation of Mattioli's famous work on medicinal plants,[3] he did not publish a single book, and even this translation was soon to be replaced by a new German edition put out by Joachim Camerarius.[4] No important medical discovery and no exciting new theory is connected with his name – not even his portrait has survived. In all his life, he was not able to establish a lucrative practice of his own nor a household. Even his appointment as a physician at the Habsburg court in Ambras near Innsbruck was less glorious than one might assume. By contemporary standards, the court was of moderate size (see Fig. 1).[5] While renowned physicians at the time were able to acquire considerable wealth, Handsch was denied such fortune. He never married and never owned his own home, living as a tenant or guest in the houses of strangers all his life. When he died, his total monetary assets amounted to only about 600 gulden. Other physicians earned this sum, and sometimes a lot more, in a year.[6]

---

[1] On the inside of the book cover of one of his notebooks (Cod. 9671) Handsch gave the date of his birth as 20 March 1529; on Leipa, its history, and the local archival documentation (which was largely destroyed by fire) see Schober/Neder, Sechshundertjahrfeier (1929); Bienert, Böhm[isch] Leipa ([around 1937]).
[2] For example, Josef Vinař, in his survey of Czech medical history, refers to Handsch in passing only as the translator of Mattioli's herbal (Vinař, Obrazy (1959), p. 111); Hlaváčková/ Svobodný, *Dějiny lékařství* (2004) do not mentioned him at all.
[3] Mattioli, Commentarii (1554); Mattioli, New Kreutterbuch (1563).
[4] Mattioli, Kreutterbuch (1586).
[5] Hirn, Ferdinand II. (1887), p. 467.
[6] Letter by Jakob Schrenck von Notzing, 15 May 1579. According to the calculations by the archducal treasurer, Handsch bequeathed 592 fl. to his heirs. From this money some debts in

Open Access. © 2022 Michael Stolberg, published by De Gruyter. This work is licensed under the Creative Commons Attribution-NonCommercial-NoDerivatives 4.0 International License.
https://doi.org/10.1515/9783110733549-203

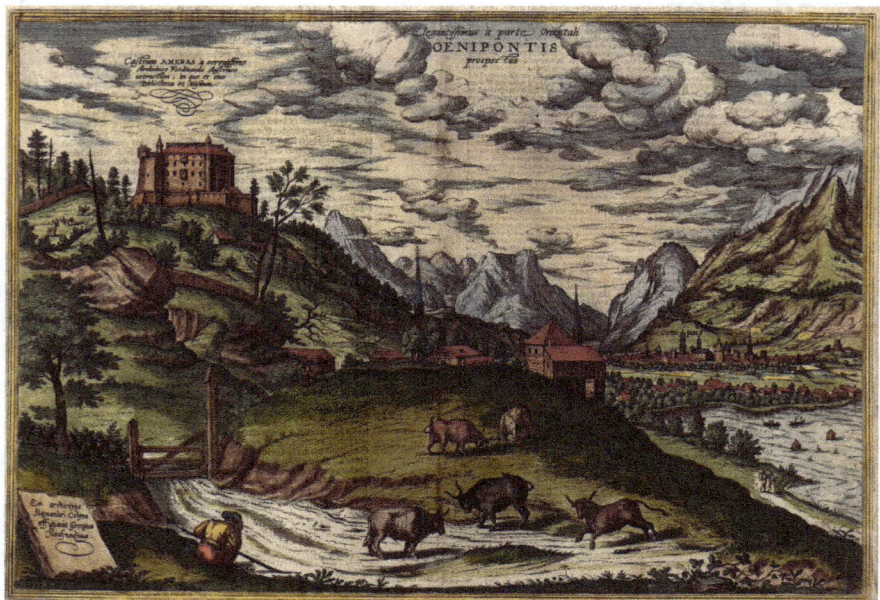

Fig. 1: Joris Hoefnagel, Innsbruck with the castle of Ambras (after Alexander Colin), in: Civitates Orbis Terrarum, part 5, Cologne 1598, n°58.

At this point, the reader may wonder: what could justify putting this clearly rather insignificant physician into the center of a monograph – and a rather voluminous one, for that matter? The question is valid but it already holds part of the answer: the major works, discoveries and theories of the leading medical authorities in the Renaissance have been quite thoroughly examined. Nancy Siraisi, Ian Maclean, Katherine Park, Jerome Bylebyl, Vivian Nutton, and Andrew Wear, to mention only some central authors, have published valuable studies: about the genesis and reception of individual ancient texts and authors, about the work of outstanding physicians and anatomists, and about the great theoretical debates of the period.[7] However, a perusal of the relevant literature also reveals a serious research gap: our knowledge about the working life of ordinary physicians, about their practice and experiences is very limited. We remain largely in the dark about the ways in which they applied the theoretical knowledge we find in the

---

Innsbruck would still have to be paid and the value of Handsch's library had to be added. Furthermore, according to Handsch's will he owned several cups made of silver or covered with gold, clothes and bedding and had inherited half of his father's house in Leipa.
7 See the bibliography.

publications of a small elite of leading authors in their daily work at the sickbed. Hardly any research has been done on how they explained and treated the most commonly diagnosed diseases and on their day-by-day interactions with their patients and with their competitors.[8]

Not least of all, this is due to the lack of suitable sources. It is only in rough outlines that we can reconstruct the working life of physicians from the medical publications of the time. And as opposed to later periods, personal notes, diaries, practice journals and similar sources that could give us more detailed insights into physicians' everyday medical practice during this period are scarce.

This brings us to the central reason for making Georg Handsch, as historically insignificant as he may be, the protagonist of this book: Handsch liked to write. He wrote a lot – a whole lot in fact – and much of what he wrote has survived. Close to thirty manuscript volumes from his pen, some of them counting more than a thousand pages, have been preserved in the Austrian National Library in Vienna.[9] Handsch's *Nachlass* comprises a broad spectrum of writings, ranging from an unpublished, multi-volume *Historia animalium* to the draft for a *Compendium medicinae*, dated 1558,[10] to a compilation of selected letters by his hand. A number of personal notebooks about the study of medicine and medical practice stand out among his manuscripts, however. On more than 4,000 pages, he wrote about all kinds of things he deemed noteworthy and worth remembering. Notes on lectures and on anatomical dissections he had

---

8 Even Laurence Brockliss and Colin Jones in their magisterial reconstruction of the "medical world of early modern France" had to limit themselves to scarce anecdotical evidence when it came to the physicians' ordinary medical practice and their interactions with patients and their families, in this early period (Brockliss/Jones, Medical world (1997), esp. pp. 284–344).
9 Codd. 9550, 9607, 9650 9666, 9671, 9821, 11006, 11130, 11141–3, 11153, 11158, 11183, 11200, 11204–11208, 11210, 11226, 11231, 11238–40 and 11251; in addition, Handsch owned student notes on Augustinus Schurff's lectures in Wittenberg in 1537 (Cod. 11228). In a supplication to the Archduke, Handsch's last servant Matheus Pärtl also mentioned two notebooks bound in green parchment which Handsch left behind in Bohemia, i.e. presumably in Leipa; according to Pärtl, they offered an "extract" from the other notebooks and Handsch valued them highly (Tiroler Landesarchiv Innsbruck, Ferdinandea, supplication, not dated but with an administrative note referring to 19 June 1578). It seems that these two notebooks are lost.
10 Cod. 11208; the title on the cover reads "Compendium medicum me authore". Handsch added a short: "Compositus est hic liber a me Doct. Georgio Handschio, Pragae, Anno 1558 ad informationem M. Georgii a Sudetis". Numerous corrections and the rather careless handwriting leave little doubt that it is a mere draft. In terms of content, the text is largely limited to dietetics, fevers and pharmaceutics. Georgius Polenta a Sudetis was dean of the philosophical faculty in Prague in 1557/58 and later turned towards medicine (Kalina von Jätenstein, Nachrichten, vol. 1 (1818), pp. 48–52). It is not known whether he ever received such a compendium from Handsch.

witnessed as a student are found next to entries relating diagnostic and therapeutic observations and experiences. Without any transition, the remarks of medical colleagues about the healing power of certain plants or the value of particular diagnostic signs are followed by notes about things he heard from barber-surgeons and lay healers or from patients and other laypeople. Not least of all, Handsch described countless clinical cases that his teachers in Prague and Padua dealt with as well as many others which he himself and his colleagues later treated in and around Prague and Innsbruck. In this way, his notebooks came to contain not only his own experiences and observations vis-à-vis his patients but also those of a whole array of famous and lesser-known colleagues around him.

For the most part, Handsch's entries are very short. Frequently they extend, at best, over half a dozen lines. Much more rarely, he went into some detail on certain topics or traced the course of a person's disease as it unfolded day by day. Some of his notebooks also contain striking other elements. In hundreds of entries, Handsch recorded verbatim, mostly in German, the terms and expressions used by physicians to explain a medical condition to patients and their families. And again and again, the notes give patients and their relatives a voice in the notes, relating their ideas about the disease process, their desires and demands, as well as their perception of the medical treatment.

What makes Handsch's notebooks all the more valuable is that they were clearly intended only for his personal use and not written with an eye to publication. Apart from several lectures he transcribed and his accounts of anatomical demonstrations, his entries are for the most part unsystematic and disorganized. Handsch simply wrote down, more or less on a daily basis it seems, what he heard and saw, learned and experienced as it happened. Some of it was clearly not intended for the eyes of others. With unsparing candor, he regularly referred to mistakes and errors he and his colleagues made in diagnosing and treating illnesses and in dealing with patients. Quite often, he even highlighted these entries in the margin, with words like "error" or "errores mei".[11] He also repeatedly mentioned his hematophobia: he could barely stand the sight of blood.[12] This was a problem for a doctor because carefully examining the blood from bloodlettings was an important and widely practiced diagnostic procedure in those days. He even described arousing sexual dreams in which he was with another man,[13] and occasionally he noted actual sexual encounters he had had with men.[14] At a

---

11 E.g. Cod. 11183, fol. 70v, fol. 77v, fol. 176v and fol. 391v; Cod. 11205, fol. 333v.
12 Cod. 11183, fol. 85r.
13 Cod. 11205, fol. 481v, "attrectationem iuvenilis membri ad meum et mihi exire sperma".
14 Cod. 11183, fol. 59v: "Ter manuduxi cum Venceslao Sseliha, in Maio".

time when same-sex sexual contact was considered a serious sin and offence, he would have had to fear grave consequences if this had become known.

Handsch did not offer an explicit explanation of what drove him to fill one notebook after the other with many thousands of entries. Despite some very personal entries, it would be rather far-retched to interpret them as evidence of the frequently invoked rise of the individual during the Renaissance period.[15] Handsch as a person – his view of the world, his social relationships or his creed – is not at the center of these records. Notes about medical observations and experiences, about things he heard and read during his studies, in his everyday work as a doctor and later in his encounters with patients and other professional healers predominate by far. It appears that the driving force behind Handsch's writing was a concrete, practical interest. His notes were meant to help him become a good and successful doctor. This emerges above all from the many detailed entries about different patients and their treatment and from his recurring attempts to derive general lessons from experiences with individual cases of illness. In their own way, as we will see, Handsch's notebooks also document the growing appreciation for empirical knowledge in sixteenth-century learned medicine.[16]

The fact that Handsch's notebooks have survived at all is thanks to a concurrence of circumstances, fortunate for historical research but less so for Handsch and his heirs. Having experienced "a severe weakness of the body" in 1576,[17] Handsch travelled from Innsbruck to his birthplace of Leipa in the winter of 1577–78, where he died on February 25, 1578.[18] Historical studies on Handsch have so far claimed that Handsch sold his library to Archduke Ferdinand II before he died,[19] but this is disproven by the surviving records. A mere eight days before his death, Handsch, while in Leipa, hundreds of miles from Innsbruck, stipulated in his will that his "Liberay" in Innsbruck be sold and the money divided up between his siblings and other named heirs.[20] Handsch did

---

15 Burckhardt, Cultur (1860), esp. pp. 131–170 (section 2, "Entwicklung des Individuums"); Burke, Individuality (1998).
16 Stolberg, Empiricism (2013).
17 Tiroler Landesarchiv Innsbruck, Kopialbuch Geschäft vom Hof, 1576, foll. 501r-502r.
18 The date of Handsch's death emerges from a letter by the mayor of Leipa, Wolff Heubner, to Archduke Ferdinand II, 6 April 1579 (Tiroler Landesarchiv Innsbruck, Ferdinandea 164).
19 Hirn, Ferdinand II., vol. 1 (1885), pp. 362–3 and vol. 2 (1885), p. 440; Beer, Philippine Welser (1950), p. 86.
20 Tiroler Landesarchiv Innsbruck, Ferdinandea 164, copy of Handsch's will, February 17. This passage is missing in the second will Handsch, which he wrote only a few days later, but he now bequeathed the "best" ten books from his "Lyberey" to a *studiosus* (ibid.); see also Panáček, Testament (2013), who only mentions this second will. Since Handsch not only left his

not sell his books and manuscripts to the Archduke. Documents from the archducal archives show that the Archduke took them for his library at Ambras Castle, paying half of their estimated value.[21] This also explains why Handsch's notebooks entered the archducal collection despite some of their very personal and compromising entries that were obviously not intended for the eyes of the ruler and his court. If Handsch had sold his books and manuscripts to the Archduke before travelling to Leipa, he could have easily separated the notebooks out.[22]

I discovered Handsch's notebooks while carrying out systematic research on early modern medical manuscripts in the Austrian National Library. A look at the older literature in the field quickly revealed, however, that the existence of these notebooks had long been known to historians who were researching the court of Archduke Ferdinand II. More than a century ago, Josef Hirn praised them as a rich source "for knowledge about the culture and courtly life of their time".[23] For good reason, no one had systematically and comprehensively read and analyzed the entire corpus, however. The handwriting of Handsch is relatively tidy and most of it is quite legible to the trained eye (see Fig. 2). His Latin is fairly easy to read and largely free of error. The abbreviations and ligatures he used, like most scholars in his day, to represent doubled letters, conjunctions, and above all common endings such as "-orum" and "-entes" usually can be decoded reliably. Only some of the proper nouns and some of the numerous marginal notes he added later pose considerable paleographic challenges. And yet, simply reading the far more than 4,000 pages of notes, along with the

---

books behind, in Innsbruck, but also his clothes and bedding he clearly intended to return to Innsbruck and had no reason to sell his library before his departure.

21 Tiroler Landesarchiv Innsbruck, Ferdinandea 164, letter from Jakob Schrenck von Notzing to Archduke Ferdinand II, dated 16 May 1579; according to Schrenck, the value of the books had been estimated at more than 200 gulden and the Archduke had "approved" to pay 100 gulden. for them, which Schrenck now listed as part of Handsch's estate. Handsch, Schrenck added, had not been able to enjoy the allowance of 200 gulden the Archduke had promised him for the time after his retirement as a court physician. According to Hirn (Hirn, Ferdinand II. (1887), p. 440 (note)), the Archduke usually had the rooms sealed when someone connected to the court died and made Schrenck come and select the books he wanted to acquire for his archducal library; on Schrenck see Heigel, Schrenck von Notzing (1891).

22 After Ferdinand's death, his son Karl sold the library to Emperor Rudolf II. In 1665, Emperor Leopold I. ordered a large part of the books and manuscripts, including those of Handsch, to be brought from Ambras to Vienna (Purš, Bibliothek (2017); Lambeck, Commentariorum liber, vol. 2 (1769), coll. 697–704, col. 926, col. 930 and col. 933).

23 Hirn, Erzherzog Ferdinand II. (1885), p. 363; in his biography of Ferdinand II, Hirn repeatedly mentions Handsch and uses his notebooks as a source but does not provide precise references; according to his own account, Hirn drew primarily from Cod. 11183 and Cod. 11204.

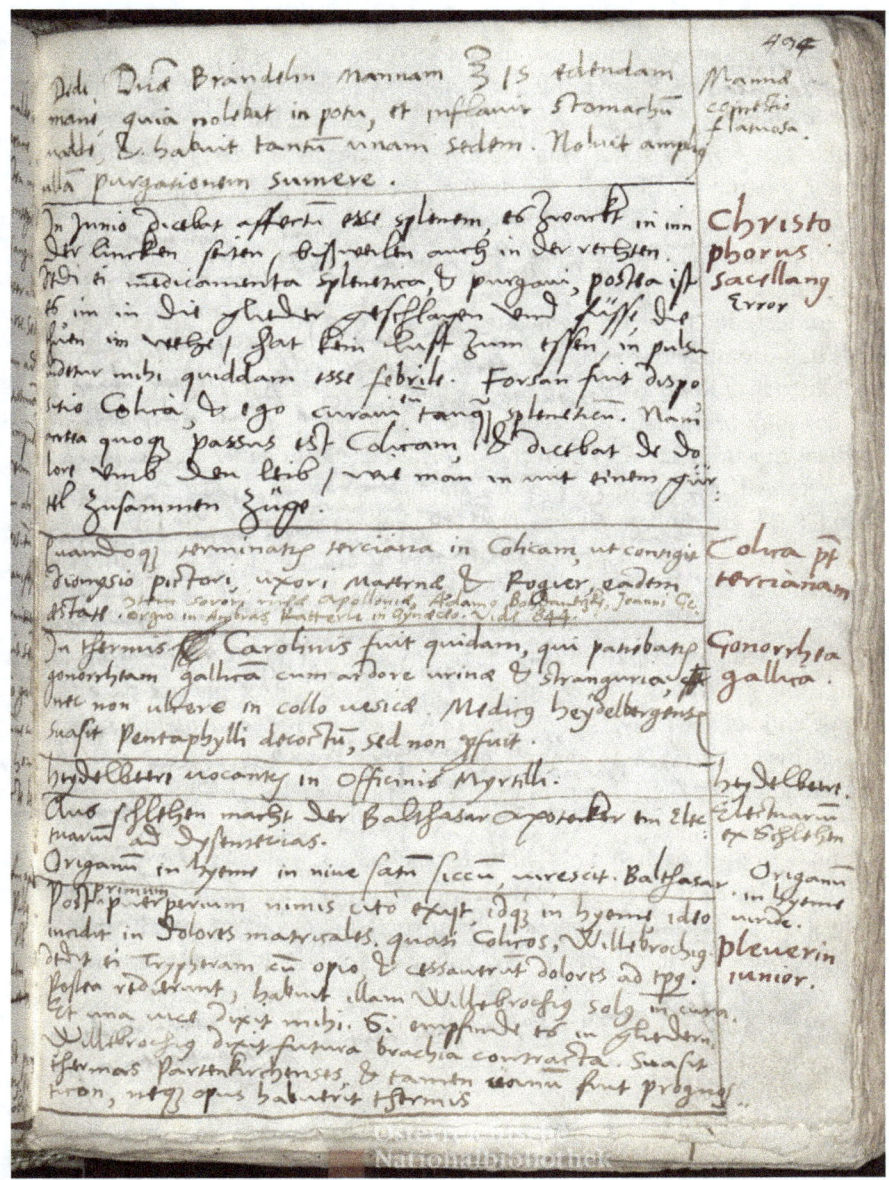

Fig. 2: Page from one of Georg Handsch's notebooks (Österreichische Nationalbibliothek, Vienna, Cod. 11183, fol. 434r).

remaining extensive handwritten texts from Handsch's *Nachlass*, is inevitably very time-consuming, even for someone who is well-versed in the material. The benefit, meanwhile, is anything but certain. As mentioned, Handsch's notes are often a motley jumble of more or less brief entries. Someone who wishes to make reliable generalizing statements about what Handsch knew or experienced concerning a particular illness or medication, for instance, would have to do what I did and read the notebooks in their entirety, collating dozens, or in some cases even hundreds, of entries made by Handsch on different occasions about the same subject.

For historians, however, who are interested not only in the great medical theories but also in their application – who seek to uncover the everyday experience and practice of Renaissance physicians, their life-world and self-conception, their relationships and interactions with patients and their families, with less learned medical practitioners, and with the medical culture in general of early modern learned medicine in all its diversity – there is more than a great challenge to be found in this colorful miscellany. The variety, the concreteness, and the closeness to everyday life are also what makes this source uniquely valuable and appealing. Handsch's notebooks give a wealth of insights into the world of learned medicine and show how young men were introduced to it and they paint a uniquely multi-facetted picture of everyday medical practice in the town and in the country, of the encounters between physicians and patients, of physicians' and laypeople's ideas about illness and how they approached it in everyday, practical ways. This picture is far richer and more detailed than that offered by the mostly printed sources on which most historical research in this area has so far had to rely.

So Georg Handsch and his singular notebooks are at the center of this book. This is definitely not a biography, however. In passing, I will also sketch out Handsch's professional career and fill in some details about his life.[24] Yet, my main aim is a different one. Taking Handsch's uniquely detailed notes as my starting point and drawing on a wide range of other handwritten and printed

---

[24] Cf. the biographical sketches by Kalina von Jätenstein, Nachrichten, vol. 2 (1819), pp. 28–43; d'Elvert, Geschichte (1868), pp. 60f.; Wolkan, Geschichte (1894), pp. 124–133; Wolkan, Handsch (1904); Senfelder, Georg Handsch (1901); Maiwald, Geschichte (1904), pp. 23–25; Rudel, Beiträge (1925), pp. 74–77; Smolka/Vaculínová, Georg Handsch (2010); Lucie Storchova, Georg Handsch (2020). Handsch is also mentioned in works on Archduke Ferdinand II and his court in Ambras (Hirn, Erzherzog Ferdinand II. (1885); Forcher, Erzherzog Ferdinand II. (2017); Haag/Sandbichler, Ferdinand II. (2017).

sources, I intend to piece together the medical world of learned physicians in the Renaissance in its manifold facets.[25]

In methodological terms, this book links micro-historical and historical anthropological perspectives with praxeological approaches. Micro-history and historical anthropology – these are two largely overlapping approaches – have become established and widely acknowledged over the past decades. Their emphasis is on the life and culture of "ordinary people", of the "common folks". Seeking to reconstruct historical realities in all their diversity, however, with the explicit inclusion of the perspective of contemporary actors, researchers have long applied microhistory and historical anthropology to social, political, and intellectual elites as well.[26] In a number of essays, Gadi Algazi, for example, has addressed the everyday life of late medieval and early modern scholars, which included academically trained physicians.[27] As the example of Algazi's work shows, these kinds of analyses may offer much more than a vivid description of everyday life. They also bring to light important insights about the learned "habitus". I use this concept in the sense given to it by Pierre Bourdieu, who defined it as an ensemble of attitudes, norms, and behavioral patterns acquired in the course of socialization that find expression in everyday life and in turn also shape it.[28]

Praxeological approaches have garnered a great deal attention in recent sociology and historiography and in areas far beyond them. They are rooted in the insight that societal structures and configurations as much as social, gender, professional and confessional identities are to a high degree created, reaffirmed, and changed through more or less routinized everyday practices about which only a limited degree of reflection takes place and which are sometimes literally incorporated or "inscribed" into the body. A central premise of these approaches is that "practical knowledge" largely follows an inherent, informal logic and needs to prove its worth time and again as it is confronted with the materiality of

---

25 I use the term "Renaissance" in a rather pragmatic fashion only, to roughly indicate the time period and because it evokes associations with phenomena such as humanism, the international republic of letters and the new anatomy which are central to my analysis. For my purposes, I can leave the hotly debated question aside whether it makes sense to talk of a "Renaissance" in the literal sense of the word (for some refreshing remarks on this issue see Starn, Postmodern Renaissance (2007)). A comprensive account of the world of the Renaissance in its manifold aspects can be found in Roeck, Morgen der Welt (2017).
26 Tanner, Historische Anthropologie (2004).
27 Algazi, Food (2002); Algazi, Scholars (2003); Algazi, Geistesabwesenheit (2007); Algazi, Habitus (2010); see also Füssel, Akademische Lebenswelt (2007).
28 Bourdieu, Esquisse (1972); cf. Raphael, Habitus (2004).

bodies and artefacts.[29] As a counterweight to the long-dominant work on the great discoveries and the theoretical conceptions of leading protagonists, approaches centered on praxis quickly acquired special significance in the history of science and the history of medicine. Here, these approaches have contributed crucially to new insights on the relation between theory and practice and have served to highlight differences and contradictions between them.

As my analysis of the interpretation, diagnosis, and treatment of illness in the Renaissance will show, a closer look at everyday practice forces us to call into question a range of well-established truths. Generations of medical historians, for example, claimed that early modern physicians rarely touched their patients and certainly did not do a systematic physical exam with their hands. It is true that physical exams are hardly mentioned in the medical textbooks of the time. Yet, the sources that describe everyday practice that I present here show clearly that the manual examination of the abdomen was a routine medical practice in the sixteenth century and that some physicians even performed manual vaginal exams on patients. To give another example from medical diagnostics: those who take at face value the copious polemical literature written by learned physicians who railed against diagnosing diseases from urine will find that this criticism was aimed chiefly at the numerous lay healers who relied, sometimes exclusively, on uroscopy. Uroscopy as such continued to be paramount also in the everyday practice of learned physicians.

In the case of disease concepts, the discrepancies are more striking still and have far-reaching implications for our understanding of early modern medicine as a whole. Not only in the media and in popular writings for a wider lay audience but even among renowned experts of early modern medicine, we still encounter the widespread notion that early modern medicine attributed diseases above all to an imbalance of the four natural humors (yellow and black bile, blood, and phlegm) and/or of their primary qualities (cold, hot, dry, and moist) and that therapy aimed at restoring a balance in the body. In fact, this notion is found in the theoretical writings of Galenic physicians, while the Paracelsians vehemently criticized the Galenists' alleged fixation on the four humors. Yet, when we turn to sources that document the diagnosis and treatment of specific cases in the everyday medical practice of the sixteenth century, we gain a completely different picture. Hardly ever were diseases explained by an imbalance of the qualities or the natural humors in the body. There was a different,

---

29 On the theoretical foundations see Schatzki/Knorr/von Savigny, Practice turn (2001); Reckwitz, Grundelemente (2003); Alkemeyer, Subjektivierung (2013); some exemplary applications of praxeological theory in writings on early modern history can be found in Alkemeyer/Budde/Freist, Selbst-Bildungen (2013) and in Brendecke, Praktiken (2015).

widely prevalent explanatory model: the vast majority of illnesses were attributed to more or less specific, impure, spoiled, foul or otherwise harmful morbid matter, which, consequently, had to be targeted specifically and evacuated.

Sources that describe everyday practice also bring to light remarkable differences between theory and praxis – in this case, more precisely, between norm and reality – when it comes to medical ethics and ideas about the professional duties of a physician. For example, the necessity of trying to help all patients equally, as proclaimed by Christian physicians, contrasted in practice with the great differences in the diagnostic and therapeutic effort made by learned physicians depending on how wealthy or poor their patients were. The widely acknowledged obligation of helping incurably ill and dying patients, to cite another example, was quite often put to the test in everyday practice when physicians, foreseeing the unfavorable course of an illness, had to fear for their reputation as successful practitioners – and sometimes preferred to leave patients to their fate.

As far as we know today, and considering the period in which they were written, the notes Handsch wrote are utterly unique with respect to how extensive, rich in detail, and close to everyday life and practice they were. I will be drawing on them throughout this book. I will complement my analysis of Handsch's notebooks extensively, however, with other handwritten and printed sources from this period. They will add to the picture painted by Handsch and will bring in some nuance where necessary and they will make it possible to assess to what degree the practice and experiences of Handsch and the physicians around him can be taken to be representative – for physicians in the German-speaking world or indeed for learned Renaissance physicians in general. A major and highly informative source for the physicians' training and for the ways in which they were introduced to the intellectual world of learned medicine are student notebooks. They have survived in substantial numbers, in handwritten and occasionally printed form and I will quote from a number of them. More rarely physicians' notebooks and practice journals are extant and provide insights into the everyday life of physicians and their clientele, and the diagnostic as well as therapeutic practice of other medical practitioners.[30] The extensive practice journal of the Zwickau town physician Hiob Finzel in particular will cross our paths more than a few times.[31] I will, of course, also take recourse to printed medical textbooks and treatises. In addition, we can gain valuable

---

[30] Historical overview in Hess/Schlegelmilch, Cornucopia (2016).
[31] Ratschulbibliothek Zwickau, Ms. QQQQ1, Ms. QQQQ1a and Ms. QQQQ1b; cf. Stolberg, A sixteenth-century physician (2019).

clues about many aspects of the medical lifeworld from physicians' correspondence, from which we learn about such things as physicians' activities outside medicine, their relationships with other scholars, the circumstances of their employment with rulers and municipal authorities, and about their private living conditions. Thousands of such letters have survived from the sixteenth century. At the Institut für Geschichte der Medizin in Würzburg, Germany, a long-term project has focused on early modern physicians' correspondence since 2009. The project has established an online database which currently offers free access to the data of more than 50,000 letters, written to and by physicians, from approximately 500 archives and libraries in Germany and abroad and for several thousand letters a detailed summary of the content as well. About 23,000 of these letters go back to the 16th-century and their number is expected to grow further over the coming years.[32] Based on these kinds of supplementary sources, I will also address subjects that do not figure prominently in Handsch's notes. For example, I will discuss the significance of holding the office of a salaried town physician. Handsch never held this office but it was an important stepping stone in the life of many physicians and a crucial factor for the spread and the establishment of learned medicine.

With its focus on real-life, everyday medical practice, this book closely connects to previous work undertaken by an international research group, funded by the German Research Foundation DFG, in which I had the honor of acting as the spokesperson.[33] In a number of research projects, each focusing on a different, well-documented case study, the twenty participating historians studied the history of medical practice in the German-speaking world between the seventeenth and the nineteenth centuries. Using practice journals as the major source and drawing on various additional sources, they looked at eight individual practices. Moreover, on the basis of these case studies they embarked on a collective, comparative analysis. In various coauthored chapters they surveyed the changes and developments that took place over time, with respect to the physicians' typical clientele, the doctor-patient relationship, the conceptions of illness that informed physicians' actions, diagnostic and therapeutic practices, the significance of the social, political, and confessional context, and many

---

[32] See www.aerztebriefe.de. This project is funded by the Union of the German Academies within the so-called "Akademienprogramm" and run under the auspices of the Bayerische Akademie der Wissenschaften in Munich.

[33] For details see https://www.medizingeschichte.uni-wuerzburg.de/aerztliche_praxis/index.html; the undertaking was initiated by Maria Ruisinger, now director of the Deutsche Medizinhistorischen Museum in Ingolstadt, and by Martin Dinges, Stuttgart, who also served as the vice-spokesperson.

other aspects of everyday medical practice.³⁴ The oldest practice examined in this context was that of Johannes Magirus in Berlin and Zerbst during the 1650s and 1660s.³⁵ In this book, I will not only take up several central questions we approached in this collective undertaking but also close the significant chronological gap in the study of early modern learned medical practice that remained for the time prior to 1650.

This book is divided into three parts. Following an introductory sketch of the figure of the "learned" physician as it developed over time, Part I offers an overview of the medical training that gave prospective physicians the rich knowledge and versatile skills that they would later put to use when treating their patients. The medical training in Padua, where Handsch – like many aspiring physicians from north of the Alps – studied, is given special attention here. The focus is not only on the lectures the medical students attended, the books they read, and the anatomical demonstrations and clinical case discussions they were allowed to attend. I will also and above all seek to reconstruct the intellectual world, the theories, and approaches with which these soon-to-be physicians familiarized themselves, which became second nature for them in the course of the years, and which they were expected to apply in their practice. I conclude this part with a discussion of the learned habitus which the future physicians acquired over many years before they entered the more narrow realm of medicine. I look at some of the characteristic humanist activities in which many physicians engaged and in which this habitus became manifest, ranging from poetry to historiography and the humanist practice of collecting and ordering excerpts in the form of *loci communes*.

Part II, the most extensive part, concerns actual medical practice in all its diversity: the diagnostic, preventative and therapeutic practices of physicians, the concepts and explanatory models on which they relied, as well as their understanding of central and widely diagnosed diseases. I will also give an in-depth description of the rise of empirical approaches in medical practice, of observational practices and sometimes experimental testing of the effects of medications, of the rise of medical casuistry, and of the practice of autopsy on deceased patients, which was already quite common in the sixteenth century.

This part of the book will necessarily be demanding for the reader. The world that we encounter here is foreign to us. Physicians and patients relied on

---

34 Dinges/ Jankrift/ Schlegelmilch/ Stolberg, Medical practice (2016).
35 DFG-research project "Ärztliche Praxis und medizinisches Weltbild um 1650: Johannes Magirus (1615–1697)"; details under https://www.medizingeschichte.uni-wuerzburg.de/aerztliche_praxis/projekt_stolberg.html; for the results of this project see Schlegelmilch, Ärztliche Praxis (2018).

concepts and images of the human body and its illnesses that often have little in common with the way we see things today. It is vital, however, if we wish to gain a historical understanding of medical thinking and acting in the past and of the way patients experienced illness, that we engage with this foreign world and its inner logic the way cultural anthropologists do when exploring foreign cultures today. If we are to understand the explanatory power and longevity of early modern disease concepts, we need to put aside the familiar view towards "progress", the search for things that were "already" known back then. From the perspective of cultural anthropology and the sociology of knowledge, medicine is a socio-cultural construct.[36] Medical practice is not successful only if healers share the theories and explanatory models of modern Western medicine. It suffices that the explanations of a given medical system are plausible and believable, that they give sick people an orientation accompanied by the promise of effective remedies. Disease concepts, as Leon Eisenberg encapsulated it years ago, are a means of creating reality and giving meaning to the experience of a chaotic world. Eisenberg here even speaks of a shared "mythopoesis" of doctor and patient.[37]

This is not to deny the reality of pathological phenomena. They are not mere figments of the imagination. Yet, which phenomena and changes we give attention to, how we interpret them, how we distinguish between different diseases, how we deal with them – all this is shaped to a high degree by culture with its specific conception of the world and the human being and by the disease concepts derived from it. Only when we make this overarching and shaping influence of culture our starting point can we understand the great diversity of medical systems and worldviews of the past and present, of which Western biomedicine is only one variant, albeit the by far most influential today. As bizarre, at times even absurd as some of the notions may strike us today, the disease concepts I will be presenting in Part II corresponded with the contemporaneous state of scientific knowledge. They satisfied the widely accepted criteria for methodologically sound, scientific insights. The diagnostic, prognostic, and therapeutic practices that were derived from these concepts were, according to the understanding at the time, rational.[38] Moreover, as we will see, these practices also seemed to prove their worth every day, over and over during medical practice: after all, most patients got better under the physicians' treatment.

---

36 Byron, Medicine (1994); Harley, Rhetoric (1999); Helman, Culture (2007).
37 Eisenberg, Physician (1981), p. 245.
38 Harley, Rhetoric (1999), pp. 417f.

Part III is devoted to the physician's everyday practice, delving into the subject of medical clientele, into what it meant for the career of many physicians to gain employment as a town or court physician, and into the interactions and conflicts between physicians and their patients. I examine the relation between the medical notions and practices of physicians and those of laypeople, unearthing a remarkable openness of learned physicians toward lay ideas and practices. Subsequently, I consider the possible reasons why, in their everyday practice, the learned physicians of the Renaissance embraced the disease concepts and practices that were preferred by laypeople when, instead of attributing illness to an imbalance of the humors and qualities, they ascribed them to impure, raw, foreign, or unnatural substances in the body.

While I will be drawing on a fair range of sources the geographical focus of my analysis will be on the situation in the Holy Roman Empire and – they overlap to a large degree – in the German-speaking areas, including large territories that are part of present-day Switzerland, Austria, the Czech Republic and Poland. Because of the marked institutional and political differences within Europe in this domain, the chapters on town and court physicians and on bath masters and barber-surgeons will indeed almost exclusively look at this area. My analysis of the medical training of future physicians, in turn, will concentrate on the universities in Northern Italy, which were widely appreciated for their superior teaching also by students from the German-speaking areas, many of whom came, like Handsch, to study or complete their medical education there. Most other chapters in this book will also draw predominantly on Handsch's notebooks from his years in Bohemia, Northern Italy and Austria and on other sources from the German- and Italian-speaking areas. However, in order to arrive at a more complete and nuanced picture, I will also draw on extant historical scholarship and to some degree on sources from other parts of Europe. Regarding the bulk of my analysis, the physicians' humanist self-fashioning and their place in the republic of letters, the prevailing explanatory concepts and theories, the diagnostic and therapeutic practices to which they resorted in their everyday practice, their interactions with patients and families and the rise of empirical approaches in learned medicine, I have not found evidence for major differences. The world of learned medicine with Latin as its common language clearly was an international phenomenon. I therefore believe that large parts of my analysis can throw a light on the world of learned medicine in Renaissance Europe as a whole.

This book is a revised English edition of my "Gelehrte Medizin und ärztlicher Alltag in der Renaissance" that came out in 2020 with De Gruyter, in German. Most of the revisions sprang from additional, new sources, such as the extensive notes of an unidentifed student or young physician who accompanied Benedetto Vittore in 1540s Bologna on his patient visits and the *consilia* of Jakob Horst, which I have only recently found and/or analyzed in detail. Some chapters draw – at times quite generously – on papers that I have previously published. I have dealt with bedside teaching and anatomical instruction in Padua in "Teaching anatomy in post-Vesalian Padua. An analysis of student notes", *Journal of medieval and early modern studies* 48 (2018), pp. 61–78, and in "Bedside teaching and the acquisition of practical skills in mid-sixteenth-century Padua", *Journal of the history of medicine and allied sciences* 69 (2014), pp. 633–661. I have studied the humanist activities and aspirations of Handsch and other Renaissance physicians in "The many uses of writing. A humanist physician in sixteenth-century Prague", in Andrew Mendelsohn, Annemarie Kinzelbach und Ruth Schilling (eds): *Civic medicine. Physician, polity, and pen in early modern Europe.* London 2019, pp. 67–87. The rise of empirical approaches in Renaissance medicine was the topic of "Empiricism in sixteenth-century medical practice. The notebooks of Georg Handsch", *Early science and medicine* 18 (2013), pp. 487–516. In ""You have no good blood in your body". Oral communication in sixteenth-century physicians' medical practice", *Medical history* 59 (2015), pp. 63–82, I have used Handsch's extensive notes to reconstruct the ways in which Renaissance physicians explained diseases and their treatment to patients and relatives. "A sixteenth-century physician and his patients: The practice journal of Hiob Finzel, 1565–1589", *Social history of medicine* 32 (2019), pp. 221–240, provides an in-depth analysis of the earliest extensive practice journal of *doctor medicinae* that is known to have survived from the sixteenth century. The interactions between physicians and patients stand at the center of my recent paper on "The doctor-patient relationship in the Renaissance", *European journal for the history of medicine and health* 1 (2021), pp. 1–29, which also draws heavily on Handsch's notes.

A final note on practical matters: To make original Latin quotations more legible, I have adapted them to modern usage with respect to capitalization, punctuation, and the use of "u"/"v" and "i"/ "j", rendering, for example, "vsus" as "usus" and "uaria" as "varia". Especially when Handsch quotes vernacular expressions used by physicians or laypeople I often provide the original German wording in the notes for the benefit of readers who are familiar with the German language. These vernacular terms and expressions are frequently endowed with a semantic richness, with metaphorical connotations and etymological connections that cannot adequately be rendered in translation. References to manuscripts with the shelf mark "Cod." without an indication of the holding institution refer to the manuscripts in the Austrian National Library in Vienna. References to letters written by or addressed to physicians that I have not analyzed personally but which I owe to the Würzburg database on Early Modern Physicians' Letters (www.aerztebriefe.de) are provided in the footnotes, citing the URL and the author(s) of the respective detailed summary.

This book is the result of years of research. Completing it would have been difficult without the various kinds of support I received. My thanks go first of all to my colleagues and collaborators at the Institut für Geschichte der Medizin in Würzburg. They helped me carve out the time for the painstaking analysis of the sources and in particular of the thousands of pages of handwritten Latin notes. I also would like to thank the staff of the National Library in Vienna, for their help and support over all these years. Alexander Pyrges and Sabine Schlegelmilch have given me valuable critical feedback on a draft of this book. My special thanks go to the Historisches Kolleg in Munich and the Fritz Thyssen Foundation, who awarded me a Senior Fellowship in 2018/19, allowing me to spend a year in the marvelous surroundings of the Kaulbach Villa, focusing almost exclusively on this book.

I dedicate this book to my wife Jackie, to whom I owe more than I will ever be able to express in words.

Part I: **Entering the World of Learned Medicine**

Prologue: The "Learned" Physician.
On the History of an Ideal

Western medicine changed fundamentally during the Middle Ages, with far-reaching effects on the development of the healing arts for centuries to come and ultimately to the present day. Medicine became an academic discipline. It established itself at the newly founded universities.[1] Today, this position is taken for granted. It is widely acknowledged that an adequate diagnosis and treatment of the various human diseases calls for a highly differentiated theoretical foundation, on the basis of a comprehensive and sophisticated knowledge of physiological and pathological processes in the body. As soon as we widen our perspective and look at the many different cultures on our planet, in the past as in the present, however, we quickly see that Western culture with its appreciation of an "academic", theory-based, scientific medicine is exceptional. In all known cultures and societies there are diseases, and there are people who concern themselves with diagnosing and treating them. And in the vast majority of cultures, medical practice is guided by more or less complex ideas of the human body and its relation to the social, the natural, and the supernatural environment, and it is in the hands of people who are believed to possess special knowledge and skill in the area. Yet, on a global scale, the conviction that medical practice requires a comprehensive, written methodological and theoretical foundation and that a true doctor must be a "learned man" is not the rule but the exception. It is found only in the few so-called "advanced civilizations" that put special emphasis on the written word and book knowledge on the whole, civilizations which moreover, it has been shown, have sometimes had a mutual influence on each other.

The German term for physician "Arzt", too, did not originally denote a studied, scholarly physician exclusively. The term likely derives from the Greek word "archiatros", which referred to a prominent member of a group of healers. Early modern physicians still sometimes used the term "Archiater" in this sense, thus giving a kind of honorary title to the leading local doctor. Even in the late Middle Ages, however, many who were honored with the title of an "Arzt" had not studied medicine. A barber-surgeon or surgeon trained in medicine as a craft, for

---

[1] For useful overviews see O'Malley, Medical Education (1970), pp. 89–102; Bylebyl, Medicine (1985); Siraisi, Medieval & early Renaissance medicine (1990), ch. 3: Medical education; Siraisi, Fakultät (1996), pp. 321–342; Siraisi, Medicine (2001); Grendler, Universities (2002), pp. 314–352; Mugnai Carrara/Forti, L'insegnamento (2008).

Open Access. © 2022 Michael Stolberg, published by De Gruyter. This work is licensed under the Creative Commons Attribution-NonCommercial-NoDerivatives 4.0 International License.
https://doi.org/10.1515/9783110733549-001

example, could also be referred to as an "Arzt".² Only in the course of the early modern period did the term "Arzt" become a term which was reserved for the academically trained "doctor medicinae" and ultimately the simple term "doctor", without the added "medicinae", came to refer to the university-educated physician. Over the early modern period, in a further twist, "doctor" became synonymous to some degree, in turn, with "medical practitioner" in general and ordinary people also began to call non-academic healers such as itinerant practitioners, hangmen, and barber-surgeons "doctors".³

Within Western culture, the ideal of "learned" medicine that rests on a scientific and philosophical foundation and on extensive reading is embedded in a millennia-old tradition.⁴ The claim that a physician also needed to be a "philosopher" is already found in the writings of Hippocrates. This was an expression of the close connection between medicine and natural philosophy. For instance, the ancient doctrine of the body's four natural humors – yellow and black bile, blood, and phlegm, with their corresponding and paired primary qualities (hot, cold, dry, moist) – was linked directly to the ancient natural-philosophical theory of the four elements and their qualities of which all things found in nature were made up, with the various combinations of elements and qualities giving rise to specific natural properties.

Of more consequence still than the transmission of specific explanatory elements was the methodological approach that had likewise been adopted from natural philosophy in antiquity. The ancient medical writers created a theoretical edifice which allowed them to explain and treat diseases in naturalistic terms. Even a disease like epilepsy, to use a famous example, which in antiquity was largely understood as supernatural, caused by the gods, was subsequently attributed in an almost mechanistic way to processes that took place inside the head, namely to the disrupted drainage of phlegm from the brain.⁵ As heirs of this tradition, we may consider a naturalistic approach to be self-evident. But it is not. In many cultures, gods and other supernatural powers that are often and to varying degrees described in anthropomorphic terms continue to be central to the interpretation and treatment of illnesses.

Even in the Western world, the naturalistic approach was for a long time rivalled by other approaches. The notion that illnesses had supernatural causes or could at least be treated with supernatural means remained alive and well, for example in Asclepian medicine, which was practiced until late antiquity,

---

2 Kintzinger, Status (2000), pp. 68f.
3 Cod. 11205, fol. 272r.
4 See Jouanna, Entstehung (1996) and Jouanna, Hippocrates (2000).
5 Temkin, Falling sickness (1971).

not only in the Greece but also in places like the Rhineland. It continued to shape the medical ideas and practices of the rural population into the nineteenth century at least. The "naturalistic" approach of Hippocratic medicine, however, informed medical writers for centuries. In the second century of our calendar, Galen of Pergamon elaborated this program of a medicine based on the theory of natural philosophy in numerous writings. He also expanded it by granting a pivotal role not only to the humors but also to the *pneuma* and the innate vital heat as well as to the individual organs and their faculties. Through his writings, he would have a leading role in the development of Western medicine for about 1500 years to come.[6]

In the late ancient and early medieval West after the collapse of the Roman Empire, learned medicine was passed on and practiced mainly in the monasteries with their libraries and scriptoria.[7] During the same period, the heritage of learned ancient medicine was cultivated and passed down to a far greater extent in the advanced cultures of the Middle East, where it was also enriched with elements of Greek, Arab, and Persian philosophy.[8] The joining of these two traditions, the European, initially predominantly monastic, and the Arab and Persian tradition, would still shape Western medicine centuries later, when, during the High Middle Ages, the first cathedral schools and universities were established.[9] Above all in the areas of contact between Western and Arab cultures, in southern Italy and Spain, extensive translation activity took place. The works of Avicenna, Averroes, and Ḥunain ibn Isḥāq (Iohannitius) took their place in libraries next to those of Hippocrates, Galen and the other Greek and Roman authorities. Initially known mostly for its successful practitioners, the famous school of Salerno, located near Montecassino with its vast library, increasingly adopted a highly differentiated theoretical and philosophical foundation.[10]

For our historical understanding it is moreover important to realize that medical subjects and especially medical theory were also discussed and taught in places other than faculties of medicine. They were taught at cathedral schools and later at universities as part of the study of the liberal arts. Even in some grammar schools, students were given the opportunity to learn from medical writings. Fourteen-year-old Isaak Keller in Strasbourg, for example, read not only excerpts

---

[6] Galen, Opera (1822); Temkin, Galenism (1973); Hankinson, Cambridge companion (2008).
[7] MacKinney, Medical education (1955), p. 844.
[8] Ullmann, Medizin (1970); Pormann/Savage Smith, Medieval Islamic medicine (2007).
[9] The history of universities in Europe has been studied by numerous scholars. For a survey of the developments in the sixteenth century see the contributions to Ridder-Symoens, University (1996).
[10] De Renzi, Collectio (1852–59).

from Cicero's speeches and the dialogue between Aeschines and Demosthenes in Greek, but also Galen's *De sanitate tuenda*.[11] This was the case even more so for the *gymnasia illustria*, founded in the sixteenth century in some cities. These institutions occupied a place between the grammar schools and the universities, and the local municipal physician often taught classes there.[12] It was sometimes physicians, in fact, who made the explicit demand for such classes to be held. In the opinion of Johann Ludwig Havenreuter of Strasbourg, medicine was to be taught at school no less than the other subjects.[13]

It was nevertheless far from obvious that learned medicine and those who taught and practiced it would gain a foothold at universities such as those of Bologna, Montpellier, Paris and Padua, which were among the earliest universities and for a long time the dominant ones. Medical knowledge, after all, was always connected to its application: to diagnosing, preventing, and treating diseases. In academic disputes over the hierarchy of disciplines, especially between physicians and jurists, the claim that medicine was a *scientia* was bitterly contested for centuries, with some saying that it only deserved the lesser rank of an art or craft (*techne*). Even leading medical teachers like Jacobus Sylvius conceded that medicine was a *scientia* only in a wider, more general sense.[14]

Ultimately decisive for medicine's successful establishment in academia was its proximity to the philosophy of Aristotle, whose position at the medieval universities towered above everything else. The Galenic writings as well as Avicenna's *Canon medicinae*, which became the leading medical textbook in the High Middle Ages,[15] were shaped by Aristotle. In fact, it was physicians more than anyone else who during the thirteenth and fourteenth centuries underlined the importance of Aristotelian philosophy.[16]

Subsuming medical subjects under the teaching of the liberal arts made a lot of sense in some respects. There was a great deal of overlap between the issues and questions of medicine and those of natural philosophy. The human being was part of nature and resembled other living beings in many respects. In *De sensu et sensatu* (436a-b) Aristotle had explicitly demanded that natural philosophy

---

11 Letter to Bonifacius Amerbach, 12 September 1544, edited in Jenny, Amerbachkorrespondenz (1967), pp. 47f. (www.aerztebriefe.de/id/00007426, S. Krauss/S. Schlegelmilch).
12 My thanks to Sabine Schlegelmilch for pointing this out to me.
13 Havenreuter, Theses (1586), thesis I.
14 Sylvius, Ordo (1548), p. 6.
15 Siraisi, Avicenna (1987).
16 Schmitt, Aristotle (1983); Schmitt, Aristotle (1985)

concern itself with the fundamentals of health and illness.[17] In the early Middle Ages, Isidore of Seville pointed out the proximity of medicine and the *artes* again. According to him, medicine was a "second philosophy" ("secunda philosophia"). While, unlike philosophy, it did not address the soul but the body, it concerned itself with the whole human being. The only reason it did not count among the individual liberal arts was that it was itself based on the liberal arts in their entirety. The physician required grammar to understand what he read and put it in his own words and he required rhetoric to make arguments, and dialectics which helped him to illuminate and consider the causes of illnesses. Arithmetic and geometry, too, were useful to the physician, for example in calculating time and the calendar. Astronomy made it possible to trace the movements of the stars, which had an immediate effect on the human body. Even music proved beneficial at times. David, for example, used his art to liberate King Saul from an impure spirit, and Asclepiades healed a raging man ("phreneticus") with "symphonia".[18]

For their part, the learned physicians of the High Middle Ages did everything they could to underline their erudition and the broad theoretical and philosophical basis of their thinking and acting. The scholastic method came to be widely adopted in medicine as it was in many other domains. Leading physicians like Taddeo Alderotti and Pietro d'Abano concerned themselves extensively with philosophical questions, were interested in solving contradictions between the medical tradition and Aristotelian philosophy, and even discussed general moral questions.[19]

In the Renaissance period, the demand that medicine be based on a philosophical foundation resonated more strongly than ever before. Galen's small treatise *Quod optimus medicus sit quoque philosophus*, translated by none other than Erasmus of Rotterdam, was widely read.[20] With great insistence, Galen demanded that a physician must also be a philosopher and have mastered the different branches of philosophy: *philosophia rationalis, philosophia naturalis* and even *philosophia moralis*. He must, based on logical observation ("logica speculatione"), recognize the nature of the body, its composition from elements, different substances ("partes similares") and organs ("partes instrumentales") as well as their functions and use for the living being. He must be familiar with different diseases and their treatment. In all that, he had to seek certain proof ("demonstratio certa"), as taught by the "ars rationalis". With regard to morality, the physician must maintain levelheadedness and must not give in to greed for money.[21]

---

17 See also Stolz, Artes-liberales-Zyklen (2004), p. 446.
18 Isidor von Sevilla, Praeclarissimum opus (1509), fol. 24r (book 4, ch. 13).
19 Siraisi, Taddeo Alderotti (1981).
20 Schmitt, Aristotle (1985), pp. 1–15 and pp. 271–279 (notes), here p. 2.
21 Galen, Optimus medicus (1547), pp. 27–31, cit. pp. 30f.

These demands were echoed by the learned physicians of the sixteenth century and reflected in university teaching. With good reason, a degree in the liberal arts was usually a prerequisite for a university degree in medicine. In some places, such as Montpellier, the pertinent knowledge was tested prior to enrollment.[22] At Italian universities, the *artes* and medicine were commonly taught in the same faculty, but here too a preparatory study of the *artes* was considered indispensable. As a minimal requirement, students had to continue with the liberal arts while studying medicine. When Ulrich Ellenbog enrolled at the university in Siena in April of 1504, he thought it common sense to first familiarize himself with the foundations of logic and philosophy before he turned to medicine. This was the way everyone did it, young and old, he found.[23] Two years later, in the spring of 1506, he reported that he had almost completed his study of logic and was now beginning his study of medicine.[24] The only philosophical subject he would continue to study was the doctrine of nature. He had already read the aphorisms of Hippocrates privately.[25] In Padua as well, sixteenth-century students of medicine did more than hear medical lectures and see anatomical demonstrations. The Zurich medical student Georg Keller, for example, studied Aristotelian logic in much detail and attended the philosophy lectures of the Padua professor Bernardino Tomitano.[26] In his letters, medical student Johannes Greiffenhagen gave as much attention to the commentary on Aristotle by Francesco Piccolomini and Jacopo Zabarella as he did to the activities at the faculty of medicine and the latest publications of Girolamo Mercuriale.[27] In the 1590s, Galileo Galilei deliberately held his lectures in mathematics at a time in the evening when no one else was lecturing, so that students of both medicine and philosophy could attend. By Galileo's account, the majority of his listeners were students of medicine.[28] Most of those students who earned their doctoral degree in Padua or at another Italian

---

22 Stolberg, Studying medicine [2022].
23 Allen, Letters (1907), pp. 740–754, here pp. 741f.; on Bologna see Simeoni, Storia (1940), p. 30.
24 On medical teaching in Siena see Piccinini, Scienza (1991).
25 Ellenbog, Briefwechsel (1938), p. 16, summary of Ellenbog's letter of 8 March 1506.
26 Schieß, Briefe (1906), p. 10.
27 Letter from Johannes Greiffenhagen to Sigismund Schnitzer, Padua, 27 June 1589, printed in: Hornung, Cista ([1626]), pp. 289f.; a preceding letter on the commentators of Aristotle's works seems to have gone lost.
28 Archivio di Stato, Venice, Riformatori allo Studio 419, letter from Galileo Galilei to the *Riformatori* in Venice (they were responsible for the administration of the university), 9 March 1609. Galileo complained that, after seventeen years of teaching, his students suddenly had to choose between his own lecture and that of Annibal Bimbiolo who had started to lecture at the same hour, without permission.

university consequently obtained a double degree, receiving the title of doctor of philosophy and medicine, which these graduates later proudly underlined in their letters and publications.

Given this situation, Georg Handsch, as we learn from his Padua notebooks, had to resort to certain tricks in order to earn his doctoral degree in medicine. While he had had thorough training in the *studia humanitatis*, he did not even have the title of a *baccalaureus* to show for himself, not to mention that of a *magister*. As his private notes tell us, he therefore had the idea of having letters sent from his home country that addressed him as "magister". Furthermore, he was going to write a panegyric for the famous professor and ducal physician Antonio Musa Brasavola (1500–1555) in Ferrara.[29] He was, by all appearances, successful. In June of 1553, he completed his studies, earning his doctoral degree in Ferrara under Brasavola.[30]

The study of the *artes* offered more than a thorough training in philosophy, rhetoric, and the art of debating, which was useful to future physicians. It also gave students some of the knowledge and skills that were useful for the study of medicine and for later professional life as a physician: natural history offered diverse insights into the world of plants, animals, and minerals, which were also used to make medicines. Mathematical skills helped with calculating birth horoscopes (nativities) and creating astrological calendars for a town (usually for the physician's place of residence), for a particular longitude and latitude. Physicians were among the major authors of astrological calendars, one of the most widely sold products of the printing press at the time.[31] Some town physicians published such a calendar for their place of activity every year.[32]

There was furthermore quite an overlap between philosophy and medicine in academic teaching in the sixteenth century, especially at the Italian universities. With medicine and the *artes* being at home in one and the same faculty, personal exchange necessarily took place. Moreover many a university career at the time led from a lesser regarded and lesser paid chair in philosophy to medicine. At the University of Bologna, for example, professors tended to first teach logic and then philosophy for a number of years before they eventually were given a chair

---

29 In Handsch's manuscript collection of his poems, there is a eulogy on Brasavola, which he recited on the occasion of his doctoral exam in 1553 (Cod. 11210, fol. 174a v; see also Cod. 9821, fol. 243v).
30 Pardi, Titoli (1901), pp. 166f.
31 Sudhoff, Iatromathematiker (1902); Herbst, Biobibliographisches Handbuch (https://www.presseforschung.uni-bremen.de/dokuwiki/doku.php?id=startseite).
32 E.g., in Zürich, Christoph Clauser (Wehrli, Clauser (1924), pp. 84–98).

of medicine.³³ Some philosophers studied medical subjects thoroughly. For example Jacopo Zabarella, one of the most influential Aristotelians of his time, sought to find ways of establishing a stringent, logical rationale to guide medical diagnostics and therapy. He put great emphasis on the significance of an analytical course of action, a *methodus resolutiva*, for medicine: from the symptoms, the physician must conclude the cause. In a second movement of thought, the physician could reverse his direction and, performing a *regressus*, arrive at an even more precise understanding of the symptoms from his knowledge of the cause of the disease.³⁴ There is much to suggest that Zabarella for his part was influenced by the Padua physicians of medicine. Most notably, Giovanni Battista da Monte, decades before Zabarella, cultivated a strict methodical procedure to be followed at the bedside and taught his students to draw from their observations of individual patients and from the changes and complaints the patient was reporting to identify and understand the pathological changes and processes that were taking place inside the body.³⁵

During the sixteenth century, philosophy and medicine were also closely linked north of the Alps, where the two disciplines were commonly taught in separate faculties. As in Italy, many a German professor of medicine started out teaching the *artes*. Philipp Melanchthon's *De anima* was among the works that reached far beyond the scope of medicine and philosophy, and it was one of the most influential treatises of the period. In formal respects, the work was conceived as a commentary on Aristotle's doctrine of the soul, yet it offered anatomical and physiological knowledge on a broad scale.³⁶ As can be seen from the repeated references to it in Handsch's Padua lecture notes, *De anima* also received an early reception in Italy.³⁷

---

33 Thus, Benedetto Vittore, taught logic in Bologna for two years and philosophy for another six before he took the chair of *medicina theorica* in 1512; like him Virgilio Gherardi and Jacopo Pacini moved from logic to philosophy and finally medicine (Mazzetti, Repertorio (1847), p. 321, p. 147, p. 230).
34 On Zabarella's logic see Mikkeli, Aristotelean response (1992); Ingegno, Astrologia (1995), pp. 85–113.
35 Da Monte, Consultationum (1554); Da Monte, Consultationum (1556); Da Monte, Consultationum (1558); Da Monte, Consultationum (1559); Da Monte, Consultationum (1565). Many of Da Monte's "consultationes" were judgements on individual patients he delivered orally and which his students recorded on paper.
36 Melanchthon, Commentarius (1540); Melanchthon, Liber (1552); cf. Helm, Galenrezeption (1996) and idem, Aristotelismus (1997).
37 E.g. Cod. 11210, fol. 4r and fol. 34r.

Choosing a Profession

At the beginning of one of Handsch's notebooks, there is a list that at first seems puzzling. It includes the words "poeta", "orator", "arithmeticus", "musicus", and also "grammaticus", "medicus", "organista" and "nigromanticus". With a different pen and different ink, Handsch added further terms such as "dialecticus" and "praestigiator".[38] On the following pages, other, more explicit entries reveal what the list is about: his "magister" intended to recommend him for work as an "arithmeticus" in the metal works of the Herr von Gendorf. God may see to it that he may become a "lector" at the university in Prague, he wrote. Other positions he named include "Stadtschreiber" (town clerk) and even "sacerdos" (priest), and teacher in the chantry ("ynn der Canterey praeceptor").[39]

There is no doubt that Handsch, who was barely twenty years old,[40] was pondering his professional future and weighing his options. It becomes clear from this list that medicine was only one of many possibilities at that point in time and by no means was it at the top. He could see himself becoming a poet, rhetor or "grammarian" – likely this meant a school teacher – a musician or organist, a town scribe or, apparently this was his favorite choice, a university lecturer. The list only appears random at first glance. Perhaps with the exception of the "career option" of "magician" or "necromancer",[41] which he was presumably not serious about, these professions had one thing in common: they required knowledge and skills of the kind that were taught in the seven liberal arts, in the *trivium* of grammar, rhetoric, and dialectics, and in the *quadrivium*, which added special knowledge and proficiencies in natural philosophy, arithmetic, geometry, and musical theory.

As Handsch's list illustrates, the cultural capital[42] of a good education in the *artes liberales* already opened up various professional prospects. A look at the medical biographies of that time shows that more than a few physicians appreciated and made use of this multitude of options. An extensive, quantitatively robust prosopography of early modern physicians in German-speaking

---

38 Cod. 9666, fol. 1r.
39 Ibid., fol. 1v.
40 The manuscript carries the date 23 September 1547 but Handsch probably added the list only later on the first pages, which he had initially left blank. Without doubt the entries date from the time before he went to Padua, however, in the autumn of 1550, to study medicine.
41 In another entry in the same notebook, Handsch mentioned that he had learned some magic tricks with cards and numbers (Ibid., foll. 134v-135r).
42 On the concept of "cultural capital" see Bourdieu, Les trois états (1979); Bourdieu, Forms (1986).

areas remains an urgent desideratum. But even a rough look at historical work done on the biographies of graduates of individual universities[43] and at the data about several thousand physicians in German-speaking areas which the Würzburg project "Frühneuzeitliche Ärztebriefe" has been amassing since 2009[44] indicates that many future physicians did not follow the straight path from Latin school to studying the liberal arts to acquiring a doctoral degree in medicine. Prior to studying medicine, many later physicians practiced other professions, some for many years. Some practicing physicians continued throughout their lives to have other sources of income that had no connection to medicine. Heinrich Stromer (1476–1542), the owner of the tavern "Auerbachs Keller" in Leipzig, is a well-known example.[45]

One obvious and relatively popular profession to take up after completing a course of studies in the *artes* – and this applied, among others, for a number of graduates of the Prague university – was that of a teacher.[46] Even some of the most renowned physicians and scholars of the time taught intermittently at a school or directed one, like Georg Agricola (1494–1555) in Zwickau. Others started out in the employ of a prince or nobleman, acting as tutor for their sons. Johann Aichholz (1520–1588), for example, travelled in France and Italy as a private teacher before earning the degree of doctor of medicine at the age of 35 and, several years later, becoming a professor at the medical faculty in Vienna.[47]

A further opportunity or way station that is commonly found in the biographies of well-known physicians, in particular, was teaching at a university. A fair number of future *doctores medicinae* first taught at an arts faculty. Heinrich Stromer lectured at the Leipzig university about the logician Petrus Hispanus (13th cent.), before turning to medicine.[48] Teaching at the Jena university in the early seventeenth century, Thomas Reinesius (1587–1667) lectured about mnemonics and other subjects before accepting the position of *Hofmeister* (private tutor) with the imperial apothecary in Prague and later with Count von Schlick. He then went on to resume his studies, earning his doctoral degree in Basel.[49]

---

43 Koch, Medizinische Fakultät (2007).
44 See www.aerztebriefe.de; the biographical data that is currently accessible online is quite rudimentary and sometimes based on secondary sources only. As part of the project work, a far more comprehensive internal biographical working database was established which will be made accessible when funding for the project terminates (probably in 2024).
45 Wustmann, Wirt (1902).
46 Truc, Aufgabe (1998), p. 205; Horský, Bedeutung (1988), pp. 279f.
47 Schrauf/Wenzel, Wiener Ärzte (1894).
48 Wustmann, Stromer (1902), p. 7; Hiob Finzel first taught in the arts before he embarked on his medical studies (Aewerdieck, Register (2010), pp. 12–21).
49 Hase, Reinesius (1858), pp. 315–6.

Even the hope of being employed as a musician was not unique to Handsch. Simon Wilde, for instance, who would later be a physician in Zwickau, initially attempted to secure a position as cantor.[50]

Clearly, many of those who eventually became physicians were not destined for a medical career from the start. The study and practice of medicine was only one of many possible options for a young *baccalaureus* of the liberal arts who hoped to find his place in society. Yet it was important to weigh this option carefully, especially in comparison to studying in one of the other higher faculties, theology or law. Physicians, who would have known best about the advantages and disadvantages of the profession, had good reason to have their sons study medicine as well, as they often did.[51] The work of a physician was respected and would become more attractive economically in the course of the sixteenth century, as we will see. Especially in cities, growing sections of the population used the services of learned physicians or indeed came to prefer them over those of other practitioners. In addition, more and more cities employed doctors of medicine as town physicians, paying them a salary that secured them a basic income. More so than theology and law, medicine promised a certain degree of freedom and independence. The physicians of that time became leading representatives of a new social phenomenon which was to play a prominent role in the centuries to come: often far from their home town and without the support of family ties, many of them were successful in establishing their livelihood thanks to their academic training alone. Some of them even achieved considerable wealth. An analysis of tax contributions along with the numerous physicians and physicians' daughters who married into the urban patriciate and in some cases even into aristocracy, reveals that many physicians were part of the urban upper classes. The most successful among them amassed extensive assets through their work and dowries and became financially powerful moneylenders.

A medical career also had its shadow sides. Young physicians in particular often struggled to hold their own and establish a successful practice in the face of the numerous competitors. Moreover, the very object that was at the center of medical practice, the human body, put the physician's reputation and dignity at risk. While university-educated physicians largely steered clear of the manual aspects of medical treatment – readily leaving bloodletting, cupping, and clystering up to the barber-surgeons – they still invariably found themselves associated with stench, corruption, putrefaction. At a time when "uncleanliness" threatened to mar one's

---

50 Buchwald, Simon Wilde (1894), p. 70.
51 For figures on Lyon and Montpellier see Lingo, Rise (1980), pp. 46f.

honor or at least one's repute, physicians had no choice but to examine human excretions as a major path to a precise diagnosis.

Contemporary critics of medicine did not mince words when bringing up this painful subject. The art of medicine, as Agrippa von Nettesheim mercilessly put it, was "filthy". It was only "because of a shameful profit" that physicians circled "around sick people's piss-pots and outhouses". They were "for the most part contagious and reeking of patients' urine and feces", "filthier than even the midwives, as they have to look at nasty and filthy things with their own eyes, and hear and smell the belching and farting of the patients."[52] Zeno Reichart was "not born for stool and urine" a befriended apothecary argued and recommended that the young man should study law rather than medicine. Although he had first wanted him to study medicine, Zeno's father now agreed.[53] Theology and jurisprudence – the latter commonly favored over medicine by the sons of nobility – did not endanger one's dignity in the same way. In addition, medicine put the physician's own health at risk, especially in times of epidemics. Many a physician fell victim to the plague, and it was commonly assumed in such cases that he had contracted it from his patients.

Apart from all that, the road to becoming a *doctor medicinae* was long and costly – though the same could be said about theology and jurisprudence. Usually following the study of the liberal arts, a medical degree took at least three or four more years, often more. This was a long time in which the young men usually continued to be a drain on their fathers' financial resources. The expense was even greater if they spent at least a part of their studies at a renowned university abroad. In addition to travel costs, enrollment fees and other tuition fees, for example for anatomical demonstrations or private courses, which played a very important role in Padua,[54] there were the costs for room and board, for clothing and books.[55]

---

52 Nettesheim, Eitelkeit (1913), p. 79.
53 Ludwig, Vater und Sohn (1999), p. 227, letter from Wolfgang Reichart to Zeno Reichart, 24 February 1524, "non ad stercora et lotia esse natum".
54 Johann Schwartz, e.g., claimed that he could make ends meet in Padua with the grant he received but only if he did not seek deeper medical knowledge ("medicinischen Sachen nicht sonderlich nachforschen") (Hauptstaatsarchiv Stuttgart, A 282, 1301, letter from Johann Schwartz to Franz Kurtz, 4 February 1573).
55 Precise figures are difficult to come by and the variety of coins and their changing value make any comparison problematic. The 70 fl. which Ulrich Ellenbog had to pay in advance at the Domus Sapientiae (University) in Siena in the early sixteenth century suggest a relatively modest price; the money bought him food, a room with bed and bedding, two tables and two chairs for a period of seven years (Ellenbog, Briefwechsel (1938), pp. 14f.). In 1553, Philipp Bech had to pay one taler and two groschen per week in Leipzig to the physician Martin

Georg Keller, in 1556, tells us about fellow students in Padua who could not make ends meet even with an annual allowance of 100 gulden[56] – and this in spite of the relatively low cost of living in Padua.[57] In Paris – expensive and in turmoil due to the French Wars of Religion and later the St. Bartholomew's Day massacre – room and board could not be obtained even for 14 gulden a month, according to a supplication by Johann Schwartz in 1572.[58]

These costs were not the only obstacle. Increasingly, having a successful medical career was tied to carrying the title of *doctor medicinae*, preferably granted by one of the leading universities of the time. Until the sixteenth century, it had been possible in many places to make a decent living as a physician without a doctoral degree. Lacking the title of *doctor medicinae*, Ulrich Lehner from the town of Kaub had a flourishing practice in Prague as late as 1550. Yet he was already an exception. In some cities, like Augsburg with its many physicians, not even a doctoral title came with a license to practice. It was merely the prerequisite to seek accreditation from the *collegium medicum*. In France, only a doctoral degree from Paris or Montpellier gave the right to practice anywhere in the country. Graduates of other universities could expect having to pass another exam if they were going to practice in a French city.[59]

A proper doctorate from a recognized university was expensive. According to Georg Keller's account, the cost in Padua in Handsch's time was twenty-four to thirty gulden, and even as much as fifty.[60] In addition to the fees paid to the professors and the custodian, students often had to pay for the banquet that was commonly hosted by doctoral candidates and for gifts in kind, such as the gloves that were given to professors in Montpellier, for example.[61] Consequently, there

---

Drembeck, in whose house he lived. The upkeep for the horse with which he wanted to ride from Leipzig back to Basel cost another taler a week; whether the amount included the cost of food and drink, is not clear (letter from Bech to Johann Ulrich Iselin, 9 September 1553, in: Jenny, Amerbachkorrespondenz (1982), pp. 140f. (www.aerztebriefe.de/id/00007930 , M. Kohler/T. Walter). Jakob Baldenberger, a medical student in Montpellier in 1551/52, spent 22 crowns or about 35 fl. in eight months (letter from Baldenberger to the town council of St. Gallen, 19 June 1552; www.aerztebriefe.de/id/00019601, A. Döll/ T. Walter). According to Johann Schwartz, in Padua in 1573, the modest meal in the *bursa* alone cost 6 crowns (Hauptstaatsarchiv Stuttgart, A 282, 1301, letter to Franz Kurtz, 4 February 1573).
56 Schieß, Briefe (1906), pp. 22f.
57 Brugi, Gli scolari (1903), p. 12.
58 HStA Stuttgart, A 282, Bü. 1301, letter from Johann Schwartz to Duke Ludwig of Württemberg, October 1572.
59 Lunel, Maison (2008), pp. 42–45.
60 Schieß, Briefe (1906), p. 23; conversion into gulden based on his own (rough) indications (ibid., p. 5).
61 Dulieu, Médecine (1979), pp. 66–69.

were many German-speaking students of universities in Northern Italy or Montpellier who opted to conclude their studies later by obtaining a doctoral degree from a different university which offered more attractive financial conditions. In the late sixteenth century, Basel was an especially popular place in this respect.

In the correspondence between medical students and their fathers, financial questions and requests for more money played a central role and were a potential source of conflict, especially when fathers suspected that their sons were not dedicated enough to their studies, or that they might even be engaging in licentious behavior or throwing money away. Johann Georg Gockel complained that the beating his father had given him had made him stop asking for money to buy new trousers, but it did not change the fact that his current trousers were riddled with holes. Going around in rags like this, he ran the risk of becoming the laughing stock among those around him.[62] Mothers and sisters, too, were sometimes approached about money. In response to his request, Gockel's mother sent her son only a pittance, and combined it with a stern admonition that he was not to waste it all on food or to mingle with bad company. If he should prove to be a wretch like his cousin, whom she had just seen, she would kick him until the dirt came out of his gullet.[63] From Siena, Ulrich Ellenbog wrote three letters in quick succession to his sister Elisabeth in Ravensburg to ask – successfully, it seems – for money for his doctorate.[64] Some medical students borrowed money from friends and fellow students, or they became indebted to their landlords for their room and board, telling them that they expected more money to be sent soon, only to make for the hills. The representatives of the *Natio germanica artistarum* in Padua – an association of the numerous German-speaking students of the arts and of medicine – had to deal on a regular basis with Padua citizens who came to them demanding the money owed them by members of the *Natio* who had left without paying.[65]

The costs of studying and gaining a doctoral degree may have been high, yet they were not prohibitive: social mobility was greater at the time than one might assume. Studying medicine was by no means open only to young men from the wealthy upper classes of European cities. The sons of ordinary craftsmen, too,

---

[62] Stadtarchv Ulm, J1 Autographen, L 74f., letter from Johann Georg Gockel to his father Balthasar, 10 May 1627.
[63] Ibid., L 76, letter from Susanna Gockel to Johann Georg Gockel, around 1627.
[64] Ellenbog, Briefwechsel (1938), p. 86, summary of a letter from Nicolaus Ellenbog to Ulrich Ellenbog, 6 January 1512.
[65] Archivio antico dell'Università di Padova, Padua, n. 476 and n. 477, Epistolario della Nazione degli Artisti, 1565–1647.

could sometimes find a way into medicine. There was, for example, Daniel Sennert, the son of a shoemaker, who studied in Wittenberg in the late sixteenth century and went on to become one of the most well-known and most recognized physicians of his time.[66] Many students were able to earn at least some of the money they required for their studies and to meet their needs. The position of assistant or *famulus* to a professor was greatly sought after. It promised not only financial rewards. Sharing a household and a place at the dinner table with a professor, students were able to establish a social bond and perhaps get to know the professor's colleagues and acquaintances, who might prove helpful further down the road. In 1572, Johann Schwartz, for instance, asked permission from his Duke to study under the famous Felix Platter, who was known to take those with whom he dined along with him when he practiced his profession.[67] Rudolf Gwalther advised the young Georg Keller, whose studies he supported financially, to try and become the assistant to a professor in Padua. Keller saw no opportunity at the time, likely because all available positions had been taken.[68] Later, when he spent more time in Padua, he did indeed have hopes of being received in the house of his revered teacher Bassiano Landi.[69] Theodor Zwinger, said Keller, was already serving Landi as his *famulus,* like other students before him. He thought that this was not a particularly toilsome position. All he had to do was write down the lectures of the professor, who would dictate them to him, go to his lectures, and generally accompany him. In exchange, this would give him the opportunity to learn Latin and Greek.[70] The path chosen by Jean Zonion, by contrast, was likely an exception. He first taught school in Basel but then married an approximately seventy-year-old woman, whose money allowed him to go to Montpellier and earn his doctoral degree. After her death, he practiced medicine in Ravensburg.[71]

More than a few young men who came from modest circumstances were able to win the support of a patron or were awarded a scholarship. In Augsburg, for example, a private endowment, the Remboldsche Stiftung, funded the medical studies of Adam Buecher and others.[72] In Jena, a privately funded scholarship was

---

66 Vita Danielis Sennerti in Sennert, Opera (1656).
67 HStA Stuttgart, A 282, Bü. 1301, letter from Johann Schwartz to Duke Ludwig of Württemberg, October 1572.
68 Schieß, Briefe (1906), p. 8.
69 Ibid., p. 20.
70 Ibid., p. 21.
71 Platter, Tagebuch (1976), p. 188; Gaudin, Platter (1892), p. 63.
72 Letter from Adam Buecher to the town authorities in Augsburg, 13 June 1603 (www.aerztebriefe.de/id/00011653, S. Herde).

available for students of medicine from Coburg.[73] A scholarship donated by the physician Johann Neefe in Chemnitz allowed Martin Cotta to study in Leipzig.[74] Some municipal authorities likewise supported the sons of their citizens with significant sums of money and enabled them to study medicine at a distinguished university, thus securing the future services of a well-trained physician for the town. Scholarships like these are known to have existed in Torgau,[75] Zurich,[76] St. Gallen,[77] and Königsberg,[78] for example. Some territorial lords supported the medical studies of their native sons for similar reasons. Johann Schwartz, for instance, received 150 gulden from Duke Ludwig of Württemberg for his medical studies in Paris.[79]

Georg Handsch, like many young men who later practiced medicine, came from a well-to-do middle-class background. His father Wenzel must have been a rather wealthy and respected man.[80] Probably he was a cloth merchant or clothier. In his botanical notes about *rubea tinctorum*, also known as "madder" or

---

73 Hase, Reinesius (1858), p. 314.
74 Letter from Cotta, who was still an arts student at the time, to Johann Neefe, 12 April 1561 (www.aerztebriefe.de/id/00030051, T. Walter).
75 Horst, Epistolae (1596), p. 70, "vestrumque studium iuvandi egestatem meam mihi [. . .] gratissimum acciderit".
76 Schieß, Briefe (1906).
77 Arbenz/Wartmann, Vadianische Briefsammlung, part 6/2 (1908), pp. 612–615, letter from Jakob Baldenberger to Joachim Vadian, Strasbourg, 31 March 1547, about fellow students and others of his age group who received a grant from the town council (www.aerztebriefe.de/id/00006766, M. Kohler/T. Walter/M. Huth).
78 See, e.g., the letter from Konrad Battus to the Elector Joachim Friedrich of Brandenburg, 10 July 1600 (www.aerztebriefe.de/id/00004069, U. Schlegelmilch); letter from Valerius Fiedler, medical student in Padua, to Duke Albrecht von Preußen, Padua, 20 August 1554, asking for his grant to be increased in order to allow him to spend a third year in Italy, inspite of the high costs (www.aerztebriefe.de/id/00020767, U. Schlegelmilch); idem, Padua, 12 January 1554, expressing his gratitude for the 200 crowns he was granted for the current, third year (www.aerztebriefe.de/id/00020768, U. Schlegelmilch).
79 Hauptstaatsarchiv Stuttgart, A 282, 1301, letter from Johann Schwartz to Duke Ludwig of Württemberg, October 1572.
80 The parish books from Leipa have survived only from the eighteenth century onwards. The "memory books" (Gedächtnisbücher) of the town mention Wenzel Handsch since 1531 (Hantschel, Heimatkunde (1911), p. 617; in the council minutes ("Stadtbuch"), Wenzel appears for the first time in 1540, as a guarantor for a new citizen (Ebelová, Pamětní (2005), p. 161; further entry in 1549, ibid., p. 168). It is possible that the family originally came from Leipzig. In the 1550s a certain Georgius Hantschius ran a printing workshop there. He may have been a relative but this is made unlikely by the fact that Handsch (according to Cod. 11205, fol. 1r) was surprised when he saw a book at Collinus' that bore the note "Lipsiae in officina Georgij Hantschij".

"dyer's madder", Handsch remarked that he had seen how the cloth makers at his father's place used the red root of the plant for dyeing.[81] His father owned a house in Leipa[82] and was a member of the town council.[83] For the burial of his son Christoph in 1557, at which various members of the nobility were present, he spent around eighteen talers.[84] He gave Georg a good schooling, first with a teacher in Leipa, whom Georg later thanked with a poem saying he had led his peasant's mind ("agrestem mentem") to higher things.[85] After this he attended the Latin school in the Silesian town of Goldberg, today's Złotoryja in Poland. This school was one of the most renowned Latin schools of the time and, under the directorship of Valentin Trotzendorf, was known far beyond the borders of the land. Among its students were Caspar Peucer and others who later rose to eminence. It offered a comprehensive education in the *studia humanitatis*, above all in the ancient languages. Classes were taught in Latin and students were admonished, under the threat of punishment, to speak only Latin among themselves.[86]

Presumably in 1544, but perhaps as late as 1545 or 1546,[87] Handsch went to Prague. There is no evidence that he was enrolled there at Charles-University to study the arts.[88] His own notes tell us that he never earned the title *magister artium* and the dean's records of the faculty in Prague do not even list him among the graduated baccalaureates.[89] His poems from that time – among them a versified autobiography – suggest that instead he attended the private-school lessons

---

81 Cod. 11205, fol. 117r.
82 Cod. 9821, fol. 80r: "Has Venceslaus Handsch renovavit sumptibus aedes/ Ista stat Italico facta labore domus".
83 Pardi, Titoli dottorali (1901), p. 166.
84 Cod. 9550, fol. 1r-v.
85 Cod. 9821, foll. 24r-27r.
86 Bauch, Valentin Trozendorf (1921); a Latin school was established in Leipa in 1627 only (Hantschel, Heimatkunde (1911), pp. 856–858). A contemporary school book based on Trozendorf's method (Ludovicus, Compendium (1572)) shows that the teaching of Latin was quite sophisticated in didactic terms.
87 In December 1544, he wrote a letter from Prague but this does not prove that he had moved there permanently (Cod. 9650, foll. 1r-3r).
88 Wolkan (Geschichte (1894), p. 126) already came to the same conclusion.
89 Liber decanorum (1832).

for "boys" taught by Magister Johannes Schentigar,[90] perhaps in preparation of a later course of study at university.

Then, however, came a caesura: it seems that Handsch's father Wenzel, who had been generous for many years, was no longer willing to continue to support the education of his son in the same manner.[91] The reasons for this remain unclear. Following the early death of Georg's mother, Wenzel had married again and had more children.[92] Numerous entries in Handsch's notebooks show, however, that he had a good rapport with his stepmother, whom he often called simply "mother" ("mater"), and with his half-siblings. When later writing his will, he specifically asked to be buried next to his father. We can only speculate about the reasons, but it appears they had a falling-out. In later times, Georg's father continued to be critical of his work and sometimes accused him of lacking earnestness, as various entries in Georg's notebooks tell us. Possibly, he was unhappy about his son's lifestyle. Georg's notebooks include numerous indications that he had a pronounced penchant for wine, even by the comparatively generous standards of the time.[93] Already as a young man in Prague, he was rebuked by his mentor Lehner and others because of his drinking. He considered these remonstrations justified and intended to remain soberer and mindful of his dignity.[94]

Georg Handsch, in any case, found himself in the position of needing to earn his own living. He asked Schentigar to commend him to Matthaeus Collinus (1516–1566), the leading mind of the Prague humanists and a teacher in the arts faculty,[95] and to ask that he be given the vacant position of assistant.[96] In 1543, Collinus had founded a private school for the sons of the Prague gentry,

---

90 Cod. 9821, fol. 130r, "Et quia Schentyarus clarus, doctusque poeta/ Privatim pueros instituebat ibi/ Huius discipulus sum factus ludimagistri"; drawing on ancient Rome as a model, "ludimagister" was a commonly used term for "teacher" at the time. In 1545, Handsch contacted Schentigar several times and asked, among other things, on behalf of the student body ("grex discipulorum") for permission to play some "honourable" games (ibid., foll. 7v-8r.); on Schentigar see Kalina von Jätenstein, Nachrichten, vol. 1 (1818), pp. 18–29; Hejnic, Dva humanisté (1957), pp. 6–16.
91 Cod. 9821, fol. 130v: "Ante meus genitor sumptus mihi suppeditarat/ Et studium largo foverat aere meum."
92 She died in 1539 (Ibid., fol. 69r and fol. 74r).
93 Feustel, Grenzgänge (2013), esp. pp. 34f.
94 Cod. 11205, fol. 292v: "Sis sobrius et serva gravitatem"; "hic peccavi q[uod] permisi me inebriari, et hoc M. Ulricus in me reprehendit"; similarly, ibid., fol. 533v.
95 Cf. Storchová, Collinus (2020); see also Jakubcová/Pernerstorfer/Reitterer, Theater (2013), pp. 123–125, and Menčik, Dopisy (1914).
96 Cod. 9821, foll. 77v-78v; the heading "Pragae Anno 1547" on the preceding page, fol. 77r, suggests that he wrote this poem like the two preceding ones in 1547.

and in 1548, he acquired the so-called Angel's Garden in Prague's New Town including its buildings for this purpose.[97] Schentigar's efforts were apparently successful and Handsch took up work as teaching assistant in Collinus's school.[98] Thanks to his excellent education, he had knowledge enough of the *studia humanitatis* and the *artes liberales* to earn a modest living even without a formal academic degree. He was able to instruct his friend Thomas Mitis not only in music and arithmetic but even in the Hebrew language.[99]

This connection with Collinus was decisive for Handsch's future. Thanks to Collinus, Handsch gained access to the circle of humanists and poets associated with the wealthy Bohemian vice judge Johannes Hoddeiovinus (Hodiejowsky of Hodiejowa), who asked them to write poems for him that would, for one thing, glorify him and his possessions. We will come back to this later. It was also Collinus who, in 1548, helped Handsch find a position as assistant with the aforementioned Prague physician Magister Ulrich Lehner.[100] At the time when he was writing poems for Hoddeiovinus, Handsch, under the tutelage of Lehner, was also striving to expand his medical knowledge, and thus he was – as he wrote in a letter – doubly following in the footsteps of Apollo, the inventor of poetry and medicine.[101]

We know little about his work for Lehner. Handsch made only infrequent notes. While two of his notebooks concern Lehner's practice during the late 1540s,[102] it appears that Handsch only copied the practice records of his teacher,[103] including many entries from years before he was under Lehner's tutelage. There are only occasional indications that he personally treated patients during his time

---

97 Jakubcová/Pernerstorfer/Reitterer, Theater (2013), p. 124.
98 Handsch called himself one of Collinus' "hypodidascali", i. e. lower ranking teachers (Cod. 9650, foll. 6r-9r, copy of a letter to Thomas Mitis, 25 July 1548).
99 Cod. 9821, fol. 77r-v, copy of a letter from Handsch to Mitis; possibly Handsch learnt Hebrew from Dominicus Nösler in Leipa, whose knowledge of Hebrew and Latin he later praised in an epitaph (ibid., foll. 80v-81v).
100 Ibid., fol. 130v.
101 Cod. 9650, foll. 6r-9r, copy of a letter to Thomas Mitis, 25 July 1548.
102 Cod. 11006, "Praxis et factitatio medicinae D. Ulrici medici Pragensis nec non D. Galli et Gerhardi regis Ferdinandi physicorum, observata et collecta exquisitissime per Georgium Handschium Lippensem germanicobohemicum Pragae An[no] 1550"; "Gerhardi" probably refers to the Habsburg court physician Gerhard Bucoldianus; Cod. 11247, "Secunda pars practicae D. Ulrici Leonori a Cauba, Medici Pragensis. Collecta per Georgium Handschium Lippensem Germanico-Bohemum Anno 1550".
103 The handwriting is very clean and uniform; repeatedly Lehner's approach is explicitly rendered in the first person ("omisi", "ordinavi").

with Lehner. For example, Handsch mentioned a formula Lehner had dictated to him for an acquaintance in Leipa.[104]

At any rate, the course had been set for the first leg of Handsch's medical journey. It appears that Handsch came to the conclusion relatively early that medicine had particularly good prospects to offer. "Recht Artzney Künst / Erlannget Günnst / Lob, Ehr unnd Gellt / Ynn aller Wellt" [Good medical art / Achieves favor / Praise, honor and money / In all the world], he rhymed at the beginning of one of his notebooks. Commenting on his verse, he wrote that medicine was a safe companion ("viaticum") in all lands.[105] Without his father's support, however, he lacked the necessary means to study medicine, all the more so because he would have to go abroad; the medical faculty at the Prague university was no longer active in Handsch's time.[106] It appears that in the end it was thanks to a benefactor that Handsch was able to study medicine. In the summer of 1549, when Handsch was already learning from Lehner, he still hoped to find employment at the court chancellery.[107] The following summer, he was still encouraging an acquaintance of his to send that man's brother to Prague, promising that he would help him learn the Czech language.[108] Yet, then in the fall of 1550, Handsch left for Padua and took up the study of medicine. He documented his journey via Salzburg in an elaborate travel poem, a *hodoeporicon*.[109] It has been supposed that a young nobleman, Karl von Dietrichstein, whom Handsch accompanied to Padua, funded his studies, but there is no explanation of what might have caused Karl von Dietrichstein (or his parents) to extend this generous support.[110] An entry in Handsch's notebooks as well as his later work in the house of the Habsburg court physician Andrea Gallo make it almost certain, in fact, that things were different: "Doctor Gallus wants to send me to Italy with his son and pay for my expenses", the succinct entry reads.[111] Gallo lived in Prague and Handsch had befriended his son Giulio.

---

104 Cod. 11006, fol. 31v; it was merely a remedy against toothache.
105 Cod. 11210, fol. 1r.
106 Svobodný, Medical faculty (2001); Hlaváčková/ Svobodný, Dějiny lékařství (2004), pp. 51–53; Hlaváčková/Svobodný/Adamec, Biografický slovník (1988/1993).
107 Cod. 9650, foll. 18v-20r, copy of a letter to Martin Hanno, 25 July 1549.
108 Cod. 9650, fol. 22r-v, copy of a letter to Martin Huber, 22 July 1550.
109 Cod. 9821, foll. 288v-297v.
110 Handsch dedicated a long poem to von Dietrichstein in which he referred to the years they spent together, first at Collinus' school in the Angel's Garden, in Prague, and later in Padua, but he did not mention any financial support or express his gratitude, something he was not usually relectant to do (ibid., foll. 248r-250r).
111 Cod. 9666, fol. 1v: "Doctor Gallus vult me mittere in Italiam cum filio suis sumptibus".

Attending an Italian university must have seemed an obvious choice in the case of Giulio Gallo. His father had studied in Padua and, before coming to Prague, had practiced in Trento.[112] To Handsch, going to Padua came with another tangible benefit: medicine was taught in Padua in the arts faculty.[113] And this meant that, unlike with other universities, students wanting to enroll did not have to show the master's degree that he had never earned.

---

112 For Gallo's biography see Span, Epicedion (1560). According to Span Gallo spent the last twelve years of his life, i.e. from about 1548, in the service of the Habsburg court; before that he practised medicine in Trento. He had two other sons, Guglielmo and Ludovico. For Gallo's correspondence with Sigismondo Thun see Quaranta, Medici-physici trentini (2019) pp. 62–73.
113 Bylebyl, Medicine (1985); only the students of law had a faculty of their own.

The Study of Medicine

In the sixteenth and seventeenth centuries, students from north of the Alps flocked to the universities of Northern Italy, mainly Padua and Bologna. Although there were quite a number of universities north of the Alps that had their own faculties of medicine, a Europe-wide comparison yields striking differences. At most of the late medieval universities in German-speaking areas – and the situation was similar in England and large parts of France[114] – the faculty of medicine played a rather insignificant role.[115] It stood in the shadow of the arts faculty and the other two higher faculties, theology and law. Some faculties of medicine employed only a single professor and even in places where there were two or three professors of medicine, they were often little known, unrenowned individuals. The number of medical students was also very modest in most cases and the number who received a medical degree was even smaller. According to the matriculation records in Cologne, for example, only about 0.4 percent of students studied medicine there in the time between the late fourteenth and the early sixteenth centuries.[116] During about the same time period in Erfurt, there was a total of sixty-four medical graduates, including those who had followed up their studies in the local arts faculty with medical studies. Medical scholars and students there did not even have their own lecture hall.[117] And even in Basel, where at the end of the sixteenth century a considerable number of medical students received their doctorates, the situation was described as unsatisfactory by Georg Keller: of the two professors, one, Johannes Huber, was considered a practitioner more than anything else and the second, Isaak Keller, did not enjoy a good reputation.[118]

At the leading universities in Italy – and the same was true in France in Montpellier and Paris – the situation was very different. There medicine was more or less on par with the two other higher faculties with respect to the number of students and lecturers, but also with respect to status, and this found expression not least of all in the remuneration of the professors. In addition, a certain degree of religious tolerance was extended, at least to foreigners.[119] Accordingly,

---

114 Lunel, Maison (2008), p. 31.
115 On medical education in the universities of the various European countries, see Siriasi, Medicine (2001); with a focus on the German universities Nutton, Medicine (1997), pp. 173–190 and on those in the Netherlands Lindeboom, Medical education (1970), pp. 201–234.
116 Abe, Medizinische Fakultät (1974), p. 26, on the figures for Cologne.
117 Ibid., p. 28.
118 Schieß, Briefe (1906), p. 11.
119 Although Johann Schwartz was full of praise for the University of Padua in the 1570s, he preferred to take his doctorate in Basel because he would have had to take a papal oath in

the aforementioned universities attracted many medical students from north of the Alps.[120] Precise numbers are lacking, but a look at physician biographies even suggests that it was more a rule than an exception for physicians from German-speaking areas to do their training (and often receive their doctorates) in Italy or the south of France until well into the sixteenth century.[121] This gradually began to change in the second half of the sixteenth century when Basel and Wittenberg increasingly attracted medical students.

By far, the most predominant form of transferring knowledge at universities across Europe throughout the entire early modern period and for all disciplines was the *lectura,* the lecture.[122] Lectures gave shape to teaching activities and set the daily, weekly, and annual rhythm of academic life. In Padua and Montpellier, but also in Ingolstadt for example, the lecture period ran from late autumn to early summer.[123] In Padua, the anatomical demonstrations were held over the Christmas holiday,[124] and the winter carnival in nearby Venice caused long interruptions. As Georg Keller complained, no *collegia* were held during his first year in Padua between January 21 and March 4.[125] Teaching activities were sometimes disturbed for even longer periods by epidemics. In times of pestilence, students found themselves needing to move to other university towns that had not yet been affected – if they were still allowed to do so. In his letters, Georg Keller described the drastic measures to which everyone, including of course students, was subjected when the plague befell Padua in 1555. Houses that were suspect were barricaded, the town gates closed. He had already experienced something similar in Paris.[126]

Generally, lectures were held in the morning and in the afternoon, five days a week. Usually no lectures were held on one workday. The university in Padua

---

Padua (HStA Stuttgart, A 282, Bü 1301, supplication by Johann Schwartz to Duke Ludwig of Württemberg, submitted 26 April 1576; ibid., letter from Schwartz' father-in-law, Samuel Heiland, 6 April 6 [1575]).
120 Cf. Germain, Les pèlerins (1878), vol. 1, pp. 161–181.
121 See also Dotzauer, Deutsches Studium (1974).
122 Overviews of medical education in the sixteenth century in O'Malley, Medical education (1970), pp. 89–102; Talbot, Medical education (1970), pp. 73–87; Siraisi, Faculty of medicine (1992), pp. 360–387; Nutton/Porter, History (1995); Nutton, Medicine (1997), pp. 173–187; Brockliss, Curricula (1996), pp. 565–567; Siraisi, Medicine (2001).
123 In Padua, the academic year was usually inaugurated on the day after All Saints' Day (Bertolaso, Ricerche (1958–59), p. 19).
124 Adam, Vitae (1620), p. 205.
125 Zentralbibliothek Zürich, Ms F 38, fol. 30bis r, letter from Keller to R. Gwalther, 10 March [1552]; cf. Schieß, Briefe (1906), pp. 7f., letter from Padua, 26 February 1551.
126 Schieß, Briefe (1906), p. 18, letter, 4 October 1555.

was unique insofar as two professors who had the same areas of specialization would give their lectures at the same hour and would thus enter into direct competition with each other. When Joachim Curaeus went to Padua in 1557, Vettore Trincavella, for example, whom Curaeus considered to be the more learned professor, was competed against Antonio Fracanzano, who according to Curaeus knew better how to attract students with his well-chosen words.[127] In these circumstances it was especially important in Padua to coordinate the times of the lectures. Statutes precisely regulated the schedule. Immediately following the tolling of the morning bells, the professors for theoretical medicine would start the morning lecture. Unlike for professors with other specializations, they were required under the threat of disciplinary action to read for at least two hours. Subsequently, associate professors lectured on *medicina practica*. In the afternoon – until Easter at the 21st hour and after Easter at the 19th hour (in Padua, the first hour started at sunset the previous evening) – the associate professors of theoretical medicine delivered their lectures followed by the full professors of *medicina practica*.[128]

The term "lecture" has endured to the present day, but for the early modern period it is to be taken quite literally. In the traditional lecture, the lecturer read from an authoritative text, explaining the meaning sentence by sentence or passage by passage. Supported by a firm grasp of Latin, a basic knowledge of natural philosophy, and critical evaluation skills acquired through training in Aristotelian logic, prospective physicians gained significant knowledge during these lectures in which a professor introduced texts, interpreted difficult passages, and weighed conflicting opinions or tried to reconcile them.

With the so-called *Articella*, a certain canon of authoritative texts had already become established in the Middle Ages. The central texts of this collection of writing, which has its origins in the Salerno medical school, remained influential in the medical teaching of the Renaissance: the Hippocratic *Aphorisms* with Galen's commentary, Hippocrates' *Book of Prognostics*, and Galen's *Ars parva* with the introduction ("Isagoge") by Ḥunain ibn Isḥāq (Iohannitius). Since the High Middle Ages, Avicenna's *Canon medicinae* had served as a further central textbook. In contrast to the loose succession of the numerous writings by Galen and the short, largely unstructured propositions of the Hippocratic *Aphorisms*, Avicenna's work offered a systematic survey of medicine as a whole and could thus serve as a first-rate textbook.[129] The curriculum that was set forth in the statutes of Padua in

---

127 Adam, Vitae (1620), pp. 204f.
128 Bertolaso, Ricerche (1958–59) gives a list of the holders of the individual chairs; the major early modern source is Facciolati, Fasti (1757).
129 Avicenna, Canon (1595); Siraisi, Avicenna (1987).

1495 largely still corresponded with this traditional canon of writings. First-year students had to read the entire first book of the *Canon,* followed in the second year by the Hippocratic aphorisms and Galen's commentary and, if time permitted, Hippocrates' writings on prognosis. In the third year, Galen's *Ars parva* was next in line.[130]

With the rise of humanism, some physicians, buttressed by their excellent knowledge of Latin and Greek, made it their mission to significantly expand the traditional teaching canon. In their investigations of old manuscripts, they discovered medical texts of ancient authorities that had remained unknown thus far, especially those from the Hippocratic school and by Galen. Toiling collectively, they went through the collected Greek works of Hippocrates and Galen, producing numerous translations of the ancient writings in elegant, humanist Latin.[131] The spectrum of available writings was thus greatly expanded, so that Jacobus Sylvius, for example, in his *Ordo et ordinis ratio in legendis Hippocratis et Galeni libris* (1548), was able to list dozens of works by Galen, Hippocrates, and other authorities in thematic order. For university teaching, however, this richness also presented new challenges. In a disclaimer to his list, Sylvius commented that it would be exceedingly protracted and onerous ("longissimum et molestissimum") to treat all of these works in medical teaching. His personal selection was already extensive enough. As one could gather from his lectures, he limited himself to certain works for each of the different areas of medicine. He named about fifteen works in particular, most of them by Galen.

For some in the medical profession, medical humanism brought with it pronounced anti-Arab sentiment.[132] Certain physicians pulled Persian and Arabic physicians to pieces along with their "barbaric" medicine, and even wanted to see them banned from the medical curriculum.[133] Others considered a deficient translation of these works to be the problem. Even some of the humanist admirers of Hippocrates and Galen had to admit, however, that the writings they

---

130 Statuta (c. 1600 [?]), book 2, XVI; this is probably a later print – the statutes are clearly dated 1495.
131 The literature on this topic is extensive; a good first orientation is provided by Durling, Census (1961); Bylebyl, Medicine (1985); Boudon-Miller/Cobolet, Lire les médecins Grecs (2004); Fortuna, Latin editions (2012). Vivian Nutton has explored various aspects of medical humanism in numerous contributions; see idem, Diffusion (2002); idem, Hippocrates (1989); idem, John Caius (1984). An excellent overview of the situation in Padua can be found in Bylebyl, School of Padua (1979).
132 Germain, La médecine arabe (1877); Baader, Medizinische Theorie (1987).
133 Cornarius, Medicina (1556), pp. 116–119.

had left behind were not nearly as extensive and thorough as Avicenna's systematic survey of the whole field of medicine in his *Canon medicinae*. It was not until the second half of the sixteenth century that the *Canon* was challenged by a serious competitor in the form of the *Universa medicina* by Jean Fernel (1497–1558). Based on Galen but developing his medicine further, Fernel gave a comprehensive overview of the entirety of theoretical and practical medicine, one that was comparable to the *Canon* but more readable, up-to-date, and succinct. His work remained very influential until well into the seventeenth century.[134]

As a result of the intensive editing and translation work of the medical humanists, the *Canon*, Rhazes's *Ad Almansorem* and other leading works of Persian and Arabic medicine gradually lost significance. In no way, however, did they become obsolete. At leading Italian universities as elsewhere, the *Canon* remained a pillar of medical teaching.[135] In Padua – and this is also shown by Handsch's extensive lecture notes – the *Canon* and *Ad Almansorem* still made up the core curriculum around 1550, along with Galen's *Ars parva* and the Hippocratic *Aphorisms*.[136]

The most important source in historical research about university teaching has traditionally been the historical statutes listing the set texts that were to be commented on in lectures. These lists, however, give an incomplete view of the actual lectures. Not only did they lag behind the actual teaching practice, frequently laying down what had actually been long established in teaching practice.[137] They also represent only a part of the teaching activity. Looking only at these lists, essential elements of medical training remain largely invisible.

A more precise and detailed picture of the medical teaching can be gained by looking at student notes. Happily, a wealth of such notes from the sixteenth century has survived, but not much of it has been systematically researched.[138] The notes vary widely with respect to the form they take. Sometimes students wrote down the lecture word for word. This went so far that they even reproduced forms of address such as "you young men" ("vos juvenes"), used by the

---

134 Fernel, Universa medicina (1644); Sherrington, Endeavour (1946); Roger, Fernel (1960); Hirai, Medical humanism (2011), pp. 46–79.
135 Siraisi, Avicenna (1987).
136 Under the heading "leguntur Paduae", Handsch explicitly listed the works mentioned – and only these (Cod. 11240, fol. 28r); even in the early seventeenth century there was still a chair in Padua with the denomination "Ad lecturam secundae fen primi Canonis Avicennae" (Bertolaso, La cattedra (1960), p. 113). On the humanistic reception of Galen's *Ars parva* see Mugnai Carrara, Epistemological problems (1999).
137 Brockliss, Curricula (1996), p. 563.
138 In the course of my research, I have so far been able to identify more than two dozen such handwritten lecture notes from Padua alone.

lecturer. It was also not unusual for them to retain the use of the first person ("ego") in their notes when the lecturer made statements about his own experience or relayed his personal opinion. At the other end of the spectrum there are short, sketchy notes only about certain aspects that struck the student as noteworthy and important to remember. In Handsch's Padua notebooks we find the whole range, from *dictata* to short, loose notes.

From Handsch's notes as well as those of other contemporary students, two important developments come to light which find only very incomplete expression in the statutes. First, the professors did much of their teaching privately, outside the official, curricular courses, with smaller groups of students. As we will see, "private" lessons given to a limited group of paying students were especially important in teaching anatomy. They were, in fact, far more important in helping students gain anatomical knowledge and skills than the large public anatomy demonstrations which have so far been the focus of historical research on anatomical instruction in the early modern period.

Second, the sixteenth century saw an increase in the significance, at least at the Italian universities, of lectures with a thematic orientation. Here the professor did not comment on one specific text. Instead he would treat a certain subject area, drawing on the works of different authors and sometimes on personal, practical experience as well. Giovanni Battista da Monte was once more among the trailblazers who, as his student Girolamo Donzellini emphasized, not only explained authoritative works, but treated important subjects separately.[139] In Padua, Handsch heard the private lectures of Fracanzano on diseases of women and took notes during private, at-home lectures about stomach diseases, which were given by Trincavella on holidays.[140] Handsch's notes on a lecture by Fracanzano about the French disease also give the distinct impression of a private lecture.[141] A couple of years later, another student in Padua took notes on Fracanzano's *lectiones extraordinariae* on fever symptoms.[142] During those years, Bellocati lectured, again "extra ordinem", about children's diseases, while Trincavella, in

---

139 Da Monte, Opuscula (1558), vol. 1, dedicatory epistle by Donzellini to Giulio Alessandrini: "Solebat enim ille, praeter seriem authorum, quos explicabat, peculiares aliquando tractationes facere, in quibus de rebus maxime necessariis auditores erudiebat, et ad authores ipsos exactius intelligendos magno eorum emolumento instituebat."
140 Cod. 11226, fol. 160v.
141 Ibid., foll. 92r-119r, from 16 December 1551; ibid., foll. 123r-140r; cf. Fracanzano, De morbo (1564) (based on student notes on Fracanzano's lectures in Bologna). Fracanzano taught in Padua from 1538, first logic and then medical theory. He went to Bologna in 1555 and returned to Padua in 1564 (Mantese, Storia (1969, pp. 64–66).
142 Biblioteca dell'Arciginnasio, Bologna, Ms. A 46, title according to the heading of the index on fol. 143r.

addition to his lectures about Avicenna's writing about fevers as well as about Rhazes's teachings on the diseases of the head and chest, taught "extra ordinem" about "worms" and "arthritis".[143]

The authors of contemporary study guides put great emphasis on attending lectures. Johannes Brettschneider (aka Placotomus, 1514–1577), for example, stressed that in no way should students choose independent study over a lecture. He held that a lesson with a living voice ("viva voce") best allowed medical doctrine to be imparted as the voice had something of a "hidden energy" ("energiae latentis"). No one could learn the *pensum* of a lesson on his own with equal success.[144]

The transcripts of good lectures were, however, valuable to students who could not attend the lecture. Some lectures were even printed and published from student notes. It seems a certain demand for them was to be expected. And students would also request handwritten copies of lecture notes from each other.[145] Such a copy of a lecture, written in another man's hand is also found among the manuscripts in Handsch's *Nachlass*. It was a lecture that Augustin Schurff had given years earlier in Wittenberg, and Handsch wrote his own supplementary notes in the margins.[146]

Not only were students urged to attend lectures; intensive preparatory and follow-up work was also recommended. Student guidebooks like the one by Brettschneider even advised students to read the passages from an authoritative text that were to be addressed in the lecture at home beforehand. After the lecture, they were then supposed to carefully go through their notes and excerpt the most important topics, theorems, problems, and questions in a *diarium*. It was also said to be useful to talk and compare notes with other students, since presenting to others what one had learned was a good schooling for the mind. At the end of the week, it was then advisable to go through the week's notes, now organized thematically, and to enter them in a second, permanent notebook, one that allowed entries on certain subjects to be looked up and the grasped material to be committed to memory. It was furthermore recommended to learn one

---

143 Adam, Vitae (1620), p. 205.
144 Placotomus [Brettschneider], De ratione (1552); Adam, Vitae (1620), p. 204 attributes the same notion to Joachim Curaeus.
145 See e.g. Planerio, Epistolae (1584), letter to Franciscus Ticinensis, 1 January 1536, responding to a request for a copy of the "lectiones ordinarias".
146 Cod. 11228, "Annotationes in Nonum Rhasis ad Almansorem dictatae a doctore Augustino Schurphio in schola Vitebergensi Anno 1537". In the back cover, we find the name "Hanns Adlerus", possibly the name of the writer; in the Corpus Inscriptorum Vitebergense, however, no student of this name can be found (https://www.civ-online.org/de/service/startseite/).

theorem by heart every day. Within just a year, one would thus gain a considerable wealth of knowledge.[147] Such recommendations were taken to heart. Georg Handsch sketched a very similar two-step process. From one's unorganized lecture notes it was advisable to first gain an overview of the subjects that had been treated and then to enter the notes in a book, organizing them under different headings.[148]

Above and beyond the lectures the students also – and this was expected of them – studied the medical literature independently. The long summer vacations in particular provided opportunity for this. Some students appear to have acquired their medical knowledge almost exclusively from reading books. This was particularly true of those who started out in other areas and earned their living doing non-medical activities. The thirty-seven-year-old humanist and poet Helius Eobanus Hessus, for example, a long-time teacher of Latin at the University of Erfurt, said he had been reading Galen's works for a long time and it seemed to him that he had gained extensive knowledge of medical theory. All he was missing, he said, was practical experience and the doctor title.[149]

Contemporary reading- and study- guides provided extensive recommendations for students on how they could work methodically and commit what they read to memory. It was important first of all to make a careful selection of authors and works. In his *De ratione discendi medicinam epigraphe*, Girolamo Mercuriale asserted that one should concentrate on the recognized authorities. Students were warned not to attain their medical knowledge from compendia or summaries. According to Mercuriale, one should even avoid reading commentary if possible; it was better to penetrate the text oneself. The only exceptions here were the works of Hippocrates, with its dark passages, and Avicenna's *Canon*.[150]

The study guides recommended concentrating on not more than a few works at the same time. As Brettschneider put it, the person who ate too many dishes at once ruined his stomach and the same was true of reading.[151] Mercuriale made the specific recommendation that only one or two authors should be studied closely at once; they should be read each day at the same time, preferably in the early

---

147 Placotomus [Brettschneider], De ratione (1552).
148 Cod. 11239, fol. 100v.
149 Hessus, Helii Eobani Hessi (1543), pp. 112–115, Brief an Georg Sturtz, 14.3.1525 (www.aerztebriefe.de/id/00013019, M. Bleistein); Hessus asked Sturtz, who had left Erfurt and settled as a physician in Annaberg, for support, just as he had given it to his student Euricius Cordus; in a subsequent letter to Sturtz, dated 5 June 1525 (ibid., pp. 118–9), Hessus also referred to his medical studies.
150 Mercuriale, De ratione (1607); see also Durling, Girolamo Mercuriale's De modo studendi (1991).
151 Placotomus, De ratione (1552), no pagination.

morning hours and in the evening.[152] It was helpful, in Johannes Brettschneider's view, to proceed from the simple and general to the more specific. Not all books required the same amount of study. Some had to be read again and again ("crebro"), while others needed to be picked up only a few times or once.[153] Despite these qualifications, the long lists of recommended authors in reading- and study guides indicate a reading load far too great to be reasonably tackled.[154] Mercuriale further underlined to prospective physicians the importance of reading the poets and historians: Homer, Hesiod, Lucretius, Virgil, Horace, Juvenal, Martial, Columella, Vitruvius, Herodotus, Strabo, Pausanias, and others. Galen for his part quoted from them repeatedly and thus, according to Mercuriale, it was appropriate to branch out and collect whatever served the enrichment and adornment of medicine.[155] Not surprisingly, when Isaac Habrecht prefixed his notebook from around 1600 with an extensive list of well over sixty ancient and contemporary works, these writings found only very limited expression in his excerpts. For the most part, his notes focused on introductory *institutiones* and surveys like those by Jean Fernel and Leonhard Fuchs.[156]

Theoretical Medicine

In *medicina theorica*, students first learned to grasp the essence of medicine, to define it and to name its various branches. One of Handsch's Padua notebooks accordingly offers an overview of the terminology and classifications as we know them from numerous printed works of the time.[157] The source of his knowledge is unclear, but the systematic approach and the occasional rejection of certain parts of academic wisdom point to a lecture, perhaps by Bassiano Landi.[158] He began with Galen's oft-cited definition of medicine: medicine was the art that protected existing health, improved impaired health, and restored lost health.[159] As Handsch noted, speaking of health that was only "impaired" – as opposed to

---

152 Mercuriale, De ratione (1607), pp. 34–35.
153 Placotomus, De ratione (1552).
154 Stainpeiss, Liber (1520); cf. Pawlik, Martin Stainpeis (1980); Pons, Medicus (1600).
155 Mercuriale, De ratione (1607), p. 25.
156 Det Kongelige Bibliotek, Copenhagen, Ms. Gl. Kongl. 4 1691, medical notes of Isaac Habrecht (1606).
157 Cod. 11210; the title which Handsch gave to it was "Compendium medicinae collectum Patavii A[nno] 1551".
158 On Landi see Ferretto, Bassiano Landi (2006–2009) and Ferretto, Maestri (2012).
159 Cod. 11210, fol. 2r: "Est ars quae sanitatem praesentem custodit, viciatam emendat, et amissam restaurat".

"existing" and "lost" health – referred to a Galenic concept that was heavily discussed at the time, that of a "neutral state" between disease and health.[160] Medicine was a "scientia" insofar as it considered the causes of illness, the nature of human beings, and the efficacy of medicines. At the same time, it was a craft or an "acting art" ("ars factiva"), insofar as it was practiced. Its subject was the human body; its goal was health.[161] This was a goal it could not always achieve, however. What was crucial was to act in such a way that health was served, even if success sometimes failed to materialize.[162] Medicine consisted of a preventative and a curative part. Curative medicine consisted of medicinal, dietetic, and surgical or manual treatment.[163]

According to Handsch's notes, this was followed by a short overview of ancient medical schools after Galen. The following distinction was another topos of contemporary medical literature: on the one hand, the "empiricists" ("empirici") treated diseases based only on their experience ("suis experimentis"), without reason ("ratio") and judgment ("iudicium").[164] The "dogmatic" ("dogmatici") or "rational" ("rationales") physicians on the other hand considered human nature and the causes and fortuities of diseases on the basis of early, present, and future signs and used remedies on patients with rationality and the most finely-attuned ability to judge ("exquisito cum iudicio").[165] According to Galen, reason ("ratio") and experience ("experientia") were the legs on which medicine stood.[166]

Essential for a rational, scientific approach as per contemporary standards were the fundamental principles of natural philosophy. Knowledge based on natural philosophy about the construction, the faculties, and the functions of the human body and its parts – which is to say, knowledge about *physiologia*, as it was already called at the time – was indeed an indispensable requirement for the understanding, the diagnosis, and the treatment of illnesses.

Aspiring physicians were told and they read that the human body was composed like everything in nature of the four elements: fire, earth, water, and air. To each of these a combination of two of the four primary qualities – hot, cold, dry, and moist – was assigned. Naturally, what was even more important in understanding the human body and its functions were the four humors, whose

---

160 Joutsivuo, Scholastic tradition (1999).
161 Cod. 11210, fol. 2r.
162 Ibid.
163 Ibid., fol. 2v; the third medical sect commonly discussed in this context were the methodists who attributed diseases to an excessive widening or narrowing of the ducts in the body.
164 Ibid.
165 Ibid.
166 Ibid.

existence ancient medicine had already postulated on the basis of the teaching of the elements: yellow and black bile, phlegm, and blood. As with the elements, each of these was assigned a pair of primary qualities. Yellow bile was hot and dry; black bile was cold and dry; phlegm was cold and moist; and blood was hot and moist. The individual combination of the four humors in the body resulted in the temperament of the person in question, or, with respect to the qualities, in the person's *complexio*. Temperament or *complexio* was often recognized in external features such as the color of the hair and face. The English word "complexion" still denotes facial color or countenance today. The humors also, however, had a far-reaching effect on what was taking place within the body and they determined not least of all the temperament as we define it today. If yellow bile predominated, the resulting "choleric" (from Greek, chole = yellow bile) temperament would lead to a tendency toward fits of anger. If, on the other hand, viscous, slimy phlegm was predominant, one could expect a thoughtful or even sleepy nature – a "phlegmatic" nature as we still say today. The individual combination of humors and qualities was innate, but it was subject to change with age and the influence of the external environment.

To properly understand the physical functions and processes within the body, it was essential to have a knowledge of the body's faculties, the so-called *facultates* or *virtutes* such as the *facultas expulsiva*, the *facultas motrix*, and the *facultas cogitativa*. From today's perspective, they may seem like a mere theoretical construct, even like empty words, but from the perspective of the time, they were indispensable to understanding human (and animal) physiology. They emerged from Aristotelian natural philosophy, according to which every motion and thus every change had an efficient cause. In the healthy human body, changes were constantly at work: matter was moved, food was assimilated, excretions were taking place, and a host of further functions were carried out, all without an identifiable source of the movement and change. Even if a movement could be traced to a person's will, there was still the question of how a decision made by the immaterial soul could have the very concrete effect of moving a finger or the leg. This gap was filled by the concept of nature in general but in particular by its concretization in the *facultates*. Handsch noted a succinct definition: "The faculty ["virtus"] is the cause that precedes the action."[167] And, conversely: "when the faculty perishes, there is no action."[168]

Three general *virtutes* or *facultates* were to be distinguished which "governed" ("gubernant") and preserved the body. Handsch made a carefully

---

167 Ibid., fol. 41v.
168 Ibid., fol. 42r: "Si facultas perit, nulla sequitur actio."

subdivided list here. First there was the mental faculty, the *facultas animalis*, which had its seat in the brain and communicated sensations and conscious, deliberate movements via the nerves. Cognitive faculties in a narrower sense were subdivided into the imagination, judgment, and memory. Second, there was the *facultas vitalis*, which had its primary seat in the heart. And third, there was the *facultas naturalis*, the natural faculty that ensured the alimentation of the body.[169]

The vital and the animal faculties – whether the natural faculty could be included here remained subject to debate – required a material instrument that would allow them to take effect not only in their particular location but throughout the whole body. This came in the form of the *spiritus*, a further key concept of contemporary physiology. The *spiritus vitalis* was, as we find in the standard definition noted by Handsch, a "subtle, airy, transparent substance that is produced from the most delicate part of the blood so that the faculties can be taken from the main parts to the other [parts], so that they can carry out their specific activities".[170] This *spiritus vitalis* was generated with the help of the innate, vital heat ("insiti et nativi caloris causa existens"). It was produced in the left chamber of the heart from delicate blood and inhaled air and it flowed through the arteries into the rest of the body.[171] Parts of this *spiritus vitalis* were refined in the brain or, as Handsch wrote, in the *plexus reticularis* to become the *spiritus animalis*, or animal spirit, which spread throughout the entire body via the nerves and was responsible for movement and sensation.[172]

A central task of the natural faculties and of vital heat, the *calor innatus*, was the assimilation of ingested food. This process had presented learned physicians with a puzzle since antiquity. How was the body able to quite literally assimilate the wild mix of comestibles that it took in daily, producing material that belonged to the body, as the growth of children and adolescents so impressively illustrated? How could milk, grits, porridge, bread, and the like be made similar to or indeed transformed into bodily substance, into muscles, bones, and individual organs? In the case of adults, the necessity of the constant assimilation of food that was foreign to the body was not quite as apparent.[173] Stories of young women who had reportedly not eaten for years lent credence to the idea that the human body was not crucially dependent on a constant intake of food. These apparent miracles of fasting were, however, a frequent subject of controversy among physicians and were sometimes exposed as frauds – for example when the woman said to be

---

169 Ibid., fol. 41v.
170 Ibid., fol. 42v.
171 Ibid.
172 Ibid., foll. 42v-43r.
173 Ibid., fol. 50r.

fasting had, as it turned out, drunk her mother's breastmilk when she came to visit.[174] Physicians assumed that the adult body, too, required constant nutrition because it was always using up or losing substance and it needed to offset this loss. Handsch noted: "Children and adolescents eat so that they may grow, [while] adults eat only to preserve their bodies".

Models explaining the process by which food was assimilated had already been developed by ancient physicians, and constituted basic knowledge that every aspiring physician in the early modern period had to learn. To summarize the essential: Galenic medicine described the assimilation of food quite literally as a cooking process. Just as food was cooked on the kitchen stove, vital heat within the body concocted the ingested food in several steps, separating that which was of use – so that it could be appropriated by the body – from the useless, which had to be excreted.[175] In a first step – and this was also learned by Handsch – food was concocted in the stomach. Useless, coarse, and dry matter was excreted as feces via the bowel. Via the abdominal veins, the more delicate matter was transported as liquid food or *chymus* to the liver, where in a second step it was concocted to become nutritious blood that made its way to all parts of the body through the veins. Unusable matter was also separated out in this second concoction process; it was transported for the most part to the gall bladder as yellow bile and ultimately emptied into the bowel. Further substances were carried to the spleen as black bile. The superfluous watery matter, finally, accompanied the blood first in the large vena cava but was then attracted by the kidneys together with some of the blood and excreted through the urinary tract.[176] The third step in the concoction process took place in the individual body parts, which took from the blood the matter that they were able to appropriate. The unusable parts, destined for excretion, which resulted also during this last concoction process, either went back to the blood and were finally excreted with the urine or they left the body as imperceptible perspiration ("transpiratio insensibilis") or as visible sweat through the numerous pores of the skin.[177]

Each organ thus fulfilled a different function. The stomach and liver primarily served to concoct food into blood. The kidneys, spleen, bladder, skin, and bowels, on the other hand, were excretory organs first and foremost. The lungs, too, belonged to the latter insofar as they not only cooled the hot heart but also freed the body of fumes. The heart and brain took prominent positions. The heart was where *spiritus vitalis* was produced, while in the brain the *spiritus animalis* was

---

174 Pulz, Nüchternes Kalkül (2007).
175 Da Monte gave a good summary in his introduction to Da Monte, Lectiones (1552).
176 Cod. 11210, fol. 80v, here in the context of the theory of the origin of urine.
177 Ibid., fol. 67r.

generated, which communicated between the immaterial soul and the body in the ventricles of the brain; they were considered the true location of the faculties of understanding.[178]

Practical Medicine

Learning the theoretical, natural-philosophical foundations of medicine was only one of the pillars of medical training. *Medicina theorica* was complemented by *medicina practica*. This division must not be misunderstood.[179] The teaching of *medicina practica* was also largely theoretical and based on lectures about authoritative texts with commentary. The difference, however, was that the lectures in *theoria* were primarily directed at general natural-philosophical and epistemological foundations, while teaching in *medicina practica* put pathology at the center, the etiology and pathogenesis of particular diseases and, based on this, diagnosis, differential diagnosis and – especially in the context of pharmacology – therapy.

In the hierarchy of the disciplines, practical professorships stood for some time below theoretical ones, something that also found expression in professors' salaries. The typical career of a successful university professor thus began with a professorship in practical medicine and led to one in theoretical medicine. Even Giovanni Battista da Monte, known today above all as a clinical teacher, followed this trajectory in Padua. In the course of the sixteenth century, however, this relationship began to reverse, indicating the effects of an overarching development that we will encounter again and again in this book, namely the growing appreciation among learned physicians of the practical knowledge and skills that were indispensable to successful diagnosis and treatment.

Handsch heard a number of lectures on the canonical texts and the specific subject areas of *medicina practica*. Over time, he complemented his notes on these lectures with many more notes, often based on actual experiences with patients or on what he heard from colleagues. Clearly, the foundation he acquired as a student proved helpful during his time as a physician. In 1551, for example, he attended a lecture by Vettore Trincavella on pathology as discussed in the ninth book of Rhazes's *Ad Almansorem*. According to Handsch's notes, which appear to relay the lecture word for word, Trincavella gave a detailed presentation

---

[178] A good, widely quoted overview was given in the early seventeenth century by Daniel Sennert (Sennert, Institutionum (1620)).
[179] Bylebyl, School of Padua (1979), pp. 337–339.

of the different forms, causes, and treatments of headaches, palsy, tremors, and melancholy. After about 160 pages, however, Handsch's notes end with catarrh. Trincavella had not even completely covered the diseases of the head up to that point.[180] To these notes Handsch added notes from lectures by Alvise Bellocati about the sections in the ninth book of Rhazes's *Ad Almansoren* on the diseases of the chest and abdomen.[181] He also included an excerpt of notes from G. B. da Monte's lecture on pathology according to Rhazes.[182] Further notes on various private lectures were included as well, for example by Fracanzano about fever, female diseases, and the *morbus gallicus,* as well as by Trincavella about stomach diseases.[183] Nevertheless, Handsch's notes in their surviving form remain piecemeal. Systematic notes by his hand or even lectures transcribed verbatim on the entire thematic spectrum of *medicina practica*, on all diseases from the head to the foot and on fevers, are not extant. Possibly to make up for this lack, Handsch obtained for himself an extensive, 250-page-long transcript, which survives in his *Nachlass*, of a lecture given by Augustin Schurff in Wittenberg in 1537. In the lecture, Schurff covered all subjects presented in the ninth book of *Ad Almansorem*.[184]

Following Galen, learned medicine in the sixteenth century defined itself as a decidedly rational undertaking. This self-image arose not only from its basis in natural philosophy but even more so from its strict methodological approach.[185] The positive experiences made by trying certain medications and other treatments on certain disease patterns might be a satisfactory basis for treatment to "empiricists", but for learned physicians who followed the Galenic motto "ratio et experientia", it was important to be able to get to the bottom of things and recognize the cause of the complaints and the disease itself. As Da Monte and other professors advised their students, it was only in this way that the disease and its cause could be eradicated, literally pulling the disease out by the roots with a "radical" treatment; the term "radical" comes from the Latin "radix" for "root". Not getting to "root", on the other hand, meant that one was contenting oneself with merely a

---

180 Cod. 11226, foll. 2r-82r.
181 Ibid., foll. 149r-175v and foll. 182r-207v.
182 Cod. 11240, foll. 9r-26r.
183 Cod. 11226, foll. 92r-119r and fol. 160v.
184 Cod. 11228.
185 Wightman, Quid sit methodus (1964). It was in this spirit that Fonseca recommended to the budding physicians in his theory of fevers to follow "prae caeteris exactissimam methodum, sine qua nihil recte vel scribi, vel operari potest" (Fonseca, Opusculum (1596), p. 4). A detailed discussion of the teaching of method and its significance for Paduan medicine can be found in Ferretto, Bassiano Lando (2006–2009) and Ferretto, Maestri (2012). On method in contemporary philosophy in general see Leinkauf, Philosophie (2020), pp. 48–81.

"palliative" treatment, that is to say with only "cloaking" (Lat. *pallium* = cloak) the symptoms.[186] "Palliare", as Handsch noted in this context, meant "covering up the disease for some time".[187] Such a treatment would leave the real causes untouched and would not prevent the progression of the disease. As we will be seeing, a "cloaking" treatment was only indicated in certain cases, particularly for the incurable and the dying. In other cases, it was considered equal to forgoing a potentially effective therapy or even doing harm.

In this vein, Antonio Fracanzano told his students the story of a gouty patrician in Venice whose feet a lay healer had treated topically with a lotion that warmed, tightened, and strengthened the skin. The podagra disappeared. But because nature was no longer able to chase away the morbid matter from the life-sustaining parts along the usual paths, it sent it to the throat and ultimately to other body parts as well. The man first got *angina* and then died in the fifth year from asphyxia.[188] As a physician, Handsch himself later criticized the numerous opiates that his colleague, the court physician Johann Willenbroch,[189] prescribed to the sick wife of a chancery scribe. This was, in his view, not a "true" but only a "palliative" treatment.[190]

Because of its significance in the understanding of disease as well as its endorsement of a successful "radical" treatment, the theory of causes assumed a preeminent position in the learned medicine of the time. It was essential that the aspiring physician first learn – and this is also shown by Handsch's lecture notes from Padua – to distinguish the different categories of causes. These were first of all the external causes, the *causae primitivae* or *procatarcticae*. They included violations of the rules of a healthy way of life and other external factors that led to illness.[191] Certain diseases, like consumption, leprosy, epilepsy, and the plague, Handsch learned, were transmitted by a specific *contagium*, which entered the body through touch or through the air, while other diseases were hereditary.[192]

---

186 Stolberg, Cura palliativa (2007), pp. 7–29.
187 Cod. 11206, fol. 135v.
188 Cod. 11238, fol. 128v.
189 So far very little is know about Willenbroch's biography (cf. the biographical sketch in Kühlmann/Telle, Frühparacelsismus, vol. 2 (2004), pp. 932–934). In his notebooks, Handsch often mentioned him as one of the physicians in his circle and both later worked together as court physicians in Ambras. Willenbroch probably came from Danzig and was younger than Handsch. He studied in Wittenberg and later in Padua. A letter dated 15 October 1586, eight years after Handsch's death, shows him still in the service of the Archduke (Universitätsbibliothek Basel, Frey-Gryn Mscr. 11, fol. 85r-v; http://doi.org/10.7891/e-manuscripta-7721).
190 Cod. 11183, fol. 483, "non praestant veram curam, sed palleativam [sic]".
191 Cod. 11210, fol. 69v.
192 Ibid., fol. 72r.

The second category, also essential for an understanding and successful treatment of diseases, was that of the *causae antecedentes* or *causae corporales*, the immediate, bodily causes, for instance pathological humors in the body or a clogged liver.[193] The distinction from the above-mentioned *causae procatarcticae* or *primitivae* roughly resembles today's distinction between "etiology", the theory of causes, and "pathogenesis", the specific pathological development and changes within the body.

More disputed was a third category, the *causae coniunctae*. Avicenna, as Handsch learned, used the term to describe the specific pathological changes in the body that were the immediate cause of the pathological disturbances to the natural body functions and thus of the observable symptoms. In the case of catarrh, for example, the *causa procatarctica* could be coldness that acted upon the head and body from the outside. A possible *causa corporalis* were the vapors that rose from the stomach, condensing to liquids in the head and then running off as such. These liquids, which would collect in the airways or in joints, for example, and make breathing difficult, cause a joint to swell, or other pathological changes to occur, was in this case the *causa coniuncta*, according to Avicenna.[194] Similarly, Peter Vietor considered the *causa coniuncta* in the suffocation of the mother to be the harmful vapors that emanated from the underlying bodily cause, the spoiled menstrual blood that collected in the womb.[195]

A further, equally controversial theoretical distinction was that between "symptom", "disease", and its "cause". Galen had attempted to delineate them clearly. All three – *symptoma*, *morbus*, and *causa* – were, according to him, *affectus*, that is deviations from the natural state of the body.[196] *Morbus*, was the central concept. It was the unnatural ("praeter naturam") disturbance to a bodily function ("actio"). The disease was preceded by a *causa*, which was not, however, identical with the disease as such. Keeping company with the disease, as shadows or companions as it were, were the *symptomata*, whose role reflected the literal sense of the word, which comes from the Greek words for "together" and "fall".[197] From his reading of Galen's *De methodo medendi*, Handsch took the example of a phlegmon of the foot: a phlegmon was an illness that impaired walking and its symptoms

---

193 Ibid., fol. 69v.
194 Ibid., foll. 69v-70r.; .
195 Vietor, De praefocatione (1610), thesis 9.
196 Galen, De morborum et symptomatum differentiis (1547), p. 80; I use a contemporary Latin translation, as Handsch and his teachers will have used it; Greek text with modern Latin translation in Galen, Opera (1822), vol. VII, pp. 42f.
197 Galen, De morborum et symptomatum differentiis (1547), p. 86; cf., Galen, Opera (1822), vol. VII, pp. 49f.

were local changes such as redness and swelling. The bodily cause, the *causa antecedens* or *corporalis*, was identified in an overabundance of blood. The external *causa procatarctica* could be an excessive consumption of food.[198]

In abstract theory, the different types causes could be defined fairly easily. When applied to actual cases, however, the distinctions often raised questions. Pains and cramps, for example, could be painfully disruptive to bodily functions and thus could be categorized according to the outline above as diseases whose immediate causes had to be addressed. But they could also be considered the symptoms of the real disease, which could have completely different causes. In his works, Galen, not surprisingly, made contradictory statements at times, which the leading authors of the sixteenth century such as Leonhard Fuchs, Giovanni Argenterio, and Jean Fernel tried to reconcile in different ways.[199]

The concept of "symptoms" was particularly problematic. In his lecture notes from Padua, Handsch wrote down the overarching, general definition: the term "symptomata", or "accidentia" in Latin, signified the pathological process, the illness as a whole. In a narrower, more specific sense, however, the "symptomata" were the actual, perceptible consequences of a disease, namely 1) the signs of abnormal sensory, motor, and cognitive faculties, 2) external physical changes perceptible by the senses such as changes to skin color as a whole or in particular regions, changes in the smell that emanated from the mouth or other orifices, or the palpable texture of the skin, for example a hardening or tightening, and 3) abnormal excretions of urine, blood, sweat, and so forth.[200]

In early modern medicine, the modern distinction between "symptoms" in the sense of the complaints of the patient and the "objective", externally perceptible "signs" that a physician could recognize was not yet firmly established. The subjective complaints as experienced and reported by patients ultimately also served as diagnostic and prognostic signs. Vice versa, the reddish urine which a physician found upon examination could be called a "symptom".[201] According to an entry in Handsch's notebook it was primarily a matter of perspective: it was said, he claimed, that what was a "symptom" to the sick person was a "sign" to the physician.[202]

Particularly important and useful was the knowledge and identification of characteristic symptoms or signs, which were specific to a particular disease and

---

[198] Cod. 11210, fol. 70r.
[199] Siraisi, Disease (2002) provides a detailed account of the complex debates, presenting the different positions of selected authors.
[200] Cod. 11210, fol. 72v.
[201] Biblioteca comunale Aurelio Saffi, Forlì, Fondo antico, Ms. 94, fol. 39v.
[202] Cod. 11210, fol. 72v, later addition.

allowed the physician to diagnose it. They were sometimes called "pathognomic" or "pathognomonic", a term that is still commonly used today. The triad of fever, breathing difficulties, and a cough, for example, allowed for a quite reliable diagnosis of pleurisy ("pleuritis"/ "pleuresia").[203]

Crucial to an understanding of the nature of each disease and to the possibility of a targeted treatment were the *causae antecedentes* or *corporales,* that is, the bodily causes in a narrower sense. As Handsch learned in Padua, these physical causes were divided into *genera*. There was, first of all, *dyscrasia* or *intemperies,* a deviation from the natural *complexio,* from the natural, individual balance of humors and qualities. Less significant deviations from the natural state that did not produce perceptible functional abnormalities were not considered diseases. According to Galen, the state of "health" was characterized by a certain range or latitude (*latitudo*). Pathological deviations could be either equal ("aequalis") or unequal ("inaequalis"). An equal *intemperies* affected all parts of the body. An illustrative example here was hectic fever, where the entire body became equally heated. An unequal *intemperies* was limited to certain organs or parts of the body. It could be "immaterial" or could accompany a merely qualitative change to the natural *complexio* of the organ or body part in question, but it could also be "material", meaning that it was caused by a pathological build-up of matter. A vivid example here was the abscess ("apostema"). Illnesses belonging to a second group were traced to the unnatural composition ("compositio") of one or more parts or organs, for example if they were too large or too small or if ducts or cavities were occluded. In everyday medical practice, such illnesses hardly played a role. The third group was composed of diseases and injuries that went hand in hand with a "dissolution of cohesion" ("solutio continuitatis"). It included for example broken bones, ulcers, torn ligaments, and other injuries which belonged first and foremost in the domain of surgery.[204]

Bedside Teaching

In the teaching of *medicina practica,* lectures, especially those about the works of Rhazes and Avicenna, had a prominent position, just as with *medicina theorica*. An awareness gradually emerged, however, both north and south of the Alps, that theoretical knowledge about the diagnosis and treatment of illnesses was insufficient for the aspiring physician who wanted to be successful in treating patients

---

203 Cod. 11183, fol. 42v, "signum pathognomicum".
204 Cod. 11210, fol. 70v-71r.

down the road. Certainly, the learned, academic physician distinguished himself through his profound knowledge of the medical literature and was able to cite important passages from the works of Hippocrates or Galen off the cuff. He had mastered logic and methodology and was conversant in physiological and pathological theories, which could be very complex. Yet medicine was not only *scientia*. It was also *ars*, the practical application of general, abstracted knowledge to individual cases of illness. And for the successful application of theoretical knowledge, experience was indispensable. Along these lines, Johannes Brettschneider warned medical students in 1552 that "Rules alone are insufficient without plentiful practice".[205] One of Handsch's student notebooks begins with the maxim, "Medicine teaches how to treat the human being [as such] but not Stephen or Peter".[206]

Practical knowledge and skills were the key to professional success. It was true that because of their academic education, physicians enjoyed more of an initial reserve of trust than other healers. Erudition was esteemed by most people, not only the learned. But in both rural and urban areas, one thing counted more than anything else in the final analysis: a good reputation. It was essential that people became convinced that the physician could diagnose illnesses with accuracy and reliability and had particularly good patient outcomes to show for himself. Medical students and physicians in training were thus well-advised to gain as much practical knowledge and skill as possible, the kind that in the judgment of the day was crucial for successful diagnosis and treatment, and that, in tandem with their theoretical knowledge, would presumably guarantee their superiority over non-academic healers.

Padua, Bologna, and Montpellier were known for the high quality of their practical training. This, along with the extensive practice of autopsy was the central reason why many students from north of the Alps commenced or continued their medical studies in northern Italy or the south of France.[207] By his own account, even after eight years of study, young Antonius Juncker's teachers recommended to him that he go to Montpellier, because there "better than anywhere else one sees the *praxis medica,* including the *res simplex* and the teaching of

---

[205] Placotomus, De ratione (1552), no pagination, "nec sola praecepta sine multo usu sufficiant".
[206] Cod. 11240, fol. 3r: "Medicina docet curare hominem sed non Stephanum, Petrum."
[207] Bylebyl, School of Padua (1979), p. 339.

anatome."[208] He followed the advice and studied there for a year and a half, under such professors as Guillaume Rondelet.[209]

The appeal of Montpellier, Padua, and other leading Northern Italian universities derived in large part from the eminence of the professors who taught medicine there. As practitioners, men like Rondelet in Montpellier, Musa Brasavola in Ferrara[210] and Da Monte, Trincavella, Mercuriale, and Capivaccia in Padua were European celebrities. Even some who were less well-known professors were valued for their good practical teaching. Explaining that he was "seeking practice" ("respiciens ad praxin"), Joachim Curaeus in 1557, for example, said he preferred Alvise Bellocati with his large practice in Padua over the young Apelatus, who was said to be very popular, especially with the *germani*.[211]

In addition to the outstanding reputation of the professors, students met with good learning conditions at these institutions. Universities north of the Alps largely confined themselves to encouraging students, through statutes and ordinances, to follow an experienced physician in his medical practice, to accompany him on his patient visits outside their regular studies. In Montpellier and at the leading Northern Italian universities, by contrast, bedside teaching was an integral part of medical training. In Montpellier as in Padua, doctoral candidates in the early seventeenth century were even required to prove their diagnostic and therapeutic skills in a bedside test with actual cases.[212] Records show a similar situation in Spain in the late sixteenth century and in Padua as early as around 1530. Girolamo Amalteo recounted how he had to discuss the case of a fever patient during his exam.[213]

Titled *Practica mea cum medicis patavinis*,[214] an account in one of Handsch's notebooks provides uniquely detailed information about the practical training of medical students in Padua. Other student notebooks, like that of Johannes

---

208 Thüringisches Hauptstaatsarchiv, Weimar, Ernestinisches Gesamtarchiv, Reg. Rr 1–316, 803, letter from Juncker, probably to Johann Wilhelm zu Sachsen-Coburg, describing his previous career, 7 December 1556; "res simplex" undoubtedly refers to the simples, i. e. to medicinal plants.
209 Afterwards he obtained a doctoral title in Valence (Archives départementales de la Drôme, Valence, D 17, list of doctoral degrees, with an entry on Juncker on fol. 7r).
210 Bacchelli, Brasavola (2008).
211 Adam, Vitae (1620), p. 205.
212 Germain, Anciennes thèses (1876), pp. 14–20; British Library, London, Ms. Sloane 727, foll. 50r-51v, G. D. Sala, *Generalis casuum recitandorum forma* and ibid., foll. 57r-70v, idem, *Modi recitandi casus in Patavino Lycæo recepti parvulum compendium*.
213 Biblioteca Marciana, Venice, Cod. lat. VII 66 (= 9684), notes by Amalteo; Clouse, Medicine (2011), p. 54.
214 Cod. 11238.

Brünsterer from 1547–48 and of Johannes Hessus from 1552–1554, also demonstrate just how much emphasis was placed by professors and students in Padua on the acquisition of practical knowledge and skill.[215] Even in their lectures, the professors took recourse to actual cases of illness so as to illustrate the practical application of medical theory to the individual patient and to provide empirical examples for the efficacy of recommended treatments.[216] In his edition of the *consilia* and letters of his father, Bernardo Trincavella also published three of his father's lectures, each focusing on individual cases of illness. They were rather common cases: a woman with irregular menstrual periods, a melancholic young man, and a *matrona* who had become paralyzed following an *apoplexia*. In his lectures, Trincavella described the medical history or read from the written report, presumably by the attending physician, and then explained the processes taking place within the body that in his view accounted for the illness.[217]

Some professors even illustrated pathological theories and treatment measures using fictitious, invented cases. In his lectures on the ninth book of Rhazes's *Ad Almansorem*, Trincavella discussed at least four such fictitious cases, which he introduced with phrases such as: "A case is being presented. Imagine a person who . . .". This was followed by a brief description of, for example, the case of a patient who lived a life of idleness and gluttony, who lost sensation in one limb, which then became paralyzed, without there having been an injury. Following this was a detailed presentation of the indicated treatment.[218]

An innovative teaching format that appears to have been developed in Padua at the time received particular attention among contemporary observers: the so-called *collegia*. Referred to occasionally as *consultationes*, the *collegia* presumably developed from the common practice of physicians consulting jointly about a patient, orally or in writing. Students highly valued this form of instruction and took detailed notes. Their notes on *collegia* were sometimes printed in collections of *consultationes* and *consilia*.[219] As a result, some historians have confused them

---

215 Universitätsbibliothek Erlangen, Ms. 911 (Brünsterer) and Ms. 910 (Hesse).
216 E.g. Cod. 11006, fol. 150v, note on Bellocati's story of his successful treatment of dropsy.
217 Trincavella, Consiliorum (1586), foll. 105v-111v; Trincavella's comments on these three cases are explicitly marked as "lectio" and Trincavella addressed his listeners directly with words like "you have heard" ("audivistis"); on Trincavella's *consilia* see also Tanfani, I consilia medica (1952).
218 Cod. 11226, foll. 2r-82r, here foll. 50r-51v: "Proponatur casus. Sit aliquis qui patiatur paralysi"; similarly ibid., foll. 72v-74r: "Proponatur casus. Sit aliquis, qui patiatur epilepsiam per essentiam a capite et inquirat praeservationem."
219 Thus, in his preface to Da Monte, Consultationum (1565), Johannes Crato wrote of the "consultationes", which were commonly called "collegia" ("quae vulgo collegia appellantur"); for example, Trincavella, Consilia (1587) documents numerous *collegia* with the respective

with epistolary consultations, but this was a very different genre.[220] During a *collegium*, several professors would come together and discuss a particular case of illness in front of students. First, one of the professors would introduce the medical history orally ("audivistis historiam") or based on a written report ("exhibita charta"), which was read aloud. Following this, he and the other professors in attendance would present their assessment one after the other. From the complaints that had been described and possibly from the externally visible signs of illness, when the patient was present, they would conclude which pathological processes were taking place within the body and which remedies were best suited to combatting the causes of the illness and healing the disease.[221]

This reviewing of cases in a shared and structured manner in front of congregated students, with professors presenting their case evaluations in turn, clearly was a very efficient didactical method, one that might in fact even be worth reviving in present-day medical teaching. Students were presented with actual cases of illness and learned the methodological approach that was to be followed at the bedside – how they were, as Vettore Trincavella put it, to arrive at an understanding of the hidden from what was manifest to the senses,[222] and so how to identify pathological changes within the body from signs and symptoms and to come to therapeutic conclusions. At the same time, students experienced how, depending on the illness and the case, even the assessments of famous luminaries could significantly diverge from one another. And all the while they were gaining a skill that would be crucial in dealing with noble patients, assuring their professional success: the ability to distinguish oneself by convincingly presenting a well-founded assessment at the bedside during a joint consultation with other physicians present.

---

statements of Trincavella, Fracanzano, Falloppia, Bellocati, Frigimelica and other Paduan professors.

220 Treating the oral statements of Da Monte and Capivaccia recorded by their students like written *consilia*, because they were published under titles such as "consultationes" and "consilia", Monica Calabritto has argued for a substantial transformation of the genre of the written *consilium* since the Middle Ages (Calabritto, Curing (2012)). However, these differences are clearly due to the difference between written *consilia* and student notes on the professors' oral pronouncements.

221 E.g. "Collegium habitum de muliere laborante cancro in dextra mamilla", with statements by Gabrielle Falloppia, Francesco Frigimelica, Vettore Trincavella and two other professors, 10 April 1552 (Universitätsbibliothek Erlangen, Ms. 910, foll. 50r-53r); the manuscript contains notes on a whole series of *collegia* as well as copies of various *consilia*, among others by Pietro Andrea Mattioli.

222 Trincavella, Consilia (1587), col. 266.

The *collegia* and the casuistic elements that came to bear in lectures were perfectly suited to teaching aspiring physicians the cognitive and argumentative skills that they would need later in practice. They imparted the systematic, methodological-analytic approach that would make it possible to recognize the true causes of disease within the body and thus to attack the disease at its roots. They pointed the way to "rational" methodological medicine, which served learned physicians as a means to distinguish themselves from the "empiricists" whose knowledge was purely experiential. But without a patient present, students could only acquire the practical, sensory, physical, and manual skills needed at the bedside to a very limited extent – skills that could determine a physician's success or failure. Without seeing what the patient looked like, it was difficult to determine his or her temperament, and they had no opportunity to ask the right questions, to inspect excretions, to examine the patient with their own hands if need be, or to adapt treatment as his or her condition changed in the course of the disease.

Padua, Montpellier, and other Northern Italian universities offered excellent conditions for the acquisition of such practical skills. Before all other "innovations in the study of medicine", contemporaries already extolled the "exceedingly praiseworthy practice" at Italian universities of discussing the nature, causes, and treatment of illnesses with students at the bedside ("circa aegrorum lectulos"), that is, during shared patient visits.[223]

This practice of bedside teaching has received a great deal of attention in historical research, undoubtedly also because of the preeminent significance of clinical teaching in modern medical training. Older generations of historians traced the beginnings of systematic teaching at the bedside to seventeenth-century Leiden, Netherlands – until evidence was found that Leiden was modelled on the much earlier example of Padua, in turn, where Dutch medical students had experienced it.[224] In Padua, already in the 1540s Giovanni Battista da Monte had taken his students with him on patient visits in the *Ospedale di San Francesco*. Unlike many other hospitals of the time, especially those north of the Alps, which served primarily as care facilities for the impoverished elderly, the infirm, or the otherwise needy, major hospitals in Northern Italian cities also provided

---

223 Solenander, Consiliorum (1609), preface to the students, "de aegrotis confabulationes quaedam, quales in visendis aegrotis solent inter medicum et discipulos haberi: qui Italiam vidit, novit morem hunc laudatissimum, quo sane cunctas alias nationes in studio medico antecedit"); similarly Trincavella, Consilia (1587), dedicatory epistle of the printer C. Waldkirch to Petrus Severinus, 1 April 1587.
224 For a detailed summary of the development of bedside teaching in Leiden see Beukers, Clinical teaching (1989).

medical care in a stricter sense.[225] For some 200 years, da Monte came to be considered the "inventor" of clinical teaching in Western medicine.[226] In recent times, some authors have once again cast doubt on this assessment, however. From their analysis of the sources, they have arrived at the conclusion that Da Monte only seldom taught at San Francesco, and when he did it was not because he was actively seeking the opportunity to teach in this way but because physicians at the hospital had called him. They concluded that there was no evidence that any systematic clinical teaching was going on.[227]

These doubts are unfounded, however.[228] Merely reading the various volumes of Da Monte's *Consilia* shows there were at least two dozen consultations at the hospital which were written down by students who participated in them, and we may assume that there were many more. Da Monte's *Consilia* alone mention ten visits with a consumptive patient with an empyema, a collection of pus in the lung,[229] and six with a febrile, dropsical boy. Da Monte dictated a consultation with a boy with scabies "at the hospital, during the sixteenth visit".[230] In a different *consilium,* a seventeenth bedside visit is documented, a call on a clergyman who was once ill with the French disease but was now suffering from the effects of mercury poisoning.[231] According to the student notes, Da Monte connected the bedside teaching with lectures. In his discussion of two patients with *pseudotertiana* during his last teaching rounds in 1543, he explicitly stated his intention of linking what he taught that day from the lectern with that which manifested itself in the patient.[232]

It seems that Da Monte was not the only one to take his students with him on clinical rounds and, as Handsch's notes clearly show, these rounds remained an established practice in Padua after Da Monte's death in May of 1551. Lorenz Gryll, who studied for almost two years in Padua, with Da Monte and Landi, later recounted how he went to the hospital in Padua with Antonio Fracanzano every day

---

225 Henderson, Renaissance hospital (2006).
226 Comparetti, Saggio (1793); Rasori, Sul metodo (1808/1809), pp. 58–62.
227 Orsolato, Prima fondazione (1872–73), pp. 127–152; Ongaro, L'insegnamento clinico (1994), pp. 357–369.
228 On the following, see my detailed account in Stolberg, Bedside teaching (2014).
229 Da Monte, Consultationum (1565), coll. 455–461, "De empyico et phthisico in hospitali, visitationes decem".
230 Ibid., col. 885, "in hospitali, in XVI. accessione".
231 Ibid., coll. 867–869: "Haec cura facta fuit [. . .] in decima septima visitatione hospitalis, quae dedit occasionem octo lectionibus de morbo Gallico"; it is not clear whether the visits took place in the same year as the above-mentioned sixteenth visit.
232 Ibid., col. 938 (wrongly paginated as 638): "Ut continuemus ea quae docemus in cathedra, cum iis quae apparent circa aegros, non abscedemus ab iis quae diximus hodie."

at a certain hour, where he witnessed the treatment of innumerable patients.[233] Along the same lines, Handsch claimed that he "went with the physicians to see the sick people at the hospital nearly every day, where, on many a day, one observed up to thirty urines."[234] He recorded, in particular and at times in great detail, cases he saw in the hospital with Antonio Fracanzano, highlighting some of his entries with headings such as "Among the patients of Doctor Fracanzano at the Hospital of San Francesco" or "A few things that I saw at the hospital with Doctor Fracanzano".[235] Like Da Monte, Fracanzano paired his bedside teaching with lectures. Handsch filled about twenty-five pages just with his notes on a lecture ("lectio") about uroscopy, which Fracanzano had given at the hospital.[236] A visit with a patient with a raw, altered voice who was experiencing asthmatic complaints and who thought he was bewitched even gave Fracanzano the opportunity to speak at length about conjurations and inflicted illnesses and about evil women who harmed others with dried menstrual blood.[237]

Whether the *Ospedale di San Francesco* was the first place in Europe where students received clinical instruction at the bedside is a different matter. At about the same time, the cases of various hospital patients in Bologna were also captured in the student notes that served as the basis for the *Processus, curationes et consilia* of Elideo Padovani (aka Helidaeus Padovanus, d. 1575). Mention is made, for example of a "paralytica in hospitali", of two dropsical patients at the hospital who, according to Padovani suffered from a hardening or occlusion of the spleen, of a man "in hospitali" with an occluded and hardened spleen and there is an especially elaborate description of a "pleuritico in hospitali". Students took note of the prescriptions that Padovani made on six different days – and thus, by all appearances,

---

228 On the following, see my detailed account in Stolberg, Bedside teaching (2014).
229 Da Monte, Consultationum (1565), coll. 455–461, "De empyico et phthisico in hospitali, visitationes decem".
230 Ibid., col. 885, "in hospitali, in XVI. accessione".
231 Ibid., coll. 867–869: "Haec cura facta fuit [. . .] in decima septima visitatione hospitalis, quae dedit occasionem octo lectionibus de morbo Gallico"; it is not clear whether the visits took place in the same year as the above-mentioned sixteenth visit.
232 Ibid., col. 938 (wrongly paginated as 638): "Ut continuemus ea quae docemus in cathedra, cum iis quae apparent circa aegros, non abscedemus ab iis quae diximus hodie."
233 Gryll, Oratio (1566), fol. 4r: "Cum Antonio autem Francazano [sic] quotidie stata hora in Xenodochio Patavino, crebris, varijs et prope infinitis curationum exemplis interfui".
234 Cod. 11206, fol. 26r.
235 Cod. 11238, fol. 119, "inter patientes D. Frankenzani in hospitali S. Francisci" (Handsch later added "anno 1551 et 52"); ibid., fol. 127r: "Pauca quae vidi in hospitali cum D. Frankenzano in vere anni 1553".
236 Cod. 11240, fol. 151r-v and foll. 80r-92v.
237 Ibid., fol. 120v.

on six different visits.[238] These medical rounds may well have taken place before Da Monte introduced the practice in Padua around 1542. Padovani received his medical doctorate in Bologna already in 1535 and cases he treated outside of the hospital are documented already for the year 1540.[239] Pieter van Foreest, who studied in Bologna from 1540 to 1543, furthermore gives an account of a kind of outpatient clinic at the hospital during that time. He describes how Padovani in the presence of students gave medical advice to the large numbers of country people who came with their urine to the local *Ospedale della Vita*.[240] There is so far no conclusive evidence that Padovani was a professor at the university. He may have been employed as a hospital physician.[241] In the title of Johannes Wittich's edition of Padovani's *Consilia*, he is explicitly called a "professor", however, and the medical students who accompanied him are mentioned. The volume also contains various lecture-like texts in which the author, as was typical for lecture notes of the time, spoke of himself in the first person and addressed his audience in the second person. Moreover, a manuscript in the *Biblioteca comunale* in Cesena, contains three treatises bei Elideo Padovani, on the diseases of women, on the diseases of children and on the simples.[242] All this strongly suggests that he was, to some degree at least, involved in formal university teaching.[243]

There is also another reason why some restraint needs to be practiced with respect to the eulogies sung for Da Monte as the "inventor" of bedside teaching: the professors did not need a hospital to do their bedside teaching. Most sick people were treated not at the hospital but at their own home. Professors of medicine commonly had their own larger or smaller private practices, and they allowed their students to accompany them on their house calls. When they walked down the street surrounded by a sizeable group of students, this even redounded to their honor and polished their reputation. Thus the opportunity frequently arose for aspiring physicians to watch experienced practitioners on the job, and this

---

238 Padovani, Processus (1607), p. 16, p. 137, p. 143 (wrongly paginated as 431) and p. 72; further hospital cases on p. 103, p. 141, p. 208, and p. 215.
239 Dondi, Elideo Padovani (1951); idem, Cenni (1975); Fantuzzi, Notizie (1788), pp. 215–218; Biblioteca comunale Aurelio Saffi, Forlì, Fondo antico, Ms. 94, fol. 7r, fol. 17r, fol. 39v, fol. and 59r (patients treated by Padovani in the spring of 1540).
240 Foreest, Uromanteia, p. 229; according to Mauro Guarino, students in Bologna regularly visited patients in the Ospedale della Morte with their professors in the fifteenth century already (Guarino, Profilo storico (2005), pp. 77–93, here p. 79); unfortunately, he does not indicate his source.
241 Dondi, Elideo Padovani (1951), pp. 139–144.
242 Biblioteca comunale, Cesena, Ms. 167–29.
243 Padovani, Processus (1607).

practice appears to have been routine at leading Italian universities in the sixteenth century.[244]

House calls provided an especially good opportunity for comprehensive instruction that was literally "clinical"; the Greek work "kline", after all, simply means "bed". At the hospital, as was doubtlessly advantageous, professors and students could visit several patients during a single call and thus could gather experiences with different disease patterns more quickly. House calls, on the other hand, allowed for a closer observation of patients' life circumstances and habits, which medicine at the time deemed of major significance when establishing the origin and development of illness. In the process, students also learned from their role models how to interact with those wealthy, upper-class patients whose endorsement and patronage would later determine their professional and economic success in their own medical practice.

In Padua, the conditions for training during house calls were quite favorable. Just within the town itself with its approximately 5,800 houses (1554),[245] there was a considerable number of potential patients. Moreover, Venice, one of the largest cities in Europe at the time, was not far away. In their notebooks, Handsch and Brünsterer recorded dozens of patients they saw, accompanying their professors. Quite frequently, they visited the same patient a number of days in a row, meaning that they were able to follow the course of the disease and observe the success of the treatment. Handsch mentioned, for example, two house calls by Gabrielle Falloppia to a child who had accidentally drunk poison, and further visits to a patient with the French disease. It appears it was common for medical students to come under the tutelage of a certain professor or at most two. In the case of Brünsterer it was Alvise Bellocati, and Lorenz Gryll also followed Bellocati, "in practice, as they call it, for several months throughout the town".[246] Handsch saw numerous patients with Fracanzano and Trincavella. As various entries in Handsch's notebooks make clear, these house calls also offered a welcome opportunity to discuss each case and the disease in question with the professor.[247]

A manuscript I recently discovered in Forlì documents the same practice for Bologna, for the years from 1540 until 1543.[248] An unknown writer described in considerable detail the cases of almost a hundred patients he saw with his

---

[244] Rath, Entwicklung (1965), pp. 8–10; Fichtner, Padova e Tübingen (1972–73), here p.54; Bylebyl, School of Padua (1979), p. 339.
[245] Brugi, Gli scolari (1903), p. 12.
[246] Gryll, Oratio (1566), fol. 4r.
[247] Cod. 11238, fol. 128v.
[248] Biblioteca comunale Aurelio Saffi, Forlì, Fondo antico, Ms. 94; the manuscript carries the title, in handwriting, "Curationes variae di Alessandro Padovani". This title is clearly

"teacher" ("praeceptor"), the Bologna professor Benedetto Vittore (Benedictus de Victoriis, Benedetto Vettori, d. 1561). Frequently they paid a whole series of daily or twice daily visits to one and the same patient. Sometimes other physicians were involved in the treatment as well and the writer learnt about their approach and their remedies – the writer mentions among others Matteo Corti (aka Curzio, 1475–1542/44), Elideo [Padovani], Lodovico Vitali (d. 1554), Jacopo Pacini (d. 1560), Virgilio Gherardi (d. 1541), and Antonio Maria Betti (d. 1562) who treated patients together with Vittore or before Vittore was called in. Occasionally, the writer also indicates that he himself took care of patients, before he consulted Vittore or the patient called him. The notes focus on the treatment and, in particular, on the professors' recipes, which the writer probably hoped to use later himself, on his own patients. He also describes, however, how they examined a patient's urine, blood or excrements together and how Vittore palpated a patient's liver.[249] At times, Vittore seems to have turned patient visits into an opportunity for more elaborate explanations. In the case of a 33-year-old patient, for example, he pointed out "the manifest signs, from Galen and others" (which showed that the young man suffered from consumption, which a colleague had doubted) and listed the four "intentions" ("intentiones") which guided his treatment, targeting the patient's pulmonary ulcer, his fever, his cough and his catarrh respectively.[250]

In Ferrara, where Handsch would later receive his doctorate, we find a similar situation. A manuscript that appears to have been composed by different medical students or physicians in training contains detailed notes on the cases of illness that were observed in Ferrara, in the 1540s, by one or several medical students or young physicians when they accompanied Antonio Musa Brasavola,

---

erroneous, however, and was added later. The manuscript has survived among the documents of the physician Alessandro Padovani (d. 1637) but many of the entries in this manuscript carry a precise date, starting in February 1540. The writer does not indicate whether other students or budding physicians were with him. There are altogether 101 cases. Vittore treated 96 of them, alone or with others. The notes on four cases only mention Matteo Corti and in one case we hear of the treatment by a certain Hieronymus de Lageris. The large majority of cases, as far as they are dated, occurred between the spring of 1540 and the spring of 1543. Three entries carry later dates, namely 2 February 1547 (addition to a previous, undated note) and 1554 (a case initally treated by the writer) and 22 April 1555 (on Vittore's treatment of a woman with suffocation of the womb); they were by all appearances added later on pages that had remained empty, at the beginning, before the index, and on the last page.
249 Ibid., fol. 97v, "vidit bis urinam"; fol. 22r, "vidit sanguinem colericum et adustum nigrum"; ibid., fol. 20r, "inspexit excrementum"; ibid., fol. 87r, "tetigit tumorem".
250 Ibid., fol. 82v-84v, 9 November 1541; "demonstravit per indicia manifesta ex Gal[en]o et ex aliis".

Antonio Maria Canani, Domenico Bondi, and Luca Riccardo on their visits to patients. Sometimes they even visited the same patient twice on the same day.[251]

In Paris, too, it was normal for the *baccalaurei* of medicine to come under the tutelage of a professor and accompany him on his house calls.[252] Professors in Montpellier invited or asked their students to accompany them on visits. In the early seventeenth century, Regensburg physician Strobelberger was emphatic in his praise for the practical "exercises" in Montpellier which he had experienced himself. In the town and in the hospitals, according to his account, students had the opportunity to visit sick people, ask them questions, and hone their skills at performing uroscopy and pulse diagnosis. In German countries, by contrast, he complained, students were not allowed to join their teachers at the bedside but had to stay outside.[253]

So far, little evidence has been found of regular bedside teaching in German-speaking areas during the sixteenth century. At the university in Tübingen, the statutes stipulated that students were to accompany their teachers on patient visits, but it remains questionable whether this was ever put into practice.[254] Of course, bedside instruction may simply not have been put on record at universities with few medical students because the professor could easily take individual students with him when he visited patients. This was especially true if students, as was often the case, boarded with their professors or at least dined with them. Soon after devoting himself to medicine in Wittenberg, Simon Wilde regularly dined at the table of Georg Curio in his house and could thus hope to accompany him on his sick visits. Curio did in fact take him along for several days "on his practice" when he travelled to the court of the Prince of Anhalt.[255] And in the extensive medical notes written by a student of Jodocus Willich in Frankfurt on the Oder in the 1550s, there are also a number of entries

---

251 Biblioteca Ariostea, Ferrara, Collezione Antonelli, Ms. 531, "Curationes Antonij Musae Brasavoli"; the title was probably added at a later point; on this manuscript see Menini, Curationes (1952) and Pomata, Sharing cases (2010), pp. 208–211. A number of entries are dated but without indicating the year. Occasionally the day of the week is given, however, (e.g. "Die lune 13. Aprilis") from which we can conclude that visits took place in and around 1545 or in and around 1551 – only in those two years April 13 fell on a Monday. Since an entry towards the end of the manuscript, which is written in the first person and apparently documents the beginning of the writer's own medical practice, is dated April 1547, the visits to the sick documented in this manuscript most likely took place in or around 1545.
252 Lunel, Maison (2008), p. 40.
253 Strobelberger, Laureationum medicarum (1628), p. 18.
254 Kuhn, Studenten (1971), p. 36.
255 Buchwald, Simon Wilde (1894), pp. 73–75.

on the way in which Willich treated a certain patient, suggesting that the unknown author had been with him at the bedside.[256]

Clear indications of systematic practical teaching by professors have so far only been found for the Northern Italian universities and Montpellier. Even there, some students would take time off to enhance their practical knowledge or would use the long summer holiday to work with a physician outside the university and gain practical experience and perhaps even treat individual patients on their own. Handsch mentions quite a few cases that he saw in the summers of 1551 and 1552 with the Padua professor for *medicina theorica* Comes de Monte (?–1587) also known as Panfilio (or Pamfilio) Pigatti – not to be confused with the more famous Giovanni Battista da Monte – in Comes de Monte's hometown of Vicenza.[257] According to his own account, Andreas Vesal treated patients in Venice under the guidance of the most well-known professors there. And J. C. Monnet, too, used the Padua university's summer break to go to Venice, where he could observe medical practice and could practice treating patients himself in individual cases ("in singularibus").[258] In Montpellier it was even expected that physicians in training would spend at least half a year working with an external physician to gain practical experience.[259]

Patient visits with professors – more than the case studies treated in lectures and the discussion of individual cases in the *collegia* – provided aspiring physicians with the knowledge and skill that they would later need in their medical practice. This is where students learned how to apply their theoretical knowledge to a specific case of illness, how they were to recognize from the symptoms and signs as well as from patient history the nature and causes of the illness in question. Based on this they furthermore learned what kind of treatment they were to prescribe, and here they also took the way of life and the temperament of the patient into consideration. But more than this, they learned to

---

256 Medical Historical Library, Yale University, New Haven, c. 1552, not inventoried; on the cover, the initials "I. M. D." are written. I have not yet been able to identify the author. Since the "D" most likely stands for "doctor", the first name probably began with an "I" or a "J" and the last name with an "M", which was very common combination of initials at the time.
257 Cod. 11238, foll. 115r-118v, "Aliquot observationes ex praxi D. Comitis de Monte Vicentini, Vincentiae factae in mense Augusto et Septembri Anno 1552", apparently continued on foll. 70r-74v and, under the explicit title "Ex praxi D. Comitis de Monte observata", on fol. 124r-v. Little is known about Comes de Monte, who gave up his professorship in 1554 and returned to Vicenza (biographical sketches in Santa Maria, Biblioteca, vol. 4 (1772), pp. CXXVI-CXXXVI, and Mantese, Storia (1969), pp. 66–71); he published an edition of Alessandro Achillini's Opera (Achillini, Opera (1545)).
258 O'Malley, Andreas Vesalius (1965), p. 75; Monnetus, Ad lectorem (1554).
259 Dulieu, La médecine (1979), p. 63.

ask the right questions, and they learned to sharpen their perception, which was only possible with the patient in the room. While it was possible to communicate orally or in writing about a patient who could not be seen by a physician, this indirect communication was a poor match for the sensory perception that was possible when a physician attended a patient, observing his or her body and its changes and making the diagnosis.

Just looking at the sick person's body could supply valuable clues. The color of the skin and hair, the person's girth, the width of the chest, bulging veins, and similar signs were helpful in determining a patient's temperament or *complexio*. Certain pathological changes were also readily visible to the naked eye. Sometimes they were pathognomic, so indicative of certain illnesses that is that they alone were enough to make a diagnosis: swollen stomachs or extremities, for example, for dropsy; red patches, pustules, and other skin conditions for certain fevers; or tumors under the skin, at times ulcerating, for cancer.

The physical presence of the patient was especially important if not indispensable for physicians in training who wanted to learn and practice the three most important diagnostic procedures of the day: uroscopy – insofar as the finding was to be compared with the physical constitution of the patient – and, more so, pulse diagnosis, and palpation, especially of the abdominal area.

Handsch took lengthy notes from a lecture about uroscopy given by Antonio Fracanzano at the hospital.[260] The performance of uroscopy required more than extensive knowledge, however. It took practice. From Handsch's notes we learn, that, according to G. B. da Monte, some were so skilled at uroscopy that they were able to say amazing things ("miranda") after having examined urine.[261] For this reason, Handsch repeatedly complemented his notes with practical tips given by Da Monte and other professors in their lectures or during patient visits. The urine of an old woman, for example, whom Handsch had visited with Trincavella in November of 1551, was of a "good" consistency with "praiseworthy" sediment and a barely visible cloudiness in the middle. The coloration, however, was more intensive than was to be expected with a woman whose vital heat was necessarily weakened due to age. The darker coloration alone, then, was enough to diagnose a fever according to Trincavella.[262]

If a patient was visited several times or even daily, as was common with both house calls and hospital consultations, students furthermore had the opportunity to observe the variation in the urine of one and the same patient. They were able

---

[260] Cod. 11210, foll. 80r-92v; according to a note which Handsch added later (ibid., fol. 80r), Fracanzano lectured again on the topic the following year.
[261] Ibid., fol. 80r.
[262] Cod. 11238, foll. 95r-96r.

to follow the changes and the course of the disease and sometimes the success of the treatment. Johannes Brünsterer wrote in his notes, for example, that the urine of a sick teacher was cloudy and reddish on the first day. Brünsterer had made several visits to the patient with Alvise Bellocati in October 1547. On the second day, the urine was greenish and at the bottom of the flask a very raw substance had collected. In keeping with the dominant conception, it was there that the morbid matter could be presumed to reside. The patient gradually felt better and the urine was less cloudy, something Bellocati interpreted as a sign that the nature of the patient had successfully evacuated the morbid matter over the past days.[263] Similarly, Handsch in his student notes described the changes in the urine of a young man with putrid fever whom he visited a number of times with Trincavella. At first, the urine was copious and thick and not particularly reddish, with whitish residual matter at the surface, which, however was blown apart by winds ("ventositates"). The following day the visible matter was more homogenous. On the third day, the two men saw the plentiful material lying in a circular shape at the bottom of the matula, looking like a thick cloud. According to Trincavella, if a disease was receding, this manifested itself in this way as nature began to separate out the burnt, ashen parts that had been produced during the putrefaction within the body. In the case at hand, however, the patient's condition deteriorated and he died.[264]

The urine could be examined in the patient's absence if necessary although in this case some important diagnostic clues might be missed that could be taken from his or her external appearance or from the answers to the physician's questions. The patient's presence was essential, however, during diagnostic procedures that relied on the sense of touch. Determining the qualities of the pulse and recognizing the subtle differences so as to draw the correct diagnostic, prognostic, and therapeutic conclusions was notoriously difficult and required a great deal of experience. Pulse diagnosis did not mean counting the number of beats during a given period of time with the help of a clock; such quantification gained importance only centuries later. Even in the simplified form that Da Monte taught his students, at least four central characteristics had to be determined: 1) the size or amplitude ("parvus", "magnus"), 2) the speed ("velocitas"), with which the individual beat reached its greatest expanse, 3) the frequency, i.e. whether the individual beats followed fast or slow upon each other, and 4) the evenness ("aequalitas"), which could be disrupted by pauses or

---

263 Universitätsbibliothek Erlangen, Ms 911, pp. 1–2, p. 11 and p. 14.
264 Cod. 11238, foll. 96r-97v; shortly afterwards, he noted the urine findings he encountered during various visits to a woman with tertian fever (ibid., fol. 99r-v).

additional beats. Some authors added further characteristics like the "strength", as measured by the force the physician needed to use to stifle the pulse.

The pulse could thus be described in great detail and diagnoses were accordingly differentiated. Da Monte, for instance, found that the pulse of a severely ill febrile and dropsical patient was hard, like a taut bow, and because of the hardness the frequency ("frequentia") was far more pronounced than the speed ("velocitas").[265] The physician, then, had to draw the right conclusions from his characterization of the pulse, which he tried to make as precise as possible. Above all, he had to consider the vital force, the vital heat, and the movement of the vital spirits whose periodic passage in the arteries was responsible for the palpable pulse according to the dominant medical teachings.[266] In the case just mentioned, it was important to decide whether the hardness of the pulse originated from the great load in the vessels ("ex materia") or from the strength of the driving force ("ex virtute").[267] At a different occasion, Da Monte taught his students that a weak and fast pulse indicated grave danger for life and limb.[268] Fracanzano, too, was very pessimistic about such cases.[269]

Professors encouraged their students to gain experience in the art of pulse diagnosis. Da Monte, for instance, visiting a patient with empyema and consumption with students, explained that the patient's pulse was quite small. "If you haven't grasped this yet, practice with your hand and reason so that you can grasp it".[270] About one of his sick visits with Fracanzano, Handsch noted, "He had me feel the pulse".[271] At such opportunities, students also learned practical tricks: "Always speak with the patient when you feel the pulse", Handsch noted, for example. This would soothe the patient and help ensure that the pulse was not changed by the patient's fear and thus that the diagnosis was not distorted.[272]

The third, central diagnostic skill that had to be acquired and that likewise involved the aspiring physician's senses was the physical examination of the patient. This claim may seem surprising at first glance. Until very recently, researchers in the history of medicine claimed that early modern physicians

---

265 Da Monte, Consultationum (1559), p. 555.
266 Handsch also pointed out the alternative explanation that the arteries pulsed on their own thanks to their *vis vitalis* (Cod. 11224, fol. 155v).
267 Da Monte, Consultationum (1559), p. 555.
268 Da Monte, Consultationum (1565), col. 460.
269 Cod. 11238, fol. 127v.
270 Da Monte, Consultationum (1565), col. 460: "Si haec nondum deprehendistis, exercete manum et mentem, ut possitis deprehendere."
271 Cod. 11238, fol. 128r.
272 Ibid., fol. 121r.

physically examined their patients only seldom or not at all.[273] Handsch's notes give us a completely different picture, however. Even as a student, he described numerous occasions when he saw his teachers put their tactile sense to use. Just touching the patient could unearth important diagnostic and prognostic clues. In the case of fevers, the skin was hot. Excessive coolness could be an indication that the vital heat was dying down: the inner heat and the vital spirits were retreating to the inside. Thus Bellocati, according to Brünsterer's account, saw how poorly an old woman was doing when he touched her cold extremities, and also felt her weak pulse. She died the next day.[274]

In medical practice, but also in medical teaching, the physical examination of the abdomen in particular played a central role. Handsch repeatedly described how his teachers examined patients with their own hands and showed their students how to diagnose properly on the basis of manual examination. He wrote, for example, "He touched the area of the liver" when describing a patient visit with Trincavella, who suspected a blocked spleen, "and in one part it was harder and in another part softer".[275] In the case of a female patient, Trincavella diagnosed an obstruction of the spleen after having touched the upper abdomen ("tetigit [. . .] hypocondria"); he later specified his diagnosis: the issue was *scirrhus*, a hardened tumor of the spleen.[276] The famous physician Vesal – this Handsch heard from Falloppia – had ridiculed those who wanted to learn the constitution of the spleen through palpation as the spleen lay too deep within the body. Falloppia countered this by saying that this was only true of healthy people, thus exposing Vesal's lack of clinical experience. An obstructed, hardened spleen, he continued, could be very large and weigh many pounds.[277] Francesco Frigimelica (1491/92–1558)[278] and Fracanzano too, examined their patients in this way in the presence of their students and sometimes repeated the examination at the next visit. In his account of Fracanzano's examination of a patient with pleurisy Handsch wrote, "He palpated the liver and then the ribs".[279] In the case of Fracanzano's

---

273 Porter, Rise (2004); see, however, my detailed analysis in Stolberg, Examining the body (2013).
274 Universitätsbibliothek Erlangen Ms. 911, p. 3.
275 Cod. 11238, foll. 98v-99r.
276 Ibid., fol. 89r.
277 Cod. 11210, fol. 4r.
278 Cod. 11183, fol. 51v and fol. 106v; Frigimelica taught in Padua first on medicinal plants and then, since 1532, on theoretical and practical medicine (Riddle, Three contributors (1979), p. 148–150; Ongaro, Medicina (2001), pp. 173f.).
279 Cod. 11183, fol. 123v: "Tangebat hepar et deinde costas".

examination of a young Englishman with a persistent fever he noted, "He palpated the upper abdomen".[280] When he accompanied Comes de Monte on his house calls in and around Vicenza, Handsch also saw how his teacher examined patients' abdomens with his hands. This was, as Handsch put it, common practice.[281]

Students were more than observers in these situations. They were allowed to literally try their hand at manual examination, at palpation, especially of the abdominal area. When Fracanzano felt for the spleen during a sick visit and said it felt hard and swollen, he also gave Handsch the opportunity to examine the patient. Unfortunately, Handsch felt nothing.[282] Student notes on Da Monte's teaching also repeatedly refer to cases involving diagnosis from palpation. They show beyond any doubt that patients' abdomens were frequently examined with the hands. In retrospect, it is difficult to determine how often this happened in the presence of students. In any case, Da Monte emphasized the significance of palpation and the findings that come from it, and taught students to correctly assess them. In the case of a young man, for instance, he diagnosed a pronounced hardening of the spleen, which could almost be called a *scirrhus*, and similarly in the case of a Milanese clergyman, he diagnosed a very hard and enlarged spleen.[283] His findings in the case of an unnamed patient from the higher nobility were especially detailed: what was initially very striking was a tenseness in the right upper abdomen in the stomach region, in the area of the false ribs. If one pressed lightly in this area, the patient felt only slight pain, but it became stronger the harder one pressed. In addition to this there was a tension in the entire abdominal area.[284]

It was not in Padua alone that students were introduced to physical examination, to the palpation of the abdomen. In Ferrara, Da Monte's teacher Musa Brasavola likewise examined patients with his own hands in the presence of students. In the case of a patient with lung empyema, for example, he found a collection of pus in the lung, a hardening in the liver area and, more importantly, in the area of the spleen. He also pressed with his fingers on the patient's lower ribs, which caused intense pain.[285] Students also documented a manual examination performed by Elideo Padovani in Bologna on a woman who believed she was

---

280 Ibid., fol. 129r, "tetigit hypocundria [sic!]" .
281 Ibid., fol. 125v, "ut mos est".
282 Ibid., fol. 130v, "ego tangens nihil sensi".
283 Da Monte, Consultationum (1554), p. 304 and p. 361.
284 Ibid., 370.
285 Biblioteca Ariostea, Ferrara, Collezione Antonelli, Ms. 531, fol. 17r.

pregnant. Her womb had felt enlarged for the past ten months. On the basis of palpation, Padovani concluded that there was a collection of fluid.[286]

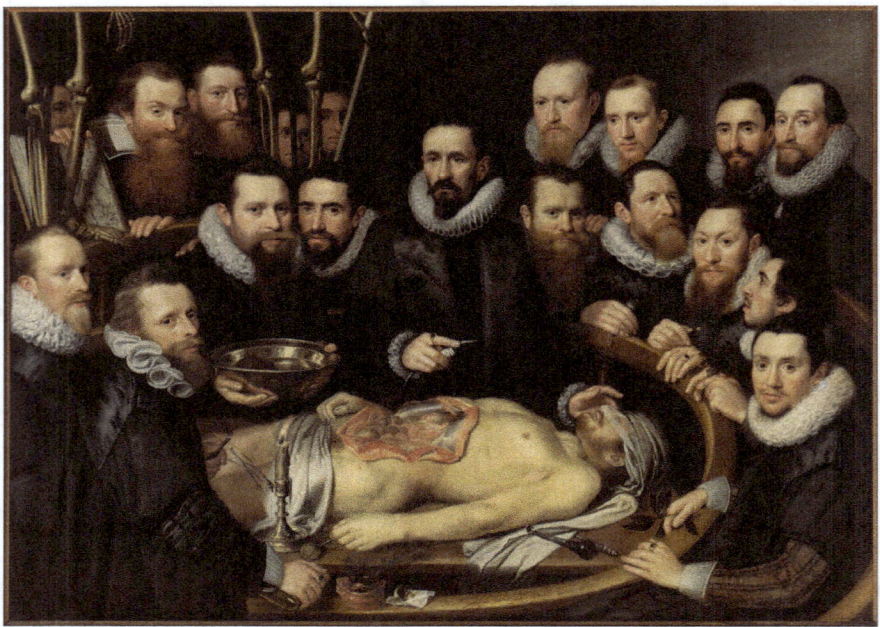

Fig. 3: Michiel Jansz van Mierevelt, Anatomy lesson of Dr Willem van der Meer, 1617, Museum Prinsenhof, Delft.

Anatomy

As we have seen, one reason why students from all over Europe were drawn to the universities in Padua, Bologna, and Montpellier was the excellent practical training offered there. This was coupled with a major second factor: the quality of the anatomical teaching at these universities. We might be tempted to ask to what extent a detailed anatomical knowledge was of use to a physician at a time when the vast majority of illnesses were not traced to pathological changes in organs or anatomical structures. Learned physicians – those practicing north of the Alps in any case – hardly concerned themselves with surgery, for which

---

[286] Welsch, Consiliorum (1676), pp. 391–2: "Helidaeus tactu aquositatem subesse deprehendit".

good anatomical knowledge was of obvious significance. Nevertheless, the anatomical Renaissance not merely reflected a natural-philosophical interest in the human body. From a contemporary medical perspective, it was very much connected to the tangible hope that diseases could be better understood, identified, and treated with the help of precise anatomical knowledge, all the more so since the anatomical teaching of the day also dealt in a wider sense with the physiological functions of the organs and body parts.[287]

Anatomical knowledge was imparted on the one hand in lectures based on authoritative texts, such as Galen's anatomical writings, the parts of Avicenna's *Canon medicinae* that were devoted to anatomy and *Anathomia* by Mondino de Luzzi (c. 1270–1326). Only scattered sixteenth-century student notes on anatomy lectures have been identified so far, however. In 1551, Handsch took extensive notes on Falloppia's lecture about Galen's work about skeletal anatomy (*De ossibus*). Falloppia went through the numerous bones systematically, from the skull – including the teeth – to the feet. He explained the various terms, described the structure and position, and sometimes the function of the bones.[288] Handsch also took some notes on a general introductory lecture by Antonio Fracanzano about the different parts of the body.[289] As those of other students, however, Handsch's notebooks give prominence to what the anatomists explained on the occasion of an anatomical demonstrations.

Historical research has so far shed little light on the details of anatomical teaching demonstrations and the specifics of what students learned there. Until very recently, the most important source for Padua was the *Acta* of the *Natio germanica*, which recorded in short minutes the events of the academic year including the anatomies that were performed.[290] As I have shown at length elsewhere,[291] student notes provide a much richer and more nuanced view of anatomical teaching. Georg Handsch took in-depth notes on anatomies, and we can also look at the extensive anatomical notes from two further medical students in Padua around the same time, Johannes Brünsterer (or Prünsterer) from Nuremberg and another who cannot be identified with certainty but may have come from Helmstedt.[292] Further

---

[287] Stolberg, Post-mortems (2017); as Handsch noted, some of the functions of the body and its part were ideally studied on the living, as Vesal had [allegedly] done on a Jew (Cod. 11210, fol. 191).
[288] Cod. 11210, foll. 34v-40v; Franciscus Michinus later published his notes on Falloppia's lecture on *De ossibus* (Falloppia, Expositio (1570)).
[289] Cod. 11210, foll. 187r-191r.
[290] Favaro, Atti (1911); the *Acta* are the principal source also for the latest comprehensive overview of anatomical teaching in Padua by Cynthia Klestinec (Klestinec, Theaters (2011)).
[291] Stolberg, Teaching anatomy (2018).
[292] Universitätsbibliothek Erlangen, Ms 909; Staats- und Universitätsbibliothek Göttingen, Ms Meibom 20; Helmstedt University was only established in 1576, however.

student notes are extant on the anatomical demonstrations of Fabrizi d'Acquapendente and Giulio Casseri in late sixteenth-century Padua.[293]

While studying in Padua, Handsch witnessed the complete, systematic dissection of a cadaver for educational purposes multiple times. Soon after he had arrived in December 1550, he included a description in his notebook of how Alessandro Sarego from Verona, who had recently taken over the surgical and anatomical instruction, dissected the body of a very corpulent woman while – in keeping with the traditional division of labor – another professor, presumably Antonio Fracanzano, expounded on what was being shown.[294] The cadaver had an unusual history. As Handsch noted in the margin, the woman was not a criminal but was herself the victim of a crime. Her husband had strangled her and thrown her into the water because she refused to earn money as a prostitute. The man was decapitated and likewise dissected.[295] In the winter of 1551–52, Gabrielle Falloppia took over the chair of anatomy and surgery. Handsch documented two anatomical demonstrations that took place that same winter.[296] As Andreas Vesal had done some years before, Falloppia combined the tasks of the lecturer, who explained and expounded upon what was being shown, with those of the *sector* who dissected and prepared the cadaver with his own hands. Handsch was also still in Padua when Falloppia, according to his own account, performed a further public demonstration on a cadaver in the winter of 1552–53.[297] In the following years, Falloppia developed a very active practice of dissection. Just in the winter of 1557–58 he dissected seven cadavers, according to Joachim Curaeus.[298]

Historical research about the anatomical practice at universities in the sixteenth century has concentrated for the most part on the public anatomical

---

293 Cf. Stolberg, Learning anatomy (2018).
294 Cf. the edition and translation of Handsch's notes on this anatomical demonstration in Mache, Anatomischer Unterricht (2019). Sarego was appointed in December 1550 and taught until Falloppia took over a year later (Facciolati, Fasti, p. 387). Handsch's notes on the other participants are contradictory. First he wrote of "D. Antonio Frankenzano legente et demonstrante" (Cod. 11210, fol. 187r), but later of "D. Appellato legente" (ibid., 191v, marginal note). Provided Handsch did not simply make a mistake here, it is most likely that Apellatus only read out an anatomical text, while Fracananzo commented on what he saw as well as on the text that had been read out and thus directed the event.
295 Cod. 11210, 191v.
296 In ibid., fol. 187r, Handsch listed the dissections he saw. He inserted his notes on subsequent dissections under Falloppia in his notes in the margins, between the lines and sometimes also on additional slips of paper.
297 Falloppia, Observationes (1561), fol. 65r. Handsch's notes do no not explicitly document this dissection.
298 Adam, Vitae (1620), p. 205.

demonstrations, which were great events in the life of the university, attracting prominent figures from inside and outside the university. Some places even had their own anatomical theaters built. Handsch's notes as well as those of other contemporary students show, however, that these public events were by no means the only opportunity students had to see the anatomical structures of the human body with their own eyes and to commit them to memory. There were also various "private" dissections ("anatomiae privatae") for a small number of – presumably paying – students. Handsch mentioned a number of such *anatomiae privatae*.[299] They often covered particular areas of the body or body parts, like the head. Unlike with the large public demonstrations, students here could observe the structures up close, rather than from up in the stands of a large anatomical theater.

Practical anatomical teaching was not limited to the dissection of human cadavers. The dissection of animals proved to be a welcome addition. Dogs and other animals, as Handsch learned, had the same physiological functions ("operationes") as human beings. It was thus thoroughly instructive to practice anatomy on a dog ("in eo exercere anatomia"), which Falloppia did with his students.[300] Observed by his students, Falloppia also dissected simian and bovine eyes and demonstrated the external eye muscles. Other students, too, documented such animal dissections, describing for example Falloppia's dissection of a dog and an ape in an *anatomia privata*.[301] Animal dissections were particularly useful in understanding fetal development and the changes of the womb during pregnancy. Pregnant women on the dissecting table were a rare occurrence. In Handsch's Padua years, Falloppia dissected at least two pregnant ewes. Students at this opportunity could see the fetus, which Falloppia likewise opened up to show the students the pulmonary vessels.[302]

As a supplement to the demonstrations with cadavers, anatomists took recourse to prepared specimens and visual media. Prepared skeletons were useful for learning the numerous bones in the human body and their spatial relation to one another. Handsch described in his Padua notes, apparently taken during a lecture on Galen's *De ossibus*, what he saw on such a skeleton ("Quae in skeleto vidi"), which was held upright by an iron rod.[303] Shortly thereafter, he worked with a real skull, taking extensive notes on the cranial bones and sutures and

---

299 Cod. 11210, fol. 21v, fol. 23v, fol. 28r and foll. 144v-145v.
300 Ibid., 191v; see also ibid., fol. 194r.
301 Staats- und Universitätsbibliothek Göttingen, Ms Meibom 20, foll. 127r-143v.
302 Ibid., fol. 11r.
303 Ibid., fol. 30v; probably on the same occasion, he made further notes on the anatomy of the spine (ibid., foll. 38v-40v).

illustrating them with a small drawing.[304] In his teaching, Falloppia also used anatomical illustrations or sketches to elucidate the complex anatomical structures such as the various layers of the eyeball and the "humors" inside it.[305]

Padua was therefore a place where prospective physicians could gain extensive, detailed anatomical knowledge with their own eyes and aided by the explanations of an experienced anatomist and surgeon. Over many pages, Handsch noted down what he was learning about the structures within the three body cavities – the cranial, thoracic, and abdominal cavities – and named the numerous bones, muscles, and tendons of which the human body is made. The anatomical demonstrations were generally connected with physiological explanations. Students not only saw the heart valves but also learned their function. According to contemporary teachings, they prevented the blood from flowing backwards, which, upon the expansion of the ventricle (*diastole*), was pulled from the large *vena cava* into the heart and pushed during systole into the lung and into the aorta, here together with the vital spirit, the *spiritus vitalis*, that was generated in the heart.[306]

Handsch's notes on the anatomy of the female genitalia are especially detailed. The "secrets of the female body" had long attracted heightened medical interest. As we will be seeing, sixteenth-century physicians also increasingly concerned themselves with diseases of women that had their sit or origin in the genitalia and above all the uterus, which marked the fundamental anatomical and physiological difference between man and woman.[307] Through his own research in the field, Falloppia distinguished himself in this regard. He was the first to provide a precise description of the parts still known today as "Fallopian tubes", which unlike the seminal vessels in man, he found, were not connected to the *testes* but ended in the space below them, widening like the opening of a trumpet or tuba – hence the name.[308] As Handsch learned, the passageways below the female "testiculi" opened, especially with the movement and warmth of coitus, allowing the female seed to enter the womb. This corresponded with the Galenic doctrine, according to which not only a male seed contributed to conception but also a female seed,[309] which served "as it

---

304 Ibid., fol. 38r-v.
305 Ibid., fol. 27r.
306 Ibid., foll. 17v-18r.
307 Cf. Stolberg, Woman (2003).
308 Falloppia, Observationes (1561), foll. 195v-196v.
309 E.g. Neefe, De missione (1548), conclusio I.1: "Corpora nostra ex sanguine, et maris foeminaeque semine conflata esse constat."

were as nutrition for the male [seed]".[310] Falloppia also explained to Handsch and to his fellow students that accounts of a "virgin's membrane" ("hymen") belonged to the realms of fantasy. He had, he said, dissected three virgins and found no hymen. Bleeding during the first act of intercourse was due to the narrowness of the vagina and was from burst veins.[311] He would later correct himself, however: with certain virgins one could find a "membrana nervosa", with a hole in the middle large enough to allow menstrual blood to pass.[312]

The principal purpose of anatomical teaching was to convey anatomical knowledge that was, where appropriate, supplemented by references to physiological and pathological contexts and their diagnostic and therapeutic significance. Beyond this, students had the opportunity to gain the manual skills, the craftsmanship that they would require later when they wanted or had to dissect a corpse themselves, possibly in front of colleagues or a larger audience. They knew only too well from the anatomical demonstrations of their experienced teachers how difficult it was to identify, separate and distinguish the various anatomical structures. For good reasons, Handsch added a reference from Galen to his anatomical notes who had admonished physicians to practice anatomy on animals first to develop the necessary skills.[313] Vesal, on his part, had emphasized how valuable it was for students to try their hand at the task.[314]

Handsch made note of a few well-known basic rules, for example that the dissection of a cadaver was best begun with the abdominal organs because the entrails began to rot particularly quickly.[315] But not only this; he also noted down the various instruments needed: from the different scalpels to the small knife Falloppia preferred, the probe used to explore vessel openings, the sponges to absorb fluids, the oil that made it easier to separate the muscles from one another, and even the burning candles which generally served as a light source at the time (cf. Fig. 3).[316] Handsch also wrote down the practical procedure: removing the hair (or fur in the case of animals), the two long, cross-shaped cuts used to open the abdomen, longitudinally from the sternum over the navel to the pubic bone and then across the navel on both sides, followed by folding back of the abdominal wall, initially only

---

310 Cod. 11210, fol. 9v.
311 Ibid., fol. 10r.
312 Falloppia, Observationes (1561), fol. 194r-v.
313 Ibid., fol. 193r.
314 Vesal, De humani corporis (1543), p. 547; cf. Carlino, Books (1999), pp. 188f.
315 Cod. 11210, 192v.
316 Ibid.

on one side.[317] And he learned little practical tricks, for example that when dissecting the liver, one could first tie up the veins with thread to prevent bleeding.[318]

The anatomical instruction in Padua and other Northern Italian universities such as Bologna and Ferrara[319] was of such a quality that abroad only the universities in Paris and Montpellier – at best – could keep pace. The one in Montpellier regularly practiced educational anatomies already in the early sixteenth century. For just the time between 1526 and 1535, records of twenty-nine dissections are extant.[320] The university even had its own anatomical theater.[321] As in Padua, not only the corpses of executed criminals were dissected[322] but also those of people who died in accidents[323] and of deceased hospital occupants.[324] Dissections continued to be actively practiced later on as well. In his memoir, Felix Platter, who studied in Montpellier in the 1550s, told of several human dissections, but also of one ape dissection.[325]

At German universities, the practice of anatomical teaching was by far less intensive. Anatomical demonstrations only took place every few years, if at all.[326] As late as 1572, Johann Schwartz explained that in "Germany" it was only possible to learn anatomy on cadavers in Basel, under Felix Platter.[327] There are extant reports of earlier anatomical demonstrations at German universities. At the university in Wittenberg, for example, the first public anatomy took place in

---

317 Ibid., 194r.
318 Ibid., 192v. In her detailed analysis of anatomical education in Padua in the sixteenth century, Cynthia Klestinec described the teaching of concrete practical anatomical skills, especially in the context of private anatomies, and the students' interest in them as a new phenomenon, which she attributed to institutional and professional changes in the last two decades of the sixteenth century (Klestinec, Theaters (2011), pp. 153–155 and p. 225, note). Handsch's notes make it clear, however, that this development began much earlier. It is just not well documented in Klestinec's principal source, the *Acta* of the German Nation (Favaro, Atti (1911)).
319 Cf. Lind, Pre-Vesalian anatomy (1975), pp. 307–316.
320 Germain, Les étudiants (1876), p. 33.
321 Bibliothèque de la Ville de Montpellier, Manuscrits Germain, Ms. 111, Liber procuratoris (copy), fol. 214r, fol. 232r, fol. 233r and fol. 234r); Dulieu, La médecine (1979), p. 180.
322 E.g. Bibliothèque de la Ville de Montpellier, Manuscrits Germain, Ms. 111, fol. 213r and fol. 229r.
323 Thus, in 1532, a woman who had drowned in a watermill outside the town (ibid., fol. 214r).
324 Ibid., fol. 220r and fol. 243r.
325 Cf. Platter, Tagebuch (1976), p. 151, p. 187, p. 193, pp. 207–8 (on the dissection of a monkey under Guillaume Rondelet), p. 235, p. 238, p. 241 (on the dissection of a woman and of a girl), p. 259 and p. 261; see also Dulieu, Félix Platter (1991), pp. 17–20.
326 Kuhn, Studenten (1971), p. 36.
327 HStA Stuttgart, A 282, Bü. 1301, letter from Johann Schwartz to Duke Ludwig of Württemberg, October 1572.

1526, with Augustin Schurff showing the anatomy of the head to an audience.[328] But as far as we can tell today, there was no regular and reliable anatomical teaching at German universities and that situation was not to change soon.

Pharmacy and Botany

Along with anatomy, the teaching of medical botany – of the numerous medicinal plants or *simplicia* – took on increasing importance in university teaching in the sixteenth century. Medicinal botany established itself as an independent subject of instruction taught by specially appointed professors.[329] A key factor in this pronounced rise in significance was once again the increased orientation in medical teaching towards the needs of medical practice. Thorough botanical and pharmaceutical knowledge was considered absolutely essential for a successful medical practice. And there were other developments that supported and encouraged this renewed appreciation of medical botany. The humanists rediscovered Galen's work on medicinal plants (*De simplicibus*) and the great pharmacological treatise by Dioscorides (*Res medica*). The commentary on Dioscorides by Handsch's later mentor Mattioli became the central pharmacological reference work in the second half of the sixteenth century.[330] Since the Middle Ages, trade had also been bringing with it increasing numbers of exotic plants, and north of the Alps, physicians and apothecaries were discovering a native flora that found no mention in the works of Galen, Pliny, and other authorities who had practiced in more southern climes. With the traditional classification of healing plants according to qualities (cold, hot, dry, and moist) as a starting point, there also developed an awareness and an appreciation of the empirically observable "specific" effects of medicinal plants on particular organs or humors and against specific illnesses or complaints.[331] Handsch reported that, in one instance, his professor Fracanzano even prescribed a sick patient black hellebore specifically "so that we would see its effects".[332]

---

328 Koch, Anatomie (2003), p. 169.
329 Overview in Reeds, Botany (1991).
330 Mattioli, Commentarii (1554; 1565; 1570); Ferri, Dioscoride (1997); Fausti, Complessa scienza (2001); Ciancio, Many gardens (2015); cf. Reeds, Botany (1991), pp. 21f.; biographical surveys in Fabiani, Mattioli (1872), with an edition of relevant sources; Ferri, Mattioli (1997); Hejnová, Mattioli (2001).
331 See my discussion of drug effects in the chapter on empirical knowledge.
332 Cod. 11238, fol. 121r, "ut nos videremus eius operationem".

A physician was expected to know what the plants he was prescribing looked like. Insufficient experience in this respect could quickly lead to disgrace, a humiliating experience that Handsch was not spared. He repeatedly made note of errors he made in the identification of plants, for example when he mistook storksbill (*erodium*) for Venus' comb (*pecten veneris*) and had to endure the lecture of someone who knew better.[333] He noted elsewhere that he wanted to protect himself in the future from a similar "disgraceful error" ("turpis error"), after having falsely declared a common field plant to be Alexanders (*smyrnium*) in front of a Wittenberg student.[334] He also failed to impress Collinus on numerous occasions when he misidentified plants.[335] But even the famous Mattioli – and this Handsch seems to have noted with a certain sense of satisfaction – was sometimes unable to identify plants correctly.[336]

If future physicians wanted to appear capable in the eyes of their patients, they had to acquire a broad and practice-oriented knowledge of the numerous known medicinal plants and the various ways they were to be administered. Some of this could be gained from lectures and books. In one of his Padua notebooks, Handsch took extensive notes based on Matteo Cortis's explanations of pharmacological indications, dosage forms, and dosages. His notes include references to syrups that were used for a hot, cold, dry, or moist *intemperies,* followed by syrups, waters, and numerous healing plants (*simplicia*) as well as mixtures of herbs (*composita*) that served the intended digestion, dissolution, mobilization and evacuation of bilious, black-bilious, and phlegmatic matter. After this, he listed remedies that were said to strengthen, warm, or cool specific organs or body parts like the head, as well as instructions on how to apply enemas and ablutions and use poultices and plasters. These explanations were accompanied by numerous formulas for prescriptions and dosage information.[337]

Herbal books furthermore provided prospective physicians with entries about a host of medicinal plants introduced one after the other, with their characteristics and effects.[338] Handsch made notes of such works as Leonhard Fuchs's *De historia stirpium,* which, already in its early editions, covered well over 300 plants, listing them in order with their Greek, Latin, and German names. It further included their

---

333 Cod. 11210, fol. 121v; similarly Cod. 11183, fol. 40v: "Turpe me dedi."
334 Cod. 11210, fol. 125v.
335 Ibid., fol. 120v: "Turpiter me dedi coram Collino".
336 Ibid., fol. 124v.
337 Cod. 11210, foll. 94r-114r. Corti (or Curzio) was the author of a treatise *De dosibus,* of which only an edition of 1561 is known (Brambilla, Scuola Longobarda (1781), pp. 1–4). Perhaps Handsch had access to lecture notes.
338 Overview in Arber, Herbals (1986).

external appearance, the preferred habitat, the blooming period, the individual mixture of the four basic qualities (*temperies*), and the medicinal properties ascribed to them by Dioscorides, Galen, Pliny, Theophrastus, and other ancient authors.[339]

Herbal books were valuable as the source of theoretical knowledge and they could be useful for reference. But even when they featured – as did Fuchs's work – illustrations of the healing plants that were more or less true to nature, they only gave the physician a limited ability to recognize and name the plants in question. The illustrations were black and white woodcuts that at best were colored, on occasion, by the owner of the book or by somebody commissioned to do the coloring by hand (and by no means necessarily from nature). The student's own visual inspection and experience with real plants remained indispensable. The great significance that was attached at the time to a precise knowledge of the numerous medicinal plants for a successful medical practice was thus also decisive in the emergence of an important innovation, which still shapes the cityscape of some university cities today: the establishment of botanical gardens for educational purposes. This new development had its beginnings in Italy and soon spread to all of Europe.[340]

There was a large and famous botanical garden in Padua. The *Orto dei semplici* was founded in 1545, a few years before Handsch's arrival.[341] Handsch's notes show just how much the medical students made use of the opportunity to familiarize themselves with the various medicinal plants. Under the heading "Plants I got to know in the garden in Padua", Handsch in one of his Padua notebooks presented dozens of plants that he had seen in the botanical garden, and sometimes at other occasions. With varying degrees of detail, he described the appearance of many plants, their blossoms and leaves, and sometimes also mentioned the taste, as with bitter absinth. He even described many well-known native plants, like chamomile, borage, and common bugloss in this way. And he occasionally drew the outline of a leaf, to show, for example how it was elongated or heart-shaped or had a serrated edge. Only in rare instances, in the case of moneywort or houseleek, for example, did he find it enough to simply write "nota", meaning "known". His notes were limited to botanical characteristics; he made no mention of the particular illnesses for which the plants were used nor did he even indicate their *temperies*. Evidently, his notes were primarily meant to help him memorize the appearance of the plants and plant parts that he had seen

---

339 Fuchs, Historia stirpium (1542).
340 Bedini, L'orto (2007).
341 Minelli, L'orto botanico (1995); Cappelletti, Le piante (1995).

with his own eyes; he was training his ability to identify and distinguish plants and plant parts rather than addressing their therapeutic application.[342]

Establishing botanical gardens for the purpose of teaching students was a painstaking and costly task, and this impressively underscores just how much significance was now being attached to arriving at a medical knowledge of medicinal plants through personal observation. But the significance of these botanical gardens in teaching students must not be overstated either. Even in Padua, physicians in training found other ways of experiencing plants and thus acquiring botanical knowledge. By implication, this means that even when no botanical garden was available at a university, botanical knowledge could still be imparted in ways other than through books.

One obvious possibility here – one that has so far found little consideration in historical research – is that students visited private gardens.[343] There are countless indications from Padua and Prague, but also from Augsburg, Nuremberg, and other cities, that the owners of private gardens – especially apothecaries and physicians – grew native and exotic plants and showed them to others.[344] Handsch in his Padua notes repeatedly mentioned native and exotic plants that he had seen in the garden of his professor Antonio Fracanzano.[345] In the garden of a certain Daniel or Daniele – possibly an apothecary – he found gladiolas and lemon balm.[346] In the same entry – though he might have added this later – he referred to *clematis flammula Jovis* shown to him by a certain Thaddeus "in his garden" ("in suo horto").[347] One of the plants he saw when visiting a certain Cetterius was Spanish chamomile root (*piretrum*).[348]

Students furthermore sought to deepen their knowledge of botany in the wild. With acquaintances, Felix Platter went on botanical excursions near Montpellier.[349] Strobelberger later praised the wealth of plants in the fields, olive groves, vineyards, woods, mountains, hills, rivers, lagoons, and the sea there.[350]

---

342 Cod. 11210, foll. 115r-120v: "Herbae quas didici in horto Paduano".
343 See, however, Ciancio, Many gardens (2016), p. 37, on Pietro Andrea Mattioli, who praised the garden of Maffeo de Maffei in Venice in this respect.
344 Lorenz Scholz even devoted a separate publication to a simple list of all the plants in his garden in Breslau (Scholz, Catalogus (1594)), which he had established seven year before; see also Rindfleisch et alii, Epigrammata (1594).
345 Cod. 11210, fol. 117r: "Vidi in horto Frankenzanii".
346 Ibid. The entry is followed by: "Item in apotheca monstravit lapatum, item hyacinthum." One of Handsch's fellow students was called Daniel Cellarius.
347 Cod. 11210, fol. 120v.
348 Cod. 11183, fol. 40v.
349 Platter, Tagebuch (1976), p. 219 and p. 222.
350 Strobelberger, Laureationem (1628).

Handsch, too, reported how went to the country ("in agro") with some people and documented the herbs that he saw on this occasion,[351] along with the plants that Fracanzano had pointed out to them at the riverside.[352] The repeated mention of Fracanzano in this context also shows that students by no means only learned about the various healing plants from the professor who was responsible for teaching about the *simplicia;* in Handsch's time this was Falloppia.

In his early years in Padua, Handsch also learned how to press and dry plants and then collect them in a book. He saw this when visiting a certain Ladislaus, who was presumably a fellow student who showed him various plants in the botanical garden. Thus he knew that one could not simply put fresh plants in such a book but had to press and dry them first; otherwise they would rot.[353] The production of such "herbaria viva" was a relatively new technique. Their invention is generally attributed to Luca Ghini (1490–1556), who taught medical botany in Bologna and Pisa and founded the botanical gardens in Pisa and Florence.[354] The herbaria soon spread beyond the Alps. In the late sixteenth century, Caspar Ratzenberger compiled two magnificent, multi-volume herbaria within just a few years.[355]

Aspiring physicians in Padua and other places did not only have to familiarize themselves with a multitude of medicinal plants and more generally with all sorts of plant-, animal- and mineral-derived medicinal substances; they also had to be able to recognize them in a processed form and learn how medications were produced. As a rule, medications were manufactured or at least blended at the physician's behest by apothecaries and their assistants. Basic pharmaceutical knowledge was, however, essential for physicians. In the case of herbal infusions or decoctions, brewing the plant in hot water might be enough. But even here, and most definitely when prescribing syrups and electuaries, pills or tablets (we may imagine them like small cookies), the physician had to bear in mind the taste and possibly consistency. Otherwise, as we will see, physicians could expect to meet with considerable resistance from the patient. It was also important for the physician to know how the different ingredients interacted with one another, and which ingredients he had to add to achieve the desired consistency and taste. Not least of all, he had to ensure that the prescribed medicinal mixture would not quickly decompose or spoil.

---

351 Cod. 11210, fol. 119v.
352 Ibid., fol. 117v.
353 Ibid., fol. 115r.
354 Arber, Herbals (1986), pp. 138–143; Findlen, Death (2017).
355 Forschungsbibliothek Gotha, Chart. A 152–155; Stolberg, Konservierte Pflanzen (2019); on the second *herbarium vivum*, which today is in Kassel, see Schaffrath, Läuse (2012).

The apothecary were artisans, they learned a trade. As a rule, they did not go to university. Many of them were educated, however,[356] and, most crucially, they could draw on a wealth of experience in dealing with medicinal substances. They knew how to judge the qualities of ingredients, and they had the necessary practical skills in producing medicines in their various forms. Physicians increasingly demanded and were granted the power to supervise apothecaries. But in practical matters, physicians stood to learn a great deal from them. In his later years, Handsch still often took note of what he had learned from apothecaries about certain medicinal plants and about the production of medications, and he even occasionally took guidance from them.[357]

For medical students, apothecaries played an even greater role. In some university towns, apothecaries were even involved in university teaching to a certain extent. During Handsch's Padua days, Antonio Fracanzano took his students not only to the botanical gardens to look at living plants, but also to apothecaries, where they could learn to identify and evaluate the blossoms, leaves and roots of medicinal plants in a dried and processed state, for example grated guaiacum wood.[358] In his Padua notes, Handsch repeatedly named the plants and plant parts he had seen at the apothecary's, such as the leaf of a mandragora, shown to him by an *apothecarius*.[359] In Montpellier, Strobelberger praised the local apothecaries, chief among them Laurentius Catellanus, who were very learned ("doctissimos"). They presented the entire *materia medica* privately and publicly, showed native and exotic plants, and demonstrated the production of complex medicinal products such as theriac, mithridate, and alkermes.[360] Felix Platter during his time in Montpellier made a point of lodging with Catellanus and would profit very much from this. He was learning a lot, he wrote to his father in 1553, and that he would "lodge in the pharmacy, in which my master has much to do, so much that he needs four or five servants," and would "learn about everything there daily."[361]

Prospective physicians were also well-advised to continue cultivating their botanical knowledge after they had completed their studies. Handsch as a young physician compiled further lists of "simplicia" that he had seen himself, beginning with a list of "simples I learned about in Prague in 1554".[362] There were no

---

356 Hoppe, Bildungshungrige Apotheker (1992).
357 Cod. 11183, foll. 147r-152v; Handsch used the word "docuit", "he taught".
358 Cod. 11210, fol. 140r.
359 Ibid., fol. 117r.
360 Strobelberger, Laureationem (1628), p. 18.
361 Platter, Tagebuch (1976), p. 157.
362 Cod. 11210, fol. 120v-125r: "Simplicia quae Pragae didici".

botanical gardens there, but private gardens offered ample material to be viewed. He repeatedly mentioned the garden of Collinus, for example, and noted that Collinus showed him *aristolochia rotunda* there.[363] It is possible that he was referring to the Angel's Garden, where Collinus had established his school, but Handsch also hinted at the existence of a second, possibly private garden belonging to Collinus. His medical teachers too, Lehner and Gallo, had their own gardens in which Handsch saw noteworthy plants such as loosestrife (*lysimachia*) and savory (*satureja*).[364] References to further private gardens may be surmised from entries such as "at old Wenzel's I saw *florem Martii* [hyacinth? common narcissus?]", "I saw meadowsweet at Klaus's", and "I saw lavender at Blasius's".[365]

The young Handsch moreover went on botanical excursions in the company of Mattioli. In 1555, he listed a good dozen plants under the title "Cum Matthioli et aliis ivimus herbatum"[366] and he explicitly mentioned M. Thadeus and M. Iacobus Camenicenus.[367] As late as 1563, he went on a botanical excursion ("herbatio") with Mattioli and an apothecary.[368] In his Innsbruck years as well, he continued his student notes about *simplicia* and described among other things several plants in the Archduke's garden in Ambras.[369]

Surgery

Another feature that distinguished the universities in Northern Italy and Montpellier from those north of the Alps was the importance they gave to the surgical training of prospective physicians. In Italy – and the same holds for Spain[370] – surgery had been firmly established at the universities since the Middle Ages.[371]

---

363 Cod. 11205, fol. 564v.
364 Cod. 11210, foll. 124r-125v.
365 Ibid., fol. 121r: "Paeoniam vix cognovi in horto D. Ulrici"; "vidi apud Adamum" (ibid. fol. 122v); "filipendulam vidi apud Claudium" (ibid., fol. 123r); "gariophyllam in horto Collini optime vidi" (ibid.); "apud presbyteram Venceslaum vidi florem Martii" (ibid., fol. 125r).
366 Ibid., foll. 123v-124r.
367 Probably Handsch was referring to the physician and clergyman Jacobus Camenicenus († 1565), whom he mentioned repeatedly.
368 Ibid., fol. 126r; according to Handsch, their destination was the "Devil's hole" ("foramen diaboli"); possibly this refers to the Průrva Ploučnice, an artificial, partly underground canal at the end of a reservoir in the area around the former Wartenberg (Stráž pod Ralskem) on Rollberg, not far from Handsch's home town Leipa.
369 Ibid., fol. 127r.
370 López Pinero, Ciencia (1979), pp. 360–368.
371 Siraisi, Faculty of Medicine (1992), pp. 381f.; Fischer, Hartmann Schedel (1996), p. 54.

In Bologna, for example, set texts for surgery, which the professors had to read from and comment on, were listed in the statutes as early as 1405, and leading medical authors like the Florentine Dino del Garbo (1280–1327) concerned themselves with surgical topics.[372] In sixteenth-century Italy, there were already quite a number of professorships for surgery, usually connected with anatomy and botany. Leading professors practiced surgery in all its aspects. Himself the son of a surgeon, Berengario da Carpi in Bologna, for example, was not only a famous anatomist but for twenty-five years occupied the chair of surgery there and was known as much as a surgeon as for treating internal diseases.[373] Some graduates of Italian universities – including those from north of the Alps – later proudly carried the title of a doctor in medicine and surgery. Hartmann Schedel, for instance, who earned his doctoral degree in Padua in 1466, already practiced medicine under the title "Doctor utriusque medicinae".[374] Paracelsus, too, called himself a "doctor of both medicines". Allegedly he studied in Italy for some time[375] but the doctorate he is said to have earned in Ferrara cannot be verified.[376] Some Italian universities, including Bologna and Padua, even offered a shorter course of studies that enabled students to earn only the title of *doctor chirurgiae*.[377]

In academic medicine north of the Alps, by contrast, surgery continued to live in the shadows.[378] Some physicians bemoaned this state of affairs. "Contrary to the doctrine of the old physicians", the Chemnitz doctor Caspar Neefe (1514–1579) lamented in 1548, surgery had been separated from "physica medicina".[379] At the University of Leipzig, Duke Moritz established a surgical lectureship in 1542. At first, the university used the money for other purposes but in 1554 Moritz' successor August insisted and Gregor Schett, doctor "in both medicines" was

---

372 Later published as *Chirurgia cum tractatu eiusdem de ponderibus et mensuris nec non de emplastris et unguentis* (Ferrara 1485; Venice 1536).
373 Bylebyl, Cardiovascular physiology (1969), p. 111.
374 Fischer, Hartmann Schedel (1996), p. 54.
375 Paracelsus, Grosse Wundartzney (1536), preface to the reader.
376 Ibid., dedicatory epistle to Emperor Ferdinand, 7 May 1536.
377 Nutton, Humanist surgery (1985), p. 80. Thus we find in Padua and Venice in the 1540s the "doctor chirurgiae" Franciscus Litigotus, and in April 1549 a doctorate in surgery is documented for a certain Paolo Casiccio, who had his fees waived because of his poverty (Bernardi, Prospetto (1797), p. 39 and p. 22).
378 Schlegelmilch, Surgical disputations (2021), esp. pp. 255–260; see also Schütte, Medizin (2017), pp. 272–276.
379 Neefe, De missione (1548), problema I.

appointed. It is worth pointing out, in our context, that the professor was not only to teach medical students but also, in German, non-academic barber-surgeons.[380]

Two main causes of this marginal role of surgery in the learned medicine north of the Alps may be identified. For one thing, academically trained physicians were concerned that the manual aspects of surgery might be damaging to their scholarly dignity. The word "Chirurgie" in German and French or "chirurgia" in Italian – as with "surgery" in English – derives from the Greek terms for "hand" and "work", and the surgeon necessarily had to dirty his hands. In Italy, such reservations were apparently less widespread, perhaps because academic physicians had occupied an uncontested place there in the healthcare of even smaller towns since the late Middle Ages and did not feel the same need to set themselves apart from the manual aspects of medicine. In many Italian towns, they were even employed as *medici condotti* and paid a regular salary.[381] The other reason was that, in German-speaking areas, barber-surgeons had been successful in broadening the scope of their activity to include not only hair and body care but minor surgery. They were organized in guilds and asserted their monopoly when it came to surgical cases, even against learned physicians.[382]

In Padua, Handsch met with conditions that favored the acquisition of surgical knowledge and skills.[383] For good reason, Conrad Gessner recommended to the town of Zurich that the young Georg Keller be given a scholarship so he could study in Padua and gain surgical knowledge in particular.[384] As in other Italian universities, the dual chair of anatomy and surgery in Padua, which linked the two fields, was advantageous to both. Presumably, Vesal was not particularly proficient at surgery considering his relatively young age and his limited bedside experience. However, Gabrielle Falloppia, Giulio Casseri,[385] and Girolamo Fabrizi d'Acquapendente, who succeeded him in shaping the anatomical and surgical teaching in Padua, enjoyed excellent reputations as practicing surgeons and as anatomists.

---

380 Zaunick, Beiträge (1924/25).
381 Nutton, Continuity (1981).
382 Cf. Jütte, Ärzte (1991), pp. 20–22; Kinzelbach, Sozial- und Alltagsgeschichte (1994); see also below the chapter on bath-masters and barber-surgeons.
383 Nutton, Humanist surgery (1985).
384 Zentralbibliothek Zürich, Ms. S 85, N. 11, letter from Gessner to the town authorities in Zürich (I owe this information to Tilmann Walter).
385 On Casseri see Sterzi, Giulio Casseri (1909); Cunsolo, Giulio Casserio (2008); on Fabrizi see among others Favaro, Contributi (1922); Scipio, Girolamo Fabrizi (1978); Fossati, Girolamo Fabrizi (1988).

Regardless of the paramount significance of manual work, of practical technical skills in surgery, university teaching in this field relied heavily on commenting on authoritative works. Professors were able to draw on a remarkable corpus of ancient, Arabic, and medieval works. Book Six of Paul of Aegina's compendium of medicine, which treated a broad range of surgical procedures in detail,[386] served as an important foundation, along with Galen's *Methodus medendi*. The Hippocratic text on injuries of the head, the relevant passages of Aëtius of Amida and Oribasius, and the exhaustive treatment of Greek and Roman surgery in Celsus received less attention in the sixteenth century.[387]

No notes from surgery lectures in Handsch's hand have survived. On a few occasions, however, he wrote down what he learned about particular surgical procedures in the anatomy lessons taught by Gabrielle Falloppia, because Falloppia sometimes recounted his own experiences in surgery to his students.

Concerning the throat and esophagus, Falloppia discussed the removal of swallowed fish bones. Some, he explained, advised the use of a piece of dry sponge that was coated with sugar and lowered into the throat on a string. When, meeting with humidity, the sugar became liquid, the sponge expanded and could be pulled out, taking the fish bone with it.[388]

On the basis of anatomy, Falloppia gave his students an exact description of where to place the incision to drain the liquid accumulated in the abdomen in patients with massive abdominal dropsy (*ascites*).[389] He explained that this procedure, called *paracentesis* was carried out by surgeons when drug therapy failed. He warned, however, that great caution was required as the procedure was dangerous. He himself had performed it on three patients and all three had died, one of them within a month. His listeners were therefore not to carry out a paracentesis of their own accord, but only if their patient explicitly demanded the procedure. The incision must not be made directly under the navel because this would damage the sinews of the straight abdominal muscles (*musculi recti*) which connected to the pubic bone. These were very sensitive to pain and would contract, which could result in fainting, and they also healed badly. It was better to place the incision in the fleshier parts to the left or right below the navel, keeping a distance of approximately three finger-widths from the pelvic bone. Here too, Handsch drew a small sketch. The procedure in this area was less painful

---

386 Paulos von Aegina, Sieben Bücher (1914), pp. 466–604.
387 On the following see also the excellent survey in Nutton, Humanist surgery (1985).
388 Cod. 11210, fol. 202r.
389 Ibid., fol. 144v-145v; Michinus, the editor of Falloppia's *Observationes anathomicae*, also described how Falloppia used the dissection of a dog to show him and other students how to proceed on humans (Falloppia, Expositio (1570), foll. 71r-76r).

and the opening would heal better. The incision could be made lengthwise but Falloppia recommended doing a transverse cut. With dropsical patients, he said, the danger of damaging the intestines was not great. However, the incision should be made in such a way that the opening into the depth of the body would be covered again by superficial skin following the procedure. Furthermore, it was important to drain the liquid not in one sitting but in several steps. From a note in the margin we may surmise that Falloppia demonstrated the procedure for the students, using a dog ("in cane"): he first used a small knife to make a lateral incision in the skin before perforating the muscles below the incision and inserting a silver cannula ("cannula argentea").[390] Falloppia illustrated his explanations with cases from his own practice. He told of a dropsical peasant ("rusticus"), for example, in whose case simply scoring the abdominal skin was enough to produce two bowls full of liquid and to eliminate the pain in the tight, bulging belly.[391]

As part of his teaching on the anatomy of the abdomen, Falloppia also showed his students what the anatomical preconditions were for the development of an inguinal hernia. Hernias or intestinal hernias were common at the time and feared, and they could become monstrous in size.[392] Hernias were also considered a major cause of male infertility and could critically jeopardize a man's marriage prospects. Falloppia's students were allowed to feel for the hole in the groin of a corpse through which the spermatic cord went to the scrotum – the most common opening for hernias in boys and men. They also learned about the different layers that had to be cut during such an operation. The anatomist gave his students a precise description of his procedure, which did not involve the commonly practiced removal of the testicle. The surgeon had to push the intestines back as far as possible, cut through the scrotum and its inner covering and then burn the region with a red-hot iron in such a way that the intestine could no longer move down. He warned against excessive optimism, however. He had healed some patients in this way, but with others the operation had not been beneficial. Similarly, he had successfully performed couching on one patient, but had destroyed the eye in the case of two others.[393]

Handsch even made notes on the technique of suturing. This is noteworthy because, given the circumstances at the time, Handsch could be quite sure he would never be assigned this task north of the Alps. He described at length how,

---

390 Cod. 11210, fol. 145v; a note above it, "D. Gallus Augustae", probably refers to a case of dropsy that Andrea Gallo had treated in Augsburg, which is not further outlined here.
391 Cod. 11251, foll. 29v-30r.
392 See e.g. Baillou, Consiliorum medicinalium (1635), vol. 2, pp. 244–46, on the case of a man who carried large parts of his intestines in his scrotum.
393 Cod. 11210, fol. 195r-v, inserted leaf "De herniae curatione".

according to Falloppia, deep, penetrating abdominal wounds had to be sutured and illustrated the line of the suture with two small sketches. The common suture, he said, was the one which Albucasis called the furrier's suture ("pelliparorum"). Here, the muscles and the peritoneum were simply stitched back together as one. In Falloppia's eyes, however, this method was coarse and unsuitable. A far better suture was one that Galen had mentioned, albeit in obscure words, where muscle was sutured to muscle and peritoneum to peritoneum – in other words, working with the layers.[394] At another occasion, responding to a student's request, Falloppia described the use of ants in the treatment of intestinal injuries. According to the old teachings, ants had to be set on the joined edges of the wound and their abdomens squeezed, causing them to bite. Then they were cut through in the middle and the process was repeated with more ants until the wound was closed up. He had never done this himself, however. Rather, he had sutured two patients with abdominal wounds using the (abovementioned) "furrier's suture", that is using one continuous thread. The thread could later be removed all at once in its entirety, though he did not think that leaving the thread behind would do great damage. Both patients had died, but there had reportedly been several men in the encampments who survived such intestinal wounds.[395]

Falloppia seems to have had quite an extensive surgical practice in Padua. Thus students who came with him on visits had the opportunity to familiarize themselves with surgical methods, to observe him doing the many small maneuvers that were decisive for the success of the treatment. From students' accounts we know that Falloppia not only treated a young man with a genital ulcer and "spermatic flux" and used a probe to find a bladder stone on another patient.[396] According to Vettore Trincavella, Falloppia also used such a probe on a woman with a hard ulcer of the uterus ("scirrhus"). She subsequently died, reportedly because Falloppia accidentally punctured the uterus.[397] Handsch further described in detail how Falloppia, in June of 1552, proceeded in the case of a grossly swollen lymph node in the groin of a twenty-year-old. The swelling, it was assumed, derived from a venereal disease ("ex coitu"). Here, Falloppia used a special double-layered dressing with four loose ends that made it possible to attach it to the thighs and belly. He applied an ointment that was supposed to bring the lymph node to "maturity". When the growth had softened

---

394 Ibid., fol. 144r.
395 Ibid., fol. 198r, inserted leaf "De vulnere intestinorum".
396 Padovani, Processus (1607), p. 166 and p. 165.
397 Ibid., p. 148; by all appearances, the notes were written by a German-speaking student who studied both in Bologna with Padovani and in Padua among others with Trincavella who told his students about Falloppia's misfortune.

after a couple of days, Falloppia cut it open in the presence of Handsch, and blood and pus issued from it. Subsequently, Falloppia covered the wound with egg white and several layers of bandaging.[398] Handsch furthermore observed how Falloppia cleaned a deep abdominal wound using a small cannula ("syphunculum") and then reapplied the dressing,[399] and how, treating another young man, he lanced a phlegmon.[400] He watched as the anatomist washed a head wound, closed it with two or three stitches, applied egg white against inflammation and then a very sticky, pitch-like substance made from barberry (*berberis*), which held the edges of the wound together.[401]

In Bologna and Ferrara as well, students were able to observe the treatment of surgical patients. One of Elideo Padovani's students in Bologna, for instance, learned about hemorrhoids that they would only heal when cut and cauterized, as he witnessed himself at the hospital ("ut in hospitali vidi").[402] Among the patients visited by prospective physicians and their teachers in Ferrara during the 1540s were also several who were treated surgically, some of them by both a physician and a surgeon at once. One approximately thirty-year-old man had injuries on his head and leg from the blows of a sword; the shin and muscle of the lower-leg were almost completely severed. He was visited first by a surgeon, who let his blood and treated the injuries with egg white and rose oil, and applied a hemostatic powder. Two days later, the professor – presumably Musa Brasavola – was called in to see the patient. The patient died several days later, however. With his *praeceptor*, the anonymous student note-taker also saw less serious surgical cases, for example that of a girl who had fallen and hit her head but was not even bleeding; another was a load carrier who had broken through an attic floor with a sack of flour on his shoulders and came to the *praeceptor* eight days later to seek advice about his painful ribcage.[403]

To date, there are no known sources for universities outside Italy that describe a surgical training program anywhere near as intensive as in Italy. Montpellier at least enjoyed a good reputation with respect to surgery, among other things. At the time when the Zurich city council opened the way for Georg Keller to go to

---

[398] Cod. 11238, foll. 113v-114v; the treatment lasted for several weeks and initially the patient was visited twice a day. Handsch made detailed notes on seven such visits but was probably present at others as well.
[399] Ibid., fol. 126v, "cum Falloppia". The treatment lasted one month. Handsch's notes do not indicate how often he saw the patient himself.
[400] Cod. 11205, fol. 570v.
[401] Cod. 11238, fol. 131v.
[402] Padovani, Processus (1607), p. 133.
[403] Biblioteca Ariostea, Ferrara Ms Collezione Antonelli, Ms. 531, fol. 31r-v and fol. 47r-v.

Padua, it gave the young Kaspar Wolff a scholarship to go to Montpellier. The instructions written for the two by Conrad Gessner say that both were to go to two lectures on internal medicine and one on surgery. They were to "accompany the physicians of internal medicine and surgery in their practice every day" and finally "become physicians of internal medicine and surgery." Gessner himself had studied in Montpellier and therefore was familiar with the local conditions.[404]

In German-speaking areas, surgery in the sixteenth and seventeenth centuries remained largely in the hands of barber-surgeons. Accordingly, the first comprehensive surgical textbooks in German-speaking areas – notably written in German, not in Latin, the language of scholars – were penned by surgeons like Hieronymus Brunschwig (c. 1450–1512)[405] and Hans von Gersdorff (c. 1455–1529),[406] who had been trained as craftsmen, not by academics. The most famous surgeons of Europe during the late sixteenth century, Wilhelm Fabry von Hilden[407] and Ambroise Paré in France,[408] did not carry the title of a medical doctor and did not teach at universities. As noted above, it is not certain either that Paracelsus, who published his *Große Wundartzney* (Great Book of Surgery) in 1536,[409] had an academic degree.

It was the physicians who had studied in Italy who, in the course of the sixteenth century, increasingly added surgery to academic medicine north of the Alps. Following a study visit in Bologna, Ferrara, and Padua, Johannes Lange, as early as 1550, advocated for a greater appreciation of surgery within learned, academic medicine in Germany. A number of his treatise-like *Epistolae medicinales* were dedicated to surgical subjects such as skull fractures, eye injuries, war wounds, and questions of bloodletting, and he also published a number of surgical case histories.[410] In the late sixteenth century, the town physician of Alkmaar, Pieter van Foreest, who had also studied in Italy, even compiled a five-volume collection of surgical case histories from his own practice.[411] However, a close reading reveals that both Lange and Foreest essentially only gave advice and perhaps applied ointments and dressings in these surgical cases. There is no conclusive evidence that they personally put their hand to the task.

---

404 "Ordnung" for Wolff and Keller, 22 May 1555, cit. in Schieß, Briefe (1906), pp. 16–18.
405 Brunschwig, Buch der Cirurgia (1497).
406 Gersdorff, Feldtbuch (1517).
407 Fabricius, Opera (1646).
408 Paré, Opera (1594); biographical sketch in Dumaître, Ambroise Paré (1986).
409 Paracelsus, Grosse Wundartzney (1536); cf. Vekerdy, Great Wound Surgery (2005), pp. 77–99.
410 Lange, Medicinalium epistolarum (1554), pp. 12–36, and idem, Secunda medicinalium epistolarum (1560), pp. 33–38.
411 Foreest, Observationum (1601).

As late as 1600, surgery continued to occupy no more than a marginal position in academic medicine north of the Alps. The fact that autopsy was practiced at universities to a much lesser degree there – autopsies required keen surgical skills – went hand in hand with physicians' greater reserve about any hands-on practice on the dead or the living body. As late as the middle of the seventeenth century, the surgeon Tobias Geiger – he was originally trained as a craftsman but later earned his doctorate – felt compelled to write a passionate call for surgery to be given a more prominent place in medical training.[412] At this point, the interest in surgery among German-speaking physicians had already grown, however, likely not least of all thanks to the numerous students from north of the Alps who had gone to Italy and experienced the considerably higher status of surgery at the universities there. The example of Johann Konrad Zinn in Oettingen serves well to illustrate this point. Having studied in Padua, where he would have heard Fabrizi's lectures on surgery, he earned his doctoral degree in Basel defending a thesis on head wounds, clearly a surgical topic. He declared in a dedicatory letter that if you wanted to rightly call yourself a physician, you had to master all of medicine. Surgery was not only an essential part of medicine but it took precedence over the other parts because with internal diseases the physician had to serve nature, while in the case of surgical procedures he was her equal, and at times her superior.[413]

---

412 Bayerische Staatsbibliothek München, Cgm 3733, Tobias Geiger, *Discursus medicus und politicus* (1656); cf. Schlegelmilch, Selbstbewußtsein (2020); Meyer, Discursus (2021).
413 Zinn, Disputatio (1595), dedicatory epistle to Graf Wolfgang von Hohenlohe: "Chirurgia vero medicinae non modo pars essentialis est, sed prae caeteris insuper omnibus cum antiquitatis, tum artis (proprie quidem et seorsim absque naturae commercio consideratae) praerogativam obtinet."

Learned Habitus

At some universities, future physicians received a licentiate degree upon completing their medical studies, a first step toward the doctoral degree. In Montpellier, they then had to give medical lectures before they could receive their doctorate. At other universities, students could become a *doctor medicinae* directly. We have found evidence that in Montpellier, Padua, and elsewhere, practical experience was mandatory and even that candidates were required to demonstrate their practical knowledge and abilities in an exam on a specific case. But prospective physicians in Padua and Montpellier also had to master the art of disputation. They had to be able to defend specific statements or "theses" in an oral exam.

Still today, different European languages reflect this tradition, referring to a doctoral "thesis", "thèse", "tesi" and so forth – the "dissertation" as it is known in Germany and elsewhere – that is "defended" in an oral exam. Doctoral dissertations as we know them today – systematic, written studies devoted to a certain topic – were not yet common in the sixteenth century. The theses or *puncta* which the candidate was to discuss were, however, occasionally published as early as this time period. In German-speaking areas, this custom began to find a broader reach in the 1540s, first with titles like *Disputatio medica*[414] and then in the 1560s with the explicit characterization as *Theses*.[415] This kind of public disputation required practice.[416] Felix Platter recounted from his time in Montpellier that students toward the end of their studies even spent a good deal of their time teaching one another in this art. In Padua, Handsch formulated, presumably also as an exercise, various counterarguments ("contradictoria") against the theses ("axiomata") of his fellow student and friend Daniel Cellarius, which concerned, among other things, the function of the kidneys.[417] The outline of a lecture he wrote for his own doctoral examination indicates that for his doctoral degree in Ferrara, Handsch likely had to discuss a passage from Galen's *Ars medica* and a Hippocratic aphorism about the indications for bloodletting or for an evacuative treatment at the beginning of acute illness. Musa Brasavola, his promotor, had written a famous commentary on the aphorisms. If the outline is at all a reflection of the content of the examination, the

---

414 Drembach, De atra bile (1548); Horst, Enarratio (1563), with the *Themata disputationis de latitudine sanitatis*.
415 Early examples are Havenreuter, Theses (1568); Oetheus, Theses (1569); Planer, Theses (1577); on France see Germain, Thèses (1886).
416 An early example of a printed practice disputation is Kegler, [Quaestiones] (c. 1500).
417 Cod. 11210, foll. 166r-174v.

scope of the examination was rather modest but, of course, his draft may only have been the basis for an ensuing oral disputation and debate.[418]

With the awarding of the doctoral degree, the formal medical education of future physicians reached its conclusion. The study of medicine was in some respects only the final phase of their long professional and intellectual socialization, however. Beginning in their youth, these men had been exposed to the contemporary culture of erudition and its practices. In the course of many years in Latin school and in their study of the *artes*, they had been adopting the habitus of the learned man.[419] It was only in the course of medical studies that the more specific habitus of the learned doctor came in addition. Academically-trained physicians of the Renaissance differed markedly in this respect from today's physicians. Their identity and social status were shaped and determined to a far lesser extent by their medical activities. In their respective social and (mostly) urban environments the majority of *doctores medicinae* were doubtlessly perceived primarily as practitioners of the healing arts. However, they also understood themselves throughout their lives as members of an interdisciplinary, humanist *res publica literaria*, a cosmopolitan world of learned men in which they played a prominent role.[420]

Just how much the humanist education of Renaissance physicians shaped their self-conception and habitus, just how much it became the stuff they were made of, finds striking expression in their use of language. Not only in their letters to colleagues at home and abroad, but also in their practice journals and personal notebooks, physicians wrote principally in Latin. In the books that belonged to physicians we also find handwritten notes and supplements – sometimes very many of them – written in Latin almost exclusively. Latin, and not their mother tongue, was evidently very literally the physician's language of thought as soon as the subject at hand was the least bit medical or philosophical. Georg Handsch was

---

418 Ibid., foll. 174b r-174c v. For early seventeenth-century Padua, Giovanni Domenico Sala's *Forma recitandorum punctorum et casuum* (British Library, London, Ms. Sloane 727, foll. 47r-50r) suggests similarly modest dimensions. The exemplary text Sala offered to the doctoral candidates comprised altogether some six pages, half of which were dedicated to the philosophical doctorate. The medical part comprised not even three pages and was limited to a discussion of a phrase from Galen's *Ars parva*. In addition, a medical case briefly had to be discussed (ibid., foll. 50r-51v, *Generalis casuum recitandorum forma*); here Sala used the example of a young man with a double tertian fever and headache.
419 On the learned, humanist habitus see Müller, Specimen eruditionis (2010); Algazi, Food (2002); idem, Lebensweise (2007), pp. 107–118.
420 Neumeister/Wiedemann, Res publica litteraria (1987); Jaumann, Iatrophilologia (2001); Siraisi, Oratory (2004); on the place of learned physicians in early humanism see Schnell, Arzt und Literat (1991).

no exception here. He filled thousands of pages with his Latin notes. When he did exceptionally avail himself of the German, or, even more rarely, the Czech language, he did so almost exclusively to relay phrases and terms that physicians and patients used when speaking with each other.

Latin was also the language of most publications written by learned physicians. With publications on medicine and natural history – the latter was also largely the domain of university-trained physicians[421] – the authors presented themselves as preeminent scholars. They could hope that their works would secure the goodwill and support of the princes and members of the municipal governments to whom they usually dedicated these writings. There were even proper guidebooks explaining how to compose such dedicatory letters in Latin.[422] By writing books, physicians could hope to prompt educated and wealthy patients into seeking their counsel in person or by letter, or even that a count or a prince would appoint them his court physician.[423] Scholarly publications could also be advantageous when it came to applying for a salaried position. Marcus Banzer (1592–1664), for example, when applying to the Augsburg city council for the position of municipal physician, pointed out that not only had he studied in Montpellier, Padua, and other places, but he had also published a prescription guidebook, a *Fabrica receptarum*.[424]

Beyond this, the scholarly self-conception of physicians found expression in a broad range of non-medical activities and humanist practices of writing, publishing, and communicating. These activities were shared with others within the European republic of letters, and at the same time they marked the physicians' place in this republic. I will outline them in the following.[425]

Poetry

Of all the writings produced by learned physicians during the Renaissance, the most numerous were by all appearances not medical treatises, but poems. Physicians here were availing themselves of a genre that played a preeminent

---

[421] Cf. Eamon, Science (1994); Findlen, Possessing (1994); Friedrich, Naturgeschichte (1995); Ogilvie, Science (2006); Findlen/Smith, Merchants (2002); famous examples are Rondelet, De piscibus (1554); Agricola, De ortu (1546).
[422] Santoro, Uso (2006).
[423] For a well-documented case study see De Renzi, Career (2011).
[424] Letter from Banzer, 7 March 1624 (www.aerztebriefe.de/id/00001778, S. Herde); Banzer, Fabrica (1622).
[425] See also Stolberg, The many uses of writing (2019).

role in the humanism of the Renaissance in general.[426] Some physicians even achieved remarkable fame or were awarded the imperial title of *poeta laureatus*. Joachim Vadian (1494–1551), Konrad Celtis (1459–1508), Johannes Posthius (1537–1597), and Petrus Lotichius (1501–1567) are well-known examples.[427] Other physicians, like Handsch's Bohemian compatriot Lorenz Span, at least received some renown as poets during their time.[428]

If we want to do justice to the intention and function of this poetry and if we want to properly assess its quality and significance, we must apply the standards that were in play at the time. Poetry today is considered above all a medium that allows very personal, individual perceptions and sensibilities, feelings and states of mind to be expressed in a crystallized form with the help of powerful turns of phrase, images, and metaphors. In the Renaissance by contrast, poetry was considered a skill to be learned and perfected through practice, "a practical accomplishment rather than an inspired act", as Kristian Jensen has put it.[429] Beginning in Latin school, students were not only familiarized with poems by ancient authors such as Horace and Virgil, but were also expected to practice composing poems, in Latin, in different genres, and using different meters. The prerequisite for this was an excellent command of the Latin language. The poet furthermore had to be well-versed in the complicated rules of Latin metrics, with the stressed and unstressed syllables which gave rise to the typical rhythm of the different meters. And not least of all, he required a comprehensive knowledge of ancient cultural heritage so as to adorn his poems with numerous allusions to mythological and historical figures and events.

Most poems by physicians during this period pertained to what is commonly termed "occasional" poetry. Prime examples are countless dedicatory poems.[430] It was common practice when publishing a medical work to preface it with a poem by other learned men who would generally heap praise upon the work and its author. Even as students, future physicians worked to develop their skill in this practice. When it was time to print their dissertations or the theses they were defending, they would sometimes ask fellow students or

---

426 A wide-ranging survey of neo-Latin poetry and its many genres can be found in Ijsewein, Companion (1998), pp. 21–138.
427 On the *poetae laureati* of the sixteenth century see Schirrmeister, Triumph (2003); Mertens, Sozialgeschichte (1996); Schmid, Poeta (1989); Schmidt, Mediziner (1992).
428 Wondrák, Arzt (1983).
429 Jensen, Humanist reform (1996), p. 74.
430 A dedicatory poem by Handsch appeared in a treatise on the plague by Petrus Sibyllenus (Handsch, Ad lectorem (1564)); on the importance of humanistic occasional poetry and its distinct communicative function in the Bohemian context, see Storchová, School humanism (2014), pp. 36–43.

professors for an appraisal in verse and/or composed panegyrics themselves on their teachers or patrons.[431] Someone like Lorenz Scholz in Breslau could get no less than sixteen of his colleagues (as well as various other scholars) to contribute a poem that celebrated his garden in Breslau.[432] Hundreds if not thousands of poems from the pens of practicing or future physicians went into print in this way in the sixteenth century. With their theatrical language and frequent comparisons to mythological figures, they tend to strike modern readers as hopelessly magniloquent, but their authors at the time were demonstrating their mastery of the poetic craft and their ability to draw on a rich historical, biblical, and mythological treasure trove.

Georg Handsch took up poetry early and immersed himself quite deeply in it compared to other physicians.[433] Some of his poems were printed,[434] and others he collected in a handwritten volume of poetry.[435] Many of Handsch's poems, too, were written for some occasion like a wedding, a death, the arrival of a ruler, or a fellow student passing an exam. Like his contemporaries, he availed himself of a broad spectrum of poetic genres, from elegies, idylls, and panegyrics to distiches, and playful forms like chronograms in which the letters M, D, C, L, X, V, and I, capitalized and legible as Roman numerals, produced a date that had significance in the context of the poem or for the person to whom it was addressed. Acrostics were another playful variation, in which the first letters of each line, read from top to bottom, formed a word or phrase. In *hodeoporica,* he recounted his travels in poetic form. He composed *epithalamia* at the occasion of upcoming weddings, and he wrote epitaphs.[436] The final poem in his handwritten poetry collection is such a poem, written in Latin for his own grave.[437]

---

431 Early examples are three detailed *carmina gratulataria* dedicated to Jakob Horst on the occasion of his doctoral examination (Horst, Brevis et dilucida enarratio (1563)) and Hubner, Disputationis (1578), here for Henricus Husanus).
432 Rindfleisch et alii, Epigrammata (1594).
433 The work of Czech historians on Handsch has concentrated on his poetic work; cf. Nováková, Rytmické (1966); Martínek, Jan Hodějovský (2012); more recently, Lucie Storchová has dealt with Handsch in greater detail (Storchová, Paupertate (2011); eadem, Handsch (2020).
434 Besides the *Farragines* of 1561/62, which Handsch compiled and which also contain poems by himself (see the list in Kalina von Jätenstein, Nachrichten, vol. 2 (1819), pp. 40–43), Handsch's poetic work includes: Handsch, Calendarium (1550); idem, Dedicatory poem (1554); idem, Ad lectorem (1564); idem, In effigiem (1562); idem, In icona (1562).
435 Cod. 9821.
436 E.g. Cod. 9821, fol. 216v, on the Emperor Charles.
437 Ibid., fol. 321v: "Vivere si dulce est, sit quoque dulce mori". "Christe resurgentium princeps, ardentibus oro votis, te nobis adsere, nosque tibi." "Nam quem fraus mundi, mors Christi, gloria coeli commovet, hinc totus laetus in astra migrat."

There was a relationship in the Renaissance between poetry and another humanist field of activity, namely the art of letter writing, which we will be returning to. Numerous poems by Handsch were addressed to a specific recipient and, like letters, were given a date and place of composition. They quite often carried personal messages or referred to the relationship between Handsch and the addressee. With good reason Handsch referred to them as his "poetic letters" ("epistolas meas poeticas").[438] He often wrote them for proponents of Bohemian humanism such as his teachers Matthaeus Collinus and Johannes Schentigar, and his classmates Martin Hanno and Thomas Mitis.[439] His epistolary poems at the same time vividly illustrate how poetry could be instrumentalized for the benefit of one's career and financial situation.[440] Before his medical studies, when Handsch was in Prague, he jumped at the opportunity opened to him by Collinus to become involved with the circle of humanist poets surrounding the rich judge and patron Johannes Hoddeiovinus.[441] He approached Hoddeiovinus with letter-poems and was able to get into his good graces. He subsequently wrote numerous poems for Hoddeiovinus. Around 1560, years after receiving his medical doctorate, he spent several months at Hoddeiovinus country residence in Rzepice[442] putting together a four-volume poetry anthology titled *Farragines poematum*,[443] The work was dedicated to Hoddeiovinus and featured Handsch's own poems as well as those of Matthaeus Collinus, Johannes Schentigar, Thomas Mitis, Martin Hanno, and other Prague humanists.

Handsch and his fellow poets gained no glory from this enterprise. A later critic called the *Farragines* "nothing but miserable mess-making, and yet put together by 43 bunglers who hatched their monstrosities at the same time". He went on to criticize the publication's "flat, often barbaric Latin, without style,

---

438 Cod. 9650, frontispiece.
439 Cod. 9807, fol. 63r.
440 Cf. Storchová, Humanist occasional poetry ([in print]); I am grateful to the author who allowed me to see a preliminary draft of this contribution.
441 On Hoddeiovinus and his circle see Martínek, Jan Hodějovský (2012); Storchová, Bohemian school humanism (2014), pp. 40–43.
442 Cod. 9650, foll. 35v-36r, copy of a letter to Matthaeus Collinus, Rzepice, 8 September 1557; Cod. 9821, foll. 285r-287r, epistolary poem, October 17, 1557; Cod. 9650, foll. 39v-40v, copy of a letter to Simon Ennius, Rzepice, 26 December 1557; on the duration of his stay see Handsch, Secunda farrago, foll. 192v-193r: "Cras sum discessurus ab arce/ In qua novem menses fui" ("Tomorrow I will leave the castle where I spent nine months"); however, Handsch also spent some time in Rzepice in 1559 and since the *Farrago* did not appear until 1561, he may have completed the work later.
443 Collinus et alii, Prima farrago ([1561]); Handsch, Secunda farrago (1561); Collinus et alii, Tertia farrago (1561); idem et alii, Quarta farrago (1562).

without salt".[444] This could be owed to a change in taste. It is probably fair to say, however, that the poems even by contemporary standards were too obviously suffused with flattery. The task of the poets in the judge's entourage was, above all, to create myriad variations of poetic praise for the patron, for his estates, and achievements. In return, they could hope to receive material and immaterial compensation.[445] It was doubtlessly through Hoddeiovinus's intercession that Handsch and his friend Thomas Mitis were awarded titles of nobility in 1556.[446] Handsch now called himself "von Limus" after one of his patron's estates. He was clearly proud of this, writing in large letters on the first page of one of his notebooks "Georgius Handschius a Limuso. Artium et Medicinae D[octor]".[447] At the same time, a distinct uneasiness about such commissioned poetry is discernible in his personal notes and letters and even in some of his letter-poems to Hoddeiovinus. At the risk of disgruntling the patron, he sometimes hesitated to deliver poems that had been requested.

As several entries in Handsch's notebooks make clear, poetic skills, demonstrated in an oral presentation, could sometimes also be the means for public self-fashioning as a learned man in the local urban society and at the court. Under headings such as "In convivio proponebatur" and "In coena proponebatur", Handsch mentioned small poetic competitions taking place at banquets and other social gatherings. The guests were asked to compose and present a Latin poem ad hoc on a given subject or motto, such as "Nature does nothing in vain"[448] and "If it be God's will, envy can accomplish nothing".[449]

---

444 Review, signed "O." in Neue Literatur 1 (1771), n° 19, pp. 294–299, "lauter elende Schmiereyen, und doch von 43. Stümpern, die ihre Missgeburten zu gleicher Zeit ausheckten, zusammengetragen"; "plattes, oft barbarisches Latein, ohne Styl, ohne Salz".
445 In an epistolary poem, Handsch thanked Hoddeiovinus, for example, for his gift of a silver object ("ex aere lunari") (Cod. 9821, fol. 255r-v); see also Collinus et alii, Quarta farrago (1562), foll. 617v-618v.
446 The repertory on the *Adelsakten* in the Staatsarchiv in Vienna lists a title of nobility that was awarded to "Georg Hanczl" on 4 May 1556. This is clearly a spelling mistake. Handsch's compatriot Lorenz Span, also received a title of nobility, in 1558, probably thanks to the intercession of Christian von Lobkowitz, to whom he dedicated some of his poems (Wondrák, Span (1983), p. 239).
447 Cod. 9821.
448 Ibid., fol. 254r: "Ex tempore apud coenam" – "Natura nihil facit frustra". Handsch arrived at: "Omnia quae peperit rerum natura genitrix/Haec nec fine suo, nec ratione carent" ("Whatever nature gives birth to as the creator of things lacks neither goal nor purpose").
449 Ibid., fol. 252v: "Volente Deo nihil valet invidia"; another poem entitled "De coralia extemporanea" probably was written on the same kind of occasion, in this case during Handsch's stay in Trento (ibid., fol. 245v).

The *album amicorum*

The humanist identity of medical students and physicians found further expression in the rapidly growing popularity of another humanist practice, one that in some respects was closely related to the practice of poetry: the creation of friendship books or *alba amicorum*.[450] Beginning in the mid-sixteenth century, the practice became increasingly popular among students in German-speaking areas and throughout the Republic of Letters.[451] Usually a person would have a small album made for himself, one that was easy to hold and whose pages were blank, that is white (Latin "albus"). Some students and scholars also used interleaved copies of printed books for this purpose, meaning that they had blank pages bound in between the printed pages or at the beginning and/or end of the book, thus making room for entries. Especially emblem books like the one by Andrea Alciati with its illustrations and adages were used for this purpose.[452] The owner of the album asked *amici*, "friends" in the broad definition of the time, to immortalize themselves with an entry – fellow students, colleagues, professors, and other scholars but, on occasion, also members of the aristocracy or indeed ruling princes. Students in particular carried these *alba amicorum* with them during their *peregrinatio academica*. When they arrived in a new place, they would pay a visit to physicians, scholars, and other influential figures who might help advance their careers, and ask them for an entry.

There is no extant *album amicorum* from Georg Handsch, and unlike in the cases of Stephan Laureus, like Handsch a court physician to the Archduke,[453] Handsch's university friend Daniel Cellarius,[454] and his mentor Mattioli,[455] no entry has been found in Handsch's hand in the album of a contemporary. The *album amicorum* put together by the Zurich city physician Conrad Gessner in 1555 counts on the other hand as one of the oldest surviving friendship books altogether.[456] Gessner had made a name for himself through his work in natural

---

450 On the history of *alba amicorum* see Rosenheim, Album amicorum (1910); Gemert, van/ Bots, Introduction (1975); Ludwig, Stammbuch (2006); Schwarz, Studien (2002). In many cases, the term "album amicorum" is somewhat misleading insofar as the owners also asked princes and other powerful and influential personalities for an entry, who even by the generous standards of the time could not be considered as "friends".
451 The practice probably originated from students in Wittenberg (Klose, Corpus (1988)).
452 Alciati, Emblematum (1531); on the genre see Henkel/Schöne (Hrg.), Emblemata (1996).
453 National Library of Medicine, Bethesda, Ms. E 77, n° 6.
454 Ibid., n° 98, 9 April 1559.
455 Neuser, Stammbuch (1964), p. 116 (reproduction).
456 National Library of Medicine, Bethesda, Ms. E 77; see also Durling, Liber amicorum (1965), with a list of the names and dates.

history and many students and scholars who were passing through Zurich made a point of paying him a visit. Among the album's contributors are numerous physicians, well-known names like Achilles Pirmin Gasser, Thomas Erastus (1524–1583), Theodor Zwinger, and Adolph Occo, and lesser-known men like Johannes Cosmas Holzach, Johannes Erhard Stürmlin, and Ortolf Marold.[457] Another early *album amicorum* has survived from the belongings of the Augsburg medical student and later physician David Wirsung. Dating between 1565 and 1583, it contains numerous entries, including by members of the nobility, one of whom was Handsch's patron and employer Archduke Ferdinand II, as well as by other high-ranking people, and it features many colorful illustrations.[458] In Basel, *alba amicorum* from the late sixteenth and early seventeenth centuries have survived from the two medical professors Caspar Bauhin and Thomas Platter. They, too, were visited by many travelling students and scholars who paid their respects.[459]

The *alba amicorum* of medical students and physicians from the sixteenth and early seventeenth centuries and the entries they made in those of others are not fundamentally different from those of students and professionals in other disciplines. By keeping an *album amicorum* themselves and in the way they contributed to those of others, medical students and physicians were again underlining their humanist education and their participation in the *res publica literaria*. To start with, like other learned contributors, medical students and physicians generally used Latin, the scholarly language *par excellence*. Some even immortalized themselves with entries in Greek or Hebrew script.[460] The entries of medical students and physicians by and large corresponded with those of other scholars also with respect to content. For the most part, they addressed religious or moral subjects, quoted from the Bible or from works by ancient poets, historians, and philosophers. Philipp Wirsung in his contribution to Gessner's album wrote "The fear of God is the beginning of wisdom".[461] Caspar Bauhin's choice was "All is vanity except love for God".[462] With "If the snake does not eat others, it will not become a dragon", Justinus Mylius relayed a well-known adage about the nature

---

[457] Gessner sometimes also asked pharmacists for an entry, e.g. National Library of Medicine, Bethesda, Ms. E 77, n° 158.
[458] Anna Amalia Bibliothek Weimar, Stb 134 (https://haab-digital.klassik-stiftung.de/viewer/epnresolver?id=1297966422, accessed 5 June 2021); the library catalogue in Weimar also lists an *album amicorum* of Sigismund Schnitzer (Stb 143 V), which is now lost, from his time as a medical student in Altdorf and Bologna around 1579, with entries, among others, by Caspar Bauhin, Ulysses Aldrovandi and Julius Caesar Arantius.
[459] Vischer, Stammbücher (1949), pp. 247–264.
[460] E.g. National Library of Medicine, Bethesda, Ms. E 77, n° 130, Bauhin and n° 174, Funccius.
[461] Ibid., n° 99: "Timor domini initium sapientiae".
[462] Reproduced in Hild, Stammbuch (1991), p. 203: "Omnia vanitas praeter DEUM amare".

of political power,[463] which he had perhaps heard as a student in Wittenberg from Philipp Melanchthon. Altdorf professor Caspar Hofmann chose "May what is right take place, not what I want".[464] The Flemish medical student Nicolaus Espillet opted for "Sensual pleasure is the enemy of virtue".[465] "Have trust, but be cautious in whom you place it" wrote Thomas Platter in the *album amicorum* of the Bohemian Paracelsian and poet Daniel Stoltz – a motto also used by scholars of other disciplines in their friendship albums.[466]

Only on occasion did the entries refer to medical subjects in a stricter sense. Even here, however, the contributors followed a convention that had developed in the blossoming culture of *alba amicorum*: the entries were tailored to the owner of the album. In the albums of students and scholars from other disciplines, too, the contributors took up topics relating to the album owner's field of knowledge and activity, especially if it was also their own. Much like in speeches, dedicatory letters, and encomia, medical contributors praised medicine in particular and the physician, and distinguished the learned physician from the less educated competition. One of the four adages written in the friendship book of the French student Isaac Perusset by fellow medical student Johann Christoph Cherler was "In the hands of the uneducated ["indocti"], medicine is like a sword in the hands of a madman".[467] Next to it are quotes from or allusions to the writings of ancient medical authorities. In the Hippocratic spirit, Johannes Benzius wrote in Gessner's album, "Nature is the healer of diseases, the physician her servant".[468] There were also warnings and moralizing adages with a medical connotations. "Nothing is so difficult that it cannot be examined with questions", wrote

---

463 National Library of Medicine, Bethesda, Ms. E 77, n° 157: "Serpens nisi devoret serpentem non fit draco."
464 Marienbibliothek Halle, Ms. 92, *album amicorum* of Joachim Oelhafen, Altdorf, 13 July 1625: "Contingat id, quod expedit, non quod volo."
465 National Library of Medicine, Bethesda, Ms. E 77, n° 163, 1 October 1562: "Virtuti inimica voluptas."
466 Hild, Stammbuch (1991), p. 204 and p. 201 (photographic reproduction of the page): "Fide, sed cui vide"; on Stoltzius see also Kühlmann, Poet (1991).
467 Bibliothèque municipale, Avignon, Ms. 1998, fol. 84, Montpellier, 26 March 1620: "Medicamentum in manibus indocti est ut ensis in manibus furiosi." Somewhat less polemically Valentin Dryander in National Library of Medicine, Bethesda, Ms. E 77, n° 131, (9 July 1560) wrote: "If Quintilian calls that speaker a good man who knows how to talk, the doctor who knows how to cure can all the more be defined as a good man."
468 National Library of Medicine, Bethesda, Ms. E 77, n° 153, Johannes Benzius [October 1561, on his way to Padua]: "Morborum medica natura, medicus minister." Laurentius Helandus used a Greek quotation from Hippocrates in Marienbibliothek, Halle, Ms. 92, *album amicorum* of J. Oelhafen, 2 February 1621.

Hieronymus Brixinus in Gessner's *album amicorum*.[469] Felix Platter drew on a motto borrowed from the Roman poet Juvenal, which is still known today, when he wrote, "May a healthy mind be in a healthy body".[470] "We practice medicine not to avoid death, but so that we may wait for it in preserved health", Christian Rumpf, court physician to Frederick V of the Palatinate, chose for his entry in Joachim Ölhafen's *album amicorum*.[471] Rumpf also used the same phrase a few years later for his entry in the *album* of Daniel Stoltzius.[472]

Letter Writing

In the *res publica literaria* of the Renaissance, letters were an essential means of communication[473] and at the same time a central element of humanist self-presentation.[474] Medical students and physicians were very active participants in this letter writing culture. Some physicians – well-known examples here would be Crato von Krafftheim (1519–1585) and Caspar Peucer (1525–1602) – corresponded so actively that a significant portion of their day was, it seems, taken up with letter writing.[475] Their correspondence was certainly not limited to medical colleagues. The Würzburg project "Frühneuzeitliche Ärztebriefe" ("Early Modern Physicians' Letters") has so far identified about 18,000 letters from the German speaking areas alone that were composed in Latin by physicians or addressed to physicians in the sixteenth century. Without a doubt, they represent only a fraction of the epistolary correspondence in which physicians were involved; the vast majority have surely been lost.[476] Of the letters that

---

469 National Library of Medicine, Bethesda, Ms. E 77, n° 149, [around 1561]: "Nihil tam difficile quin quaerendo investigari possit",
470 Folger Library, Washington, Bd.w. 158–133q, *album amicorum* of Johann Ulrich Höcklin, entry made on 5 August 1566: "Orandum ut sit mens sana in corpore sano"; in Gessner's *album amicorum* Platter wrote more shortly: "Mens sana in corpore sano" (National Library of Medicine, Bethesda, Ms. E 77, n° 143, 28 March 1561).
471 Marienbibliothek, Halle, Ms. 92, *album amicorum* of J. Oelhafen, Küstrin, 2 March 1621: "Medicinam facimus non ut mortem vitemus, sed ut eam integra sanitate expectemus."
472 According to Hild, Stammbuch (1991), p. 206.
473 The literature on humanist letter writing is very extensive. For a useful introduction see Worstbrock, Brief (1983).
474 See the programmatic title of van Houdt et alii, Self-presentation (2002); an exemplary case study, on Felix Platter, is Walter, Ärztliche Selbstdarstellung (2013).
475 Gillet, Crato von Crafftheim (1860); Hasse/Wartenberg, Caspar Peucer (2004).
476 Especially with municipal authorities but also with some of their patients the physicians communicated in German.

have been processed so far, only about 5,000 were exchanged between physicians but about 8,700 letters were written to a physician by or addressed by a physician to someone who had a humanist education but was not a medical professional.[477]

With their letters, physicians maintained and demonstrated – as did other humanist scholars – their place in the *res publica literaria,* and they upheld the humanist ideal of *amicitia,* friendship among peers and like-minded people.[478] Even compatriots who spoke the same language generally corresponded in cultivated Latin. Learned letter writers addressed one another with "tu," "tibi," or "te" and followed established conventions, from superlative forms of address like "clarissime" and "praestantissime", to the frequent apology for a late reply due to various other obligations, to requests to pass on greetings to shared acquaintances, to a *captatio benevolentiae,* for example the reference to the immediate departure of the messenger, which forced the writer to send the letter as it was, in all its brevity and incompletion. As a result of the humanist predilection for *miscellanea,* learned letter writers would often string together short discussions of completely different topics in a more or less disjointed manner.[479] So physicians certainly did not correspond about medical questions alone. Like other scholars of the day, they wrote about a broad spectrum of subjects that in a wider sense were commensurate with humanist erudition, everything from genealogy to local history to linguistic research to numismatics.[480]

Letter writing was an important, acquired skill. In fact, in the words of Franz Josef Worstbrock, the "art and culture of the letter [became] the most noble measure of the skill of writing as such."[481] As with poetry, the art of letter writing was already imparted in Latin school. Towering role models were Marcus Tullius Cicero and Pliny the Younger, whose letters went through endless editions,[482] as well as Petrarch, who dynamized humanist epistolary culture.[483] Various epistolographic

---

[477] The data is from December 2020. In addition, the database documents thousands of letters written by and to patients, princes, authorities and institutions, in Latin or German.
[478] See e.g. Quaranta, Medici trentini (2018), on the correspondence of Mattioli, Alessandrini and other physicians from Trento.
[479] Siriasi, Communities (2013), p. 8.
[480] Adolph Occo III. (1524–1606), for example, cultivated extensive numismatic interests. In numerous letters, he discussed numismatic topics (see www.aerztebriefe.de).
[481] Worstbrock, Brief (1983), preface, p. 5.
[482] Cicero, Epistulae (1471); Plinius, Epistolarum (1539); in a dedicatory epistle to Charles V, Juan Luis Vives also referred to these two great models (Vives, De conscribendis epistolis (1536)).
[483] Enenkel, Grundlegung (2002).

handbooks were on the market, which taught the reader the art of letter writing. The numerous reprints suggest that they met a great demand.[484]

In one of his notebooks, Georg Handsch compiled this kind of advice on writing letters. He noted how to correctly write the date and appropriate salutations, he cited the abovementioned reference to the waiting messenger.[485] As a model for his own letters, Handsch sometimes turned to the missives of well-known letter writers such as Johannes Crato and Aeneas Sylvius.[486] Elsewhere he noted various vernacular phrases that were appropriate in correspondence with less educated contemporaries and authorities. The body of the letter could begin with a simple "Amicably at your service, with greetings",[487] but could also use a more elaborate salutation. Expressions of gratitude might follow, often with promises of services to be rendered in return, for example, "I give my thanks for all your friendship and honor" and "I will be very happy to do for you what I can, Sir, when the opportunity arises, and my deeds shall surpass my words etc.", and "I am very pleased and have received your letter with great thanks, and I must admit that I owe you my humble services for this, which I am always willing to extend to you."[488] At the end of the letter, a pious phrase was appropriate such as, "This is what I would like to answer to your letter with my obedient opinion, wishing you God's blessing and that you may be well in body and soul. Amen."[489]

Handsch collected a selection of his own correspondence in a volume of copied letters.[490] In it, he added many small corrections, hoping perhaps for an

---

484 Influential examples are Erasmus, De conscribendis epistolis (1521); Vives, De conscribendis epistolis (1536).
485 Cod. 9550, foll. 570r-587r.
486 Ibid., foll. 578v and 587r.
487 "Mein freundlichen Dienst und Gruß".
488 "Ich bedanck mich gegen euch aller Freundschafft und Ehren" – "Was ich dem Herrn nach Gebung der Gelegenheit und meines Vermögens dienen kan, wil ich herzlich gern thuen, und die Werck sollen die Wort übertreffen etc." – "So habe ich solche euer Schreiben, und das des ir euch in Sonderheit gegen mir entbiettet, in großem Wolgefallen und sonderem Danck von euch auffgenommen, und bekenne mich selbs schuldig sein, solchs umb euch zuverdienen mit meinen armen Diensten, die ich allzeit zu erzeigen willig sein wil."
489 Cod. 9671, foll. 192r-210r: "Solchs alles hab ich auff ewer an mich gethan Schreiben dienstlicher Meinung hinwider berichten wöllen, mit Wunschung Gottes Segen und alles, so euch an Leib und Sehl gutt ist. Amen."
490 Cod. 9650; summaries of the contents by Ulrich Schlegelmilch can be found in the database of the Würzburg project on "Early Modern Physicians' Letters" (www.aerztebriefe.de). Two letters to Simon Ennius and one to Collinus were published in 1913 in Latin editions (Handsch, Two letters (1913), pp. 167–169 and p. 179); Dana Martínková made Czech translations of several letters (Martínková, Poselství (1975)). As Handsch explained (Cod. 9650, fol.

eventual publication. Or maybe he was simply following the example of his patron and engaging in another established humanist practice, that of "collecting letters and binding them into a book, as Hodd[eiovinus] did".[491]

Handsch's letters illustrate in an exemplary fashion the conventions of epistolary exchange in the Republic of Letters. Handsch emphasized his friendships effusively. "Dearest" ("charissime") he used to addressed the book merchant Hieronymus of Trento, who, as Handsch stated, had written him in a manner that was as learned as it was amiable.[492] He spared no words in commenting on and lamenting the silence of his friend Thomas Mitis and evoked the "love" ("amor") between them, the tie that was not to dissolve because this was what befitted men of cultivated education ("politioris doctrinae").[493] He also interspersed his missives with references to ancient writings and figures and wrote the occasional passage in Greek.[494] The content of a letter by Handsch could range from his relationship to the addressee (which he brought up very often) to personal messages to scientific subjects and news, for example a conflagration in the city, the punishment of a heretic, or a man who had abused his daughter for twelve years.[495] And even when Handsch was a *doctor medicinae*, only few of the letters he deemed worthy to be preserved were devoted mainly to medical matters.[496]

Alongside the overarching humanist features I have mentioned, the correspondence between physicians and naturalists was also marked by certain specific characteristics. To be pointed out first of all is the outstanding significance of "gift exchange", to use a term from cultural anthropology coined by Marcel Mauss.[497] In very different cultures, gift exchange plays an important role and

---

24r), he had lost drafts of many other letters he had addressed to his teachers and mentors Andrea Gallo and Ulrich Lehner; letters to Johannes Schentigar, Ludovicus Tremenus and Winkelmann were also missing (ibid., foll. 27v-28, on letters to Tremenus in Poland; ibid., fol. 30v, on letters to Schentigar and Winkelmann).
491 Cod. 11205, fol. 360r.
492 Cod. 9650, fol. 24r-v.
493 Ibid., foll. 6r-9r, copy of a letter to Thomas Mitis, 25 July 1548.
494 E.g. ibid., fol. 36r-v, copy of a letter to Matthaeus Collinus, 8 September 1557; ibid. foll. 63v-67v, copy of a letter to the pastor in Leipa (around 1561/62).
495 Cod. 9650, foll. 6r-9r, copy of a letter to Thomas Mitis, 25 July 1548, here fol. 9r.
496 Only one letter to Handsch is known to have survived, from Mattioli, who later published it (Mattioli, Epistolarum (1564), pp. 343–346). Here, Handsch basically only acted as an intermediary, however. Mattioli answered an inquiry by the well-known Saxon physician Johann Neefe, with whom he was not personally acquainted, about the way he prepared medicinal hellebore.
497 Mauss, Gabe (1990).

generally involves the expectation that gifts will be answered with goods or services in return. But it is not based, as with bartering or trading, on immediate reciprocity. This form of material and immaterial exchange played an important role in the *res publica literaria* as a whole. It made a very befitting component of the humanist culture of *amicitia*. At a basic level, this gift economy began with the only seemingly banal expectation that the letter writer would be answered with a letter as a "gift in return". Whenever someone asked the recipient of his letter to lend support to an acquaintance or student or to send a newly published book his way, he was most definitely implicitly obligating himself to reciprocate with a similar act as soon as his counterpart brought a similar wish to his attention.[498]

Among physicians and naturalists – who were generally also physicians – the phenomenon of gift exchange took on further dimensions. They not only exchanged letters and lent or otherwise procured books for one another;[499] they also sent each other interesting medical case histories and formulas for medications that had proven successful in their practice. Not only this, but letter correspondence could also serve as a means of exchanging plants and seeds, and other objects of natural history.[500] In his time in Padua, Handsch promised the book merchant Hieronymus in Trento that he would send him plants from the botanical garden in Padua.[501] Some physicians had their own gardens and would request that plants or their seeds be sent by mail so that they could cultivate them. Others, like Caspar Ratzenberger (1533–1603), received rare and exotic plants for their herbaria in the same way.[502] The great botanical undertakings of the time would have been unthinkable without the tightly-knit network of correspondence. The famous herbal book by Pietro Andrea Mattioli, which presented increasing numbers of plants as it went through its various, relied heavily on the legwork of numerous contributors who provided Mattioli with information and plants from near and far. As Andrew Wear put it bluntly:

---

498 On early modern gift culture and its complex codes, see Algazi/Groebner/Jussen, Negotiating the gift (2003).
499 Cf. e.g. Planerio, Epistolae (1584, separate pagination), fol. 49r, letter to Aloysius Mundella, 1 August 1546, requesting that he return the *Historia naturalis* of Pliny and other books, which Planerio had left with him. Handsch, for example, promised Sigismund Carcinus in a letter to send him the requested book on algebra, which he so far had not yet seen in print, however (Cod. 9650, foll. 1r-3r, copy of a letter, 31 December 1544).
500 See also Olmi, Molti amici (1991); Agasse, Introduction (2016), pp. 25–27.
501 Cod. 9650, fol. 24r-v, undated letter from Padua; since the botanical garden was still closed in order to protect the plants, Handsch had to wait until after Easter.
502 Forschungsbibliothek Gotha, Chart. A 152–155; see also Schaffrath, Läuse (2012) on a second herbal Ratzeberger compiled, which is today in Kassel.

"Mattioli did no botanical work of his own but, bolstered by the Emperor's money, published the work of others who sent their results to his house in Prague and then later in Innsbruck."[503] The contributors, who included apothecaries and other non-academically trained professionals, could hope that in return they might appear in the work's introduction or might be given credit in the relevant chapter(s).[504]

In the correspondence among physicians, significant attention was given to medical or related naturalist topics – to concrete, practical questions like the efficacy and application of certain medications, or cases of illness from their own practice. Such letters with their strong focus on medical questions, on the author's own observations, and his discussion of them can be understood in many respects as a form of publication. Scientific journals in which physicians could have presented their observations and considerations did not yet exist. If a physician wanted to make his insights and ideas public, he had to put them into book form and find a publisher who was willing to take the financial risk of printing the book, or the physician had to pay for the printing himself. At universities, professors at least had lectures as a way of presenting their insights. In the disputes about who discovered which individual anatomical structures first, something that became a widespread phenomenon at the time, the testimony of students could be decisive when a physician wanted to assert his preeminence in the matter. In this situation, letters offered a welcome alternative for professors, but also for others, all the more so since one could count on the message being shared not only orally but also insofar as the addressee would, following a widespread contemporary practice, circulate the letter.

It was not long before the composers, recipients, and collectors of letters on specific medical and medically-relevant naturalist subjects began making these letters available to a wider public in printed form. It appears that, as a rule, the letters were edited with respect to language use and style before they were published. Through publication, the authors of medical letters wanted to heighten their profile as physicians by highlighting their linguistic confidence, their elegant style, and perhaps also their familiarity with ancient authors by weaving in allusions and quotes. But not only this: when correspondence with an illustrious figure – and this could be either the author or the addressee – was published, this served to underline one's own rank, one's preeminent position within

---

503 Wear, Medicine (1995), p. 303.
504 Findlen, Formation (1999).

the *res publica literaria*. As was plain for anyone to see, the correspondent was interacting with the leading minds of the time, was enjoying their friendship.[505] For less well-known physicians in particular, letters to famous contemporaries offered an excellent opportunity to not only demonstrate one's scintillating medical erudition but also to make one's place among the distinguished experts known to a wide public. The letters were proof that these physicians were engaging in exchange with the leading specialists, even if a closer look sometimes reveals that all they had done was to ask them for advice on the case (and in the name) of a wealthy patient.

In the sixteenth century, physicians – mainly those from Italian and German-speaking areas – began printing and publishing collected *epistolae*.[506] It was a particularly attractive means to boost one's status in the medical republic letters. For, as Nancy Siraisi, put it "a published volume of *epistolae medicinales* doubtless served as valuable evidence of the breadth of his learning, his professional status, and the distinction of at least some of his professional contacts".[507] Some of the best-known printed *epistolae medicinales* had little in common with the everyday medical correspondence, however, that has survived in manuscript. The form of the letter was excellently suited to the discussion of specific scientific questions and findings and to the presentation of pointed personal opinions and interpretations as they were published by later generations in the scholarly periodicals, which did not yet exist at the time. *Epistolae medicinales* of this type might be formally addressed to a colleague or indeed mention their previous correspondence, like a letter by the addressee on the same subject or the addressee's explicit request that the writer state his opinion on the matter.[508] But with respect to their content, they were often dedicated to a clearly outlined medical subject, as announced in the heading, and they were often considerably longer than was common in contemporary letter correspondence.[509] On its 275 pages in quarto format, the *Epistolae et consilia* by the Spanish physician Antonio Alvarez, for example, offered only nine letters, each dedicated to a very specific medical subject, and a *consilium*.[510] Such letters were obviously destined for publication in print from the beginning and it remains doubtful whether they were ever even sent to those they formally

---

505 Olmi, Molti amici (1991); van Houdt et alii, Self-presentation (2002).
506 Cf. Maclean, Medical republic (2008); Siraisi, Communities (2013).
507 Siraisi, Baudouin Ronsse (2016), p. 139.
508 E.g. Erastus, Disputationum (1595), foll. 1r-2v: "Quaestionem mihi proponis discutiendam".
509 Theodosius, Medicinales epistolae (1553), for example, frequently indicated the topic of the respective letter already in the title.
510 Alvarez, Epistolarum (1585).

addressed. The authors in these cases were simply using the letter as a literary form.

A famous and influential printed collection of medical letters – one on which further collections would be modeled – was Giovanni Manardi's (1462–1534) *Epistolae medicinales*.[511] Manardi was a leading proponent of medical humanism and a successor of Niccolò Leoniceno (1428–1524) in Ferrara,[512] and his collection of twenty-three letters, first published in 1521, went through numerous editions. In the role that they played, his addressees were similar to the dedicatees of books. The treatment of specific subjects was front and center. Typical headings for the letters are "To the most learned Caelius Calcagninus on the stomach" or "To Hippolytus Roscius on what 'albesed' means in Avicenna".[513] The *Epistolae medicinales* of Johannes Lange (1485–1565), court physician of the Palatine Elector, a collection of approximately 150 small treatises in epistolary form, is even considered to be his principal medical work.[514] The *Epistolae* of Thomas Erastus (1524–1583)[515] and Orazio Augenio (1527–1603),[516] too, offer a series of shorter scientific treatises; only to a very limited extent can they be considered to represent true correspondence. In their epistolary collections, Lange, Erastus, and Balduin Ronsse (1525–1597)[517] at times did not even name an addressee. The *Epistolae medicinales* by Handsch's mentor Pietro Andrea Mattioli exhibit a greater concordance with the common and everyday medical correspondence of the day, but they too offer brief scientific treatises on a variety of subjects, along with polemical responses to critics,[518] who had reproached Mattioli for erroneous botanical classifications.[519]

Historiography and Ethnography

Historiography and ethnography were two further fields that were at the center of humanist endeavor, and some physicians engaged very actively with them. The historical interests and activities of physicians, like those of other contemporaries,

---

511 Manardi, Epistolae medicinales (1521).
512 Premuda, Discepolo (1963); Dell'Acqua, Giovanni Manardo (1963).
513 Manardi, Epistolae medicinales (1521), fol. 18 and fol. 27.
514 Lange, Medicinalium epistolarum (1554); idem, Secunda medicinalium (1560).
515 Erastus, Disputationum (1595).
516 Augenio, Epistolarum (1602).
517 Ronsseus, Miscellanea (1590); Siraisi, Baudouin Ronsse (2016).
518 Mattioli, Epistolarum medicinalium (1561); idem, Epistolarum medicinalium (1564).
519 On Mattioli's vitriolic dispute with Gessner see Delisle, Letter (2004).

could take various forms. Among the works of Achilles Pirmin Gasser, for example, were a chronicle of the world from its very beginnings,[520] which went through multiple editions, a catalogue of the emperors and kings of the countries of Christian Europe,[521] and a treatise about the kings of Jerusalem.[522] Some physicians, like Paolo Giulio in Rome, even shifted their activities almost entirely to this area. Others continued practicing as physicians but devoted considerable attention to historical matters on the side and sometimes even, like Hartmann Schedel, became famous first and foremost as historians and chroniclers.[523]

Occasionally, physicians became chroniclers of their times, especially if it fell to them to bear witness to epidemics. An illustrative example here is Georg Handsch's account of the plague epidemic which raged in and around Prague from the autumn of 1562 to February of 1563.[524] While the entire royal court left Prague, Handsch stayed behind in the city with an acquaintance and a maidservant. Again and again, they saw funeral processions – three, four, five, even seven in a day. A total of nine people died in a single house, and within a week there were 200 or even more pestilence-related deaths, according to Handsch. He named a whole series of deceased individuals by name, most of whom he appears to have known from the court: several physicians, a painter, a jurist. He also gave the names of various plague victims who fled Prague in vain, falling victim to the disease in the countryside or on their way there. Among them were a treasurer and his wife, the Archduke's tailor, Handsch's former teacher Johannes Schentigar, and Mattioli's assistant Paulus.

Giovanni Planerio gave an impressive account of the plague epidemic that befell his native Northern Italian town of Quinzano d'Oglio in 1529. He described the wailing and moaning and finally how people became accustomed to ever-present death, the absence of funerals as people were buried in mass graves that were covered by so little earth that the stench of the corpses seemed to be quite literally poisoning the air.[525] During the great plague epidemic in Basel in 1610/11, Felix Platter (1536–1614) even compiled some of the earliest detailed plague statistics, tracing not only the number of sick and dead over the course of time, but also

---

520 Gasser, Historiarum (1532).
521 Gasser, Catalogus (1552).
522 Gasser, De regibus (1555).
523 Cf. Siraisi, Anatomizing (2000); eadem, History (2007); see also Pomata/Siraisi, Historia (2005).
524 Cod. 11183, foll. 143r-146r.
525 Planerio, Brevis patriae (1584), fol. 6r-v.

giving a very detailed presentation of the distribution of cases of illness and death within the city and in the outskirts.[526]

Closely related to historiography were the fields of topography and ethnography. Here, humanist interests went hand in hand with patriotism, with pride in one's hometown, one's land, one's nation. This patriotism found literary expression in descriptions of cities and countries in particular. They constituted an important area of activity for humanists, and many are extant, surviving in the form of prose and poetry, here especially in the form of panegyrics of cities.[527] As a rule, they connected a historical depiction – an outline of the town's glorious past and a presentation of its famous sons (and much more rarely daughters) – with a description of its present-day merits. Among the composers of such accounts we again find multiple physicians. Michele Savonarola (1384–1464), for example, the author of a well-known textbook on medical practice, also wrote a work about Padua's famous personages.[528] In his *Brevis patriae suae descriptio* from 1564, Giovanni Planerio presented among other things the various learned men his native town of Quinzano d'Oglio had produced.[529] Achilles Pirmin Gasser (1505–1577) wrote an extensive chronicle of his native city of Augsburg.[530] In Handsch's closer Bohemian environment, the genre of poetic town descriptions in particular enjoyed great popularity.[531] His teacher Johannes Schentigar composed a poem about Joachimstal,[532] his friend Thomas Mitis wrote an *idyllion* about the thermal baths of Teplitz,[533] the Olomouc physician Lorenz Span glorified an archducal palace not far from Prague in a poem.[534] Pietro Andrea Mattioli composed a thorough, though in his case Italian, poem about the palace of his then employer Bernardo Cles in Trento.[535] In a poem to Thomas Mitis, Handsch

---

526 Platter, Beschreibung (1987).
527 Cf. Thurn, Städtelobgedichte (2002).
528 Savonarola, Practica (1502); Siraisi, History (2007), p. 14.
529 Planerio, Brevis patriae (1584) (separate pagination).
530 This work appeared post-humously in a German edition under the title *Chronica der weitberuempten keyserlichen freyen und deß H. Reichs Statt Augspurg in Schwaben*, vol. 2, Basel 1595.
531 Martínková, Beschreibungen (1993); eadem, Literární druh (2012).
532 Collinus et alii, Tertia farrago (1561), foll. 132v-133r.
533 Guth, Idyll (1930).
534 Martínková, Beschreibungen (1993), p. 28.
535 Mattioli, Il Magno Palazzo (1539).

himself, very much in the tradition of this genre, praised his Prague, the capital of the kingdom located on the Vltava river and greatly blessed with wine and crops.[536]

A further essential element of "patriotic" historiography and topography was a concern with the native language and culture, with the way of life and the character of the people at present.[537] An influential pioneer of this kind of ethnology *ante litteram* was the poet and historian Konrad Celtis (1459–1508). In his description of Nuremberg and in his poetic comparison of Prague with ancient Rome, he foregrounded his connectedness with his own landscape and culture. While some might be inclined to boast about their travels in distant lands, he, a learned German man, knew the language of his home, the rites, laws, dialects ("linguas"), and confessions, the physical build of the people, their diseases, and their appearance.[538]

In the descriptions of towns, the statements about the character and customs of the people who lived in them was usually limited to very short, generalizing characterizations such as references to people's strong work ethic and modesty. In this regard, Handsch, especially with his "Weltbüchle" ("Little World Book"),[539] was quite extraordinary. He described the German-speaking culture in which he had grown up and continued to move in great detail.[540] Handsch learned the Czech language and even taught it to others. His loyalty was clear, however. In his manuscripts he repeatedly and emphatically called himself a "Germano-Bohemus".[541] He collected numerous German proverbs, sayings, aphorisms, and anecdotes, which it appears he learned in oral exchanges with people, first in Bohemia and later in Tyrol. Numerous entries made with different inks and quills demonstrate that these manifestations of popular culture were dear to his heart and that this interest stayed with him throughout his life. Handsch's

---

[536] Cod. 9821, foll. 65r; according to Storchová, Handsch (2020), Handsch also penned a small prose text about Prague, which was printed in a broad-sheet in Prague in 1562.
[537] Schmidt, Deutsche Volkskunde (1904) (ch. 2, § 1).
[538] Celtis, Quattuor libri (1934), p. 7, preface, "qui patriae suae linguae fines et terminos gentiumque in ea diversos ritus, leges, linguas, religiones, habitum denique et affectiones corporumque varia lineamenta et figura viderit et observavit"; cf. Wiegand, Volkskunde (2004).
[539] Cod. 9671.
[540] National "identities", based on linguistic difference, were of particular relevance in Handsch's home country. In Prague and the surrounding Bohemia, representatives of "Czech" culture and language lived side by side with those of German culture and language. Many merchants and craftsmen and also large parts of the nobility spoke predominantly or exclusively Czech. Parts of the population and especially the members of the Habsburg court preferred German (Glück, Deutsch (2002), pp. 345–350).
[541] E.g. Cod. 11006, frontispiece.

notes only rarely take an evaluative stance, following instead a primarily documentary approach, and thus they provide valuable insights into the language and convey the images that characterized people's experience of life in Bohemia and Tyrol – and presumably across wide stretches of the German-speaking regions as well. From today's perspective, this makes Handsch a pioneer of ethnology.

A prominent feature in Handsch's notes were the many figures of speech and metaphors used to express feelings. The heart, which in the learned medical discourse about affects played a leading and very specific, physiological role,[542] also took a central place in colloquial language, in phrases such as, "I don't have a heart of stone".[543] Expressing joy were idioms such as, "My heart is swelling"[544] and "His heart is laughing in his body".[545] In the case of "Herzeleid" ("heartache") a person might say, "my heart cries in my body" or the heart "hurt",[546] "he's eating himself up"[547] or "with a bitter heart".[548] The saying "A drop of blood falls from my heart when I think of it"[549] is reminiscent of the expression "my heart is bleeding", which is still in use in German today. Wrath and anger, on the other hand, were associated more with the liver, the primary location of yellow bile. If someone was angered easily, he would say, according to Handsch, "My liver overflows from time to time" or "My bile overflows from time to time".[550] One could also be more vivid and say that spiders were running over the liver.[551]

Other sayings reflect the great importance of drinking in contemporary social life. Under the heading "Drunkenness" ("ebrietas") Handsch made note of expressions like "He's so full he takes a white dog for a miller's knave" or "He's drunk to the point of staring, he's blind-drunk". Sayings like "When he could not drink wine, he thought he'd go to pieces" imply the experience of dependence.[552]

---

542 Stolberg, Emotions (2019).
543 Cod. 9671, fol. 53v: "Ich hab nicht eyn steynern Herz."
544 Ibid., fol. 60r: "Es wechst mirs Herz"; similarly ibid., fol. 34v.
545 Ibid., fol. 53v, "das Herze lacht y[h]m ym Leib".
546 Ibid., fol. 34v and fol. 53v.
547 Ibid., fol. 167r.
548 Ibid., fol. 177r.
549 Ibid., fol. 174r: "Ein Bluttstropff fellt mir vom Herzen, wenn ich daran gedenck."
550 Ibid., fol. 170r: "Es laufft mir auch bißweilen über die Leber." – "Die Gall gehet mir auch bißweilen über."
551 Ibid., fol. 56v.
552 Ibid., fol. 38v: "Er ist so vol, das er eyn weissen Hundt vor eynen Müllerknecht ansehe" – "Er ist starrend vol, blindvol" – "Wenn er nicht solt Weyn trincken, er meynet, er muste zerfallen".

And a drinker might be characterized and denigrated as an "relentless toaster", as a "real wine spigot" or a "beer donkey".[553] Sexuality, too, could not be left out. Under the heading "Libido. Fornication" ("Libido. Scortari") he noted sayings like, "If a nanny-goat were wearing a veil, he would court her" and "He's got as many whores as a beggar has flies" or "as a dog has fleas".[554] Handsch even found curse words and insults, whether said in earnest or in jest, to be noteworthy, including, "You stinking [heap of] filth", "You dirt sack" or "You arse cap".[555]

Loci Communes

A further practice that was characteristic of Renaissance humanism and which many physicians adopted was the compilation of personal collections of *loci communes*.[556] The term and the associated practice originated with Aristotelean rhetoric. The "loci", or in Greek "topoi", were the "places" or "seats" of arguments within a subject area of which the orator or rhetor could avail himself. Certain generic, overarching terms such as *genus, species,* and *proprium* were "common" *loci*, thus literally *loci communes*, headings under which various narrower terms could be subsumed. During humanism however, the term "loci communes" was increasingly used for a general, thematically-organized collection of quotes and collectanea.

The technique of *loci communes* was the apotheosis of the humanist art of excerpting and ranked among the fundamental learned cultural techniques of the time.[557] Beginning in school, students learned to organize their collectanea in this form. These were often quotations and aphorisms that were common knowledge among scholars, a circumstance that led to the rather disparaging meaning of the term "commonplace", the literal translation of "locus communis", today. Over time, handbooks on the art of reading and excerpting, in which the *loci communes* technique played an important role, found a large readership.[558] Leading humanists like Erasmus of Rotterdam praised the practice of

---

553 Ibid., "unbarmherziger Zutrincker", "rechter Weinzapff", "Biresel".
554 Ibid., fol. 42v: "Wenn ein Geis eyn Schleier auff hett, er wurde yr bulen" – "Er ist mit Huren befangen, wie eyn Bettler mit Moschen."
555 Ibid., fol. 40v and fol. 170r: "Du stinckender Unflat", "Du Drecksack", "Du Arschkappeln".
556 On the following, see also Stolberg, Medizinische Loci communes (2013); Stolberg, Medical note-taking (2016).
557 Schmidt-Biggemann, Topica universalis (1983); Moss, Printed commonplace-books (1996); Moss, Power (2011).
558 Sacchini, De ratione (1614); Drexel, Aurifodina artium (1638).

collecting *loci communes* as a first-rate means of learning to express oneself in elegant Latin and as an inexhaustible source of *copia*, of a wealth of ideas and expressions on which one could draw for one's own writing and speech.[559] As banal and predictable as the use of well-known quotes from the works of Latin poets and historians was, it was considered essential for certain occasions. If a medical doctor, for example, dared to get straight to the point in an academic oration, he had to be prepared to be booed.[560]

Georg Handsch was very well-versed in the technique of *loci communes*. An extensive, 1,100-page-long *Promptuarium sive loci communes latinitatis* from his pen has survived from the time before he studied medicine. It includes numerous aphorisms, definitions, and sometimes lengthy quotes from works by well-known classical authors. He carefully organized a wide range of topics according to categories and sub-categories, covering everything from God, Heaven and Earth to medicine, geography, and meteorology, and all the way to agricultural machinery.[561] In a second manuscript, titled *Rhapsodia seu loci communes*, he likewise compiled quotes and phrases from the works of ancient poets. Several dozen pages with unsystematic entries on subjects such as *triumphus*, *pericula*, and *coelum*, are followed by entries in alphabetical order.[562] Other future physicians, too, assembled *loci communes*, collecting passages and quotes from the works of ancient poets, philosophers, and historians for the purpose of using them later in their letters, poems, forewords, and so forth. Salomon Alberti (1540–1600), for example, who later became a physician and a professor of anatomy in Wittenberg, produced a collection, organized alphabetically according to keywords, of quotes and phrases from the works of Cicero, Plautus, Terence, Livy, and other authors.[563]

As Handsch's *Promptuarium* impressively illustrates, extensive collections of *loci communes*, in their effort to cover all areas of knowledge and all the important standard subjects, bring to mind encyclopedias, that is thematically organized collections of the existing knowledge. Indeed, certain physicians of the sixteenth and seventeenth centuries did not limit themselves to producing *loci*

---

559 Erasmus, De duplici copia (1514).
560 Siraisi, Oratory (2004), p. 201.
561 Cod. 9550. The manuscript is dated 1549. Since Handsch addressed the reader ("lector") directly and called himself explicitly the "author", he may have hoped for its publication. Perhaps he was thinking more specifically of Collinus's school in the Angel's Garden in Prague. In the introduction to the Latin language he wrote for his pupils, Collinus printed a *cisioanus* Handsch had composed, i. e. a poetic annual calendar that made it easier for the pupils to remember the many different holidays (Handsch, Calendarium novum (1550); cf. also Cod. 9550, foll. 626r-630v).
562 Cod. 9607.
563 Staatsbibliothek Berlin, Ms. Lat. Qu. 41.

communes for private use alone. As Handsch himself may have planned to do, too, they published printed comprehensive, encyclopedic collections of quotes and excerpts on all areas of knowledge.[564] The authors or compilers of two of the most important encyclopedic collections of this kind were physicians. In 1545, Zurich's city physician Conrad Gessner brought out his *Bibliotheca universalis*. The approximately 12,000 entries list the Latin, Greek, and Hebrew works of about 3,000 authors, some with biographical details and critical annotations by Gessner. Building on the *Bibliotheca universalis*, Gessner published his *Pandectae* a few years later, which was organized by keywords.[565] While Gessner concentrated on presenting knowledge along bibliographical lines,[566] the Basel physician Theodor Zwinger (1533–1588) with his *Theatrum vitae humanae* offered a comprehensive and widely read thematic overview of the knowledge of his time.[567]

The technique of *loci communes* also allowed collectanea and generally anything that was worth knowing from different disciplines and fields to be compiled and structured thematically. A leader in this domain was Philipp Melanchthon (1497–1560), who made the genre popular in theology. In his *Loci communes rerum theologicarum* of 1521, he departed from the familiar practice of presenting and commenting on sentences and passages from a book of the Holy Scriptures one after the other, as they occurred in the text. Instead, Melanchthon collated what he found on major theological topics in the various books of the Bible under about two dozen headings such as "Creation", "Men", "Vice", "Punishment", "Faith", and "Hope".[568] In law as well, collectanea and generally anything worth knowing about a specific fact or matter could be drawn together from various legal sources.[569]

A similar practice suggested itself for medicine. Instructional books on the study of medicine explicitly recommended that students organize their *collectanea* in the form of *loci communes*.[570] In 1596, Jakob Horst (1537–1600) emphasized to his listeners (and later to his readers) in an academic speech that because the human memory was weak, students ("tyrones artis") were well advised to create the true guardians of memory for themselves, which were commonly called "loci communes". According to Horst, well-ordered titles or headings were to represent

---

564 Zwinger, Theatrum vitae (1586).
565 Gessner, Pandectae (1548); cf. Nelles, Reading (2009).
566 See also Spach, Nomenclator (1591).
567 Zwinger, Theatrum vitae (1586).
568 Melanchthon, Loci communes (1521).
569 See e.g. the legal encyclopaedia of almost 1,200 pages by Sole/Schultes, Loci (1607).
570 Kijper, Medicinam (1643), pp. 265–267.

the essential teachings of medicine and to serve, as it were, as small nests to which the students could accordingly allot everything they read, heard, or saw. In this way, they would create for themselves a corpus of medicine as a whole and could draw what they needed from it as necessary.[571] Thomas Bartholin (1616–1680), too, praised the merits of medical *loci communes* and recommended to those starting out in their careers that they keep a *compendium novorum titulorum* in which they devote a volume to each discipline, briefly ("brevissime") writing down everything noteworthy in its proper place ("suo loco").[572]

When these authors gave their readers this advice, it was likely the advice which professors often gave students, not only in writing but orally too, and it reflected a widespread practice. The instrument of the *loci* also proved useful to students who were preparing for disputations on detailed and specific medical matters and who were studying the passages in the authoritative works that provided the basis for examinations and tests at many universities. Through this practice, students could bring together the relevant statements of authorities so as to commit them to memory in context and perhaps as a means of comparing and weighing them against one another in a discussion.[573]

Dozens of such medical notebooks are extant in European libraries.[574] In student *loci communes*, systematic organization of the notes as in the chapters of a book predominates, and most of them share another striking feature: at some point in time, the compiler gave up. Joachim Camerarius (1534–1598), for example, following in the footsteps of his father, a well-known humanist, who had published philosophical *loci communes* himself,[575] embarked on a systematically organized *Mnemoneutikon* of medical practice. He earmarked pages to be used for generic diseases ("De morborum generibus"), causes of disease ("De morborum causis"), symptoms ("De signis morborum"), and signs of the location of disease in the body ("De signis loci affecti"). Further pages were reserved for such things as the individual humors, as well as pulse diagnosis and uroscopy. Yet, under many of the neatly arranged headings there is not a single entry; the pages are blank.[576] Things are hardly any better in the case of the *Memoriale practicum* by Erasmus Reinhold the Younger (1538–1592). Here too, filled pages dedicated to specific types of medication such as purging agents or to particular illnesses like

---

571 Horst, Oratio (1596), p. 565.
572 Bartholinus, De libris legendis (1711), p. 149 (posthumous edition with a preface Bartholinus wrote in 1672).
573 My thanks to Sabine Schlegelmilch for pointing out this specific use to me.
574 See the bibliography in Stolberg, Medizinische Loci communes (2013).
575 Camerarius, Arithmologia (1552).
576 Universitätsbibliothek Erlangen, Ms. 935.

epilepsy neighbor pages that lack any sort of entry.[577] The failure of such efforts is particularly striking in the case of a magnificently bound book of medical *loci communes* that is extant in St Gall.[578] Some of the pages are filled in. Under the heading "Of Fevers and Unnatural Heat in General",[579] the unknown author collected about twenty references and quotes from works by ancient and recent writers, from Galen and Hippocrates to Avicenna to Emanuel Stupanus, Leonhard Fuchs, Jean Fernel, and Girolamo Mercuriale, and he added an oral statement made by Caspar Bauhin during an examination.[580] The majority of the pages, however, apart from the headings, are mostly or completely empty.[581] The extensive *Volumen locorum communium conscriptorum,* created by an unknown medical professional around 1600, which is extant at the university library in Leipzig, is another case in point. Some pages, for example on the pulse ("pulsus"), are filled, while others, like the one on natural laughter ("risus naturalis") have only a single entry, and others still, like the one about "the diseases of pregnant women" ("praegnantium morbi") remain entirely blank.[582]

There is likely a banal reason for this failure. With their systematic approach, the authors were aiming at completeness. This was the goal of Isaac Habrecht (1589–1633) when he by his own admission wanted to thematically organize the entire medical theory of his time by collecting excerpts from works by Jean Fernel, Leonhard Fuchs, Johannes Heurne, Jean Riolan, and others.[583] Erasmus Reinhold (1511–1553) aimed to note at least that which was to be generally heeded in medical practice.[584] Isaac Habrecht had just turned seventeen when he began his *loci communes*; Erasmus Reinhold was twenty-two and a medical student in his fourth year. But not only was it a mammoth undertaking to systematically note down by hand the entirety of medical knowledge in the manner of a

---

577 Staatsbibliothek Bamberg, Bamberger Sammlung, Msc. misc. 385.
578 Kantonsbibliothek Vadiana St. Gallen, Ms. 408.
579 "De febribus et cal[ore] p[raeter]n[aturali] in genere" (or: "p[raeter] n[aturam]").
580 Kantonsbibliothek St. Gallen, Ms. 408, coll. 600–602.
581 Ibid., col. 1114 and coll. 1031f.
582 Universitätsbibliothek Leipzig, Ms. 2494. Caspar Weckerlins *loci communes* (Det Kongelige Bibliotek Copenhagen, Ms. Gl. kongl. S. 4° 1694) probably survived only because he later used the empty pages for notes on various cases from his practice, recipes and outstanding payments that had nothing to do with headings such as *mala*, *morbus* and *motus*, to which the pages were originally assigned. The author was probably the later Strasbourg physician of the same name, who was awarded a doctorate in Leiden in 1613.
583 Det Kongelige Bibliotek Copenhagen, Ms. Gl. Kongl. 4° 1691: "Dispositio totius medicinae theoricae".
584 Staatsbibliothek Bamberg, Bamberger Sammlung, Msc. misc. 385: "Generalia in omni praxi medicinae observanda".

textbook: it was also not worth the trouble, because alternatives were available for purchase. They came in the form of the *Theses seu communes loci totius rei medicae* by Otto Brunfels and the close to 700 folio pages of comprehensive *Loci medicinae communes* by François Valleriola (1504–1580), which was especially widely circulated and went through many editions. These printed collections compiled the medical knowledge of the time with a systematicity and completeness that the average medical student or young physician could not dream of approaching.[585]

Not only this, but in the course of the sixteenth century, there was a significant increase in the private ownership of books, including by physicians and medical students, which largely rendered the painstaking work of systematically noting down medical collectanea an avoidable task. This statement contradicts a widely shared and accepted view in recent work on the history of note-taking and thus demands explanation. Drawing on the note-taking that was the basis for comprehensive printed encyclopedic works like Theodor Zwinger's *Theatrum vitae humanae* and Jean Bodin's *Universae naturae theatrum*, historians have come to a very different conclusion. They have interpreted the rise of *loci communes* as a response to an early modern "information overload", to the flood of books that was indeed bewailed by some contemporaries.[586] Printed encyclopedias that follow the principle *loci communes* can only be compared to the handwritten *loci communes* to a limited extent, however. They were not working tools, but scholarly publications that were geared toward providing a comprehensive overview. For the common physician and scholar, by contrast, books were not only the source of an overload of knowledge but, at the same time, also the key to mastering it. If you owned a few general textbooks or reference works, you could make notes in the margins or at least add a "nota bene" or other marks so that you could return to the book later and quickly absorb the subject matter that was important. This was also the advice of early modern reading and guides to excerpting.[587] And it was how readers went about things in practice, as is shown by extant copies of books that were originally owned by medical students, physicians, and other educated readers.[588] It was a much more efficient method than laboriously making excerpts, and when they were looking for entries on a certain subject, all the book owners

---

[585] Brunfels, Theses (1532); Valleriola, Loci medicinae (1562); idem, Loci (1563); idem, Loci medicinae (1589).
[586] Rosenberg, Information (2003); Blair, Reading strategies (2003); Blair, Too much too know (2010).
[587] Kijper, Medicinam (1643), pp. 266f.
[588] Sherman, Used books (2008).

had to do was go to the table of contents or index, find the right chapter or page and read the passage in question.

As opposed to the systematic and structured approach that Camerarius, Haprecht and Reinhold adopted in their early years, sequential *loci communes* were very useful paper tool, especially in the hands of physicians and naturalists. Sequential *loci communes* did not aim for completeness and they followed no a systematic or alphabetical[589] order. They simply contained collectanea or empirical observations in the order the author encountered them. In this way they largely resembled common notebooks, also known as *adversaria* at the time, except for one important difference: the individual entries were given keywords, as was typical for humanist *loci communes*, and in this way, they were assigned to larger subject categories. Leafing through later on, the authors could quickly identify the entries about a subject or *locus* which was their present concern. Sometimes they made their search easier by adding an index of keywords. We will be returning to this form of *loci communes* in the context of the rise of empirical perspectives.

Scholarly Self-Fashioning

Taken together, the learned habitus, the use of Latin, and the various humanist practices in which medical students and physicians engaged during the Renaissance can be understood as a substantial component of their "self-fashioning". Here I am making use of a concept introduced into historical research by the literary theorist and Shakespeare scholar Stephen Greenblatt.[590] In the field of history, self-fashioning was sometimes reduced to the presentation of a "false" self and likened to theatrical acting, even to lying or dissimulation.[591] In Greenblatt's approach, however, self-fashioning combines two aspects which, while they are often conceptualized and studied independently of each other, are closely related both historically and in the present day, and have a mutual in-

---

[589] Ambrosius Prechtl (1533–1569), who later served as a town physician in Straubing, used this procedure quite successfully, from 1557 onwards and thus presumably at the beginning of his medical practice, to make concrete entries on medical practice based on alphabetically arranged keywords such as "abortus", "dissenteria", and "epar" (Universitätsbibliothek Erlangen, Ms. 1206).
[590] Greenblatt, Renaissance self-fashioning (1980); see also Buschmann, Persönlichkeit (2013), pp. 125–149; Stolberg, Identitätsbildung (2015).
[591] On the uses of the concept by historians, see Pieters/Rogiest, Self-fashioning (2009).

fluence on each other. These are the self-conception of historical individuals on the one hand and their outward self-presentation on the other.[592]

Adopting this approach, the concept of self-fashioning may contribute substantially to a historical understanding of the relationship between the self-presentation and the identity of an entire professional group, in our case learned physicians.[593] The use of Latin, the practice of poetry, the correspondence with other learned men including those outside medicine, humanist practices such as the creation of *loci communes* and *alba amicorum* – all of this gave expression – and not only outward, public expression – to the deeply entrenched humanist self-conception that was acquired from a very young age.[594] The learned habitus had become second nature to the physicians; it was an essential part of their identity.

This humanist self-conception was, however, intrinsically linked to self-presentation towards the outside world – indeed, to what we can call self-staging.[595] Engaging in educated, humanist practices and underlining one's own erudition also served as a way of drawing a line between oneself and lesser-educated, non-academic competitors – the barber-surgeons and lay healers. And not least of all, a public presentation of oneself as a man of letters served well to counterbalance the less glorious aspects of medical practice. In the sickroom, at the sickbed, physicians inhabited a world which was drastically removed from that of academic learning. Everything revolved around the creaturely body and the effort to relieve sick patients of their suffering. Physicians were confronted every single day with complaints and wails of pain. Worse still was that, in a time when contact with "impure" matter was greatly stigmatized, they constantly had to deal with disgusting discharge, with ulcers, skin rashes, and abscesses, and with patients' foul-smelling excretions. When asked to treat cases of the French disease, as well as fractures, tumors, and other external damage, Janus Cornarius (1500–1558), a leading proponent of medical humanism, emphatically refused to do so, saying that such maladies were not part of internal medicine and that "lovers of cleanliness" would not want to put their hands on such patients.[596]

The learned self-conception of physicians and their efforts to create an effective corresponding self-presentation for the public find striking expression in contemporary physician portraits. When genre painters of the sixteenth and seventeenth centuries painted an academically trained physician, they

---

592 Greenblatt, Renaissance self-fashioning (1980), p. 3.
593 On collective self-fashioning, see also Kirwan, Introduction (2013), pp. 8–11.
594 On the self-fashioning of humanists in general, see Enenkel, Self-representation (2003).
595 Cf. Stolberg, Identitätsbildung (2015).
596 Employment contract, quoting Cornarius, 18 September 1546. (www.aerztebriefe.de/id/00014028, A. Döll/T. Walter).

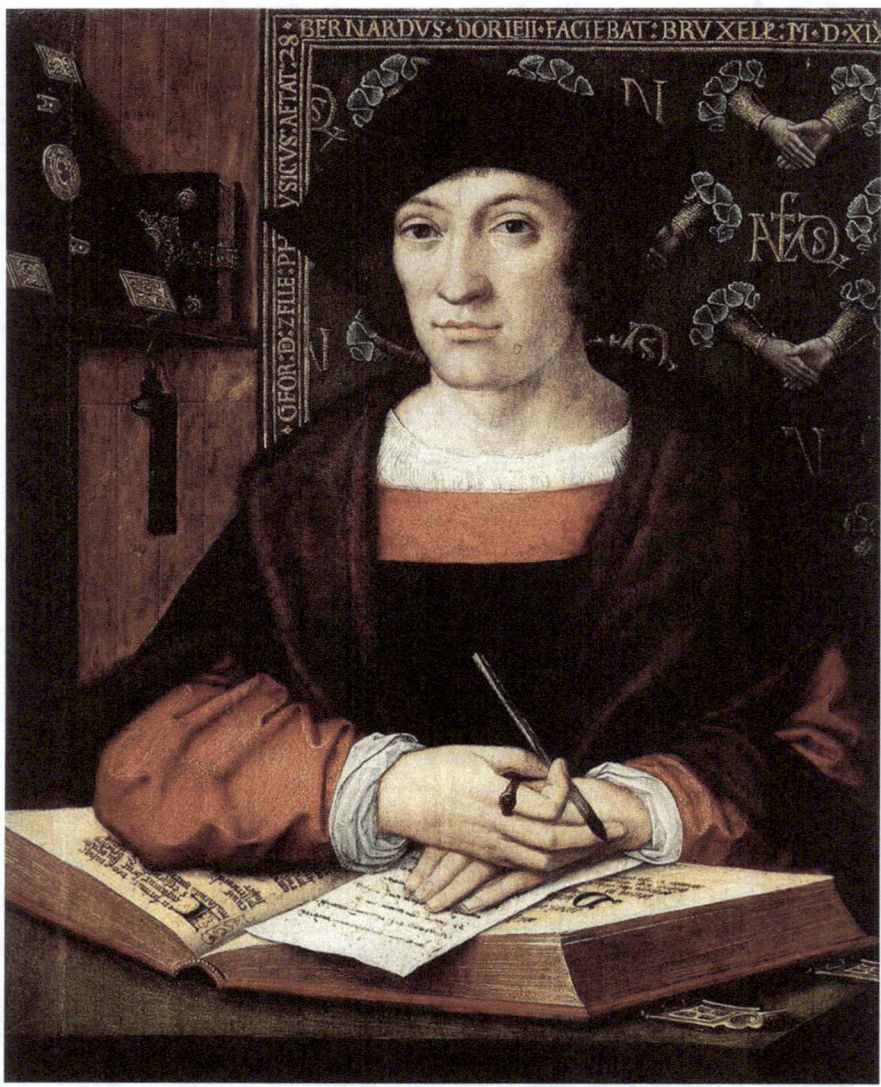

Fig. 4: Bernard van Orley, Portrait of the physician Joris van Zeile, Musées royaux des Beaux-Arts de Belgique, Brussels.

usually showed him as a practitioner in a sickroom, often with a matula in hand, sometimes taking a patient's pulse. Completely different representational conventions applied, however, to portraits of physicians who were identified by name and who presumably had a say in the composition of the portrait. Here, the physician is almost always shown in his *musaeum,* his study, possibly with an open book or a handwritten text in front of him and further books nearby or on a shelf in the background. His clothing is dignified. Fine gloves and rings on his fingers point out to the viewer that he or she is not looking at a manual laborer or a craftsman. At most plants, skulls, and bones, stuffed animals, astronomical instruments, and similar attributes point to the new empirically-oriented erudition of the medical naturalist. The familiar attribute of the matula is missing, however, and, as a rule, no patients are present either. Unless the painter included books with legible author names like "Hippocrates" or "Galen", often all that identifies the sitter as a physician is an inscription that gives his name and profession (see Fig. 4).[597]

---

[597] Kitti, Quacksalber (1985); Fürst, Arztporträt (2009); contemporary collection of physicians' portraits in Reusnerus, Icones (1590).

―――
Part II: **Learned Medical Practice**

From theory to practice

As we saw in Part I, the numerous aspiring physicians who studied, like Handsch, at one of the leading Italian or French universities profited from comprehensive training. They not only studied the central, authoritative works of ancient and recent writers in great depth, but they also had various opportunities to acquire the practical knowledge and skill they would need later when diagnosing and treating their patients. Professors even worked specific case histories into their lectures. In Padua, the *collegia* offered valuable insights into the ways in which the discipline's leading authorities followed a strictly methodical process when identifying pathological changes inside the body and devising treatment. Accompanying their professors during patient visits at the hospital or on house calls brought future physicians face to face with actual patients and witness how the professor interacted with patients of diverse social status.

We know little, however, about how physicians later applied what they had learned in their own practice, how they diagnosed and treated medical conditions in everyday life. Much historical research has focused on the general concepts and theories of learned medicine, on individual elaborations and interpretations of the ideas of leading medical authors and on the lively debates that were sparked by some theoretical questions.[1] Practical medicine, by contrast, has received much less attention, and the few studies that have been published in this area rely largely on theoretical statements about different illnesses, not on casuistic sources describing everyday practice.[2]

In the first part of this book, we discussed the essential concepts and theories that, with some variation, were taught at universities. At the center of orthodox, Galenic academic medicine was the concept of *intemperies* or *dyscrasia*, of an imbalance or disproportion of the four primary qualities (cold, hot, dry, and moist) and/or the four humors (yellow and black bile, blood and phlegm). A therapy that followed this explanatory model consequently needed to aim at evacuating the humor or the two humors that were overabundant and/or to restore the proper relation of the primary qualities. In the case of a hot illness, for example, this would have been done with medicinal plants with a cooling effect. As the familiar, oft

---

[1] See the surveys by Bylebyl, Medicine (1985); Siraisi, Avicenna (1987); Siraisi, Medieval & early Renaissance medicine (1990); Wear, Medicine (1995); Maclean, Logic (2002); Wear/French/Lonie, Medical Renaissance (1985); Cook, Medicine (2006).
[2] Wear, Explorations (2000); Maclean, Logic (2002), pp. 234–332; Calabritto, Medicina practica (2006); Siraisi, Medicina practica (2008); on English medicine see Wear, Knowledge (2000); on the fifteenth century, Jacquart, Theory (1990).

Open Access. © 2022 Michael Stolberg, published by De Gruyter. This work is licensed under the Creative Commons Attribution-NonCommercial-NoDerivatives 4.0 International License.
https://doi.org/10.1515/9783110733549-005

reiterated master narrative has it, this orthodox, Galenic medicine widely prevailed during the sixteenth century. It also holds that the radical alternative model was Paracelsism, which had a certain following in the sixteenth century but always remained in a minority position. Until very recently, academic as well as popular historical depictions have thus essentially reduced sixteenth-century medicine to the concept of an imbalance of the humors and qualities in the body, which physicians had to diagnose and equalize.[3] Even first-rate experts on the learned medical theory of the sixteenth century like Ian Maclean, arrive at the conclusion that the learned physicians of the day ascribed diseases to "asymmetric or unbalanced states of the body".[4]

Generalizations such as this disregard one essential question, however: to what degree was the concept of an imbalance of the humors and qualities actually applied in everyday practice? To what degree did it inform the way in which physicians diagnosed and treated their patients? Theory and praxis, as we know, can be worlds apart, not only in medicine. For good reason, Iain M. Lonie cautioned years ago that "without some kind of access to practical medicine and its teaching, we are in danger of ending with a history of medicine which includes everything except the craft of medicine itself."[5] This reminder remains as relevant as ever and especially when it comes to understanding sixteenth-century medicine. As I have already indicated in my introduction, a detailed study of everyday medical practice reveals profound differences between the concepts that prevailed in the theoretical writing and those that guided the diagnostic and therapeutic practice of physicians: the often-invoked doctrine that illness arose from an imbalance of the humors and qualities in the body proves to have been largely irrelevant in everyday medical practice.

A major reason why historians have largely ignored the marked differences between theory and practice is no doubt that the study of everyday medical practice is attended by great challenges. Theoretical concepts and the debates on them can be studied relatively easily in the numerous medical publications from that time. By contrast, sources for everyday medical practice in the sixteenth century that reflect how physicians applied the theoretical knowledge at the bedside are much more difficult to come by.

---

3 Jütte, Ärzte (1991), p. 42.
4 Maclean, Logic (2002), p. 260; in addition, Maclean mentions the two other categories which Galen had described but which were irrelevant for most cases of illness physicians encountered in their everyday practice, namely the "mala compositio" of individual organs and the traumatic "solutio continuitatis" (ibid.) which was primarily the domain of surgeons. For an early nuanced account, which focuses more on actual practice see Wear, Popularized ideas (1989).
5 Lonie, Paris Hippocratics (2000), p. 157.

Among printed sources, published medical case histories offer some important insights at least. Beginning in the middle of the sixteenth century, more and more collections of *curationes* and medical *observationes* were published. The genre quickly became very popular among students and physicians.[6] Like the medical *consilia*, which met with great interest in the late Middle Ages already,[7] they gave medical readers an opportunity to learn from the experiences of others and to apply them to their own practice. As a genre, collections medical *observationes* have garnered some attention in historical research.[8] So far, however, there are hardly any systematic studies of medical case histories as documents of ordinary medical practice.[9]

To be sure, the problems with this kind of analysis are considerable. It is difficult to draw general conclusions from countless individual cases, especially because many published case histories focus on therapy, on the treatment with various medicines and the respective recipes. Moreover, there is always the question as to whether the published case histories adequately reflect the author's everyday practice – not to mention the everyday practice of most physicians. The authors were mostly very successful and had a large practice. On top of that, they usually made a more or less narrow selection from the numerous cases they had seen. Some limited themselves to publishing *observationes rarae* to begin with, to extraordinary or unique observations of unusual cases of illness, deformities, and so forth.[10] Even authors and publishers of collected case histories who asserted that they were presenting cases from the own practice had good reasons to prefer and select those that were complicated and difficult.[11] Medical readers would not have had much to gain from reports of everyday, banal cases

---

6 The earliest larger collection of this kind were the *Curationes* of Amatus Lusitanus; the first *centuria* appeared in 1551 (Lusitanus, Curationum (1551)).
7 Agrimi and Crisciani, Consilia (1994); see also Lockwood, Benzi (1951); Crisciani, L'individuale (1996).
8 Temkin, Studien (1929); Laín Entralgo, Historia clinica (1961); Stolberg, Formen (2007); Pomata, Sharing cases (2010); eadem, Observation rising (2011); eadem, Word (2011).
9 Huber, Felix Platters "Observationes" (2003); some of my doctoral students in Würzburg and Regensburg have examined how physicians understood and dealt with certain diseases in more detail; cf. Mayer, Verständnis und Darstellung des Skorbuts (2012); Reger, Affectio hypochondriaca (2015); Gößwein, Mater puerorum (2016).
10 Dodoens, Medicinalium observationum (1581); Schenck, Observationum (1600); Hochstetter, Rararum observationum (1624); early examples are the stories of "wondrous" cases and cures of Antonio Benivieni and Girolamo Cardano (Siraisi, L'individuale (1996)).
11 François Valleriola, for example, published 60 case histories, in 1573, and added that he had collected another 600 stories of "more serious" cases. If we add the less serious cases in his practice, his published cases thus clearly represent only a tiny selection of those he had dealt with (Valleriola, Observationum (1573), p. 263).

and they did not allow the author to show off his extraordinary diagnostic acumen and therapeutic know-how either. For the same reasons admissions of errors and mistakes are few and far between and we find hardly any histories of patients whose treatment ultimately failed or ended with death.[12] Since they threatened to put the author into a bad light, they were unsuited for publication, although readers could have learned much from the mistakes. Last but not least authors may have embellished stories in order to highlight their skill and success and quite possibly may have invented some of them completely.

Physicians' personal notes and practice journals that were not intended for publication allow for a much better, more realistic view of common medical practice. Unfortunately, very few are extant. My most important source for the following discussion will therefore again be Handsch's notes. In their ability to shed light on everyday medical practice in the sixteenth century, they are unparalleled. In his extensive notes on the numerous cases that he or physicians from his professional environment treated, Handsch frequently included the reasons for the physicians' diagnostic and therapeutic conclusions and decision making. The medical understanding of disease that informed the practice of these physicians becomes especially clear and is most explicit in the hundreds of entries in which Handsch, writing in German, recorded how he and his fellow physicians explained (or could in future explain) medical conditions and the treatments they recommended to patients and their relatives.[13] I will also draw on other sources, so as to arrive at generalizable statements. The practice journals of Hiob Finzel and Ulrich Lehner will feature prominently here. Detailed explanations about the nature and cause of widespread and common diseases can further be found in handwritten letters which physicians, communicating in the vernacular, sent to patients and their relatives in response to a request for counsel.[14]

---

12 Unless the responsibility could be attributed to other healers or to the patients themselves; see e.g. Foreest, Observationum (1603–1606), pp. 482–486, on the fatal outcome of various cases of breast cases after they had been treated by empirics.
13 Numerous phrases of this kind can be found in particular in Cod. 11206; for further details see Stolberg, "You have no good blood" (2015).
14 See, in particular, the collection of about 80 *consilia* by Jacob Horst from the 1570s and 1580s in Staats- und Universitätsbibliothek Göttingen, Ms. Meibom 146.

Pathology

In their publications as much as in their personal notes, and to a limited extent in their communication with patients and their relatives as well, physicians made use of a whole range of established disease names. Most of them derived from medieval works on medical practice,[15] and some of them even had ancient origins. When it came to printed collections of *observationes* and *consilia*, they were often organized by disease name or at least these names served as headings for individual case histories. Handsch, too, often captioned his entries with disease names such as "hydrops" or "epilepsia". Disease names played an even more important role in the remedy books of physicians and laypeople, for example when remedies for the "bloody flux" [dysentery] or "stroke" were noted. In other words, the idea that there were different diseases and that each was marked by a specific clinical picture was well established in the sixteenth century.

At the sickbed – that is, during the encounter with a specific case of illness – naming the disease was but one aspect of medical diagnostics, however. Physicians first and foremost strove to grasp the disease process at work inside the body as precisely as possible. As described above, the future *doctores medicinae* in Padua were taught the required method at the sickbed and in the *collegia*. They had to determine the immediate *causa corporalis* and to understand the specific pathological processes and changes in the body. It was this search for the immediate, inner causes or processes, giving rise to subjectively experienced symptoms and externally recognizable pathological changes that distinguished rational and, in the judgement of that time, scientific medicine. Learned medical practice stood on the foundation of this precise analysis, and it was only possible to carry out a causal treatment that started at the root when supported in this way. It was the only way to effectively combat an illness instead of simply removing its symptoms. With these rational, causal explanations of the disease process as their gold standard, learned physicians also distinguished themselves from the numerous less educated competition: the barber surgeons, and lay healers. If we were to believe the learned polemics, these practitioners administered their medicines on a wing and a prayer, without a system or a method.

But this was about more than the scholarly standards of the physicians. It becomes abundantly clear from Handsch's notes about the oral diagnoses made by physicians that patients and their relatives demanded these kinds of explanations of disease processes. "They always want to know where the disease comes

---

15 Demaitre, Medieval medicine (2013).

Open Access. © 2022 Michael Stolberg, published by De Gruyter. This work is licensed under the Creative Commons Attribution-NonCommercial-NoDerivatives 4.0 International License.
https://doi.org/10.1515/9783110733549-006

from", he explained.[16] They expected the physician to tell them what was happening inside them and why they should endure the treatment he recommended. The disease name, by contrast, was apparently not of primary interest to patients and their relatives. In his notes on diagnoses communicated to patients, Handsch often did not even give the name of the disease.

The medical pathology of the time was complex and its application to specific patients was demanding. Studying it more closely reveals a world that may be foreign, even strange to today's readers – but it was a world that was consistent within itself and followed its own logic. Therefore, the following brief survey of the central concepts and explanatory elements will demand quite a lot from readers. However, a basic knowledge of the subject is necessary to develop a historical understanding of the prevalent diagnostic and therapeutic practices of the time, the images and concepts that were connected with different clinical pictures and, not least, of the interactions and conflicts between physicians and patients. Without this knowledge, essential elements and aspects of sixteenth-century medical practice and medical culture would remain impenetrable.

Morbid Matter, Fluxes, and Obstructions

For both early modern physicians and lay people, the notion of impure, harmful morbid matter at work was central to an understanding of the vast majority of diseases. It led to pathological changes in the body and produced the patient's symptoms. There were two main sources of morbid matter. First, the body was always ingesting foreign, impure, and potentially harmful substances with the food. Second, even the body's own, natural substances could spoil and fester over time, especially if they remained stagnant for a longer period in a certain part of the body.

The notion of morbid matter which accumulated in certain parts of the body combined with the growing interest in anatomy to effect a marked shift of focus.[17] Galen had already underlined the importance of local lesions. Renaissance physicians now came to see it as one of their major tasks to identify the site of the disease in the body. In the genesis of many diseases one organ in particular played a paramount role: the stomach. In a vast majority of cases it was causally involved, though often further organs such as the liver, spleen, intestine, lung, and brain played a part as well. The reason for this was the stomach's importance in Galenic

---

16 Cod. 11205, fol. 428r, "semper volunt scire unde morbus".
17 Cf. Temkin, Galenism (1973), pp. 134–141.

physiology. As we have seen, it was considered crucial for the successful concoction and assimilation of the raw, foreign matter that the human being ingested daily with food and drink. It sifted out the useless parts of the food, passing them on to the intestine. The usable rest it concocted in a first step, in which it became chyme. The chyme moved on to the liver, which concocted it to nutritious blood and discharged the remaining parts that could not be assimilated in the form of urine, yellow bile and, as some authors surmised, black bile as well. In a language that was accessible to laypeople, Handsch summed up: "The stomach is the food chest. The liver is the blood chest".[18] The nutritious blood then travelled from the liver to the individual body parts via the veins. In a third phase of concoction, the body parts absorbed and assimilated the elements that served to nourish them, while the useless rest was excreted in the form of sweat or reached the kidneys as *serum* and was excreted by the bladder.

If this first step, the concoction of food in the stomach, was disrupted, this necessarily had far-reaching consequences for the person's health. If the stomach was too weak and did not have "its natural digestion",[19] it could not concoct the ingested food properly. Likewise, the stomach and the vital heat could be overtaxed by the sheer amount and/or by the raw, cold nature of the ingested food. In both cases, raw, viscous mucus would collect in the stomach. This mucus or slime is not to be confused with the *phlegma,* the natural humor of similar mucous consistency (though pathological mucus was also sometimes described as *phlegma*). In such cases, the physician could say, as Handsch noted, "If the stomach does not digest naturally, which serves to feed the body, the result is usually mucus".[20] "A foul mucus is lying in his stomach", we read elsewhere.[21]

The same ideas can be found in a handwritten *Formula loquendi vulgariter in iudicio urinali,* compiled several decades earlier by the physician and clergyman Dr. Michael Braun. As indicated by the title, Braun offered the reader phrases he could use when examining someone's urine and that would be understood by laypeople, explaining to them the nature and causes of a disease. "Dear friend", he might say, "as the urine shows me, the basis and primary cause of the person's disease is in the stomach, in which a lot of mucus has collected and settled [. . .], which is why the stomach has gone bad and is unable to digest or turn

---

18 Cod. 11206, fol. 22r: "Der Magen ist der Futterkasten. Die Leber der Bluttkasten."
19 Ibid., fol. 126v, "nicht sein natürliche Dewung".
20 Ibid., fol. 20v: "Der Magen thut kein naturliche Dewung, was dem Leib sol Narung geben, wirt das meyst zu einem Schleim."
21 Ibid., fol. 23v: "Ein fauler Schleim ligt i[h]m im Magen."

food into nourishment for the body. [. . .] The food is further not turned into good humor but only to mucus and dirt."[22]

The notion of the stomach being congested with slimy matter was widespread and certainly not limited to physicians. A lay healer, whom Handsch's pregnant stepmother in Leipa asked for advice, also found that her stomach was "congested with mucus".[23] When the concoction in the stomach was insufficient for a longer time, producing phlegmy matter, this led to a vicious cycle. The sticky slime would attach to the stomach wall – Handsch compared it with hide glue as was used to glue wood.[24] This cool, moist phlegm that covered the stomach wall, gumming up the stomach and finally beginning to fill it, added to the cooling of the stomach and further hindered the concocting effect of vital heat on ingested food. More phlegm was produced and kept building up in the stomach.

Due to an insufficient concoction of food, chyme that was raw, viscous, and phlegmy reached the liver and threatened to obstruct it. "Your disease comes entirely from the stomach", Handsch explained to a patient. An insufficient concoction of food had not only caused him to lose weight but also led to an "obstruction of the liver" and "what should become nourishment turns into mucus."[25] If this went on long enough, chyme could flow back into the stomach. When the aging Anna Welser suffered from a febrile "rawness" ("cruditas") of the stomach, Handsch explained, "The liver is obstructed, so the food from the stomach cannot be received, has no way to pass through and therefore remains stuck in the stomach."[26] "You are obstructed around the liver, in the

---

[22] Bayerische Staatsbibliothek München, Clm 25087, foll. 5v-6r: "Lieber Freundt, also mir der Urin anzeigt, so hat die Person ihr Krancheit von erste alß von einem Fundament und ersten Ursprung uß dem Magen, in welchem sich etlich Schleim gesamelet unnd in die Feld gelegt hat, dorumb der Magen vorderpt und nicht verdewen oder zu Narung des Leibs die Speiß verkeren mag. [. . .] Es wirt auch die Speiß nit zu guter Feuchtickait verkert sonder allein zu Schleim und Dreck." According to the manuscript, the author was a physician by the name of "Micha Braun", a "plebanus" from Krems. This was probably the physician Michael Braun, who moved to Krems in 1526 to work there as a *plebanus*, i.e. as a clergyman, but also continued to practice medicine; cf. Wiedemann, Geschichte (1882), p. 60.
[23] Cod. 11205, fol. 124r, "verschleimpt". He also diagnosed an "obstruction" and a suppressed menstruation.
[24] Cod. 11206, fol. 129r.
[25] Ibid., fol. 23v.
[26] Ibid., fol. 20v: "Die Leber ist verstopfft, kan die Speiß vom Magen nicht annemen, hat kein Durchgang, bleibt also im Magen stecken." Since Handsch wrote of the "Domina Welserin" he was probably referring to the old Anna Welser and not to her daughter Philippine, the wife of the Archduke.

stomach or between the two", Dr. Kunstat explained to a sick captain.²⁷ The apothecary Balthasar, who also treated patients, employed this concept as well. From the urine of a patient, he concluded that there was a "rawness" and "obstruction" of the liver. If he didn't watch out and didn't take care of himself, he would have a fever.²⁸

Having to work with raw, insufficiently concocted *chymus,* the liver could only create imperfect, viscous, and less nutritious blood. If the first concoction was deficient and produced mucus, the second and third concoctions could not compensate, Gallo explained in the case of the sick brother of an administrative official.²⁹ The stomach and the liver were "so weakened and spoiled", the physician told the relatives of another patient, that "everything he eats is turned into mucus and bad humor."³⁰ In the same vein, Handsch told a bookkeeper that he was "overburdened with cold, viscous fluxes and mucus". What he ate and drank, was turned "for the most part into mucus and fluxes".³¹ "The blood has become viscous", Willenbroch told the wife of a guard.³² And the patients shared this idea: "In my opinion, the main cause of my ailments is bad digestion, and the stomach and liver", the sick Christoph Hasenstein wrote in a letter; "with me, all the food that is supposed to be turned into blood is turned to mucus and phlegma".³³

At times the problem was found in the liver itself, which did not produce good blood even though the stomach delivered well concocted *chymus.* A Dutch physician, for example, – this is what Handsch was told by one patient – saw the cause of that patient's disease in the liver, which was too cold and therefore unable to produce good blood.³⁴ In the case of a sick girl from Rott, Handsch even declared that the liver was the reason for the stomach's poor concoction of food. For it was the liver's task to heat the stomach above it like the coal fire heated the kettle. The weak liver, however, failed to do so and most of the food

---

27 Ibid., fol. 25r; Cod. 11205, fol. 195v: "Yr seyt verstopfft umb aber [oder, M.S.] zwischen der Leber und umb den Magen."
28 Cod. 11206, fol. 27r-v; probably Handsch was referring to the archducal pharmacist Balthasar Klössl, whom he often mentioned in his notes.
29 Cod. 11207, fol. 119v.
30 Cod. 11206, fol. 172v, "dermassen geschwecht und verterbt"; "alles, was er isset, in einen Schleim und böse Feuchtickeit verkert wirt."
31 Ibid., fol. 18v, "mit kalten, zähen Flüssen und Schleijm überladen".
32 Ibid., fol. 38r: "Das Geblütt ist verschleimpt."
33 Ibid., fol. 17v: "Ich bedenck sovil, das die Heuptursach aller meiner Gebrechen ist die böse De[u]ung, Magen, und Leber"; "alle mein Speiß, so in Blutt verwandlet werden sol, die wirt bei mir in Schleim und Phlegma verwandlet."
34 Ibid., fol. 17v.

turned into mucus instead of nutritious blood.[35] At times, physicians also suspected other pathological changes of the liver, for example a shrunken liver[36] or an induration.[37] In extreme cases, the physician might even claim that the liver was literally consumed and shrunken to the size of a chicken egg, even a walnut.[38]

If the liver produced raw, viscous, and impure blood, the rest of the body could be affected in a number of ways. One direct result was an insufficient supply of nutritious blood to the different body parts. This presented a logical explanation when patients, as was typical for many chronic illnesses, became emaciated. The patient had "no good blood in his body" Handsch judged during his time in Innsbruck after examining a farmer's urine:

"This is an old illness that has built up in him over a long time and has needed different medications, which have made him worse instead of helping him. And now his stomach has become filled with mucus, congested, and spoiled so that it can no longer serve the body. He does not feel like eating and what he eats is not properly digested and does not agree with him, and so the body loses its strength and substance. When the stomach is not well, the other body parts suffer want, just as when a landlord is sick and unable to care for the household and [therefore] no one in the house will be well; and so, the stomach is like a landlord in the body who is supposed to supply all parts with food. [. . .] Therefore, if one is to help him, one must give medicines that clear the stomach, clean and strengthen it and make it right again."[39]

Insufficiently concocted, watery and viscous blood was also a recognized cause of dropsy. Handsch explained to the girl from Rott, for example, that her belly and legs became swollen because her stomach turned most of the food to mucus instead of good blood.[40]

---

35 Ibid., fol. 39v.
36 Ibid., fol. 21v, copy of a letter by D. Phaedrus to a sick young woman.
37 Ibid., fol. 132v.
38 Ibid., fol. 14v.
39 Ibid., foll. 16v-17r: "Es ist ein alte Kranckheit, hat sich ein lange Zeit bei i[h]m gesamlet, hat auch mancherley Arzney gebraucht, die haben i[h]n mehr verterbet denn gholfffen, und ist nu[n] an dem, das im der Magen gar verschleimpt, verstopft und verderbt ist, das er dem Leib nicht mehr dienen kan, hat kein Lust zum essen, und was er isset, das wirt nicht recht verdeuet, und gedeyet i[h]m auch nicht, also kompt der Leib von seinen Kräfften und nimpt ab. Den wenn der Magen nicht gutt ist, so müssen die andern Glieder Not leiden, gleich als wenn ein Haußwirt kranck ligt, und kan die Wirtschafft nicht versorgen, so gehets im ganzen Hause nicht wol zu, also ist der Magen wie ein Haußwirt im Leib, sol alle Glieder mit Narung versorgen. [. . .] Derhalben sol man im helffen, so muß man Arzney[en] geben, die den Magen reumen, reinigen, stercken, und widerumb zu recht bringen."
40 Ibid., fol. 39v.

Another frequently observed consequence of insufficient concoction in the stomach and/or the liver were "fluxes". Physicians and laypeople understood these as the presence of liquid morbid matter that moved through the body – usually but not always following gravity – and ultimately accumulated in certain places. In the populace, fluxes counted among the ailments that were assumed or diagnosed most often until far into the nineteenth century. A flux, in early modern medical lay culture, was a disease *sui generis*. Thus, there was no question in the mind of a young church musician, for example, that his headache on one side "was fluxes".[41] A servant had the same explanation for his headache.[42] In a letter, a young merchant suffering from "buzzing in his ears" complained about the "fluxes" that woke him up.[43]

"Fluxes" also played a central role for academically trained physicians. However, they used this term not so much as a disease name but to describe causes. Many different diseases were ultimately ascribed to a local accumulation of pathological, raw, or impure matter. Fluxes in this sense were by far the most important explanation for local symptoms.

One of the most common manifestations of a "flux" was the "catarrh". The term derives from the Greek words "kata" ("down") and "rrheo" ("to flow"). "Catarrh" was understood at the time not only as the result of a cold but in a much more general sense as pathological accumulations of a watery, viscous or otherwise pathological or rotten fluid matter that flowed from the upper regions of the body, especially from the head, downward. According to Handsch, a physician could say in such cases, "It's fluxes. You have a liquid head. Cold and heavy fluxes are sinking down."[44] Explaining the complaints of a hunter, Handsch wrote, "The fluxes are flowing down from his head, have settled in his chest and are constricting his breathing".[45] Morbid matter that flowed down was also a plausible explanation for painful, swollen joints.[46] Even the dislocation of vertebrae – which could have grave consequences when a vertebra pressed on the spinal cord – could be attributed to a "catarrh", because, over a longer period of time, it dissolved the tendons that held the vertebrae together.[47]

---

41 Cod. 11183, fol. 76r-v; Handsch suspected the French disease.
42 Cod. 11206, fol. 344r.
43 Cod. 11205, fol. 102v.
44 Cod. 11206, fol. 22r: "Es sindt Flüsse. Yr habt ein flüssigen Kopff. Kalte und schwere Flüsse sezen sich herab."
45 Ibid., fol. 21v: "Die Flüsse fallen im von dem Kopff, sindt im in die Brust gesessen, machen im ein engen Athem."
46 Ibid., fol. 151r.
47 Staatsbibliothek Berlin, Hdschr. 311, fol. 18r.

As we see indicated here, fluxes were often found to accumulate in individual body parts or organs. "You have a liquid head", Handsch explained to an older man who had difficulty breathing, "and the fluxes are flowing down into your chest and lungs".[48] "You have a weak, poorly digesting stomach", he told the sick Frau von Schwanberg, "which makes mostly fluxes and mucus from food and drink. From the stomach it spreads to all other body parts. Firstly, it goes to the head as vapor; toward the heart, [causing] tiredness. To the loin [it brings] sand and stones; [moves] to the uterus, polluting it; to the feet, making them heavy; to the chest, causing difficulty breathing."[49] Even the heart could be "burdened by fluxes".[50]

A further commonly suspected and feared consequence of incomplete concoction of food to blood was that the quality and thereby the mobility of the blood changed. Here, we encounter an explanatory element that has so far been insufficiently appreciated in the history of medicine: Renaissance physicians widely also relied on mechanistic, hydraulic explanations of the kind that medical historiography traditionally described only for the iatromechanical theories of the seventeenth and early eighteenth centuries. Blood that was permeated by mucilaginous, sticky matter moved more slowly, clogged up vessels, and, in the worst case, disrupted the movement of the blood altogether: "the blood cannot move freely, it is all pain and narrowness. The nourishment cannot get through", Handsch noted down as a possible phrase to use with patients.[51] Or: "The blood is soiled, spoiled, filled with mucus and clogged; it lacks its natural flow, gets stuck and is constricted in the veins like water in the pipes."[52] Or: "The blood cannot move freely, is congested, mucous, and soiled."[53] Or: "The mucus sticks to the veins, in the liver, to the liver

---

48 Cod. 11205, fol. 424v: "Yr habt ein flussig Haupt unnd die Fluß fallen euch hinab ynn die Brust, ynn die Lungen."
49 Cod. 11206, fol. 33r: "Ir habt ein blöden, ubeldewenden Magen, der do auß der Speiß und Tranck am meysten Flüß und Schleim macht. Auß dem Magen teylet es sich in alle Glieder. Erstlich dempffts ins Haupt, gegen dem Hertzen, Matikeit. In die Lenden, Sandt und Stein, in die Mutter, verunreinigt dieselbe, in die Füsse, werden die Füsse schwer, in die Brust, schwerer Athem."
50 Ibid., fol. 183v, "von Flüssen bedrengt".
51 Ibid., fol. 24r, "das Geblütt hat keinen freien Gang, es ist alles Qual und Angst. Die Narung kan nicht durchkommen."
52 Ibid., fol. 15r: "Das Geblüt ist verunreinigt, verterbt, verschleimpt, verstopft, hat seinen natürlichen Gang nicht, steckt und engstiget sich in dem Geäder wie ein Wasser in der Roren." The German term "engstiget sich" clearly is to be understood literally here in the sense of "narrowed". As we will see, the German term "Angst" could then also refer to the physical sensation of pressure on the chest, which continues to be associated with the emotion "angst".
53 Ibid., fol. 20v: "Das Blutt hat keinen freien Gang, ist verstopfft, verschleimpt, verunreingt."

ducts like glue to a board."[54] Consequently, it was possible to justify the treatment by saying that the veins or the blood were "congested and soiled with coarse viscous mucus" and "if one cleanses the blood and opens up the clogged blood vessels, you will be healthy."[55]

Lay healers as well relied on such explanations, and patients and their relatives were receptive to them in Handsch's experience. A consumptive woman who had been in Handsch's treatment for some time told of an *empiricus* who had seen her once when Handsch was away. "It is your stomach", he had said, "and your blood vessels are congested so that the blood cannot move freely into the arms and feet." The sick woman had agreed.[56]

Similar to the way the stomach wall could gum up with mucous substance, the insufficiently concocted, viscous and mucous blood could cling to the walls of vessels like glue or pitch and constrict the vessels. One could explain, according to Handsch, that, in the same way that water did not flow well if dung or excrement lay in the water pipe, blood could not move freely, and "therefore it has to work to get through, which gives you bodily complaints."[57] One could also make a comparison with lime scale: just as calcified water pipes slowed down and diminished the flow of water, catarrhal matter clogged up the veins.[58] The doctrine of "tartar", which Paracelsian physicians began to popularize at the time, offered an analogous explanation. People knew from experience that tartar formed a sediment in wine barrels. Willenbroch, in the account of the patient, literally attributed the disease of Mathias Zobell to the sedimentation of tartar in his vessels. The overburdened stomach, said Willenbroch, had allowed the ingested wine to move on to the liver and the vessels unconcocted, where it had hardened to tartar.[59]

Viscous, glutinous, and mucous blood could obstruct not only the vessels but also the organs.[60] Organ obstructions were feared by physicians and laypeople alike, and they were one of the most common diagnoses of all. Other organs besides the liver that were particularly at risk were the spleen and the

---

54 Ibid., fol. 19r: "Der Schleim klebt im Geäder, in der Lebern, an Leberrören, wie ein Leym am Brete."
55 Ibid., fol. 15r, "mit grobem zähem Schleim verstopfft, verunreinigt"; "so man das Geblütt wider reinigt, und die verstopffte Adern öffnet, seydt ir gesundt."
56 Cod. 11205, fol. 533r: "Es ligt euch bei dem Magen und die Adern syndt euch verstopfft, das das Geblütt nicht ein freien Gang hat ynn Armen und Füßen."
57 Cod. 11206, foll. 26v-27r, "so arbeitet es zum Durchdringen, das ir must Beschwernüß im Leib empfinden."
58 Ibid., fol. 121v.
59 Ibid., fol. 146v.
60 Ibid., fol. 23v.

uterus. Obstructions hindered or interrupted the natural movement of the blood that was produced by the liver, which, according to Galenic doctrine, slowly flowed through the veins to the individual organs and body parts, which fed on it. Obstructions might also disrupt the elimination of excremental or pathological matter. When an organ became obstructed the blood accumulated inside and in front of it. Therefore, an obstruction often led to a swelling of the organ, a tumor, and, if the blood or the humors dried out, it could ultimately lead to an induration of the organ in question, which would hinder the flow of the humors even more. As we have seen, the detection of such swellings and indurations was the main reason why students of medicine in Italy learnt to routinely practice the manual examination of the abdomen.

There was moreover a risk – and this was true with regard to the obstruction of both the vessels and organs – that the slowed down or completely halted movement would produce a qualitative change in the blood. It became even more viscous and could spoil easily, might perhaps become putrid or take on other harmful properties. There was even more danger when obstructions interfered with or interrupted the movement and elimination of excremental matter. This matter was in itself already impure, putrid, and spoiled. If it accumulated in or just outside an organ or in an obstructed vessel for a longer time, it could take on even more dangerous, harmful properties. The prime example here was the obstruction of the uterus. It interfered with or prevented the elimination of spoiled menstrual blood and was considered one of the primary causes of disease in women. We will return to this later.

By now, the imagery that served as a basis for this medical thinking and for the explanatory elements as sketched out above will have become clear. In the vast majority of cases, physicians – and to all appearances their patients as well – took recourse to images of dirt, of raw waste matter, of putrefaction and rot. They explained the disease processes that were taking place within the body with an analogy to the processes of decay and putrefaction which they observed in everyday life. Animal and plant matter such as fruit, vegetables, and meat, and even pure water if it remained stagnant, turned putrid and spoiled. Quite often, these things also assumed a slimy quality, began to stink and would pass on the rot to other foodstuff or substances that came into contact with them or were only close by.

Considering all the waste matter that entered the human body or accrued there even when a person was in perfect health, the body was constantly at risk of decaying, at risk of inner putrefaction. Handsch wrote down numerous phrases that could be used by physicians to explain this to patients or their relatives. They ranged from drastic, sweeping statements that would likely be used only in front of the relatives, including "He is completely rotting out from the inside",[61] and "He is rotted on the inside, a living carrion",[62] all the way to attempts at specifying the place of putrefaction, using phrases such as "A putrid mucus is lying in his stomach",[63] "His lung and liver are rotting",[64] or, "The liver has turned to manure",[65] or "His liver is half rotten"[66] or, "His spleen has become polluted".[67] A lay healer in Leipa also told Handsch's brother-in-law Heinrich, "Your lung and liver are rotting".[68] Michael Braun explained in his *Formula loquendi vulgariter* that, with women, it could principally be added that one could see from the urine "a great impurity of the uterus that has accumulated over a long time" and "when this kind of mucus gets out of hand, headaches, fainting, and a weakness of the whole body follow, and the breath falls shallow as if she were suffocating and losing control of all limbs."[69]

Another widespread medical conviction was that a faltering blood flow and localized accumulations of liquid matter in general could release fumes and vapors. According to Braun's *Formula loquendi vulgariter,* one could illustrate this with a comparison to the steam that rose from a dunghill in the morning.[70] Along these lines, Handsch wrote, "the stomach is not digesting well, therefore clogged blood enters the veins, and it hurts wherever it goes and vapors rise as well."[71] With women, the "bad vapors" from the uterus were of central importance. They originated in the spoiled, unclean menstrual blood that flowed into it every month.[72] "Her uterus is polluted and congested with mucus", Handsch concluded from the urine of a sick woman, "bad vapors and winds rise from it to the heart, stomach,

---

61 Ibid., fol. 20r: "Er faulet inwendig gar aus."
62 Ibid., fol. 170r: "Er ist inwendig faul, ein lebendigs Oß [Aas, M.S.]." Similarly ibid., fol. 114r.
63 Ibid., fol. 23v: "Ein fauler Schleim ligt im im Magen."
64 Ibid., fol. 14v: "Lung und Leber faulet ym."
65 Ibid., fol. 126v: "Die Leber veriaucht."
66 Ibid., fol. 114r: "Die Leber ist ym halbfaul."
67 Ibid., fol. 22v: "Die Milz ist im verunreiniget."
68 Cod. 11205, fol. 196v: "Lung und Leber faulet ym."
69 Bayerische Staatsbibliothek München, Clm 25087, fol. 5v, "etlich Unrainkeit der Muter [= Gebärmutter, i.e. uterus, M.S.], die sich lange Zeyt gesamlet hat"; "wan solcher Schleim uberhand nimpt, so kumpt Haupt We[h], Onmacht, Bledikait deß gantzen Leibß unnd legt sich der Athem alß mueß sie erstecken und sind i[h]m alle Glider erschlagen."
70 Ibid., fol. 5r.
71 Cod. 11183, fol. 41, "der Magen der deuet nicht wol, darumb kompt verstopfft Blutt ynn das Geeder, unnd wo es also hinkomet, da thut es wehe, unnd steigen auch Dempff auff."
72 Cod. 11206, fol. 20v.

and head, so that she feels weariness – the stomach is bungling and listless – and sometimes it goes to her head."[73] "It is a raw humor, indigestion, and excess that fumes up into the head", a physician might say.[74] As we will see, harmful fumes that rose up from menstrual blood (or from spoiled female semen) also served as a widespread explanation of the frequently diagnosed "suffocation of the womb".

People were familiar with fumes and "vapors" that formed in the body from the everyday experience of winds in the intestines. If these did not find quick egress, they could cause severe abdominal pain. They were considered the central cause of colic. "When mucus swells up, it turns into winds that stretch the gut, the bowels", Handsch wrote on the subject.[75] "It is indigestion", one of Handsch's colleagues explained to a patient who had a stomachache, "if we don't get rid of it, it will swell and one would have to worry that worse might come of it."[76] From the intestines, fumes could move into the rest of the body. Under the action of heat, viscous, incompletely concocted matter could even give off billowing smoke. "The stomach is not digesting well", the physician might say in such cases, "if the fire in the oven is not strong enough to consume the wood, there is a lot of smoke, and in the same way vapors rise from the stomach into the head if the natural heat in the stomach is weak and it digests badly."[77]

Preternatural Heat

Images of raw, slimy matter, mucus, impurity, and putrefaction are linked repeatedly in these and similar explanations. Even if they released fumes, mucus and raw matter were usually thought of as being cool or even cold. This corresponded with the common experience that rotting animal and plant matter as well as

---

73 Ibid., fol. 35v: "Die Mutter ist ir verunreinigt und verschleimpt"; "davon steigen die bösen Dempffe und Auffblähung zum Herzen, Magen, ins Heupt, fulet also Matikeit, der Magen ist ungeschickt und unlustig, es kompt ir auch bisweilen ins Haupt."
74 Ibid., fol. 19v: "Es ist ein rohe Feuchtickeit, Undeulikeit, Uberflussickeit, die dempfft ins Haupt."
75 Ibid., fol. 19r: "Der Schleym, wenn er sich auffblähet, werden Winde darauß, die spannen die Derme, das Gedärm."
76 Ibid., fol. 16r-v: "Es ist ein Undewlichkeit"; "wirt man sie nicht hinweg thuen, so wirt sie sich auff blähen, und ist zubesorgen, es möchte was ergers daraus entstehen." Handsch gave only the colleague's first name, Andreas, probably referring to Andrea Gallo.
77 Ibid., fol. 28v: "Der Magen dewet nicht wol"; "wo das Fewer im Ofen nicht starck genug ist, das Holtz zu verzeren, so gibt es grossen Rauch, also auch dempffet es aus dem Magen ins Haupt, wenn die naturliche Werme im Magen schwach ist, und ubel dewet."

foods often showed a slimy decay or an unappetizing surface, without giving off heat. However, some diseases, above all many fevers, were typically accompanied by heat. According to the *Canon medicinae* by Avicenna, who continued to be the central authority in learned fever theory, fevers sprang from a "foreign", "extrinsic heat" (*calor extraneus*) that, starting from the heart, seized the entire body.[78] This extrinsic heat was not the same as the powerful, implanted, natural heat that was present at birth, the *calor innatus,* which vitalized the body. With a fever, it was not the natural heat that became stronger or more intense. The source of the fever's heat was different and pathological.

Here, too, one could refer to everyday life experience. Some processes of decay and rot involved heat development. Fermenting refuse and even baled-up hay generated heat. This could be transferred to pathological, unclean, and spoiled substances heating up inside the body due to rot. Patients, too, took recourse to such explanations. One patient wrote in a letter, some of which Handsch copied, "This phlegma pervades my entire body and all my limbs instead of the blood, and it clogs up the liver and all other parts with their natural passages, giving rise to an unnatural heat of the liver, kidneys, and similar parts".[79]

The foreign, pathological heat could lead to various pathological changes, if, combined with the natural heat, it affected the blood, the natural humors, or insufficiently concocted, pathological, or excremental substances:

First, the fluid matter could dry out and harden, even literally bake like bricks. As we will see later, this was the principal explanation for kidney stones, which were thought to develop from mucous matter, which could be observed in the urine of patients who suffered from stones.

Second, they could literally burn from the great heat. In extreme cases, they turned completely black as if charred. Burned yellow bile (and not only the natural black bile), for example, was seen as an important cause of *melancholia* as an illness. Excessively heated matter was further widely described as being particularly acrid, and this was true of natural humors like yellow and black bile but also of the body's other moistures and humors. They acquired a sharp, caustic quality that explained why skin ulcers and cancerous ulcers ate into the surrounding tissue.

Third, hot vapors could be released and rise up inside the body. A physician diagnosing a patient with fever and a headache might say, "A mucus is clogging

---

78 For a survey of sixteenth-century fever theories see Lonie, Fever pathology (1981).
79 Cod. 11206, foll. 17v-18r, excerpt from an undated letter by Christoph von Hasistein: "Solch Phlegma zeucht sich mir durch den ganzen Leib und in alle Glieder an stadt des Blutts und davon wirt die Leber und alle andere Glieder und derselben naturliche Genge verstopfft, darauß die unnatürliche Hitze der Leber, Nieren, und dergleichen Glieder entstehet."

up the veins. When it heats up, the fumes rise up into the head."[80] And Andrea Gallo talked to Handsch's great aunt about the "inner flames", that could rise into her head.[81] Complex causal chains could be constructed in this way. If the physician had diagnosed that mucus was accumulating in the stomach or the uterus, he could warn the patient by saying, for example, "If this mucus heats up, it will cause vapor to rise and move to the heart, make the heart tired, and to move also to the stomach and weigh on the chest. It will further rise or steam up into the head and make head complaints. It will also cause complaints in the loins and thighs."[82] "Your disease is nothing but an excessive, raw and badly corrupted humor in the veins and blood", Handsch explained to the Lord of Gilemnitz. If "the same begins to stir and rises as vapor to the head, it will cause headache and fluxes, which will fall, drop down into the chest, leading to weariness and vaporousness. Similarly, they will sink down into the thigh and bring about the nasty scabby skin change with a tearing pain. [. . .] It is only fluxes that pollute the blood. You are a fluxile person."[83] Explaining the "labored breathing", the "languor", and the "dizziness" of a female patient, Ulrich Lehner said that "from the uterus, vapors are going up against her chest, heart, [. . .] into the head".[84]

Patients were apparently familiar with such explanations and images. Archduke Ferdinand II spoke quite naturally about "flying vapors" that moved now to the heart, now to the head.[85] The idea is also found frequently in letters of patients who sought counsel. Some early modern patients even claimed they could literally feel hot vapors rising up inside them.[86]

---

80 Ibid., fol. 19r: "Ein Schleym steckt im Geäder"; "wenn derselbe erhitzt, steigen die Dunste uber sich ins Haupt."
81 Ibid., fol. 25v, "ynwendigen Brünste". Handsch did not explicity name Gallo, but in this notebook it was usually Gallo he meant, when he wrote about the "doctor".
82 Ibid., fol. 23r: "Wenn sich derselbe Schleim erhitzet, dempfft er uber sich, streicht zum Herzen, macht dem Herzen ein Mattikeit, streicht auch gegen dem [sic!] Magen, macht schwer umb die Brust, ferner steigt oder dempfft er ins Haupt, bringt dem Haupt auch Beschwerung. Also auch in Lenden und Schenckeln macht er Beschwerung."
83 Ibid., foll. 15v-16r: "Euer Kranckheit ist nichts anders, denn ein ubrige, rohe böse verterbte Feuchtigkeit im Geäder und Geblüt"; "[wenn] die selbige erregt und auffdemp[f]t ins Haupt, macht sie das Hauptwehe und Flüsse, dieselbe fallen, schießen denn herab auff die Brust, davon die Matikeit und Dampffi[g]keit. Item sie sincken hinunter in den Schenckel, und machen den bösen grindigen Schaden mit Reissen. [. . .] Es sindt nur Flüsse, die verunreinigen das Geblütt. Yr seydt ein flüssiger Mensch."
84 Ibid., fol. 30r: "Von der Mutter kommen yr Dempfe kegen der Brust, Hertz, [. . .] yns Haupt."
85 Ibid., fol. 19v, "fliegenden Dempffen".
86 For a detailed account see Stolberg, Experiencing illness (2011), pp. 142–144 and pp. 164–178.

Infection

Morbid matter, to which physicians ascribed most diseases, was characterized, albeit to different degrees, by a property that was central to an understanding of epidemics: it was able to bring about pathological changes in substances and bodies with which it came into contact. Physicians described this with the term "infection" ("infectio"), which is still part of the standard medical vocabulary today, though the meaning has changed. The term combines the Latin preposition "in", meaning "in" or "into", with the verb "facere", "to make" or "to do", in the sense of "to put into". It has its origins in the trade of the dyer. As any dyer knew from experience, a small amount of dye was able to communicate its properties – specifically its color – to a volume of liquid that was many times larger, thus "infecting" it.[87]

Everyday life experience showed that rotting, decaying, or fermenting substances could transmit their properties to their surroundings. So Handsch wrote that one could illustrate the processes in the human body by drawing a comparison with a rotting apple that "infected" other apples by touching them.[88] Elsewhere, he compared the tenacious mucus in the veins and body parts with sourdough. It clung to the walls of the veins like pitch or glue, began to move at some time and spoiled other fluids next to it.[89]

Sometimes the morbid matter was so powerful that, like in the dye-works, even a minimal amount could lead to far-reaching changes. In this case, the term "contagium" was used, derived from the Latin "tangere" ("touch") and the disease was called "contagious". Centuries before the discovery of bacteria and viruses, this explained familial aggregations of cases or household clusters as much as epidemic outbreaks. When in the house of a certain Nicolai, for example, several people fell sick with a fever within a short time, Handsch surmised that a school child or university student ("scholasticus") had infected the house ("infecit domum hanc").[90] In the time of an epidemic, large numbers of people fell sick and showed a similar disease pattern after they had come into contact with the morbid matter, or so it was believed. This could happen through direct contact with a sick person or through air "infected" with minute amounts of the morbid matter ("ex contagione aeris").[91]

---

87 Temkin, Historical analysis (1968).
88 Cod. 11206, fol. 121r: "Sicut pomum putridum ex contactu alia poma inficit."
89 Ibid., foll. 18v-19r.
90 Cod. 11205, fol. 18r.
91 Cod. 11239, fol. 19r.

The physicians of the Renaissance described a number of diseases that were generally recognized as being passed on by a contagium, and this was also confirmed by their experience. In the case of leprosy, the fear of contagion was taken to justify the systematic exclusion and isolation of the sick.[92] Likewise in the case of scabies, there was little doubt that it was contagious.[93] Handsch learned from his colleagues that dysentery ("dysenteria") was contagious as well. They had observed it with their patients.[94] Elideo Padovani also warned his students in Bologna that dysentery was dangerous to physicians and bystanders. It was common to see people who got sick simply from a badly cleaned enema syringe that had previously been used on a dysenteric patient.[95] Later on, we will be discussing two further diseases at length that were widespread at the time and were thought of as contagious by Handsch and his colleagues: consumption and the French disease.

In the case of scurvy or *scorbutus*, too, some suspected a contagium, one which was active primarily inside the body, however. Beginning in the sixteenth century, scurvy became a much discussed and widely diagnosed illness.[96] The only commonality between the "Scharbock" of the sixteenth century and today's understanding of scurvy as the consequence of a vitamin C deficiency is essentially the massive alteration of the gums, followed by a loss of teeth. Johannes Schröter, in the late sixteenth century, called *scorbutus* a "highly impure" ("impurissimus") disease and warned of the risk of deterioration and putrefaction of the blood.[97] Handsch declared scurvy more broadly as a kind of French disease ("speciem morbi gallici")[98] that originated in the spleen. When vile, liquid waste matter ("foeda humorum colluvies") flowed from there to the stomach, it "infected", by way of "contagion", the teeth and the gums.[99] Whether this implied that the disease could possibly be transferred to others is not clear from Handsch's notes.

---

92 On late medieval debates on the contagious nature of leprosy, see Demaitre, Leprosy (2007), pp. 132–155.
93 Cod. 11238, fol. 127r; Cod. 11239, fol. 19v; Handsch mentioned here as a further *morbus contagiosus* the *lippitudo*, then a term for an eye disease that was usually accompanied by secretions.
94 Cod. 11205, fol. 3r, "dysenteria contagiosa"; Cod. 11237, fol. 147r.
95 Padovani, Processus (1607), pp. 104–112, *Discursus de dysenteria*, here p. 104.
96 Mayer, Verständnis (2012); Horst, Büchlein (1615) offers a systematic contemporary treatise.
97 Brendel, Consilia (1615), pp. 190–196, cit. p. 190, undated *consilium* for the son of an unnamed nobleman.
98 Cod. 11207, fol. 143v.
99 Cod. 11183, fol. 209r, "contagione quadam dentes ac gingivas inficit". At that time, it was widely assumed that the spleen emptied the atrabiliary matter that was useless for its own nutrition into the stomach by means of a vessel whose existence modern anatomy no longer recognizes; for the anatomical and physiological ideas about the spleen, see Wear, Spleen (1977).

The devastating pestilential fevers that swept across Europe in ever new waves beginning in the late Middle Ages gained special attention for obvious reasons. Other than in times of epidemics, however, the plague did not play much of a role in the everyday practice of most physicians when compared to consumption, the French disease, dysentery, and scabies. Handsch himself survived a severe plague epidemic in Prague, but not a single case of a plague patient he or his colleagues treated is documented in his extensive notes. When patients or town governments requested their advice on preventing and combatting the plague, however, physicians had to take a stand. The plague was contagious; this they knew from experience. Even the blood let from plague patients and the washing water from cloths that were used to clean plague spots were considered very dangerous in Handsch's time.[100]

There was already an established arsenal of measures to counter the plague in the sixteenth century. Based on the assumption of a contagium whose spread could be contained by preventing direct contact with the sick or with their transpiration, measures included ship quarantines and isolation hospitals. Especially in very exposed harbor cities such as Venice, these measures were developed and enforced by medical laypeople working in the town government.[101]

Handsch lamented, however, that skepticism about the contagiousness of the plague was widespread among the population. It baffled him because people certainly separated their cattle and sheep when they suspected that a contagious disease was going around. Why did these "coarse people" and "oafs" deny the existence of a contagium with humans?[102] People had good reasons to doubt, of course. Some people fell victim to the epidemic, though it could not be shown that they had come into contact with anyone suffering from the plague. This was also recognized among physicians: at the university in Padua, Handsch learned that pestilential fevers indeed did not only begin with a contagium but could also originate in powerful inner putrefaction.[103] Further, some people remained healthy although they had come into close contact with a plague patient. Leaning on established medical doctrine, Handsch explained this with respect to one's personal physical constitution, the temperament which could cause a person to be more or

---

100 Cod. 11183, fol. 382r.
101 Vanzan-Marchini, Mali (1995).
102 Cod. 11205, fol. 280r.
103 Cod. 11238, fol. 127v; in the case of the plague, in the modern sense of an infection with *Yersinia pestis*, transmission by fleas is today considered far more important than transmission through direct contact.

less susceptible. In Handsch's experience the population referred to the will of God, however, who afflicted some with the illness but not others: "It's not that the pestilence goes from one to the other", they said, "God our Lord gives it to whomever he pleases."[104]

Obstructed Excretions

The central place of unnatural morbid matter in the pathology of the time found an immediate and powerful expression in the great appreciation of excretion. Physicians and laypeople alike considered excretion absolutely essential to maintaining health and recovering from illnesses. With its help, the body, in times of health, freed itself from the raw, impure matter that inevitably accrued during the concoction of food; even in times of health, excretion that was impeded or "obstructed" therefore signaled danger. During sickness, a fortiori, the successful excretion of morbid matter was seen as a prerequisite for recovery. According to the old teachings, a "critical" excretion changed the disease process for the good, especially on the so-called "critical" days, the seventh, fourteenth, twentieth or twenty-first, and forty-second day of the illness.[105]

From the contemporary viewpoint, excretions and the pathways they took when leaving the body were much more diverse than we would assume. For the head alone, physicians and laypeople alike considered a number of specific excretions and excretory paths. Not uncommonly, mucus of varying color and consistency ran off from the nose. The eyes constantly emitted a certain amount of moisture, sometimes tears, and, when a person was sick, also a yellowish, somewhat thick liquid. The ears led excretions outside the body in the form of earwax. A coated tongue, too, indicated that waste matter was being excreted. Barber-surgeons even had special tools made of iron or willow wood to scrape coated tongues,[106] and in some cases Handsch explicitly requested for the patient's tongue to be cleaned of viscous substance.[107] The head, respiratory tracts, and

---

104 Cod. 11205, fol. 280r.
105 Sudhoff, Zur Geschichte (1929); on the theoretical debates about the astrological or natural causes see Pennuto, Debate (2008) and Cooper, Approaches (2013).
106 Cod. 11183, fol. 63v, "quam barbitonsor mundat ferramento"; Cod. 11205, fol. 522v, "instrumento vel ferreo vel saligno"; see also Widmann/Mörgeli, Bader (1996), p. 118.
107 Cod. 11205, fol. 522 and fol. 561v.

stomach could be freed from extraneous or morbid matter via the mouth, that is through coughing, spitting, and vomiting. Some authors even thought of the hair and the beard as solidified excreta.[108]

Further excretions left the body in other ways. Via the bowels, the body freed itself of coarse waste matter from the first concoction as well as of yellow bile, which was produced in the liver during the second concoction and entered the small intestine via the bile duct. Some called the stool a "beneficium ventris".[109] Urine helped excrete the watery remains from the second and, in part, from the third concoction. This watery substance was excreted mainly by invisible transpiration and sweat, however. In this sense, Handsch termed the pores of the skin "Dempflöcher", literally "vapor holes".[110] "He is working [so hard] that his skin is smoking", he put it elsewhere.[111]

With women, menstruation was a crucial pathway for the evacuation of impure, harmful substances, and an "obstructed" menstruation ranked among the principal causes of female diseases.[112] Women therefore paid close attention to even minor irregularities in their periods, noting them with great concern.[113] "Her time comes but is nevertheless not quite right, the way it should be", the physicians heard in such cases.[114] In both men and women – as mentioned, Galenic medicine held that women possessed semen, too – seminal fluid was discharged via the genitals. Sometimes, impure, unnaturally colored, and malodorous substances issued forth, as with *gonorrhoea* in men and *fluor albus,* the common milky discharge in women.

If necessary, nature was also able to open supplementary, vicarious excretory pathways, mainly in the form of nose bleeds and hemorrhoidal bleeding. Handsch noted down that nose bleeds had a positive effect on obstructions of the brain and catarrhs.[115] Hemorrhoidal bleeding protected the body from various diseases, ranging from side stitches and pneumonia to ulcers, furuncles, and leprosy, and it also had beneficial effects with respect to kidney complaints.[116] There therefore had to

---

108 For a more detailed treatment of this matter see Stolberg, Keeping the body open (2020).
109 Biblioteca comunale Aurelio Saffi, Forlì, Fondo antico, Ms. 94, e.g. fol. 6v, fol. 31r, fol. 54r, and fol. 61r.
110 Cod. 9671, fol. 179r.
111 Ibid., fol. 164r; see also Stolberg, Sweat (2012).
112 See below the chapter on disordered menstruation.
113 The term "period" ("periodus") was already in use but referred to the regular recurrence in temporal terms (Cod. 11205, fol. 454r, "quoties venit periodus"; ibid., fol. 455v, fol. 457v and fol. 633v, "servent periodum"; Cod. 11183, fol. 392v).
114 Cod. 11183, fol. 139r, cit.; similarly ibid., fol. 10v.
115 Cod. 11210, fol. 65r.
116 Ibid., fol. 66r.

be pressing reasons before a physician would try to stanch the bleeding. Many people, wrote Handsch, whose hemorrhoidal bleeding had been treated at the wrong time fell ill soon after.[117]

The Myth of Humoral Imbalance

The disease concepts and explanatory elements we encounter here may seem foreign to the modern reader at first, but they were easy to grasp and close to people's experience of their own bodies. They had very little in common, by contrast, with the familiar doctrine of unbalanced humors and/or qualities that has often been described as the basis of early modern nosology and pathology.

In order to avoid misunderstandings, we must differentiate here: physicians and laypeople, Handsch's notes and countless other sources make clear, did believe that the temperament and the physical constitution of individuals were indeed shaped by the specific, individual blend of humors and qualities in a person's body. Physicians were therefore well advised to make this individual constitution part of their diagnostic and therapeutic considerations. Diseases as such, however, were hardly ever interpreted as deviations by degree from an ideal state of humoral balance in the body. A disease was in essence something that was exterior to the body, and in most cases, it was closely linked to exogenous, insufficiently assimilated, or spoiled substances. The treatment therefore had aim at cleansing the body, at freeing it from waste matter – and not at restoring the balance of humors and qualities.

Accordingly, in sources that reflect actual everyday medical practice we find only scattered references to the notion that diseases developed from an imbalance of the humors. Occasionally, physicians suspected a pathological accumulation of one of the four humors to be the cause of the disease. However, the close examination of such cases most often reveals that this accumulation did not apply to the body as a whole but to a specific organ or body part. Further, physicians usually suspected a concurrent pathological change of the humor in question, which now was no longer "natural". "The bile has gone into his stomach", we read in Handsch's notes about such cases,[118] or "A thick bile is stuck in his stomach."[119] "You have thick bile in your stomach, which gives you fire

---

117 Ibid.
118 Cod. 11206, fol. 177r: "Die Gall ist im in Magen gangen."
119 Ibid., fol. 28r: "Ein dicke Galle steckt i[h]m im Magen."

and heat and a lack of appetite", the patient of another healer was told.[120] "The bile is spoiled and no longer able to serve the liver; it spoils the liver and the blood," explained a Paracelsian physician to the sick Tucher.[121] This was obviously not simply about a disproportionate quantity of yellow bile compared with the other natural humors but about localized processes and qualitatis changes.

Not least of all, the fact that many physicians appreciated autopsies on deceased patients as an important source of insight underscores the power of such notions of local pathological change as opposed to the idea of humoral imbalance, which could not be seen in post-mortems. We will take a close look at this later.[122]

Certain overlaps between the explanatory models that guided everyday medical practice and the traditional theory of humoral balance can be found in the concept of *intemperies,* that is in the assumption that there could be an excess of one or two primary qualities. When physicians sought to explain a disease process, they hardly ever applied this theory to the body as a whole. But they did sometimes bring into play an *intemperies* of individual organs. As a student in Padua, Handsch attended Bassiano Landi's lecture on Galen's *Ars medica* twice and filled around 200 pages with the professor's explanations of the signs of the different forms of *intemperies* of individual organs, from the brain to the genitals. Landi discussed in detail how to identify, for example, a hot, cold, dry, or moist liver by its impaired function and the associated disease symptoms.[123]

In the sources pertaining to ordinary medical practice that I am drawing on, however, the majority of the different *intemperies* of individual organs that were thinkable in theory played no role whatsoever. There are two deviations from the ideal of an organ's well-balanced qualities, however, that we encounter repeatedly in Handsch's notes and other sources that describe everyday practice: a cold stomach and a hot liver. A sick patient named Adam Bohdanski, for example, felt that he had a "cold stomach" ("frigidum stomachum") and asked Handsch to apply an external, presumably warming and invigorating,

---

120 Ibid., fol. 23r.
121 Ibid., fol. 15r-v: "Die Gall ist verterbt, das sie der Lebern nicht mehr dienen kan, verterbt die Leber und das Geblütt."
122 See the chapter on autopsies.
123 Cod. 11224, *Dictata in artem parvam Galeni*; in Erlangen, a further set of notes on a lecture by Landi on *Ars parva,* written by Johannes Brünsterer of Nürnberg has survived. (Universitätsbibliothek Erlangen, Ms. 909, foll. 224–228).

stomach ointment.[124] An Italian physician explained to the febrile Johann Georg by contrast that his liver was overheated and that that same heat had also gone to his blood and had led to the fever.[125] Even in cases as these, the question remains whether, from the physician's point of view, the organ's *intemperies* caused the condition or whether it was only a secondary consequence. In other words: was the stomach too cold and thus unable to concoct the food sufficiently, which led to an accumulation of mucus? Or did the cold slime cool the stomach, preventing it from concocting food sufficiently?

A cold stomach did not preclude a hot liver. A hot *intemperies* of the liver could in itself, in the estimation of physicians, indicate the insufficient concoction of food in the stomach, which lead to tenacious mucus obstructing the liver, spoiling it, and giving rise to heat. Physicians in fact observed quite frequently that both occurred at the same time, which made treatment more difficult. "This is a difficult matter", the physician could say in this case, "the stomach is cold, the liver is heated". "If we give something warming for the stomach, this will harm the liver."[126] "I have a bad cold stomach and a heated liver along with much moisture, that is to say too much liquid", a sick chancery clerk explained to Handsch, likely echoing the diagnosis of another physician.[127]

On the whole, the explanatory models that informed everyday medical practice in the sources I have studied are markedly different from the pathology that, according to the notes Handsch took in Padua, was taught at universities. While it is true, on the one hand, that most of the explanatory elements mentioned earlier, above all the theory of an unnatural morbid matter, a *materia peccans*, were discussed more or less at length and explicitly in the writings of Galen and Avicenna, it is also true that in the interpretation of specific illnesses and in the everyday approach to them, the weight they were given in the sixteenth century was of an altogether different order.

At this point, the question might arise as to whether my sources offer a sufficient foundation for such generalizing statements. One could argue that the concepts applied in practice by Handsch and other physicians in Prague and Innsbruck were a specific, local manifestation of the medical practice of that time. Further, one might criticize that I lean heavily on the phrases that physicians

---

124 Cod. 11183, fol. 96r and fol. 98v.
125 Cod. 11206, fol. 23v.
126 Cod. 11205, fol. 195r: "Es ist ein schwer Ding, der Magen ist kalt, die Leber ist hitzig"; "gibt man hitzendt Ding dem Magen, so schadet es der Leber".
127 Cod. 11206, fol. 23r: "Ich habe ein bösen kalten Magen, und ein hitzige Leber, und vil Feuchtigkeit sc[ilicet] Überflüssigkeit."

considered suitable to explain disease processes to laypeople. Physicians may have used explanations and images that were not so much grounded in their own ideas as in the desire, the necessity even, to express themselves to patients and their relatives in a way that made sense to them, that corresponded to their experience.

The latter point especially is a significant objection. Handsch himself as well as the physicians in his professional environment indeed tried to make themselves understood by the sick – we will take this up again later. I will even make the case that images of impurity and waste matter in the body, which showed the necessity of evacuating and purging them, were central to learned medical practice in part because they aligned in a particularly striking manner with the expectations, the ideas, and the physical experiences of patients. When we look at other sources that describe everyday practice during the same period, however, what we see is that physicians who practiced in other geographic locations used the described concepts and images very similarly in their everyday diagnosis and treatment of the sick. And they did so even when writing in Latin and not communicating with patients and their relatives.

A clear case in point is the practice journal of the municipal physician Hiob Finzel in Zwickau.[128] Between 1572 and 1588, he documented his diagnostic assessments for approximately 4000 patients. In most cases, these were terse. Finzel usually limited himself to one or at most two diagnoses that, in the causal-analytical sense described above, aimed at identifying disease processes at work inside the body.[129] Typical examples, originally written in Latin, are, "obstruction of the mesenteric veins with febrile heat", "rawness from an obstruction", "catarrh to the sciatic [nerve/tendon?]", "weak stomach with catarrh", and "suffocation of the womb and white discharge". In about 500 cases, Finzel's main diagnosis was *cruditas,* or "crudities", that is raw, unconcocted substance. In around 160 cases, he identified a cold and/or weak stomach, sometimes connected to *cruditas* or an assumed obstruction of the mesenteric veins or the liver. The total number of patients he suspected suffered from such an obstruction of the mesenteric veins, the liver and, less often, the spleen was around 160. With about 70 patients, he determined a hot liver, sometimes connected to a cold stomach. In a dozen cases, he deemed the blood burned. With

---

128 For a detailed characterisation and analysis of this journal, see Stolberg, A sixteenth-century physician (2019).
129 The total number of diagnoses is thus significantly higher than that of the patients concerned.

more than 100 patients, he identified a catarrh, apparently in the sense of a local accumulation of morbid matter, in the area of the head, the chest, in the arm, the back, the pelvis or in the foot. Roughly 145 patients diagnosed with pleurisy, bladder and kidney stones, cough or *podagra* may, in a broader sense, also be included in this group of illnesses for which he assumed a local accumulation of raw, pathogenic matter. The two most common and often not more closely specified diagnoses were, with more than 1000 cases, suffocation of the womb and, with roughly 500 cases, fevers. Suffocation of the womb was understood to have its principal cause in the harmful vapors that rose from spoiled menstrual blood or female semen. The fevers were closely associated with the notion of an extrinsic heat. By contrast, Finzel made explicit mention of an *intemperies* only twice, one hot *intemperies* of the liver, and one hot *intemperies* that he did not describe more closely, with a patient suffering from red murrain of the foot. In two further cases, he diagnosed a *plethora*, that is to say an abundance of blood or, as the cause of epilepsy, a *plenitudo*, whereby the chosen terminology already illustrates that even in these cases, the diagnosis was not about the relation of the four humors to one another but rather about a disproportion with respect to the available space in the body, more specifically in the vessels. Finzel had studied in Wittenberg and Jena. He moved in academic and social circles that stood completely apart from those of Handsch, yet his diagnostic categories and therefore his conception of disease processes agree to a great extent with those documented by Handsch.

In surviving vernacular letter consultations, in which learned physicians explained disease processes and the hoped-for effects of their treatment to patients and their relatives, the idea of an imbalance of humors and qualities in the body likewise proves to be of peripheral importance. The roughly eighty consultations from the time around 1580, which Jakob Horst wrote to patients and their families illustrate this well. Horst did not study in Italy but in Wittenberg and Frankfurt an der Oder, and practiced in Krems (Austria), Schleidnitz and Liegnitz (Silesia), Iglau (Moravia), and Helmstedt (Principality of Braunschweig-Wolfenbüttel). Yet, Horst, too, ultimately attributed most diseases to raw, slimy, spoilt, rotten, acrid, or otherwise preternatural, pathological matter that spread out in the blood or accumulated in specific organs or places in the body. And in the same way as described above, he linked this concept to the risk of an obstruction of the vessels and organs and to an impeded or completely interrupted excretion, which required treatment. One of his favored diagnoses was that the stomach had cooled down and begun to accumulate mucus, which reached the liver and possibly also the kidneys, thus obstructing these organs. The liver and kidneys heated up even more due to the obstruction and burned the mucus, which could become acrid and caustic. Only the *intemperies* of individual organs plays a somewhat larger role in his consultations than in the sources from Handsch's circle and in Finzel's journal. Horst repeatedly linked diseases not just to a hot liver but also to a hot heart and sometimes hot kidneys and, especially in women, he sometimes found that not only the stomach but also the uterus was too cold.[130]

---

[130] Staats- und Universitätsbibliothek Göttingen, Ms Meibom 146.

External Causes of Illness

If an illness was to be understood, diagnosed, and treated, it was crucial in medical practice to identify its cause within the body, above all the nature and location of the morbid matter in question. However, contemporary medicine also paid great heed to external causes that could trigger or promote a disease. Such causes helped explain what had set a pathological process in motion in the first place. Particularly in the case of chronic illness, the seed of the sickness in a specific body part had already been present early on, indeed perhaps since birth, as people believed. When, however, it was met with, to use Handsch's words, "disorder [...] be it with eating, drinking, anger, insult, chagrin, or other symptoms", the disease became manifest.[131] In Handsch's experience, patients and their relatives demanded such an explanation. They wanted the physician to explain to them where the disease had come from and they expressed their own assumptions in ways such as, "He has eaten or drunk it" or he "had a sudden drink when [he was] heated, and so harmed the liver"; it "came to him when he got a fright", he "crossed an evil trail", or "it was done to him".[132]

Environment and Lifestyle

Physicians considered environmental influences and an individual's way of life to play a key role in the development of disease. According to the well-established doctrine of the six "non-natural things" or "res non naturales", there were six particular factors relating to an individual's life circumstances that physicians considered the triggers or "first causes" of disease: air and environment, eating and drinking, sleep and rest, exertion and leisure, the passions, and excretions. We will be coming back to these in the chapter on dietetics as it was crucial to control these factors to maintain health and fight diseases. The focus of this current chapter is on their etiological role, on their importance as causes of disease.

The famous Hippocratic treatise *De aere, aquis et locis* had already lent great weight to the influence of the air and the local environment on human health. In the sixteenth century, numerous Greek and Latin editions of the work

---

[131] Cod. 11206, fol. 125r, "es sei mit Essen, Trincken, Zorn, Harm, Bekummernuß, oder anderen Zufellen".
[132] Cod. 11205, fol. 425v: "Er hat es gessen, aber [oder, M.S.] getruncken"; "auf Hitz gehling [jäh, M.S.] getruncken, das er der Leber geschadet"; "ym aus Schrecken kommen"; "eyn böse Spur ubergangen"; "es ym gethan".

Open Access. © 2022 Michael Stolberg, published by De Gruyter. This work is licensed under the Creative Commons Attribution-NonCommercial-NoDerivatives 4.0 International License.
https://doi.org/10.1515/9783110733549-007

appeared in print.[133] As Handsch learned as a student in Padua, air was particularly important because it contributed to the production of the vital spirits and the spirits of the soul and thus had a significant influence on their quality. Healthy air was clear, delicate, and moved easily. Foggy and turbid or spoiled air and fumes, on the other hand, particularly when emanating from swamps, sewers, and burial chambers, were considered to be significant causes of individual illnesses and epidemics.[134] Certain occupations too, especially mining and metalworking, exposed the body to harmful, poisonous air. If a goldsmith fell ill, it was appropriate to say, according to Handsch's notes, "You have harmed yourself with gilding, which is a concern because of the mercury", or in the case of an ill cloth dyer, "You have harmed yourself with dyeing; the steam from the kettle went into your mouth".[135]

The fact that food first had to be concocted and assimilated already implied that its quantity and quality played a central role in health. The excessive consumption of food and the enjoyment of raw, cool, slimy food, or anything that for any other reason was difficult to concoct overtaxed the stomach and the vital heat and contributed to an accumulation of mucous, potentially pathological matter. A physician in this situation could say, "He overate. Overburdened his stomach",[136] or "Eating cold dishes makes for a disorderly stomach".[137] When asked, he could explain more closely that the disease in question came from "disorder in eating and drinking, and especially in drinking", in the course of which "bad moistures" accumulated and ultimately emptied like an overflowing pond into the body.[138] Certain kinds of food and drink on the other hand – red wine especially – were considered to have a heating effect instead and could thus amplify the effects of the extrinsic heat of a fever. In this case, the physician could explain that the blood was "heated, inflamed, burnt, spoilt due to excessive drinking".[139]

Experience taught that a moderate degree of physical exertion and movement, which did not excessively heat and exhaust the body, strengthened the limbs and enhanced the natural vital heat which then more effectively concocted

---

133 Hippocrates, De aere (1529).
134 Cod. 11210, fol. 43v.
135 Cod. 11205, fol. 192r: "Yr habt euch mit dem Übergulden verterbt, denn solchs ist sorglich wegen des Quecksilbers." "Yr habt euch mit dem Ferben verterbt, das euch der Dampff vom Kessel ynns Maul gangen."
136 Cod. 11206, fol. 171r: "Er hat sich übergessen. Den Magen überladen."
137 Ibid., fol. 172r: "Kalt Speiß essen macht ein ungeschickten Magen."
138 Ibid., fol. 119r.
139 Ibid., fol. 185v, "erhitzt, entzundt, verbrennet, verterbet, auß überflüssigem Trincken".

the food into good, invigorating blood. Moreover physical exercise stimulated the vital spirits, opened the pores of the skin, and perspiration was increased.[140]

While a person slept, the vital heat was able to concentrate entirely on the concoction of food.[141] Handsch's succinct comment on this is, "Sleep helps digestion".[142] Furthermore, the mental faculties ("facultates animales") found rest during sleep. Not getting enough sleep, on the other hand, weakened the faculties of the senses and the mind and led to the generation of raw matter ("cruditatem"). Possible consequences could even be delirium and frenzy ("phrenesis").[143]

Excretions occupied a special position.[144] In the discussions of the *res non naturales*, they often occupied the most central position, as they do in Handsch's student notes on the subject.[145] By way of introduction, he referred to the chapter about them as "a long, useful, and necessary chapter".[146] With the relatively rare exception of a very excessive loss of excremental matter, in particular of menstrual blood, excretions did not rank as a major cause of diseases, however. Not the excretions per se but their obstruction was the major issue, since they were considered the most important means by which the body could fight diseases. Moreover, leaving medicines aside, they were subject to human control to a very limited extent only, mostly through the choice of suitable foodstuffs, i.e. through one of the other non-naturals.

The emotions, finally, or, in the learned terminology of the time, the affects of the mind ("affectus animi") or passions or accidents of the soul ("accidentia animae"), were thought to have a particularly great and powerful influence on the body and on health,[147] and laypeople widely shared this belief. In Handsch's experience, patients often said that worries, grief, or fear had weakened them.[148] When sick people wanted to know the cause of their suffering, as they so often did, the physician, Handsch found, could therefore hardly be wrong when he said, "You have stirred it awake with worries and concern or fright."[149]

---

140 Cod. 11210, fol. 50v.
141 Ibid., fol. 52r.
142 Cod. 11206, fol. 185r: "Der Schlaff hilfft zur Dewung."
143 Cod. 11210, fol. 52v.
144 On what follows, see also Stolberg, Keeping the body open (2020).
145 Cod. 11210, foll. 53v-67v.
146 Ibid., fol. 53v.
147 Cf. Stolberg, Zorn (2005); idem, Emotions (2019).
148 Cod. 11205, fol. 542r.
149 Ibid., fol. 434r: "Yr habt es zum ersten Mal aus Bekummernus und Anfechtungen aber [oder, M.S.] Erschrecken erwecket."

The prominent place of the emotions in 16th-century disease theory calls for some explanation. Renaissance physicians – and early modern medicine in general, for that matter – I largely interpreted emotions to be physical phenomena.[150] Handsch's Padua notes on this echo the contemporary doctrine well, albeit with a few slight variations. In the common interpretation, which Handsch adopted, fear caused the vital heat, blood, and vital spirits to withdraw into the body's interior. The extremities and the skin became cold, the pulse weak and sometimes the "retentive faculty", the *facultas retentiva,* was so weakened by the lack of vital heat that the affected person would not be able to hold in urine and feces.[151] This was at the origin of the expression "He was so afraid that he soiled and wet himself", Handsch added.[152] Shame was a lighter form of fear. As with fear, the heat withdrew into the inside at first but was then sent in the opposite direction, making the cheeks flush.[153] In the case of anger, very hot blood gushed into the heart, and the vital spirits that streamed to the rest of the body and heated it were accordingly hot,[154] which, in the worst case, could have pathological consequences. Here, the physician might say, "His disease comes from his irritation". With joy, the vital spirits likewise streamed to the outside, and in the extreme case this would be so sudden and violent that the person would fall down dead on the spot.[155] With sadness, the heart became constricted.[156] Grief but also dread, and fear could, according to Handsch's notes, likewise have deadly consequences because the heart literally suffocated.[157]

Other contemporary texts explained this at greater length. They commonly associated not only dread but also fear with a distinct physical sensation – one which we can still relate to today – of constriction and pressure in the chest, in the area around the heart. The German word "Angst" and the English word "anguish" still show this connection: both come from the Latin word "angustia" ("tightness") or "angustus" ("narrow"). This feeling of tightness and pressure lent support to the notion that blood and vital spirits were withdrawing from the rest of the body and accumulating in the limited space of the heart and the surrounding area. The connection between fear and the feeling of tightness or

---

150 Argenterio, De morbis (1556), p. 218.
151 Cod. 11210, fol. 68r.
152 Ibid., fol. 68r: "Er hat sich vor Furcht beschissen unnd beseicht."
153 Ibid.
154 Ibid.
155 Ibid.: "Sein Kranckheit kompt im von Unmutt."
156 Cod. 11210, fol. 68r.
157 Ibid.

narrowness was so strong at the time that both physicians and laypeople sometimes spoke of "Angst", in German, when they were clearly not trying to describe the emotion but rather the physical sensation of tightness and pressure, as might occur with dropsy, for example.[158] In sum: because the emotions were explained and experienced primarily as physical phenomena it was plausible to assume that they could act as a major cause of diseases.

The Moon, Stars, and Seasons

Astrology was an important branch of early modern natural history, and learned physicians played an important role in it.[159] Medical astrology could look back on a long tradition. Medieval medicine, drawing on the ancient authorities, considered the stars and planets to have a great influence on health and human life in general. The Zurich city physician Christoph Clauser explained that "Through experience I know that the work of a physician is incomplete without considering the stars".[160] Among Renaissance scholars, however, there was lively discussion about the status and scope of astrological predictions. Some astrologers claimed that the planets directly determined the life of the individual and all future occurrences on Earth. Others rejected the idea not least of all on religious grounds. For critics, such a predetermination did not seem compatible with divine omnipotence. Less problematic and thus more palatable was the assumption that the stars merely announced the future as determined by God, even if this raised questions as to the role of man's will, which allowed for actions that ran counter to the divine plan as signaled by the stars.[161]

In the sixteenth century, astrology also played an important role among laypeople. In the upper classes, including kings and princes, so-called nativities were very popular. Based on the precise time and place in which an individual was born, they predicted the course that person's life would take, including the dangers to his or her health.[162] Wealthy contemporaries paid a fair penny when

---

158 Cod. 11206, fol. 15r.
159 See e.g. the extensive astromedical lecture by Georg Tannstetter in 1531 (Tannstetter, Artificium (2006)).
160 Wehrli, Clauser (1924), pp. 94f.
161 Kusukawa, Aspectio (1993); Brosseder, Bann (2004); Cooper, Approaches (2013); Hirai, New astral medicine (2014).
162 For an exemplary analysis of a nativity from the middle of the seventeenth century see Miller, Astrological diagnosis (1953).

commissioning such personal nativities.¹⁶³ Astrological calendars were among the most widespread kinds of printed matter, not only among the learned but among the population at large. By reading them, the reader could learn, depending on the constellations, which days were most favorable for certain activities such as sowing and harvesting, but also bloodletting, cupping, and other medical procedures.¹⁶⁴

It appears that some physicians earned considerable supplementary income by producing an astrological calendar for their native town or region each year, or by giving astrological prognoses to wealthy individuals.¹⁶⁵ Both required extensive knowledge and considerable mathematical skill. General astronomical tables which displayed the course of the planets were available. Knowing how to read them required training, however. And calculations had to be adjusted to take the specific location into account – the location where the person in question was born or the area for which the calendar was to be valid.¹⁶⁶

Some physicians became renowned for their astrological abilities. Girolamo Cardano is a well-known example.¹⁶⁷ In the practice of most physicians, however, astrology played only a very modest role, at least as we can gather from the extant sources. In the numerous medical case histories, for example, which were being published at the time, planetary constellations are mentioned only rarely. The extensive astrological practice that John Napier and Simon Forman ran in the late sixteenth and early seventeenth century was very exceptional in this respect – they based their diagnoses on the constellation of the planets at the time of consultation. Both, Napier and Forman were learned laymen, however, not academically trained physicians.¹⁶⁸ To date, no *doctor medicinae* with a halfway comparably substantial astrological practice has been identified for the time period in question, neither from England nor from German-speaking areas.¹⁶⁹

---

163 Bauer, Rolle (1989).
164 Herbst, Arzt (2019).
165 In the 1490s, for example, Johann Roman Wonnecker sent an "almanac" to the Basel authorities, which he had prepared following the regulations (www.aerztebriefe.de/id/00038998, T. Walter).
166 E.g. Melhofer, Lasstafel (1543).
167 Grafton, Cardano's cosmos (1999); Siraisi, Clock (1997).
168 On Forman's and Napier's astrological practice, see MacDonald, Mystical Bedlam (1981); Sawyer, Patients (1986); Traister, Notorious astrological physician (2001); Kassell, Medicine (2005); see also https://casebooks.lib.cam.ac.uk/.
169 For the extensive astrological activities of Johannes Magirus, who practiced around 1650 in Berlin and Zerbst, see Schlegelmilch, Ärztliche Praxis (2018).

The marginal significance of astrology in the physicians' everyday practice is also evidenced by Handsch's notebooks. The influence of the planetary constellations is explicitly discussed a handful of times only and some of these entries are mere excerpts from the works of others.[170] Thus, without naming his source, he noted in a collection of poetic *loci communes* that people who had Venus and Mars in the sixth of the twelve houses of the classical nativity were exceptional in medicine.[171] Elsewhere he remarked that three predictions of an astrologer had indeed come true for his mentor Gallo: that Gallo would embark on long, futile journeys (he had to accompany the Archduke on his travels), that he would need to be wary of a servant (one of them made off with fifteen talers), and that his wife would become pregnant and suffer a miscarriage.[172] In other entries, he expressed skepticism. The more one became an astrologer, the more one turned away from Hippocrates; this Handsch gleaned from letters he read by Giovanni Manardi (1462–1536).[173] He was moreover aware of the widely read and discussed attack on astrology that had been launched by Pico della Mirandola (1463–1494).[174] Handsch also gave a thorough account of the answer to a question he had posed to the astrologer and physician Winkelmann as to whether astrology was useful in medical practice. Handsch wrote that Winkelmann had admitted to him privately that he, Winkelmann, had only wasted his time with it. If others were defending astrology, then it was only because they did not want to admit that all their efforts had been in vain. Handsch's sober conclusion was that astrology did not contribute anything to medicine.[175]

Handsch's extensive notes on the numerous patients treated by his medical colleagues and himself over the years allow for a more precise determination of the place of astrology in everyday medical practice. It becomes clear that the physicians Handsch knew and worked with paid consistent attention to only one "planet": the moon. It was much bigger in the sky compared to the other planets and, considering the tides, its influence on the sublunary world was indisputable. At most, physicians supplemented this by considering the additional influence of the signs of the zodiac or planets. Mattioli, for instance, declared bloodletting to be particularly effective when the moon was in a wet

---

170 Cod. 11240, foll. 83v-85r, excerpts on astrology from Gaudenzio Merula's *Opus memorabilium*; cf. Merula, Memorabilium (1556).
171 Cod. 9821, fol. 259v.
172 Cod. 11205, fol. 191v.
173 Cod. 11200, fol. 126r, with a reference to Manardi, Epistolae (1557), p. 603 (book 15, letter 5); Cod. 11205, fol. 9r and fol. 564v.
174 Cod. 9666, fol. 114r-115r.
175 Cod. 11205, fol. 253r-v; so far I have not been able to identfy this Winkelmann.

zodiac sign.[176] From experience, physicians believed they knew the influence of the moon on the body and on the course of a disease, and laypeople were also familiar with this. It was observed, for example, that the goiter from which the daughter of Heinrich Hirschperger had suffered for a number of years swelled when the moon was waxing and shrank when it was waning.[177] One mother noticed that her son had his peculiar fits at new moon, full moon, and half-moon, when he would turn pale, scream, and move his right hand without saying a word.[178] The daughter of Herr von Gendorf regularly took medications at the turn of the moon, when the moon was "im Bruch" ("breaking") as people said at the time, as a preventative measure against epileptic seizures.[179] From experience, she knew that her condition would worsen then.[180] It was apparently general knowledge that epilepsy was closely connected to the phases of the moon; Handsch in this regard wrote of a "symmetria". The seizures, he wrote, were most likely to happen at new moon, full moon, and half-moon, and for this reason, epilepsy was also referred to as moon sickness ("morbus lunaticus").[181]

According to Handsch's notes, the court physicians Pietro Andrea Mattioli, Andrea Gallo, and Johannes Willenbroch considered the new moon to have particularly noticeable and generally unfavorable effects, and sometimes they even declared it to be a "contributing cause" ("concausa") of an illness.[182] In some cases, this was backed up by empirical evidence, for example when a monk suffering from pleurisy or when a febrile gardener in Ambras died precisely on the day of the new moon.[183] In the case of the severely ill wife of a chancery clerk, her convulsive fevers coincided with her monthly period at new moon.[184] The heart tremble ("tremor cordis") of Maximilian II as well tended to occur at new moon and full moon.[185] When the condition of his patients worsened, Mattioli consoled them by saying it was due to the new moon, thus characterizing it as temporary.[186]

---

176 Cod. 11207, fol. 93v; in another entry, on the administration of a purgative during an ultimately fatal course of disease, Handsch mentioned the conjunction of the moon with a planet (Cod. 11183, fol. 92r). Of course, the modern English word "lunatic" derives from the Latin word for "moon", "luna".
177 Cod. 11183, fol. 140v.
178 Cod. 11205, fol. 241v.
179 Cod. 11206, fol. 178r.
180 Cod. 11205, fol. 293v.
181 Cod. 9650, fol. 36r-39r, copy of a letter from Handsch to Adam Lehner, 11 December 1559.
182 Cod. 11183, fol. 334r, fol. 339r and fol. 404r.
183 Ibid., fol. 339r and fol. 404r-v.
184 Ibid., fol. 484r.
185 Cod. 11158.
186 Cod. 11207, fol. 97r.

When treating patients or prescribing bloodlettings or purging agents or other remedies, physicians likewise primarily took the new moon or the full moon into account, or, at most, considered whether the moon was waxing or waning. As a rule, Gallo prescribed his anti-epileptic powder the day before the new moon and in a serious case also before the full or half-moon.[187] Mattioli declined to give the old Anna Welser a purgative because the moon was exactly at half, justifying this with the opinion of common people ("propter opinionem vulgi").[188]

Insofar as the application of astrological ideas in the everyday medical practice of learned physicians was largely limited to the effects of the moon, the assumed influence of the stars had its place in the wider context of the impact of cyclical natural changes. Lunar phases essentially only differed from the seasons insofar as the latter were accompanied by perceptible changes in the air, temperature, and humidity.

Physicians considered the seasons to have great effects on internal physical processes. The winter produced bad humors and preserved them, Handsch noted. They also arose in the summer, but in the summer heat they could be more easily eliminated through dissolution ("per resolutionem").[189] With phrases such as, "The body closes itself off against the winter" and "nature and the blood close themselves off", a physician could explain to a patient seeking counsel why it was more difficult to rid him- or herself of morbid matter in the winter.[190] One basic rule in therapeutic practice, which Handsch also saw his mentor Gallo apply, was that, in the case of chronic illnesses, one should wait until the weather was warmer before administering purging agents. When it got warmer, bad humors could more easily be mobilized and evacuated.[191]

The change of seasons in March was considered especially hazardous to health.[192] This was because, as Handsch put it, just as the soil opens up in the springtime, a "mislaid bad humor" could break fresh ground within the body.[193] The canicules, too, were associated with very unfavorable effects.[194] As Handsch learned from a captain, wounds did not heal as well then and even mild injuries could have fatal consequences.[195]

---

[187] Ibid., fol. 169r.
[188] Cod. 11183, fol. 361v; Handsch wrote of quarter moons but what he meant by this was undoubtedly a quarter of a full moon cycle, i.e. half moon.
[189] Ibid., fol. 457v.
[190] Cod. 11206, fol. 176v and fol. 177r.
[191] Cod. 11205, fol. 249r.
[192] Cod. 11206, fol. 184r.
[193] Ibid., fol. 185r, "verlegene böse Feuchtickeit".
[194] Cod. 11205, fol. 249r.
[195] Ibid., fol. 150r.

Diagnosis

Within the framework of the doctrine of diseases as outlined above, the principal goal of medical diagnostics was to determine with precision the physical causes of a disease, the disease process, and the nature of the morbid matter within the body so as to target, fight, and eliminate the morbid matter in question. By contrast, the act of labeling an illness with a specific name, something that is often taken to be at the heart of diagnostics today, was of secondary importance at the time. Writing in his practice journal, Hiob Finzel often took no recourse to a specific disease name. For his purposes, it was sufficient to refer to the suspected causes of the complaints, such as rawness ("cruditas"), an obstruction of the mesenteric veins, and so on. Further, when Finzel did use established disease names – and the same is true of Handsch – these were predominantly terms like "catarrh", "suffocation of the womb", and "tertiana" (literally: "third-day fever") and "quartana" ("fourth-day fever"). These, as we will see, were closely connected with specific ideas about the underlying disease processes.

The Patient's Narrative

Except in the case of serious injuries, the physicians could not look inside the patient's body, in this time long before x-ray imaging, endoscopy, ultrasound, MRI, and other modern medical imaging techniques. For this reason, a physician's conversation with patients and, depending on the situation, with relatives, was in some respects even more important than it is today.[196] The patients' account of the history of their illness and of their current complaints provided the physician with crucial information about the nature of their disease. The physician therefore had to listen to the patient's narrative "patiently and attentively", as young Handsch learnt from one of his textbooks.[197] Supplemented by the physical appearance of the patient, what the physician learned in conversation about the patient's earlier illnesses and how they had been treated, about the patient's present way of life and exposure to potentially disease-causing external influences, helped him gauge the person's susceptibility to certain diseases as well as the likelihood of success with different types of treatment. Thus, according to Amatus Lusitanus, the "good practitioner" ("bonus practicus") had to ask

---

[196] For contemporary advice on how the physician should take the patient's history see e.g. Capivaccia, De modo interrogandi (1603).
[197] Cod. 11200, fol. 56v.

Open Access. © 2022 Michael Stolberg, published by De Gruyter. This work is licensed under the Creative Commons Attribution-NonCommercial-NoDerivatives 4.0 International License.
https://doi.org/10.1515/9783110733549-008

about the duration of past diseases and whether they had been acute or intermittent, about medications the patient had taken and the effect they had had, whether his bowel movements were easy or whether he suffered from constipation, whether he had had bloodletting done and, if so, whether he had tolerated it well or had fainted. All of this was to make sure that he would not weaken or indeed kill him with purgatives that were too strong or with excessive bloodletting.[198] At the sickbed, Handsch not only inquired about current complaints such as the quality of a patient's headache, but also about previous diseases and the person's way of life. He was very clear in his opinion that this kind of knowledge made it easier to identify a given disease and morbid matter.[199]

In his notebooks, Handsch wrote down the sometimes very detailed questions which his teachers, colleagues, and he himself asked. In some cases, he even recorded short conversations between the physician and patient or relatives, with both questions and answers. When he was consulted by an old man who had suffered from genital discharge ("gonorrhea") for fourteen years and, at the beginning, from hair loss as well, Fracanzano, for example, inquired not only about the general symptoms of the French disease but also about the color the discharge left behind on the man's shirt, which was sometimes yellow, sometimes green. He wanted to know whether the man sometimes felt a burning sensation on the palms of his hands or on the soles of his feet, whether his complains worsened in the summer and whether he sometimes coughed up blood.[200] In the case of acute fevers, the physician could ask: "Do you sometimes feel a sting or pressure in your sides?" or: "Do you feel something in your sides?" to check for the symptoms of pleurisy.[201] Especially with head complaints, Handsch intended to always ask whether it sometimes "came up" against the patient's eyes and whether she or he sometimes heard a "whistling" in the ear.[202] If kidney or bladder stones were suspected, he not only asked about pain and about sand or small stones in the urine, but also about a frequent urge to urinate, a burning sensation during urination, and reddish urine.[203] The answer in such cases could be, for example, "It's in my loins, and sometimes there is a jerking pain toward the front, too".[204] With women, asking about their period, whether it was regular and what color, was a cardinal point. And the physician might hear as an

---

198 Amatus Lusitanus, Introitus (1552), pp. 1–6.
199 Cod. 11205, fol. 265r; Cod. 11238, fol. 125r.
200 Cod. 11238, fol. 130v; presumably on the same case: Cod. 11206, fol. 78v.
201 Cod. 11205, fol. 258v; similarly ibid., fol. 265r.
202 Ibid., fol. 325r.
203 Ibid., fol 262v and fol. 403r.
204 Cod. 11206, fol. 32r.

answer, "It's not red but grayish, whitish; if it came as red blood, I'd be comforted".[205] With older women, it was important to know for how long they had not had their period.[206] If a woman suffered from white discharge, Handsch would ask about further signs of a phlegmy, obstructed or "spoiled" uterus, about swollen, heavy feet, for example, heaviness in the belly, pain in the loins, shortness of breath when climbing stairs, and a tingling sensation in the arms or legs.[207] Handsch learned from Lehner that if the physician suspected worms in a child, he could ask whether the child rubbed his nose or had bad breath.[208]

Physicians even attributed diagnostic meaning to the dreams their patients told them. Following Galen, they believed that some dreams came from the humors and the movement of humors within the body.[209] When the Baroness of Hungerkasten dreamed of soft cheese under her bed from which maggots came crawling out and into her bed, Handsch interpreted this as a sign of impurities in her body.[210] When the mother of Thomas Mitis, who suffered from an eye complaint, dreamed of water, he considered this an indication that her head was filled predominantly with watery, phlegmy matter.[211] Handsch sometimes specifically asked patients to tell him their dreams,[212] and some patients told him their dreams without being prompted, that they had dreamed of fire and fish, for example.[213]

Conversations with sick people and their relatives could also be helpful to earn the patients' trust: when the physician asked about complaints the patient had not even mentioned, this demonstrated the physician's diagnostic acumen. Yet we must not overestimate the significance of the conversation for early modern diagnostics in a stricter sense, the way medical historiography has so often done in the past.[214] Quite consistently, the diagnosis was also or indeed primarily based on "objective" procedures. Such procedures provided physicians with valuable information beyond the scope of patients' oral or written communication. They could even be employed against the patient's will, when he or she wanted to keep something secret, a possible pregnancy, for example. Today, we

---

205 Ibid., fol. 475v.
206 Ibid., fol. 448v.
207 Ibid., fol. 31v, fol. 107r and fol. 289r.
208 Ibid., fol. 245r.
209 Ibid., fol. 448v, referring to Galen's treatise *Quod animi mores corporis temperiem sequantur*; Cod. 11183, fol. 265r.
210 Cod. 11205, fol. 499r.
211 Ibid., fol. 583r.
212 Ibid., fol. 554v.
213 Cod. 11183, fol. 139v.
214 See, e.g., the influential paper N. Jewson (Jewson, Disappearance (1976)).

may consider most of the "objective" diagnostic procedures that were common at the time to be of little value. From the perspective of the day, however, they promised crucial insights.

Uroscopy

By far, the most important objective diagnostic procedure was uroscopy (Fig. 5). Usually when people fell ill in the sixteenth century, the first thing they or their relatives would do was send urine to a physician or another healer. By looking very carefully at the urine, the uroscopist, at most assisted by the report of a messenger, was to make his diagnosis and prescribe a suitable treatment. When a physician was called to attend a patient, it was likewise expected that he examine the urine very closely at the bedside, then and at follow-up visits as well.[215]

Uroscopy takes up considerable space in Handsch's notes about medical practice. He brought it up in hundreds of entries – sometimes only marginally, but frequently in connection with diagnostic and prognostic assessments that vary in their degree of detail. As we have seen, students at the leading universities of the time such as in Padua and Bologna were given extensive training in the art of uroscopy. In the early seventeenth century, Antonio Negro in Padua was even obliged by decree to take his students to the Ospedale di San Francesco after his lectures to examine the urine of patients with them.[216]

It is important to realize that uroscopy did not merely serve to diagnose diseases of the efferent urinary tract. Rather, it was considered the royal road in diagnostics and could be used to pinpoint all kinds of illnesses. According to the teaching of that period, all diseases, or at least nearly all inner diseases, with the possible exception of epilepsy and a few other outliers, could be identified from the urine. From the way urine changed with time, physicians could furthermore draw important conclusions about the development of a disease and the effect of the treatment. And so, Handsch's message to sick people and their relatives was, "A physician cannot correctly judge from the urine unless he observes it several days in a row, because the urine often changes".[217]

The general principles of uroscopy were taught in lectures and scholarly treatises, which were sometimes aided by color plates that provided a succinct summary of the diagnostic significance of the different color shades. There were

---

215 For a detailed treatment of this topic see Stolberg, Harnschau (2009).
216 Bertolaso, Cattedra (1960), p. 113.
217 Cod. 11206, fol. 20r.

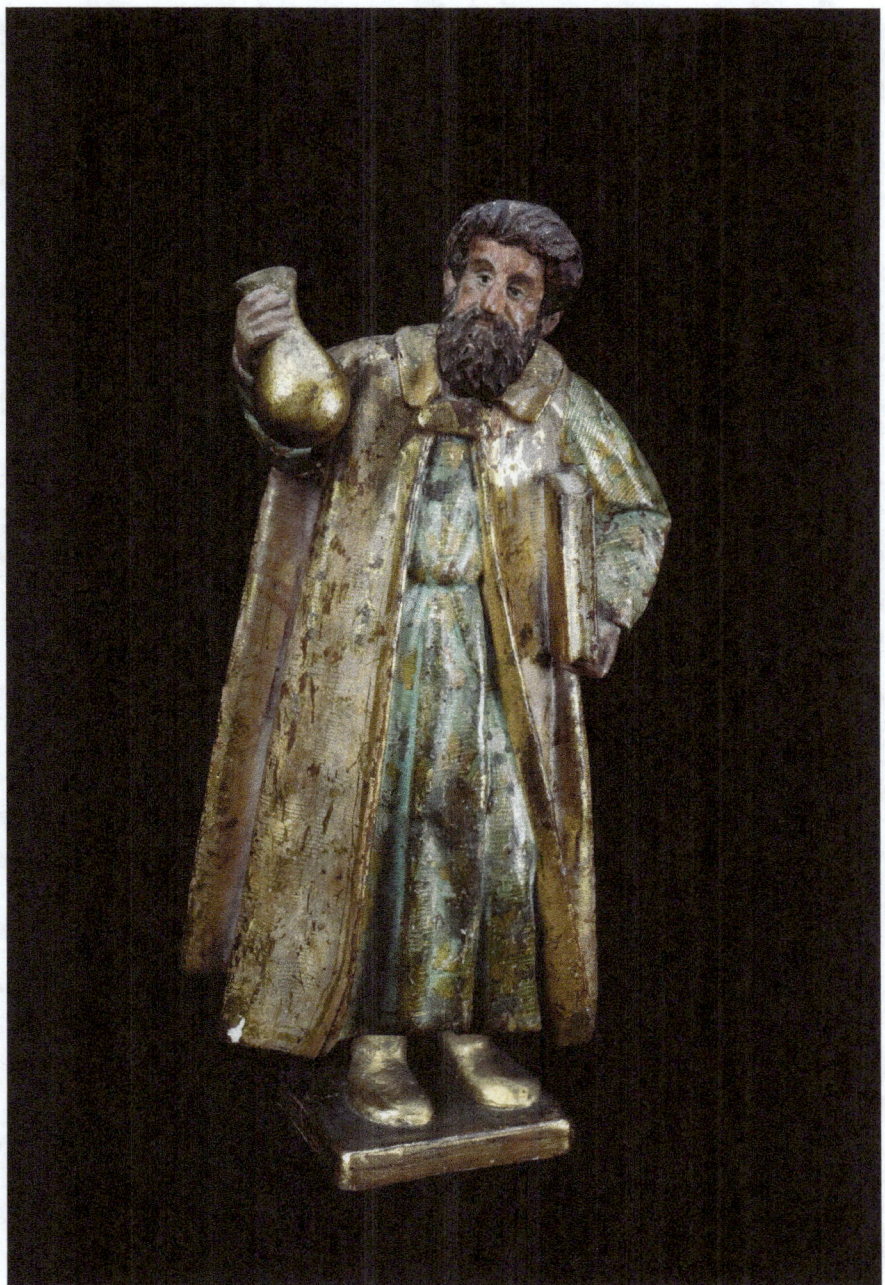
Fig. 5: Statue of St Cosmas, with urine glass, Wellcome Collection, London.

three urinary properties that needed to be determined: color, consistency or density, and visible admixtures.

Consistency and density were closely linked. Physicians could observe how thin or thick, and thereby also how transparent the urine was, by holding the urine flask up toward the window. If, looking through the full matula, the crown glass in the window ("orbiculi", "circuli") could not be made out, the urine was considered thick ("crassus").[218] The physician could also compare the urine with other liquids. Handsch filled a glass with light-colored beer from Prague and placed it next to a female patient's urine. Looking through the beer, the crown glass was much more difficult to make out than looking through the urine.[219]

An experienced uroscopist had to be able to distinguish and correctly interpret at least twenty different colors. They ranged from white or transparent like spring water to saffron yellow all the way to cabbage green, leaden, and black. Combined with the consistency, the color was thought to indicate mainly the degree of the urine's "concoction". This in turn was a reflection of the strength of the person's vital heat, which was decisive for a successful assimilation of nourishment and, as the case may be, for the concoction and excretion of morbid matter. Light-colored, thin, "raw" urine, or even urine that looked like "well water"[220] indicated a weak concoction and thus weakened inner heat, which caused impure, raw, and phlegmy substances to accumulate in the body. Dark and in extreme cases black urine, by contrast, was considered an unmistakable sign of excessive heat in the urine. The primary cause for this was the unnatural, pathological heat of fever. It could, however, also result from excessive heat that had developed in individual organs, above all the liver. The urine in this case was a vivid illustration of what was simultaneously going on in the blood and the humors: they were burning or at least assuming a harmful, caustic acridity from the heat.

Not uncommonly, admixtures could be seen in the urine with the naked eye. Settling on the bottom of the urine flask were blood, sand or small rocks, or pus; pus, an important indicator of an ulcer in the efferent urinary tract, formed a deposit more easily than phlegm.[221] Bellocati referred to a thick sediment as "burnt matter".[222] Sometimes a cloudy or stringy haze could be seen or, when the light was dim, tiny grains, also called *atomi*.[223] Volatile, vaporous

---

218 Cod. 11205, fol. 68v, fol. 263v, and fol. 264v.
219 Ibid., fol. 264v.
220 Cod. 11183, fol. 108r.
221 Cod. 11205, fol. 230r.
222 Ibid., fol. 159v.
223 Ibid., fol. 242v.

substances settled as foam on the surface. To gain better insight, especially about the sediment, physicians would swirl the urine in a circular motion. In the case of a patient who experienced pain in her shoulders and loins, this made it easier to see the sandy admixtures.[224] When Handsch found some rather coarse elements ("puncta") in his own urine, he used a circular motion to get them to settle as red sand at the bottom.[225] Handsch saw how Lehner used brushwood from broommaking to stir the urine, presumably to test if mucus would cling to it.[226] If necessary, physicians poured the liquid portion out and examined the sediment more closely, stirring it with a stick[227] or rubbing it between thumb and forefinger to better assess its consistency.[228]

The physician's findings were often finely nuanced. With a young man who suffered from a strong fever, Handsch repeatedly observed "inflamed", red urine, sometimes with foam on the surface.[229] The urine of a nobleman who suffered from colic had a "beautiful, correct color", but there seemed to be small mucous particles floating in it.[230] And his colleague Bacchus said about the urine of a patient that it was "a bad water", to which Handsch added for clarification that the blood was "spoiled, phlegmy, burnt, thickened".[231]

In the contemporary understanding, sediment could indicate the successful concoction and excretion of waste and morbid matter. Its presence was not necessarily a bad sign. Rather, clean, pure sediment in combination with a healthy, strawlike urine color indicated strong vital heat that was able to concoct food and other preternatural matter sufficiently.[232] Especially on the so-called "critical" days, physicians were hoping to find sediment, an indication that morbid matter was being successfully excreted. Lehner thus asked the young Handsch to check the urine of a patient carefully for sediment on the seventh day of the patient's illness.[233]

The uroscopist further had to take the temperament and the physical constitution of the patient into account. With a hot temperament that was governed by yellow bile, for example, somewhat pale, thin urine could already indicate a massive, pathological weakening of vital heat. With an older woman dominated

---

224 Ibid., fol. 264r.
225 Ibid., fol. 227r.
226 Ibid., fol. 257r.
227 Ibid., fol. 230r.
228 Cod. 11210, fol. 92v.
229 Cod. 11183, fol. 78v.
230 Ibid., fol. 454v.
231 Cod. 11206, fol. 25v.
232 Cod. 11205, fol. 69r.
233 Ibid., fol. 12v.

by phlegm, the same kind of urine was not thought to signal danger because of the different temperament.

Not least of all, the uroscopist had to be familiar with findings that might be deceiving. He had to know that some foodstuffs changed the color of urine. And he needed to account for external factors that might cause changes: if the urine flask was not clean, residues from an earlier use could lead to a misdiagnosis. Handsch noted that matulas had to be cleaned with lye ("lixivium") or one could put ashes in them and then wipe them clean with a small bundle of straw.[234] Urine could also be spoiled by cold temperatures. In the worst case, it could freeze.[235] If the urine was taken from the patient's house to the physician, it was inevitably shaken up. In such a case, the physician had to be careful not to mistake the foam on the surface as an indication of a disease. Moreover, according to Handsch, some women were embarrassed when they passed water "like a cow". They would send only some of their urine and pour the rest out.[236] If the physician was unsure of his assessment, factors like these that compromised the results could of course serve as a welcome excuse. "The glass was left open, the vapors have gone out", he could say if urine was delivered in an open vessel, and "furthermore you travelled yesterday; nothing clear and discriminate can be seen because it is mixed together from shaking."[237]

The diagnostic judgment which Handsch and his colleagues made based on examining urine usually corresponded to uroscopic textbook knowledge. If urine was pale, Handsch concluded that there was raw, insufficiently concocted matter in the stomach, and perhaps this would be corroborated if the patient brought up slimy vomit.[238] If pale urine had foam on its surface, this pointed to raw, unconcocted matter and vapors that rose from it, liquifying in the head and producing catarrh.[239] Considering the pale and phlegmy urine of a Prague patient, Handsch ventured to diagnose not only unconcocted matter in the stomach but also the white genital discharge that was often bashfully concealed by women, which the patient quickly admitted.[240] By contrast, when urine became cloudy only in the course of a disease, this indicated the successful concoction and excretion of morbid matter.[241]

---

234 Cod. 11183, fol. 333v.
235 Ibid., fol. 399r.
236 Cod. 11205, fol. 676v.
237 Ibid., fol. 109r.
238 Cod. 11183, fol. 40v.
239 Cod. 11206, fol. 29v.
240 Cod. 11206, fol. 33v.
241 Cod. 11183, fol. 494v.

One practical detail that we do not find as such in the standard uroscopy treatises of the time but is frequently mentioned by Handsch is the importance of collecting samples of urine at different times of the day.[242] While, in Italy, people used smaller matulas and had the physician make his diagnosis based on only one flask, Handsch found that patients in Germany used more appropriate flasks and collected separate urine samples. And so, Handsch repeatedly described two matulas with urine from the same patient, which he compared with each other, one containing the evening urine, collected before midnight, and one with the morning urine.[243] Sometimes, he even made an explicit note if a patient's urine had been delivered or shown to him in only one flask.[244] In these cases, he resolved to tell people that it "should be two flasks; one before midnight, the other after [midnight]."[245] He would add that his uroscopic examination would be incomplete if they emptied everything in one vessel.[246]

Morning urine promised more reliable information about the strength of a person's vital heat. As, during the night, the vital heat could for the most part concentrate on concoction, physicians could expect that morning urine was well concocted by comparison and therefore took on a stronger coloration.[247] Sometimes, Handsch described the urine in both flasks as identical, for example as thick, whitish, and slimy (which suggested kidney or stone complaints). Sometimes physicians observed significant differences. For example, the urine could be light and clear in one flask but cloudy in the other,[248] or the first urine was colorless and showed foam on the surface, while the second had an intense coloration and showed a lot of reddish sand at the bottom.[249]

On the basis of the urinary findings, physicians and patients sometimes engaged in a lively communication, which helped the physician further refine his diagnosis. With one patient, for example, Handsch observed a red, quite thick, almost buttery urine. Looking through the urine at the bottom of the matula, he could make out no more than the whitish outlines of his fingernail, and he found no admixtures. He explained to the patient, "your liver is obstructed; this

---

242 Ibid., fol. 87v.
243 Occasionally, for example in the case of Philippine Welser, Handsch mentioned three glasses, perhaps because patients also got up in the middle of the night (Cod. 11204, fol. 1v, "vidi urinam in tribus vitris"); in the case of a nobleman with fever Handsch even referred to four glasses (Cod. 11205, fol. 637v).
244 E.g. Cod. 11205, fol. 448r.
245 Ibid., fol. 210v.
246 Ibid., fol. 19v.
247 Ibid., fol. 17r.
248 Cod. 11183, fol. 450r.
249 Cod. 11205, fol. 257v.

is one root of your disease. This is why you sometimes have complaints in the pit of your stomach as well as in your side". The woman answered in the affirmative, "yesterday I almost suffocated and today I have stitches in my right side, and sometimes between the shoulders", which, to Handsch's mind, confirmed his diagnosis. The sick woman added, "I'm coughing and my chest feels weighed down; I can't expectorate", which led Handsch to conclude that vapors also rose from the liver to the windpipe, taking her breath.[250]

Uroscopy also allowed physicians to offer their patients visual proof of pathological changes in their bodies. Handsch wrote that one could tell women that their uterus or blood had become polluted and could ask them to collect their urine in a matula for three days. When the urine then became foul and spoiled, he could explain that this impurity was found in their blood. His sister Sabina had in fact asked him to come see her so she could show him.[251] Other physicians, too, so he heard, sometimes showed bystanders a patient's urine, if only so they could see that it was sufficiently "concocted".[252]

This brief overview already shows us that the diagnosis of an illness based on urine was a demanding process. It required a great deal of experience to identify the many natural and pathological variations and from there to correctly conclude which disease processes were happening in the body. Learned physicians agreed that, even with a lot of experience, errors in judgment happened easily. The contemporary medical literature warned emphatically of the dangers involved in a shameful false diagnosis and prognosis.

Researchers in the history of medicine have sometimes misunderstood these warnings as a blanket criticism of uroscopy as such and have concluded that uroscopy had fallen into disrepute among physicians. The skepticism and criticism were, however, not aimed at uroscopy per se, but rather at the widespread practice of diagnosing diseases based on an examination of urine alone, without seeing the patient, even without taking into account any additional information about his or her physical condition, medical history, and present symptoms.

Pieter van Foreest complained that if you asked the peasants who brought the urine about the sick person in question, they simply stood "like a stick, just as if they were mute". When they did say something after a while, they explained that they had wanted to hear it from him, had hoped "you would see it in the water, and this is why we came to see you."[253] Handsch took the same line: "The cow doctors and itinerant practitioners have gotten the common

---

250 Ibid., fol. 78r.
251 Cod. 11206, fol. 32r.
252 Cod. 11205, fol. 566v, on a certain doctor Abraham.
253 Foreest, Uromanteia (1620), pp. 228f.

people used to thinking nothing but that one can see this and that and the other thing in the water, but people like us, who have spent their money at high schools for many years and stay at one place, have to go by reason instead of pulling the wool over people's eyes and then moving on the following day like the itinerants do."[254]

In Handsch's experience, messengers sometimes even lied to the physician and deliberately obscured the patient's identity, for instance, when women were unsure whether or not they were pregnant or when widows were embarrassed to consult a physician because people might say, if she "had a young man, she'd soon be well again."[255] Handsch thought that he had to be on high alert when messengers claimed that the urine was "from the country", "from the village", or had been "dropped off". Physicians even had to consider the possibility that patients were pretending to be the messenger only when really they were bringing in their own urine.[256]

Handsch experienced these kinds of deceptive maneuvers personally. For several days, he had been treating the Baroness of Hungerkasten, who suffered from the symptoms of *suffocatio uteri*. When he visited again, he was handed some urine with the demand: "See if it is a man's or a woman's". He knew that his patient's son was also sick, and the urine seemed to him of a deeper color and "more feverish" than that of the female patient, so he stated that it was the urine of a man. The women laughed at him, because it was the urine of the mistress after all. Commenting on the event, Handsch wrote, "I turned very red". At least he had a chance to get his revenge. The next day, following his request, his stepmother got a woman to take her urine to a lay healer, a converted Jew, and had her tell him that the urine was from a farmer in the village. The healer concluded that the supposed patient had a whole range of serious complaints and conditions and noted them down on a piece of paper: "the water shows a disease that he has had for a long time and that is still stubborn, not wanting to let off; he has complaints of the stomach, which is burdened with bad humor of the phlegmatic kind; he also has pain in his left side, is short of breath, has consumption of the lung, of the spleen, is sad and strangely dim in the head because of the vapors that rise from the stomach into the head, like a daze; the fluxes also fall back into the arms and legs, cause him pain; he has a fever and chills [?], which is soon followed by heat, tightness, fainting and he is even getting very thin." Handsch's stepmother did not suffer from any of these complaints.[257]

---

254 Cod. 11205, fol. 408r.
255 Ibid., fol. 326r; for the context see the chapter on the suffocation of the womb.
256 Ibid., fol. 326r and fol. 436r.
257 Ibid., foll. 437r–438r and foll. 441v–442r.

When Handsch's brother-in-law once sent only his urine, Handsch replied that he had a "stitch in his left side", adding, however: "Examining the water is only half of what needs to be done; you have to add in the oral account. [. . .] I certainly see something in the water but also tell me what ails you and I will be all the more able to counsel you thoroughly and, with God's mercy, help you."[258] Handsch remarked disparagingly of the uroscopic diagnoses – silly and worthless in his eyes – which his colleague Johann Willenbroch made without any knowledge of the symptoms and the particular circumstances.[259]

Yet, a physician had to think twice about whether he could afford to deny giving a diagnosis based on urine alone, while many lesser educated healers did so every day, satisfying their clients. It might easily be interpreted as incompetence if he refused. Patients and their relatives could expect a good physician to be able to identify a person's sex and diseases from the urine alone. Even a renowned court physician like Andrea Gallo was sometimes willing to diagnose diseases based on nothing but the urine that was sent to him.[260] It was Handsch's firm intention to make no judgment without knowing whose urine he was examining.[261] But he, too, repeatedly gave in to the wishes of his patients and their relatives. For example, he concluded from a whitish urine alone that the "person" had a "bad stomach" and "complaints in the limbs".[262] In another case, he stated, "The water shows that the person has an unclean stomach and does not feel like eating".[263] As we will see, he sometimes even just pretended that he was making a diagnosis based on the urine.[264]

Apart from all of this, it is evident that we must not assume, based on their objections, that physicians were universally contending with a refusal on the part of messengers to give them information. We can see from Handsch's notes that many relatives were quite willing to tell the physician the patient's identity and symptoms. For example, a worried husband who took his wife's urine to Handsch told him she had "pain in the body and in the area of the loins". She had not eaten in three days and felt hot at times. She was wondering if she might perhaps be pregnant.[265] And a messenger who delivered the urine of a young husband with a suspected case of the French disease said that, starting a year ago, the

---

258 Cod. 11206, fol. 12r.
259 Cod. 11205, fol. 459r.
260 Ibid., fol. 210v.
261 Ibid., fol. 459r.
262 Ibid., fol. 210v.
263 Cod. 11206, fol. 25r.
264 See Part III.
265 Cod. 11183, fol. 11v.

patient had suffered particularly at night "from pains in the limbs and around the hips". The following day, the patient even appeared in person.[266] In some cases, patients would also send a short letter along with their urine.[267]

At the sickbed, when they had the patient in front of them, learned physicians continued to value uroscopy as one of the very best diagnostic procedures. This is amply illustrated by the countless urinary findings preserved in Handsch's notes. Handsch thought that physicians were well advised, even if there was no medical reason, to inspect the urine very carefully when in the presence of laypeople, to swirl the liquid in a circular motion and to examine the sediment. This would increase the esteem for their uroscopic abilities.[268] He wrote about a Paracelsian who inspected the urine of a patient again and again in the course of half an hour, apparently entering the sick room with the matula in his hand and exiting the same way.[269]

The importance of uroscopy in everyday medical practice declined only slowly in the early modern period. It was still in widespread use even among eighteenth-century physicians.[270]

Coproscopy

Urine was especially well suited for diagnostic purposes because it was voided regularly several times a day and was transparent, allowing for easy detection of changes and admixtures. In many cases, however, an inspection of other excretions also promised important insights. Ranking first here was stool. Known as coproscopy, the diagnostic inspection of feces had a long tradition. Its value had been pointed out as early as in the Hippocratic writings.[271] In the early modern period it was among the aspects of medical practice that physicians experienced as particularly unpleasant and a threat to their dignity. Yet, coproscopy was also a recognized procedure, one that was valued as revealing diagnostic tool in many cases. Stool, too, showed many shades of color, varied more strongly than urine in its consistency, and, like urine, could exhibit admixtures that shed light on the nature of a disease.

---

266 Ibid., fol. 460v.
267 Ibid., fol. 139v.
268 Cod. 11205, fol. 324r.
269 Cod. 11183, fol. 158r.
270 Stolberg, Decline (2007); Kinzelbach/Neuner/Nolte, Medicine (2016), p. 112.
271 Knoedler, De egestionibus (1979).

As a student, Handsch noted succinctly: "We have to examine the excrements."[272] And in Brünsterer's student notes we read, "We inspected the excrements."[273] We thus must picture the professor and his students standing in a circle around a sick person's chamber pot, solemnly inspecting its contents. Dark stool that was blackened by black blood, Handsch wrote in his notes from Padua, was a very bad sign.[274] Mucous admixtures or worms sometimes made the cause of the disease immediately apparent.[275] "He inspected the stool and recognized a weakness of the stomach", a student of Benedetto Vittore's noted.[276]

Coproscopy was a diagnostic procedure that patients and their relatives expected their physician to do. Without being prompted, they kept their stool – sometimes several stools[277] – in a bowl or chamber pot, or put a sample on a piece of paper for the physician to inspect during his next visit.[278] If any instruction was needed at all about the best way to collect the stool, Mattioli had to tell a patient explicitly to stop putting his stool in water in future but instead into a clean vessel to allow for a better assessment.[279] With an "ad cautelas", Handsch highlighted how a sick tutor had praised his physician with the words, "I like that you inspect the stool". If necessary, physicians could request a twig to lift the stool and could state, for example, that it looked like frog or toad spawn.[280]

Lay healers looked at their patients' stool as well. Apparently finding the wording useful, Handsch even noted down what one of them, a monk, had said to a man with a cold stomach: when the stool was lifted with a twig, it began to "jiggle".[281] At the court of Ambras, old Anna Welser, too, used coproscopy. She made a knot at the end of a piece of brushwood that she used to stir the stool, which made it easier to lift the mucus from it.[282] And so, even venerable professors like Handsch's teacher Comes de Monte alias Panfilio Monti were unable to forgo inspecting feces, stirring the stool, as we learn from Handsch's detailed

---

272 Cod. 11210, fol. 59v.
273 Universitätsbibliothek Erlangen, Ms 911, fol. 36: "Inspiciebamus excrementa".
274 Cod. 11210, fol. 59v.
275 Cod. 11238, fol. 74r-v; the doctrine of the so-called "spontaneous generation", of the emergence of (lowly) creatures from putrefaction, was still widely accepted at the time, even though Handsch, already as a student, noted the doubts that Aristotle had expressed (ibid., fol. 74v).
276 Biblioteca comunale Aurelio Saffi, Forlì, Fondo antico, Ms. 94, fol. 21r.
277 E.g. Cod. 11205, fol. 460r: "Vidimus singulas sedes in pelvi".
278 Cod. 11206, fol. 169v; Cod. 11205, fol. 524a r, "in charta, erat mera viscida pituita".
279 Cod. 11207, fol. 139v.
280 E.g. ibid., fol. 17v, fol. 83v, and fol. 202r; Cod. 11205, fol. 460r.
281 Cod. 11205, fol. 124v.
282 Cod. 11204, fol. 71v.

description, with a small stick or brushwood and lifting a part of it to check if it contained mucus.[283]

In his extensive notes about the treatment of sick people in Prague, and later Innsbruck, Handsch brought up coproscopy less often than uroscopy. Nevertheless, it was firmly established in everyday medical practice. Handsch relied on coproscopy as much as the court physicians Andrea Gallo and Johann Willenbroch. He would note down, "We inspected a stool; it was rather large, dense, and yellow".[284] In the case of a jaundiced patient, Handsch checked if the stool was white. Still today, this is considered an important clinical sign for an occlusion of the bile duct, one of the main causes of jaundice.[285]

Like uroscopy, coproscopy made it possible for physicians to trace the course of a disease along with the effects of their treatment, especially after they administered a laxative. We learn from Handsch's notes, for example, that Adamus Bohdanzky, after he ingested rhubarb, produced a voluminous stool shot through with seed-like grains. A subsequent stool, by contrast, was liquid, and when they lifted it with a forked twig, a lot of mucous matter clung to it.[286]

Sputum and other Excretions

In the contemporary understanding, urine and stool were part of a whole spectrum of excretions whose appearance and/or smell offered important insights into the internal bodily processes of a sick person in general and into the nature of the morbid matter in question in particular. As we have seen, physicians at the time linked a number of secretions and excretions and even hair to the function of ridding the body of impure, harmful substances during times of health, and of morbid matter in times of sickness. Some of them could also be used for diagnostic purposes. A rather unappetizing coated tongue, for example, was a further recognized route of excretion for morbid matter and also contributed to the diagnosis.[287]

In patients with diseases of the respiratory organs, the sputum held much information about the nature of the disease. Purulent sputum, for example, pointed to an ulcer in the lung. The explanation was that the sick body used this pathway to rid itself of the morbid matter. As Hippocrates and Galen had

---

[283] Cod. 11238, fol. 88v, on a visit to an old patient he made together with Comes de Monte: "Prima visitatione aspexit feces et cum baculo movit ad marginem".
[284] Cod. 11205, fol. 555r.
[285] Ibid., fol. 575v.
[286] Cod. 11183, fol. 90r.
[287] Ibid., fol. 120r.

stressed, Handsch wrote, physicians needed to observe and know how to classify nuances and changes in the sputum. To do this correctly required years of experience. The sputum of a consumptive patient, for example, whom Da Monte visited with his students at the hospital, proved to be "non-uniform, foamy, delicate, and partly concocted". The thicker, greenish, purulent part came from one side of the lung, explained Da Monte, the foamy part from the other. Da Monte also claimed that the foam arose from an admixture of the vital spirits, which were unable to enter the thicker, foul, and purulent portions. The green color indicated that the substance was of a raw and malignant nature.[288] During a visit to a patient with an *empyema*, a localized collection of pus in the lungs, Musa Brasavola taught his students in Ferrara a little trick that helped determine whether the sputum contained pus, which, he explained, was mostly the case with consumptive patients. The students were to have the patient spit his sputum into a glass filled with water. If the sputum consisted only of phlegm, it would float on the surface. Pus, however, would soon sink to the bottom, even if it was mixed in with mucus.[289] Handsch found this "experimentum" in Musa Brasavola's commentaries on the Hippocratic aphorisms.[290]

Hematoscopy

In the prevalent conception of the day, one could expect that with many diseases morbid matter was getting mixed in with the blood or that the blood itself was pathologically altered. Blood could normally not be observed by physicians, except when it left the body in the form of a nosebleed or other bleeds. However, when a physician had bloodletting done on a patient in his presence or was shown the blood in a bowl afterward, he could examine it thoroughly and draw his diagnostic conclusions.[291]

Handsch learned early as a student that the constituent parts of blood could be distinguished if one let the blood sit in a vessel for some time. The serum, which was somewhat similar to urine, rose to the top. Yellow bile formed a foam, black bile sank to the bottom, blood and phlegm remained in the middle.[292]

---

288 Da Monte, Consultationum (1565), coll. 459f.
289 Biblioteca Ariostea, Ferrara, Collezione Antonelli, Ms. 531, foll. 17v–20r.
290 Cod. 11205, fol. 164v, "sputum pthisicorum"; cf. Brasavola, In octo libros (1541), p. 776 (commentary on book 5, aph. 11).
291 On hematoscopy in the seventeenth-century medical practice see Schlegelmilch, Magnificent work (2016), p. 157.
292 Cod. 11210, fol. 54v.

When a disease was in progress, certain changes could become visible. For example, Handsch described the blood of one of Trincavella's patients who had tertian fever as "black", which indicated pathological heat in the body. The patient was a peasant ("rusticus") who had worked in the hot sun. After the blood had sat for a while, a small amount of a light, grayish liquid became visible, and it seemed as if a little pus had settled on the coagulated blood.[293] At such occasions, students also learned some practical tricks. In the case of a young melancholic man, for example, Handsch noticed that Comes de Monte poured off the watery portions that had collected in the upper part of the vessel. He showed Handsch some yellow-tinted foam on the remaining blackish mass, which he interpreted as an admixture of yellow bile. Separating the black, coagulated mass, he was able to see something "atrabiliary" in it.[294]

It was with good reason that Handsch was already instructed in the art of hematoscopy when he was a student. In everyday practice, a close examination of let blood promised important insights which, in some cases, could go significantly beyond what could be observed in the urine and feces.

As bloodletting was usually performed by a barber, physicians were often absent and did not have the opportunity to inspect the blood personally. Nevertheless, Handsch in his notebooks wrote down hematoscopic findings for a whole array of patients, some of which he had observed personally and some of which were based on the reports of others. The color of the blood already yielded important information. The topmost portion of let blood could be "yellow and watery",[295] whitish,[296] grayish,[297] or greenish.[298] Blood that was too watery could indicate impending dropsy.[299] But most importantly, if blood looked "burnt", blackish ("subniger") and in individual cases even pitch black, this pointed to an excessive heat in the blood and the inside of the body as a whole, something that was especially typical for someone ill with fever.[300] Blood taken from the gravely ill Katharina von Loxan was even collected in three portions, each in a separate small bowl, to ascertain possible differences in color, apparently between the

---

293 Cod. 11238, fol. 71r.
294 Ibid., fol. 125r.
295 Cod. 11207, fol. 210v.
296 Cod. 11183, fol. 433v.
297 Ibid., fol. 399r.
298 Cod. 11205, fol. 138r.
299 Cod. 11206, fol. 177r.
300 Cod. 11183, fol. 46v, fol. 72r, fol. 450v; ibid., fol. 453r, "erat niger, nam calebat febriliter"; Cod. 11205, fol. 668v; Cod. 11207, fol. 92v; ibid., fol 152v, on the black blood of Martinus, the teacher of noble boys, which, according to his own account, was evacuated by bloody cupping.

blood that came from the area near the bloodletting site and the blood that subsequently flowed from deeper inside the body.[301]

As in coproscopy, practitioners also commonly dipped brushwood, small twigs, or a piece of wood into the bowls with blood. They wanted to see how the blood stuck to it, which allowed them to conclude how "viscous", "phlegmy", or "congested" the blood was in the body.[302] When the Duke of Ferrara had bloodletting done on himself during his stay in Innsbruck, his court physician, as Handsch noted with interest, caught the draining blood on pieces of paper to judge its color and consistency.[303]

Sometimes admixtures and coatings could be noticed, which indicated the nature of the morbid matter. A young man, for example, had very "inflamed" or "ignited" ("inflammata") urine. He said that a woman had let his blood and that it had been "as black as frogspawn", with large yellow bubbles on the surface.[304]

Another important aspect of hematoscopy, which it again shared with uroscopy, was that physicians sometimes let the blood sit for a while and observed how the different parts settled in different areas of the glass. After three hours, greenish black foam of a "repulsive" shade developed on the black blood of one sick person, for example.[305] When Jacobus Camenicenus used a piece of wood to examine the blood of a patient with a growth on his testicle, he found that the blood had developed a thick skin, as if from suet or tallow. He thought that if one were to wash out all of the liquid, the skin would remain in the vessel like a bubble.[306] With other patients, the blood assumed an unusually firm, gelatinous consistency after less than ten minutes, followed by the precipitation of a grayish watery liquid.[307]

Ideally, physicians could show patients and their relatives the pathological changes in the collected blood, describing and explaining the changes as proof that the bloodletting had been necessary and that the diagnosis was accurate. "You have a heated liver", Handsch explained to a jaundiced patient, "and the [blood] letting did you good, otherwise we would have had to worry that it

---

301 Cod. 11183, fol. 411r.
302 Handsch repeatedly metioned a diagnosis of "obstructed" blood; e.g. Cod. 11205, fol. 207v and fol. 406v.
303 Cod. 11183, fol. 470v.
304 Cod. 11207, fol. 196r.
305 Ibid., fol. 93v.
306 Cod. 11183, fol. 218r.
307 Ibid., fol. 450v.

might develop into pox or an abscess or ulcer on the liver or lungs."[308] Handsch wrote down a whole range of phrases that he could use in this situation. He might say as a warning, "This is congested blood, spoiled, very bad blood; an abscess could easily develop from it",[309] or: "The blood is heavy",[310] or calmingly: "The blood is perhaps a little liquid and phlegmy but not too much, and otherwise its color and consistency is quite good; you might well become old with it"[311] or: "The blood is not bad, only too abundant".[312]

Laypeople trusted in the possibilities of hematoscopy. They described the blood they had collected from bloodletting if the physician was unable to see for himself, or they quoted the assessment of the bloodletter. Their blood was "black", they would tell the physician, for example.[313] They even expected – as with uroscopy – that a skilled physician would be able to correctly identify the blood of a particular patient if they sent him the let blood of several different patients.[314]

Pulse Diagnosis

Feeling for the pulse of patients played an important role in medicine, beginning with the medical training of students, and with good reason. Though in the final analysis its explanatory powers were limited, pulse diagnosis had a well-established place in everyday medical practice. Physicians examined the patient's pulse not only when seeing him or her for the first time, but if possible on every subsequent visit so they could monitor the course of the disease and the effect of the treatment. Handsch underlined the importance of this approach to a noble patient, explaining that treating him without seeing him in person was very difficult because of the necessity of feeling his pulse regularly.[315]

In hundreds of entries, Handsch wrote what he and other physicians felt when they took a patient's pulse. There was "the greatest art in the pulse", he noted in one entry. Anyone could feel if it was fast or slow, but there was much more to recognizing the "steadiness", the "proportion" and similar pulse

---

308 Cod. 11205, fol. 576r.
309 Cod. 11206, fol. 121r.
310 Ibid., fol. 177r.
311 Ibid.
312 Ibid.
313 Cod. 11183, fol. 72v, "sanguinem ex aperta vena fuisse nigrum".
314 Cod. 11206, fol. 109v.
315 Ibid., fol. 94v and fol. 149r.

qualities.[316] The differentiated language used by physicians to describe pulse qualities is impressive and illustrates their efforts to register even very fine nuances. The pulse beat could be frequent ("frequens") or rare ("rarus"); it could swell quickly ("velox", "celer"), increasingly ("subceler") or slowly ("tardus"),[317] and it could be hard ("durus", "durusculus"), large ("magnus"), "high" ("altus"), full ("plenus"), broad ("latus") and strong ("validus") or small ("parvus", "parvulus"), subtle ("subtilis"), sluggish ("exilis", "languidus"), empty ("vacuus"), tiny ("exiguus") or even "quasi nullus". If the pulse was "withdrawn" ("pulsus retractus"), it hid itself, so to speak, within the body.[318] With a variable, irregular pulse ("pulsus inaequalis"), the quality of the pulse beats changed, with some being stronger or faster than others.[319] In the case of several patients, Handsch described the pulse as vermicular ("vermicularis")[320] or as "convulsive".[321] He also observed a kind of double beat ("pulsus quasi bispulsans").[322]

Pulse irregularities drew special attention. Describing the pulse of the gravely ill Johannes Kekeritz, for example, Handsch wrote that it was "sometimes slow, sometimes fast, sometimes steady, sometimes skipping a beat", and when the patient seemed to be nearing his death his pulse jumped.[323] With another patient he observed three times that there was a pause after every fifth beat.[324] In such cases, physicians could explain, "the pulse is strange and uneven, ruined".[325] Some patients complained about these kinds of irregularities of their own accord. "It seems to me as if my heart were trembling", a patient explained.[326] The pulse of Emperor Maximilian II, who suffered from palpitations, was described by the physicians who treated him as slow, rare, small, and intermittent.[327] Handsch noticed such irregularities with himself as well. It could sometimes happen that his

---

316 Ibid., fol. 103r.
317 It is not certain that Handsch and the doctors he worked with consistently distinguished between a "fast", namely rapidly swelling individual beat ("celer") from a "fast" ("frequens") pulse in the sense of an increased pulse rate.
318 Cod. 11183, fol. 457r; Cod. 11238, fol. 123r.
319 Cod. 11238, fol. 128r.
320 Cod. 11183, fol. 421r.
321 Cod. 11205, fol. 159v; Cod. 11238, fol. 123r.
322 Cod. 11183, fol. 372v.
323 Ibid., fol. 24r, "inaequalis modo tardus, modo celer, modo continuus, modo intermittens unum tactum" and ibid., fol. 27r, "saltum elevationis".
324 Ibid., fol. 269r.
325 Cod. 11206, fol. 162r.
326 Cod. 11183, fol. 99v.
327 Cod. 11158, fol. 1r.

pulse seemed to pause or that it even skipped every second beat, and sometimes he felt two fast beats in between, and then the pulse was slow again.[328]

Handsch routinely took the pulse on both arms to detect possible differences.[329] He did so in order to compare the two sides but also because he wanted to emphasize for the patients and their relatives how diligently he worked, as he admitted.[330] One time, he believed he could feel an intermittent pulse on the right arm but not on the left.[331] Another time, he was unable to feel any pulse on the right arm, but he admitted to himself that he might not have felt for it correctly.[332]

The pulse mainly gave an indication about the vital force, the *robur vitalis*[333] or *virtus vitalis*, and the power of the vital spirits, which, according to the prevailing teachings, flowed from the heart via the arteries to the rest of the body, vitalizing it.[334] As such, the pulse was especially significant for prognosis in cases of diseases with complications. If the pulse was very weak or could no longer be felt, this often was a sign of impending death.[335] Patients knew this. In the case of a sick chancery scribe, Handsch therefore refrained from feeling the pulse at great length. He did not want to give the impression that the pulse was about to disappear.[336]

To tell more accurately how strong the pulse was, and thereby the vital force, physicians increased the pressure of their finger on the vessel and checked if the pulse could still be felt.[337] It was a good sign if this was the case.[338] Physicians told an episcopal official that he would die – correctly, as it turned out – because they felt his pulse beat disappear under the pressure of the finger.[339] In the case of a gravely ill young gardener at Ambras, Willenbroch advised that he be given his last rites because his pulse was as frequent and fast as never before and disappeared under the increased pressure of the fingers.[340] Lehner shared with Handsch that, with seriously ill patients, he felt the pulse additionally at the

---

328 Cod. 11183, fol. 99v and Cod. 11205, fol. 217v.
329 Cod. 11205, fol. 319v, "utrumque s[em]p[er] exploro."
330 Cod. 11206, fol. 149: "Ad ostendendam diligentiam tange ambos pulsus."
331 Cod. 11183, fol. 137r.
332 Ibid., fol. 258r.
333 Ibid., fol. 488r.
334 Cod. 11210, fol. 80r; Handsch quoted Fracanzano.
335 Cod. 11183, fol. 123r.
336 Cod. 11205, fol. 319v.
337 Cod. 11183, fol. 406r; Cod. 11205, fol. 297v.
338 Ibid., fol. 441v.
339 Ibid., fol. 196r.
340 Cod. 11183, fol. 404r.

heel, because the parts that were farthest away from the heart died first. If he could still feel a pulse there, death was not immanent. If he could not, the patient was in great danger.[341] Handsch resolved to follow Lehner's example.[342]

Compared to uroscopy, however, feeling the pulse resulted far less often in a specific diagnosis. The fevers were the most important exception. Here, Handsch, without any additional characterization, was often content to describe a pulse as "feverish" ("pulsus febrilis", "pulsus cum febre"), or he noted explicitly that the pulse was "without fever" ("sine febre", "pulsus non febricitans").[343] The most distinguishing characteristic of a *pulsus febrilis* was that it was accelerated. Physicians could explain the reason for this to patients, saying: "When the heart is overburdened with unnatural heat, the pulse cannot keep its natural pace but goes faster".[344] In many cases, the diagnosis of a fever was beyond doubt because the symptoms were so clear, with patients being hot to the touch and complaining about exhaustion, thirst and feeling hot, or having shivers. However, sometimes physicians diagnosed a febrile disease primarily based on the pulse,[345] or pulse diagnosis allowed them to identify a specific type of fever disease, such as putrid fevers.[346]

Physical Examination

Generations of medical historians have claimed that early modern physicians did not touch their patients with their hands to examine them physically or that they did so only rarely, exceptionally. As we have seen in Part I, this is a profound misjudgment. In places like Padua and Ferrara, aspiring physicians were thoroughly trained in manual examination, in particular of the abdomen. Manual examination of the patient's abdomen was common practice elsewhere, too. Handsch's first medical teacher in Prague, Ulrich Lehner, instructed him at the sick bed that he "is to palpate the upper abdomen".[347] Later, Gallo likewise explained to him that "with all diseases, the upper abdomen has to be palpated".[348]

---

341 Cod. 11205, fol. 2r.
342 Ibid., fol. 13r and fol. 130r; Cod. 11207, fol. 15r.
343 E.g. Cod. 11183, fol. 88v, fol. 277v, fol. 282r, fol. 295r, fol. 373r, fol. 398v and fol. 409r; Cod. 11205, fol. 116r; Cod. 11207, fol. 17v.
344 Cod. 11206, fol. 129v.
345 E.g. in the case of sick Giulio Gallo (Cod. 11238, fol. 136r).
346 Cod. 11238, fol. 128r.
347 Cod. 11205, fol. 587r, "ut tangerem hypocundria".
348 Cod. 11207, fol. 236v: "In omnibus morbis exploranda tactu hypocundria".

Ultimately, Handsch resolved to examine patients with his hands as a matter of principle at the beginning of each sick call.[349] Benedetto Vittore in Bologna used his own hands to ascertain that a patient's liver was enlarged.[350] To Heinrich Wolff as well – who studied in Montpellier – it seems to have been the most natural thing to palpate a patient's upper abdomen, concluding from what he felt and from the patient's account that the man could not be saved.[351]

This appreciation of the possibilities of manual examination must be seen in the light of the contemporary doctrine of diseases, as detailed above. Localized accumulations of morbid matter as well as obstructions and indurations of individual organs were thought to play a key role in the development of numerous diseases. Insofar as the respective areas could be reached with the fingers, the manual examination was an obvious way to gain further insight.[352]

In his notebooks, Handsch wrote about many cases in which he or Mattioli, Gallo, Willenbroch, Alessandrini, and other physicians in his professional environment did physical exams, touching and palpating patients with their own hands. Sometimes, expressions like, "while palpating" ("ad tactum")[353] or a simple summary of findings allow for the possibility that physicians only referred to the account of the patient or bystanders. With occasional findings that are expressed in German, such as her "left breast" is "hard and swollen",[354] it is even quite likely that they correspond to a patient's or relative's oral account. In most cases, however, verb forms such as "I palpated" ("tetigi"), "I palpate" ("tango") or, referring to another physician, "he palpated" ("tetigit") leave no doubt that physicians did these exams personally.

With fever diseases, physicians often only touched the surface of the skin, putting their hands on the patient's head and forehead, hands, or the heart

---

349 Cod. 11205, fol. 561r.
350 Biblioteca comunale Aurelio Saffi, Forlì, Fondo antico, Ms. 94, fol. 87r-v, "tetigit tumorem" (23 November 1541); Vittore's colleague Matteo Corti found a "manifest hardening" around a patient's spleen, in turn, in addition to a large tumor which reached down to the pubic bone (Scholz, Consiliorum (1598), coll. 340–344).
351 Letter from Wolff to Johannes Posthius, 16 February 1571, ed. in Kühlmann/Telle (2001), pp. 646f.: "Tactis hypochondriis et visis urinis cum deploratum morbum esse viderem".
352 Cod. 11207, fol. 136r, "oportet eam tangere" ("one has to touch her"), on the case of a woman with upper abdominal complaints which Gallo attributed to constipation rather than pregnancy.
353 E.g. Cod. 11183, fol. 23v, on the sick Johannes Kekeritz, who complained of "gravitas ad tactum" ("heaviness on touching") on the right side of his chest; ibid., fol. 439r, on the sick janitor.
354 Cod. 11206, fol. 33v; see also Cod. 11207, fol. 211r, "si tanget, thut es ym wehe, wie es ym geschwuricht were" ("when he touches it, it hurts, as if it were ulcerous").

region to check if it was heated.[355] Sometimes Handsch could already feel the "emitted" heat when he was just approaching the skin with his hands.[356] In addition, Handsch learned from Mattioli how one could use one's sense of touch to tell measles from petechiae, the small red dots in the skin that occurred with a number of other illnesses. Measles felt uneven, while the petechiae in the skin could not be sensed with the fingers.[357]

Touching the tongue was common as well. Handsch noted that as a rule the tongue had to be not only looked at but also touched with the finger and examined to see if it was dry or moist.[358] He frequently wrote down his findings from this procedure.[359] Andrea Gallo and the court surgeon Hildebrand, too, touched patients' tongues with the finger because they wanted to know whether they were dry or rough.[360]

If dropsy was suspected, physicians squeezed the abdomen with their hands from both sides and listened for the typical gargling noise, or they analyzed the sound produced by a soft tap of the hand.[361] They also pushed one finger into the swollen limbs to see whether dimples remained visible for some time.[362] These are all clinical signs that are still recognized in medical practice today.

Depending on the clinical picture, Handsch and his colleagues touched or palpated different body regions. In the case of injuries, they could search for a bone fracture. When Collinus was gardening and it seemed to him as if something had "burst in his chest, as if a rib had broken", no fracture could be discovered by palpating the painful area.[363] When a poor woman with a growing goiter came to see Hildebrand, Handsch palpated it and found it large and hard.[364] In the case of a nineteen-year-old young man who had had sexual intercourse with a maid, Handsch not only looked at the man's penis but even

---

355 Cod. 11206, fol. 102v: "Tangere frontem ad comperiendum calorem", Handsch wrote as a motto; examples in Cod. 11183, fol. 78v; Cod. 11205, fol. 146r, fol. 159v and fol. 299r; Cod. 11206, fol. 171v; Cod. 11207, fol. 203v.
356 Cod. 11205, fol. 307r, "per evaporationem".
357 Cod. 11207, fol. 190r; the term "petechiae" is still used today for small red spots in the skin, as they occur especially in disorders of blood clotting.
358 Cod. 11206, fol. 152r, "non tantum videnda, sed etiam digito attingenda, explorandaque an sit arida vel humida."
359 Cod. 11183, fol. 196r; Cod 11205, fol. 299r.
360 Cod. 11183, fol. 341r; Cod. 11207, fol. 17r.
361 Cod. 11183, fol 443r.
362 Cod. 11207, fol. 98v, "remansit fovea post compressionem"; similarly Cod. 11183, fol. 425r and fol. 443v.
363 Cod. 11183, fol. 84r.
364 Ibid., fol. 383r.

pulled back the foreskin – apparently with his own hands ("reduxi") – and found a white, dry secretion.[365] With another patient, he palpated the painful groin area and the left testicle, which seemed to him to be larger and warmer than the right.[366] Gallo, too, did not balk at palpating patients' testes.[367]

In the majority of cases, manual examinations focused on the abdomen, occasionally on the area around the navel,[368] but mainly on the *hypochondria* just below the ribcage, that is on the upper abdomen. For this, patients had to lie down flat on their backs.[369] Sometimes Handsch simply wrote, "I palpated the upper abdomen" ("tetigi hypocundria") or simply "I palpated", or, relating to other physicians, "he palpated".[370] But often Handsch also noted down specific findings: "I palpated the right upper abdomen and when I pushed on it, he said that it hurt".[371] With another sick person, he felt a resistance as if from a drumhead.[372] A third patient felt pain when the base of his stomach was palpated and squeezed together. The physicians suspected an *apostema*, a localized accumulation of morbid matter, in the neighboring liver.[373] A "lethargic" patient moaned when Handsch palpated his right upper abdomen, saying "how much it was hurting him".[374] With some patients, the upper abdomen was tense,[375] or an induration of the upper abdomen was accompanied by a slightly swollen belly.[376] The painful, swollen left upper abdomen of a jaundiced woman was indurated toward the navel; the entire abdomen of a patient felt hard.[377] An induration might be palpated in the area of the stomach toward the left,[378] or the area of the spleen might hurt under pressure from the outside and was somewhat indurated.[379] When Mattioli fell ill himself, Willenbroch and Gallo palpated his upper abdomen thoroughly. They pressed in different places, one

---

365 Ibid., fol. 51v.
366 Cod. 11205, fol. 260r.
367 Cod. 11207, fol. 206r.
368 Ibid., fol. 196v.
369 E.g. Cod. 11205, fol. 539; Cod. 11207, fol. 75r and fol. 107v.
370 Cod. 11183, fol. 51v, fol. 118v and fol. 281r.
371 Ibid., fol. 107v; similarly ibid., fol. 296v; similarly Cod. 11205, fol. 447r, "tetigi in sinistro, iuxta fundum stomachi, ibi ad tactum dixit se dolere."
372 Cod. 11183, fol. 412v.
373 Ibid., fol. 119v, "cum tangeretur et comprimeretur ei fundum stomachi, sensit aliquam aggravationem."
374 Cod 11205, fol. 300r.
375 Cod. 11183, fol. 140r.
376 Ibid., fol. 220v.
377 Cod. 11207, fol. 201r and fol. 213r.
378 Cod. 11183, fol. 412r.
379 Cod. 11205, fol. 285r.

after the other, and compared. They arrived at the conclusion that the upper abdomen was not equally soft throughout and that a certain tension could be felt in the area of the liver.[380]

In uncertain cases, a manual exam could prove decisive in establishing a differential diagnosis. With a noblewoman, Mattioli at first suspected an *apostema* in the uterus, whereas Gallo thought the liver was obstructed. During another visit, Mattioli palpated the liver area and found pain on pressure, whereupon he assented to Gallo's assessment.[381] Negative findings as well were highly diagnostic. Handsch sometimes made a point of noting down that liver and spleen or the upper abdomen in general did not hurt during palpation, or that he had not felt an induration.[382]

Occasionally, physicians found the result of their palpation confirmed by a postmortem dissection. In the case of a dropsical woman, for example, who had complained of pressure pain in the liver area, the liver proved to be large, hard and its surface was rough, and two pea-sized stones were found in the gall bladder.[383]

Learned physicians were not the only practitioners who used their hands when diagnosing a patient. It was common practice also among the barber surgeons, and Handsch was open to learning from them. He owed the knowledge of how to sense with the fingers whether or not a swelling contained pus to one barber surgeon in particular. One had to push on the lump with one finger while holding another finger on the skin near the swelling to see if one could feel the gurgling movement of the pus flowing out.[384] Lay healers also felt for the liver or the spleen sometimes. For example, one patient recounted that an old woman had palpated his spleen, which she found obstructed and indurated, and had stated that he was becoming dropsical.[385] Patients and their relatives were very obviously familiar with the possibilities of manual examination. One patient's husband, for example, described in surprising detail a "hardening" ("quaedam duricies") that stretched out from the woman's chest cavity to below the hypochondria and all the way to her navel. Also, the belly and loins were fuller than usual. He suspected her missed period was the cause.[386]

---

380 Cod. 11183, fol. 160r-v.
381 Cod. 11207, fol. 22r.
382 Cod. 11183, fol. 80v, foll. 108v–109r, fol. 255v, and fol. 270v.
383 Ibid., fol. 289r.
384 Ibid., fol. 35v and fol. 429v.
385 Cod. 11205, foll. 220v–221r.
386 Cod. 11183, foll. 79v–80r; the husband, in his written account, may have only quoted the diagnosis of a local healer. The wife died soon afterwards.

Therapeutic Practice

Under the telling title "Good Advice and Little Medicine", Hal Cook has argued that sixteenth-century learned English physicians, setting themselves off from their lesser-educated competitors, primarily conducted themselves as advisors or counselors, indeed, as moral authorities. According to Cook, they saw their main task not in the treatment of diseases but in giving their patients detailed advice that was tailored to their individual constitution, thereby instructing them on how to lead a healthy life.[387] A completely different picture emerges from my study of continental European sources.[388] Advice on healthy living played only a modest role in everyday medical practice as soon as one looks away from royal patients or patients of very high standing. The principal task of the physician was the successful treatment of disease. Handsch's countless notes on the effectiveness (and failure) of therapeutic efforts made by himself and other physicians point in this direction, as do the preeminent place of therapy in many published *curationes* and *observationes* and the collections of *experimenta*, that is "tried and tested" recipes that physicians compiled for their own use.

Two basic approaches can be distinguished in the curative medical treatment of disease of the sixteenth century, namely a causal one and a specific one. Both approaches aimed at combatting and eradicating the illness as such, unlike "palliative" treatment, which, in the contemporary understanding of the term, only "cloaked" the complaints. The aim of a causal treatment was to counter the pathological process within the body and/or to support nature in her battle against the disease. A specific treatment, on the other hand, relied on the hidden powers that inhered – as experience had taught – in specific medicinal plants and medications.

Treatment with medicinal plants known as specifics – we will be returning to this in greater detail later on – engendered considerable problems for the physicians' public image. It put them in dangerous proximity to the medicine of the non-academically trained healers, the *empirici*, as physicians often called them, who, according the physicians' critique, relied only on their all too often

---

387 Cook, Good advice (1994).
388 For seventeenth-century England, Cook notes a striking change in the ideal, away from the physician as an advisor, and a more active therapeutic role, which threatened the professional authority of the physicians (ibid., pp. 21–29). The extent to which the conditions in England and in continental Europe were really that different in the sixteenth century – for example, due to a greater dependence of English physicians on a small number of wealthy patients – and the extent to which the printed medical sources used by Cook may convey a distorted picture of ordinary medical practice in England is open to debate.

 Open Access. © 2022 Michael Stolberg, published by De Gruyter. This work is licensed under the Creative Commons Attribution-NonCommercial-NoDerivatives 4.0 International License.
https://doi.org/10.1515/9783110733549-009

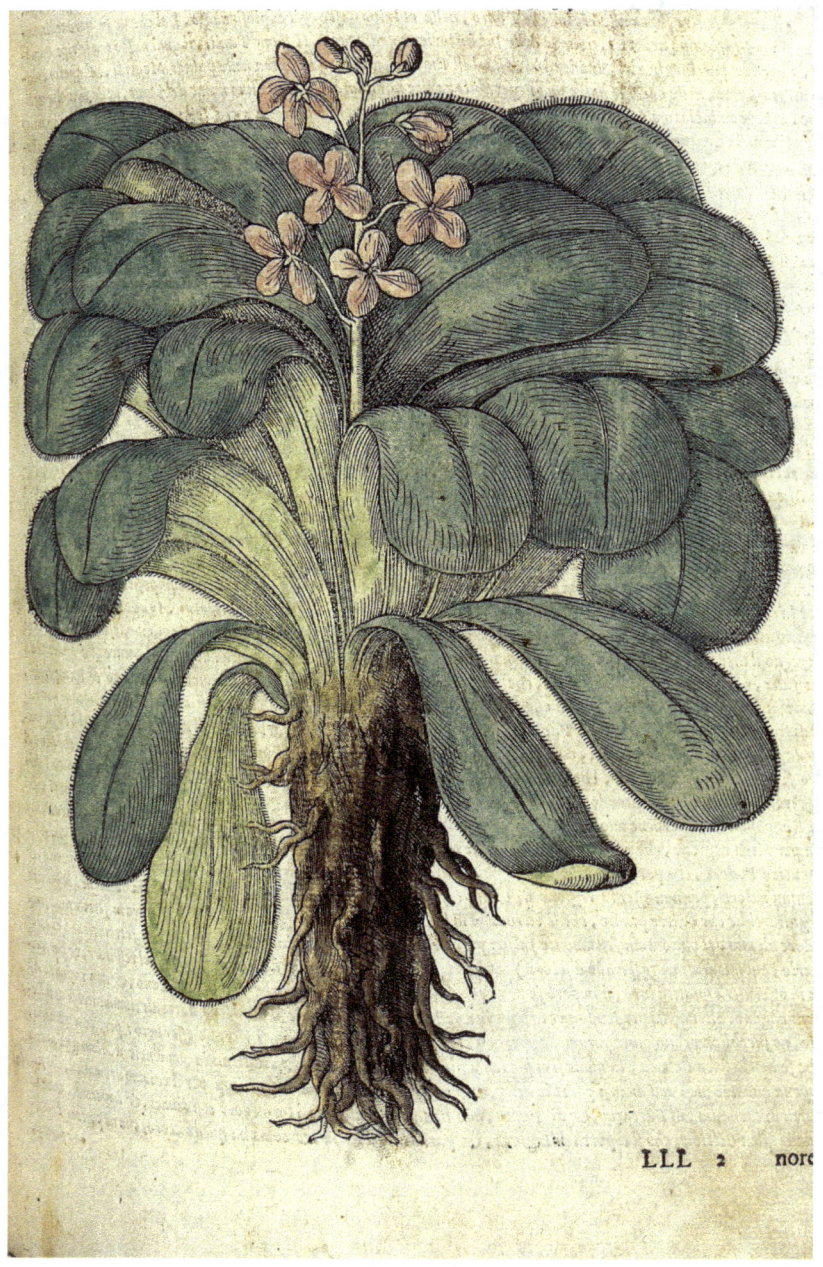

Fig. 6: Rheubabarum in: Pietro Andrea Mattioli, I discorsi nelli sei libri di Pedacio Dioscoride Anazarbeo, Venice 1568, Wellcome Collection, London.

deceptive experience when treating patients. The causal approach to treatment, on the other hand, accorded far better with the contemporary ideal of the rational physician who, thanks to his vast knowledge of the literature and his ability to decipher the mysterious pathological processes within the body, was able to target and influence the forces at work there. The causal approach was central in medical curricula and teaching activities and predominated by far in day-to-day medical practice.

Because the vast majority of illnesses were attributed to a harmful, preternatural fluid or volatile matter, efforts to treat the internal cause of an illness generally involved an emptying or purging of the morbid matter. In addition, physicians turned – especially following a successful purging of morbid matter – to remedies that would "strengthen" or "restore" (*roborativa, confortativa*) individual organs and their faculties.[389] Particularly widespread were the *cordialia,* that is heart-strengthening remedies; the term "cordial" for a fortifying remedy or stimulating preparation continues to be in use today.[390] Handsch praised sweetened wine with *amarella cerosa,* among other things.[391] Other widely-used preparations were *manus Christi,* confections, and other heavily sweetened remedies.[392] Serving as *stomachalia* were bitter substances like zedoary[393] and the aloe-containing *hiera picra,* which Gallo praised as an excellent remedy for the stomach.[394] Still today, we find traces of this tradition in the present-day use of bitters for the stomach.

Cleansing and Purgative Remedies

By far, the most common means of treating illness in the early modern period was administering purgatives. In a literal sense, these were cleansing remedies; we find the same linguistic root in "purgatory" (Latin: "purgatorium"), where the soul was cleansed of its sins.

---

389 Cod. 11183, fol. 381v.
390 Ibid., fol. 374r.
391 Cod. 11207, fol. 195r.
392 Cod. 11183, 488v; Cod. 11207, fol. 224v; at that time, "manus Christi" could refer to various medicines, including rose sugar with musk, a remedy which, according to Hieronymus Brunschwig, strengthened the heart and brain (Brunschwig, Großes Destillierbuch (1512), fol. 152r); the term was also used for castor oil.
393 Cod. 11183, fol. 478v, "Carophylli" and "Zedoaria".
394 Cod. 11207, fol. 208v.

A purgative was considered to be any remedy that promoted the evacuation of impure matter. In widespread use were cassia, manna, and rhubarb (Fig. 6), but there were numerous others. The aim in administering purgatives was to free the body – generally via the bowels, and less often via other passageways – of the raw or putrid pathological humors to which the vast majority of illnesses were ascribed.[395] Handsch, following Gallo, gave the illustrative name of "cacatorios" to remedies that emptied the bowels.[396] The central position of purgatives in the treatment of illness reflected the paramount significance of insufficiently concocted waste matter and of foul morbid matter of all kinds in the contemporary understanding of dieseases. In the rare diagnosis of *intemperies*, which did not involve morbid matter, purgatives were not indicated.[397]

If morbid waste matter had amassed in the stomach and/or intestines, one could hope to empty this matter directly. With their own eyes, people could see the stinking, slimy matter that came out.[398] As a fundamental principle, it was indicated for the bowels to be cleansed at the outset of treatment so as to get rid of the worst of the waste matter.[399] But purgatives also served to void waste matter and morbid matter found in the rest of the body. Here, a physician could explain, for example, that "The purgative will cleanse the blood".[400] In such cases – Handsch brought this up repeatedly in his notes – the physician usually had to first administer preparatory remedies, however.[401] The idea was to mobilize the morbid matter through the use of "reducing" (*minorativa*) or "softening" (*lenitiva*) remedies, to expediate its concoction as much as possible through *digestiva*, and to open the way to the bowels for it.[402] According to Handsch, one could explain, "Before the purgative, one has to give light drinks that soften, separate, and strip off the coarse blood and slime and open the obstruction" and that afterwards the purging would go well.[403] Here, physicians took recourse to warming medications in the form of sweet syrups and electuaries,

---

[395] Cod. 11210, fol. 57v.
[396] E.g. Cod. 11205, fol. 557v and fol. 593v; Cod. 11207, fol. 129v.
[397] Cod. 11207, fol. 45r, on Gallo's criticism of physicians who all too often purged; the occasion, however, was the Emperor's trembling heart, a disease which at that time could only be indirectly attributed to a morbid matter (cf. Heusinger, Das zitternde Herz [2021]).
[398] Cod. 11204, fol. 28r, "multum phlegmatis eduxerunt cum stercoribus".
[399] Cod. 11183, fol. 410v.
[400] Cod. 11206, fol. 168r: "Die Purgatz wirt das Geblütt reinigen".
[401] Cod. 11210, fol. 58r.
[402] Cod. 11205, fol. 312r, on Ulrich Lehner's "ordo curationis"; similarly, referring to Avicenna's *Canon medicinae*, Cod. 11240, fol. 2r.
[403] Cod. 11205, fol. 595r: "Man mus vor der Purgatz leichte Trenckel geben, die das grobe Blutt und Schleym erweichen, zertrennen, abstreiffen und dieVerstopffung eröffnen".

which supported the work of the vital heat.[404] Explaining this process to an elderly patient, Handsch said that they "soften and open the obstruction in the veins so that the bad humor may follow in the purging".[405] Handsch noted down how one might explain this to future patients: "The slime is caked on, glued on; before giving the purgatives one has to use the syrups to soften, detach and strip if off, like one has to use soap that eats or bites into the dirt, because without it the water washes nothing off."[406] Another formulation was: "One first has to separate and collect the bad humor that is mixed and blended into the good blood using syrups, and open up the veins inside, so the purgative will not draw out the good with the bad but only the bad, and likewise so the passageways in the veins do not remain obstructed."[407]

Physicians and patients alike measured the efficacy of a purgative above all by the number of stools it produced. It was often between five and ten. One sick young nobleman, for example, had nine "jiggly" "snaking" stools after taking a purgative.[408] For the wife of a chancery clerk, it was twelve glistening, slimy stools.[409] With powerful purgatives, patients occasionally reported significantly more bowel movements. After taking a purgative, Philippine Welser first defecated fourteen times and later twenty times more. Her stomach was subsequently in turmoil, but calmed down again after she ate and drank wine.[410] In the case of Felix Platter, aloe pills caused such "great urge" that he had sixteen bowel movements and then fell unconscious.[411] After taking a purgative, sick Toppertzer produced twenty-eight stools,[412] while in the case of Florianus, who was ill with the French disease, it was fifty.[413]

---

404 Cod. 11210, fol. 58r.
405 Cod. 11205, fol. 13v.
406 Ibid., fol. 296r: "Der Schleiym ist angebacken, angekleistert"; "ehe man die Purganzien gibt, mus man yn zuvor durch die Syrop[is] erweichen, ablösen, und abstreiffen, wie man den Unfalt zuvor mit der Seyffen ausetzen, aber [oder] ausbeysen mus, zuvor wescht das Wasser nichts ab." He added at the margin: "und die Verstopfung ynn Adern und Lebern erofnen, das die böse Feuchtikeiten mit der Pürgatz zu gange kommen mögen" ("and to open the obstruction of the vessels and of the liver, so that the evil fluids may start moving with the purgative").
407 Ibid., fol. 427v; similarly Cod. 11206, fol. 127v.
408 Cod. 11207, fol. 30r: "Man mus die böse Feuchtickait, die under das gutte Blutt gemischt und gemengt ist, zuvor mit den Sirupen absondern, zusammenbringen, unnd das Geeder inwendig eroffnen, damit die Purgatz nicht das Gutte mit dem Bösen, sondern das Böse nur allein weg ziehe, item das die Genge ym Geeder nicht gestopfft seindt."
409 Cod. 11183, fol. 458v.
410 Cod. 11204, fol. 17r.
411 Platter, Lebensbeschreibung (1976), p. 219.
412 Cod. 11205, fol. 274r.
413 Ibid., fol. 244r.

Purgatives were also administered as a precautionary measure, especially at the beginning and at the end of the winter.[414] In certain situations, it was better not to administer them, however, because they threatened to disrupt the efforts of nature to evacuate the waste and morbid matter herself. When there were indications that a "critical" evacuation via the sweat was taking place, or when a skin rash formed, or just before an expected menstruation was to take place, one ran the risk of disturbing the natural evacuations if a purgative was administered.[415] Handsch wrote that patients and their relatives would moreover sometimes resist taking a purgative because the patient had already had plenty of bowel movements and was hardly eating anything. In their opinion, there was nothing left to purge.[416] One then had to explain to them that the purgative attracted waste and morbid matter from beyond the intestines, from the rest of the body. For this reason, cleansing and emptying was most definitely still indicated.[417]

Physicians worked to adapt their prescriptions and dosages to the clinical picture and the physical constitution of the patient. Purgatives varied in strength and, as experience taught, the same remedy could produce different effects in different patients. For this reason, Handsch made a point of asking patients about their usual bowel movements and their experience with purgatives. In this way he would be better able to estimate the effects of the purgative he was about to prescribe.[418] As experience taught, excessive evacuation could strain the sick person's body tremendously, even if one ordered, as Lehner did, a fortifying remedy like rose sugar or sweet meats to be taken afterward.[419] Several times, Handsch wrote about the tragic cases of *hyperpurgatio*. After Gallo had given her a purgative, a sick patient called Marsalkowa had up to eight bowel movements every day for several days and her tongue became completely dried out. In the end she died and people said it was the physician who had killed her.[420] A young, vigorous nobleman died in the hospital after Gallo gave him a powerful purgative that produced almost thirty bowel movements and weakened him greatly.[421] The same thing had happened in the case of Handsch's patient Fröhlich. Another case was

---

414 Cod. 11207, fol. 102v.
415 Cod. 11205, fol. 334r; Cod. 11238, fol. 130r; Cod. 11240, fol. 35v.
416 Ibid., fol. 287v.
417 Cod. 11206, fol. 146r-v.
418 Cod. 11205, fol. 294r.
419 Ibid., fol. 312r.
420 Ibid., fol. 299r.
421 Cod. 11207, fol. 214v.

that of an old woman in Venice who, after taking cassia, had almost a hundred stools; she died as well.[422]

The purgative must not be too weak either. Patients desired a copious, powerful evacuation and sometimes they explicitly noted the positive effects of the purgative.[423] If the expected stool failed to materialize, the physician had made a mistake in their eyes. When Handsch gave a young female patient a purgative made with senna and she had only two bowel movements, she was dissatisfied.[424] Further, if the purgative itself was not evacuated along with the stool due to its insufficient strength, it could also produce cramps and other unpleasant abdominal complaints.[425] In the case of some diseases, like podagra, further dangers loomed. According to Gallo, if the purgative was too weak, it would merely mobilize the morbid matter without successfully voiding it. At that point, it might relocate to a new place in the body and get up to mischief there.[426]

The choice of the proper remedy was based on more than the physical constitution and the individual sensitivity of the patient. The ideal purgative would attract and evacuate the morbid matter alone.[427] In practice – and for this reason purgatives often had a weakening effect on the body – good, useful matter was often evacuated along with the "evil" matter. Concerning this, Handsch wrote, "No physician's purging only heals, From the good he also steals".[428] The physician had to at least try, however, to choose a remedy that would more or less target the morbid matter in question and evacuate it. From his reading of Galen, Handsch had gathered that a purgative would attract morbid matter that was similar to it.[429] The question remained, however, as to how, based on which criteria, the physician could determine this similarity. Ultimately, it appears that physicians relied on what they knew from experience. According to Mattioli, senna was especially well suited to emptying burnt matter.[430] Fracanzano prescribed a purgative that would target "salty humors" specifically.[431]

---

422 Ibid, fol. 152r.
423 Ibid., fol. 30v.
424 Cod. 11205, fol. 294r.
425 Ibid., fol. 294r.
426 Cod. 11207, fol. 197r.
427 Cod. 11205, fol. 396v: "Sed vera medicina est nullum alium humorem extrahere, nisi peccantem." On the contemporary discussion about the specific attraction purgatives exerted on certain types of matter, which was sometimes compared with the effect of the load stone on iron, see Temkin, Fernel (1972).
428 Cod. 11206, fol. 168v.
429 Cod. 11207, fol. 213v.
430 Cod. 11205, fol. 287v and fol. 413v.
431 Cod. 11238, fol. 121r.

An important alternative to administering purgatives were clysters, that is enemas.[432] They were especially called for in the case of intestinal colic or stones[433] but could also serve more generally as a mild means to evacuate morbid matter. Handsch and the physicians in his professional environment often employed them and Benedetto Vittore in Bologna almost routinely prescribed them.[434] When sick themselves, Mattioli and Lehner readily sought the effects of a clyster. According to Handsch, the two had had several dozen if not more than a hundred enemas done over the years.[435] Whereas purgatives always came with some risk, Handsch praised the clyster as the safest of all remedies. It could be given for any illness, to a person of any age and at any time of the year. One disadvantage was, however, that the ileocecal valve, a skin fold at the boundary between the large intestine and the small intestine, which Handsch's teacher Falloppia had only recently discovered, prevented the clyster fluid from entering the small intestine, as was known from recent anatomical research. In other words, only the large intestine could be cleansed.[436]

Depending on the quality of the stool, the physician could add different substances to the clyster. These included traditional purgatives like cassia, *hiera picra,* rhubarb and manna, herbal decoctions that stimulated evacuation, as well as oils, broths, or electuaries.[437] The fluid that was injected was certainly plentiful. Handsch repeatedly wrote of a *seidel* or a pound of fluid that the patient was to keep inside his bowels for half an hour or longer. This was not always easy for patients. Sometimes the urge was too strong and the liquid was discharged after a quarter of an hour at most.[438]

Emetics, too, were considered purgatives in a wider sense. They primarily "cleared" the stomach.[439] Sometimes patients demanded them of their own accord if they had the right symptoms. The Baroness of Hungerkasten explained, "Above the navel I kept feeling that something was lying in my stomach. [. . .] I wanted to take a stomach purgative".[440] Here too, one did not want to take things too far. Those who wanted to grow old and stay healthy, Handsch noted,

---

432 In cases of severe pain, massive diarrhoea or bloody stool, an enema with philonium and other analgesics as well as astringents could also be given to slow down the evacuation (Cod. 11183, fol. 106r, fol. 134r and fol. 439v.).
433 Cod. 11183, fol. 315v; Cod. 11205, fol. 590v.
434 Biblioteca comunale Aurelio Saffi, Forlì, Fondo antico, Ms. 94.
435 Cod. 11205, fol. 201r, fol. 236r and fol. 553v; Cod. 11206, fol. 118v; Cod. 11240, fol. 36r.
436 Cod. 11210, fol. 199v.
437 Cod. 11183, fol. 39v, fol.135r and fol. 399v; Cod. 11205, fol. 268r; Cod. 11207, fol. 205v.
438 Cod. 11183, fol. 39v, fol. 274r, fol. 414v, fol. 440r and fol. 471v.
439 Cod. 11206, fol. 172v.
440 Cod. 11205, fol. 474v.

had to avoid vomiting daily and intemperately. Otherwise, they would weaken their hearing and vision, tear veins in their chest and lungs, harm their teeth, and cause headaches.[441]

A whole series of further medications was used to promote other excretions. *Diuretica* induced urination. According to Handsch's Padua notes, they were especially useful in the case of liver obstructions or when humors accumulated near the liver.[442] *Apophlegmatica,* which were kept in the mouth and chewed, encouraged the production of saliva and attracted mucus from the rest of the head.[443] Remedies that produced the urge to sneeze, so-called *sternutatoria*, helped free the nose and head of mucus and other morbid matter.[444] "A good effect from a bad cause", Handsch noted on the subject of sneezing.[445] This ambivalence still finds reflection today when people say "Gesundheit!" ("health" in German) when somebody sneezes.

Contemporary pharmacology also ascribed "secondary" qualities to many medications. Their effect could be "softening" and "mitigating acrimonies", "dissolving" and "opening", or "astringent". These effects largely derived from the primary qualities: cold, hot, dry, and moist. They too were important for the mobilization and excretion of morbid matter insofar as they liquified hardened morbid matter and widened and softened the passageways.[446] Astringents could be used for undesirably strong excretions. Cooling substances like melon seeds served to mitigate hot, acrimonious humors.[447]

Bloodletting and Cupping

Alongside purgatives, bloodletting was the most important prophylaxis and treatment method in the early modern period. It was employed for countless illnesses. For certain diseases, such as the various fevers, the plague, and pleuritis, it was even considered indispensable. In Handsch's notebooks, there are hundreds of entries pertaining to it. Some of them come from his time as a medical student, while many others are from later years.

---

441 Cod. 11210, fol. 60r.
442 Ibid., fol. 64v.
443 Ibid., fol. 65r.
444 Ibid.
445 Cod. 9671, fol. 11r.
446 Cod., 11183, fol. 487v; Cod. 11207, fol. 157v.
447 Cod. 11183, fol. 416v.

Bloodletting was occasionally carried out as a treatment for plethora, an abundance of blood and other humors in the vessels and the body as a whole.[448] In most cases, however, the aim was to expel morbid matter or pathologically changed blood. Decades before William Harvey published his new theory of the blood circulation, which would cast increasing doubt on bloodletting,[449] Jean Fernel in the sixteenth century expressed his misgivings. Simply letting off blood only made sense, in his opinion, in the case of a plethora, an abundance of blood in the body. When, however, there was a cacochymy – when, as with most diseases, morbid matter was to be evacuated – bloodletting was useless, even harmful. It mostly meant that the body lost healthy blood and was weakened. According to Fernel, the morbid matter was to be voided with purging medications that drew out the specific *humorem peccantem*.[450]

Back when he was a student in Padua, however, Handsch had already noted down the powerful counterargument to Fernel's objection. Although not only harmful humors were evacuated during bloodletting, a voiding of harmful humors nevertheless took place. Nature was then better able to "vanquish" ("vincere") the fewer pathological humors that remained, and the good blood that was lost could easily be replenished from food.[451] This led to the conclusion that bloodletting was a most excellent ("convenientissimum") remedy for any kind of humoral excess and it was generally the indicated treatment in cases of severe illnesses like inflammations as well as burning, malicious, or persistent fevers – illnesses, that is, against which nature had to fight a vicious battle.[452] Gallo impressed upon Handsch, for example, the importance of bloodletting in the case of a jaundiced patient. There was such putrefaction in the veins that nature could not master it.[453]

When the blood as a whole was thought to be affected, bloodletting was usually done on a vein at the elbow.[454] Quite often also the small veins of the hand were bled, especially the *vena salvatella*, a small vein at the back of the hand between the base of the pinky finger and the ring finger.[455] Opening the smaller

---

448 Stengel, De venae sectione (1602) focussed on this usage.
449 Harvey, Exercitatio (1628).
450 According to Cod. 11210, fol. 55r.
451 Ibid.
452 Ibid.
453 Cod. 11205, fol. 155v.
454 Cod. 11210, fol. 56v.
455 E.g. Cod. 11193, fol. 487v; Cod. 11207, fol. 92v; Cod. 11238, fol. 132r; Cod. 11240, fol. 97v and fol. 127r.

veins was generally considered to have a less weakening effect.[456] For this reason, Handsch's teacher Lehner preferred this vein when letting the blood of noblewomen.[457]

The most important indication for bloodletting at the most accessible place, which was usually the elbow, were acute fevers. It was equally called for in the case of a pestilential fever or a tertian fever.[458] If the bloodletting could not be carried out, for example due to the age or poor condition of the patient, the disease was to be considered more dangerous.[459] Also with illnesses such as melancholy, in which the morbid matter – in this case preternatural, burnt black or yellow bile or in rarer cases burnt blood – was located in the blood, an evacuation via an easily accessible vein seemed called for.[460]

Freeing the whole body of impure, superfluous, old, or clogged blood was also the goal of prophylactic bloodletting, which many people had done, especially in the springtime and fall, even if they were in good health.[461] Emperor Ferdinand I, it appears, was bled twice a year, "cleansing" his body.[462] The danger of an accumulation of impure humors was considered to be especially great in the winter, particularly as the sweat was not able to fully carry out its cleansing function. For this reason, it made sense to begin the winter with a "cleansed" body and to empty the body of accumulated waste matter by the end of winter.

If the physician deemed that the morbid matter had accumulated either primarily or exclusively in a particular place in the body, then it was important to draw the blood from a vein that, thanks to its location, allowed the morbid matter in question to be targeted specifically. In the case of a liver or spleen obstruction, the right and respectively the left *vena salvatella* was considered the best option.[463] Letting blood from the *vena cephalica*, the vein between the thumb and

---

456 Cod. 11183, fol. 87r.
457 Cod. 11205, fol. 414v.
458 E.g. Cod. 11183, fol. 47v (pestilentlial fever), fol. 139v, fol. 294v (cases of *febris continua*) and fol. 410v (*febris tertiana*).
459 Ibid., fol. 345r.
460 Ibid., fol. 389v.
461 E.g. Cod. 11205, fol. 234v, "solet in vere mittere sanguinem"; Handsch mentioned this especially when patients had neglected a habitual preventive bloodletting and thus presumably promoted the development or progression of their disease (z.B. Cod. 11183, fol. 46v, fol. 122r and fol. 449v, "neglexit").
462 Cod. 11206, fol. 25v.
463 Cod. 11183, fol. 403r.

forefinger was, as the name suggests, particularly indicated for diseases of the head (Greek: kephalos).[464] Alternatively, one could open a vein on the head itself, at the forehead[465] for example, in the nose,[466] or under the tongue.[467]

The *vena saphena* on the leg, as Handsch learned, was often cut ("inciditur") so as to drain withheld menstrual blood. In German, this vein was also known as the "Frauenader", i.e. the "women's vein".[468] Johann Neefe advised the sick Baroness of Hungerkasten to have blood let from her *vena saphena* three days before she expected her period.[469] Mattioli tended to prescribe such bloodlettings to women in childbed.[470] Handsch had heard from a barber-surgeon that most women even had the "women's vein" opened on both legs on a regular basis.[471] Letting blood from the legs was indicated for diseases of the lower body and for uterine complaints in particular.[472]

Bloodletting did not only serve to rid the body of superfluous blood and morbid matter. A second important and widespread indication was the so-called *revulsio*. Here, bloodletting was used to give the movement of the morbid matter a different direction, to deflect it from its path towards the seat of the disease. A *revulsio* was thus advisable in cases of a local inflammation especially, as well as other pathological processes like podagra,[473] where harmfully excessive quantities of pathological blood or more or less specific morbid matter were flowing to a certain body part. When Collinus's wife was suffering from an intense attack of podagra in her left foot, Handsch thus thought the correct countermeasure was to let blood from her left arm.[474] The idea behind this was that if he had let blood from the foot instead so as to draw the morbid matter out of the body, this would have only pulled more morbid matter into the foot. When his teacher Lehner was suffering from arthritis in his left arm, he similarly had blood let from his right arm.[475] For patients with strong nosebleeds or who were coughing up blood, letting blood

---

464 Ibid., fol. 46v and fol. 67r; Cod. 11210, fol. 56v.
465 Cod. 11183, fol. 123r, in the case of a "lethargicus"; Cod. 11205, fol. 234v and fol. 237r, on hemiplegia.
466 Cod. 11205, fol. 237r.
467 Ibid., fol. 483r.
468 Ibid., fol. 450r.
469 Ibid., fol. 473r, "tribus diebus ante periodum".
470 Cod. 11183, fol. 138r.
471 Cod. 11205, fol. 473v.
472 Cod. 11210, fol. 56v.
473 Cod. 11207, fol. 22r.
474 Cod. 11205, fol. 306r-v; however, Handsch later read in Leonellus that bloodletting was indicated on the opposite side (ibid.).
475 Ibid., fol. 306v.

from the leg was thought to lessen the rush of blood to the nose and lungs.[476] In the case of a man with painfully swollen testicles, Gallo prescribed bloodletting at the arm.[477]

The decision was not always an easy one. Handsch and Mattioli both agreed that in the case of an *apostema* – an accumulation of pathological matter – of the liver, bloodletting at the opposite side, at the left arm, was indicated. With this they wanted to halt the influx of matter to the *apostema*, and they were acting on the authority of Avicenna and Jacques Despars (1380–1458). Their colleagues were of a different opinion, however. With reference to Galen and various more recent authorities, they explained that at the beginning, when the matter was still in motion, one should, just as one did with pleurisy, let blood from the affected side, thus drawing it to the outside.[478]

Physicians turned to a principle much like that of *revulsio* when they prescribed bloodletting in the case of obstructions of the vessels or organs. Their aim here was to get the stagnating, "obstructed" blood back in motion.[479] Even in the case of Gregorius, who was emaciated and haggard and showing the first signs of dropsy, Gallo prescribed bloodletting due to the strong obstruction.[480]

As with purgatives, physicians sometimes refrained from bloodletting so as not to disrupt the work of nature herself. With red murrain, or when a rash appeared on the skin in the course of the French disease or other illnesses, this indicated that nature was successfully pushing the morbid matter to the periphery, ultimately discharging it through the open pustules. If, in such cases, one attempted to evacuate the morbid matter through bloodletting, one ran the risk of pulling the matter from the surface of the body back inside.[481] For women, having blood let from the arm could disrupt the flow of menstrual blood to the uterus and thus impede health-preserving menstruation; this was because the menstrual blood would be directed upward instead of downward, as it was when blood was let from the *vena saphena*.[482]

In the case of injuries, bloodletting was controversial because of its weakening effect but Mattioli tended to see the positive sides. When there were

---

476 Cod. 11183, fol. 294r; Cod. 11205, fol. 168v.
477 Cod. 11207, fol. 206r.
478 Cod. 11183, fol. 188v
479 Cod. 11207, fol. 213v.
480 Ibid., fol. 213v.
481 Cod. 11183, fol. 129v; Cod. 11207, fol. 13r and fol. 22r.
482 Cod. 11205, fol. 490v.

injuries, especially head injuries, he would generally let blood unless there was considerable spontaneous bleeding already. His aim here was to limit the influx of blood and ward off the danger of inflammation. Handsch's colleague Tremenus held a similar view.[483]

Physicians regularly administered purgatives before bloodletting – cassia or, as was common in Italy according to Handsch, cassia with *hiera picra*.[484] Giving purgatives beforehand ran counter, as Handsch noted himself, to the recommendations of Galen and Leonhard Fuchs, who advocated for the opposite order of operations. But as Willenbroch explained, it nevertheless made sense to first clean the bowels because otherwise the bloodletting might draw excremental matter from the intestines into the blood.[485] In the case of complex disease patterns, a whole series of such evacuating measures could find application. In 1565, Handsch and Mattioli visited a woman who had been suffering for years. She described her complaints as follows: "It begins in the left side, then it goes to the stomach, then to the head, and sometimes in front of the eyes."[486] It sometimes seemed to her as if she were looking through a veil. She furthermore had lower back pain and her menstrual period was disrupted. Mattioli first gave her remedies such as fumewort and chicory to clean the blood. This was followed by bloodletting at the arm. After that she took a purgative, and then her blood was let from the *vena saphena*. At the end, she was also given sarsaparilla because it was suspected that her husband might have "infected" her. They were evidently referring to the French disease.[487]

In the vast majority of cases, a barber was entrusted with bloodletting. The wide-spread assumption in historical research has so far been that physicians avoided such manual tasks as a matter of principle. However, phrases such as "I cut", I "let his blood" ("misi ei sanguinem"), "we extracted" ("extraximus"), and "we cut" ("secuimus"), are found time and again in Handsch's notes, and they suggest that physicians may have in fact performed bloodletting themselves sometimes.[488] In Hiob Finzel's practice journal too, we find expressions

---

483 Cod. 11207, fol. 161r; Handsch mentioned again a certain Tremenus; probably referring to Dr. Ludovicus Tremenus of Trent (Tovazzi, Familiarum (2006), p. 208).
484 Cod. 11205, fol. 485v.
485 Ibid.
486 Cod. 11183, fol. 215r, "In der lincken Seiten hebts an, von dannen kompt es umb den Magen, darnach ins Haupt, bißweilen vor die Augen".
487 Ibid., "infectam esse a marito".
488 E.g. Cod. 11183, fol. 453r. This could still refer to the mere prescription of bloodletting. However, it is striking that these passages tend to refer particularly to patients from the doctor's immediate family or circle of friends; e.g. Cod. 11205, fol. 306r, on the sick wife of

such as "I cut the [vena] saphena" ("incidi saphenam"), which suggest active involvement on the part of the physician.[489]

The amount of blood that was let was quite modest in most cases. Usually, physicians were content with three to four or, at most, six or seven ounces, less than a pint in other words.[490] When a small vein was opened, the amount that was let was necessarily small. Only exceptionally, in the case of acute fevers for example, or serious mania and melancholy, did physicians see it fit to let so much blood that the sick person would faint.[491] In such cases the physician was well-advised to feel the pulse and to stop the bloodletting before there might be fatal consequences.[492]

When using smaller veins, one generally had to keep the hand or foot in question in warm water so that the blood would continue to flow. In this situation, the passing of a certain amount of time could serve as the measuring stick instead of a volume of blood. Handsch observed that a barber let blood from a hand vein for as long as it took to say three Lord's Prayers, and then he bandaged the hand.[493] He had heard that in Spain, blood was even let in a series of shorter sessions. The bloodletting was interrupted and not resumed until a few hours later.[494]

Bloodletting required skill and practice. In German the expression "die Ader schlagen" (to "hit" or "strike" the vessel) was used with respect to what was done to the vein, and with good reason. For a long time, it was to be understood literally. The bloodletter would take a so-called fleam, a sharp blade attached to a shaft, and set it down on the vein. He would then strike the fleam with his hand, opening the vein. However, Handsch generally wrote (in Latin) of "cutting" or "cutting into" the vein and mentioned as the tool a "phlebotomus", i.e. literally a vessel cutter. In contemporary sources we also find the term "flebotomator" for the bloodletter.[495] This suggests that during his time the veins were usually opened with a knife or a lancet, as we can also see in some contemporary visual representations.

Collinus, "misi ei sanguinem ex mediana"; Cod. 11206, fol. 43v, "D. Matthiolus secuit mihi venam in manu."
489 Ratsbibliothek Zwickau, Ms. QQQQ1b, p. 541.
490 Benedetto Vittore also usually ordered that from three to seven ounces be let (Biblioteca comunale Aurelio Saffi, Forlì, Fondo antico, Ms. 94, fol. 17r).
491 Cod. 11183, 389v, on the cantor Matthias who suffered from the disease melancholia; Cod. 11210, fol. 55v; Cod. 11226, fol. 79v; in the case of the melancholic Fasbinder, however, a pound of blood was deemed enough (Cod. 11183, fol. 426v).
492 Cod. 11210, fol. 55v.
493 Cod. 11183, fol. 87v.
494 Ibid., fol. 449r.
495 Biblioteca comunale Aurelio Saffi, Forlì, Fondo antico, Ms. 94, fol. 17r.

When letting blood from the arm veins, the procedure was comparatively simple. Very corpulent patients whose veins were hardly recognizable could present a challenge, however. While with Bellocati in Trento, Handsch saw how his teacher got his patient, a very corpulent monk, to hold a heavy weight in his hand so that the vein would protrude better.[496] Handsch also learned from the barber-surgeon Melchior that in the case of "fat bodies", like that of the Archduke, one should use a wide bloodletting knife.[497] Other veins were not easy to find and to strike even if the person was not corpulent. This was especially true of the veins at the back of the hand.[498] When, for example, a physician prescribed bloodletting at the *vena salvatella*, the patient was usually asked to put his or her hand in warm water, so that the vein could be found in the first place.[499] As Handsch knew from a barber, it was not easy to strike the vein without accidentally injuring the bone beneath it,[500] and this was not to mention the danger of hitting a nearby artery. It was especially difficult to let blood from the vein at the hollow of the knee, the *vena poplitea*. In some cases, bloodletting at that location could be very useful, as Handsch learned as a student. Falloppia explained to his students, however, that he had never seen the *vena poplitea* struck. Oddo Oddi claimed he had seen this done on a very thin woman. Bellocati had supposedly "cut" it once on a Greek man.[501] Willenbroch wanted to have this so-called "crural vein" opened on a patient suffering from uterine complaints and sand in her urine. The vein, however, could not be located even in warm water, so he had to make do with letting blood from the ankle vein.[502]

Even with comparatively accessible veins, barber-surgeons failed sometimes. They could not find the vein,[503] or it took them several attempts before they successfully struck it. In the case of the young wife of a very old nobleman, for example, the barber tried four or five times to no avail before opening the arm vein.[504] Of course, bloodletting necessarily left behind a small wound that needed to be bandaged well[505] and which took some time to heal. Some patients had a blue arm after the procedure.[506]

---

496 Cod. 11183, fol. 409v.
497 Ibid., fol. 444r and fol. 446r.
498 E.g. ibid., fol. 398v, on the thumb vein.
499 Ibid., fol. 46v and fol. 441r; Cod. 11240, fol. 127r.
500 Ibid., fol. 87v.
501 Cod. 11210, fol. 158v, "secuit".
502 Cod. 11183, fol. 351v.
503 Ibid., fol. 137r.
504 Cod. 11205, fol. 234v.
505 Cod. 11183, fol. 84r.
506 Ibid., fol. 333r.

Understandably, some patients awaited bloodletting with a certain amount of trepidation. The Count of Schimmern took a mouthful of strong wine to help him face his fear and the looming possibility of falling unconscious.[507] To prevent fainting, Mattioli recommended pomegranates[508] and he had Philippine Welser suck on cloves. Fearing that she would faint, Katharina von Loxan kept galangal in her mouth.[509] Handsch noted that, as a rule, it was a good idea for patients to lie in bed for a while after bloodletting to prevent fainting.[510] After having had only a good four ounces of blood let, "everything went green and yellow for Frau von Heidenreich".[511] And some patients actually did lose consciousness. In this case, one was to put them in a reclining position and moisten their face with vinegar and Malvasia wine.[512]

Bloodletting was an unpleasant and painful procedure. Nevertheless, many patients demanded it of their own accord. They believed they knew of its beneficial effects from their personal experience. Anna Gramoserin, for example, found that bloodletting at least temporarily helped with her troubled menstruation.[513] Some even felt immediately better after bloodletting. The intense abdominal pain of a patient called Tucher, for example, was initially treated with clysters, but to no avail. When his blood was let, however, the pain immediately vanished.[514]

Cupping was somewhat less painful. For dry or bloodless cupping, cupping glasses were warmed and placed on the skin. Handsch's stepmother called them "blind heads".[515] As the glass cooled, it pulled the surface of the skin inside it. One could also use, as was common in Italy according to Handsch, particularly large cupping glasses, putting burning hemp or tow ("stuppa") into them. The flame would consume the air inside the glass and the resulting "vacuum", as Handsch called it, would pull the skin into the glass with great force. It was furthermore helpful if the cupping glass had a small hole on the other side which could be sealed with wax. When one wanted to take the cupping glass off the skin, all one had to do was remove the wax. Then air would flow into the glass and it could be taken away without the use of force.[516]

---

507 Ibid., fol. 470r.
508 Ibid., fol. 444r.
509 Ibid., fol. 411r.
510 Ibid., fol. 409v.
511 Ibid., fol. 393r.
512 Ibid., fol. 473v; ibid., fol. 479r.
513 Cod. 11207, fol. 225r-v, letter from Anna Gramoserin to a "Frau Doctorin", probably to the wife of Andrea Gallo, 19 August 1550.
514 Cod. 11183, fol. 156r.
515 Cod. 11205, fol. 472v.
516 Cod. 11210, fol. 61r, note added in the margins.

This bloodless kind of cupping, which pulled fluids in the body in the direction of the glass, could be enough in the experience of medical professionals to stop a nosebleed or to suppress menstruation if this were desired.[517] In other cases, for example with phlegmons and hardened tumors, and with agonizing local pain or tension, bloody cupping was indicated. Here, one incised the surface of the skin before applying the cupping glass. In Italy knives were used to this end.[518] Later, so-called scarificators were desigend, small devices with a spring mechanism and several small blades which, operating simultaneously, would scarify the skin. When the skin was pulled into the cooling glass, liquid came out. According to Arnaud von Villanova, wet cupping could serve as an alternative to bloodletting if the patient was in a weakened condition or was shying away from having his or her blood let.[519] If the skin was cut into in such a way that blood flowed visibly, however, a considerable amount of blood could be taken in this way as well. In the case of a terminally ill archivist ("chartarius"), in Prague, the physicians had to forgo cupping because the sick man said he already had little blood.[520] The rather corpulent Archduke, on the other hand, once had ten cupping glasses applied. His physicians then weighed the blood and arrived at thirteen ounces – an average of more than an ounce per glass.[521]

Instead of wet cupping with a cupping glass, one could also use leeches, applying them to the anus or behind the ear for example, so that they would attach and fill with blood. Handsch only mentioned them peripherally[522] and above all during his time in Italy.[523] There he also observed that they were kept in glass vessels filled with water at the apothecary's.[524] Maybe their use was more common south of the Alps. Benedetto Vittore in Bologna, for example, frequently recommended their use, behind the ears or on the hemorrhoidal veins, where they would draw three to four ounces of blood.[525]

---

517 Ibid., foll. 60v-61r.
518 Cod. 11240, fol. 35v.
519 Cod. 11210, fol. 61r.
520 Cod. 11183, fol. 121v.
521 Ibid., fol. 446r.
522 Cod. 11210, fol. 61r.
523 Cod. 11226, fol. 40v; Cod. 11238, fol. 107r.
524 Cod. 11240, fol. 2v; Cod. 11210, fol. 139r.
525 Biblioteca comunale Aurelio Saffi, Forlì, Fondo antico, Ms. 94, fol. IIr, fol. 5r, fol. 6r, fol. 39r, fol. 43r, fol. 88r, fol. 100r and fol. 106r.

Bloodletting and wet cupping inevitably robbed the body of valuable natural blood and weakened it in its battle against the disease. Gallo warned that he who had his blood let often would age more quickly.[526] "Blood is the treasure of life and the favorite son of nature", Handsch wrote, repeating an Avicennian adage.[527] In another place, he noted, "He who diminishes the blood, diminishes life".[528] It was thus highly advisable for physicians to carefully consider whether the letting of blood was indeed indicated and necessary. They also had to take the patient's physical constitution into account and adapt the amount of let blood to the patient's general health. With sanguine, blood-rich patients, one could take a relatively ample amount.[529] Weakened patients, however, were only to have a small quantity let or to only have it let in small increments,[530] and sometimes it was best to forgo the procedure altogether.[531]

One had to be especially cautious with children. Handsch noted in several entries that it was best not to let the blood of children until they had reached the age of ten or even fourteen.[532] While it was true, Handsch wrote, that Averroes told of a plague-stricken three-year-old boy who was freed of the disease because his blood was let, one swallow did not make a summer.[533] At the same time, it was observed that children sometimes suffered bleeding wounds, and thus it was known that they would not necessarily be unduly weakened by a loss of blood.[534] As Handsch observed, even when the umbilical cord of a newborn had not been properly tied by the midwife, leaving the linens covered in blood the next day, the child survived.[535]

As a rule, it was also best not to perform bloodletting and wet cupping on old people.[536] Here too, the person's physical constitution had to be considered. If he or she had a strong constitution and a sanguine temperament, bloodletting could

---

526 Cod. 11207, fol. 197v.
527 Cod. 11205, fol. 398r.
528 Cod. 11204, fol. 45v: "Qui minuit sanguinem, minuit vitam."
529 However, despite his phlegmatic temperament, Ulrich Lehner also often underwent bloodletting on his arm or foot, and with good success, as he reported. He also was cupped every fortnight (Cod. 11205, fol. 235v).
530 Cod. 11210, fol. 55v.
531 Cod. 11207, fol. 51r; Cod. 11238, fol. 106v.
532 Cod. 11240, fol. 6v.
533 Cod. 11210, fol. 55r.
534 Cod. 11240, fol. 6v.
535 Cod. 11205, fol. 238v.
536 Ibid., fol. 113v.

be indicated even at an advanced age; experience taught that some seventy-year-olds tolerated it better than the odd sixty-year-old.[537] Aside from this, further factors were to be taken into consideration as they were with other treatments: the season (spring was best), the person's way of life, and even – as with prophylactic bloodletting – the time of day (preferably the morning).[538]

Cauterization

A particularly invasive and rather painful means by which morbid matter could be guided away from the site of disease and evacuated was the deliberate creation of an ulcer by means of cauterization. In the case of the socalled *cauterium actuale* this was done by means of glowing hot iron which burnt a hole into the skin and created an ulcer. A somewhat milder approach was the *cauterium potentiale*.[539] Here, the artificial ulcer was created by means of caustic substance that was applied to the skin. The ulcer would then be kept from closing by inserting foreign matter such as a little ball made of wax or silver into it. In this way, an ongoing efflux of oozing matter would be maintained. As Gabrielle Falloppia explained to his students, using a hot iron was in many ways safer because the effect of causic substances on the skin could not easily be controlled. In everyday practice, however, physicians mostly used a *cauterium potentiale*, to please their patients and also because "effeminate" patients abhorred the sight of fire.[540]

As in the case of blood-letting the choice of the site where the ulcer or "fontanella" was created could reflect two basic types of rationale. One could either cauterize close to the area where the morbid matter was thought to have accumulated and thus divert the flow and promote its direct evacuation, for example, through an ulcer on the arm when the chest was affected. Or one could use the cauter in order to direct the flow of morbid humor away from the affected part. In the case of a chest disease this could mean cauterizing a leg.[541] A further

---

537 Cod. 11210, fol. 55r.
538 Ibid., foll. 55v-56r.
539 Biblioteca comunale Aurelio Saffi, Forlì, Fondo antico, Ms. 94, fol. 99r-v.
540 Falloppia, De cauteriis (1570), fol. 71v.
541 In his detailed discussion of the cauterization, Girolamo Capivaccia added the *interceptio* as a third type of rationale to *derivatio* and *revulsio*. Here the aim was to intercept the flow of peccant humor to the affected site, e.g., when humor that descended from the head into the spine was evacuated by means of an articifial ulcer in the neck (Girolamo Capivaccia, De recta cauteriorum administratione, in: Scholz, Consiliorum medicinalium (1598), coll. 1158–1164).

use outlined by Falloppia was to dry and strengthen the very limb itself which was cauterized; it seems to have played a very minor role in ordinary medical practice, however.[542]

Handsch rarely refers to patients explicitly on whom cauterization was performed. He seems to have perceived cauterization as a treatment mostly for particularly serious cases. He does mention, however, that Gallo used it quite often.[543] In Padua, Falloppia and his fellow professors frequently recommended or at least discussed it when they offered their judgment on individual cases in a *collegium*.[544] We find the same in the practice of Benedetto Vittore in 1540s-Bologna who even convinced patients from the highest ranks of society to subject themselves to the painful procedure.[545] More resarch is needed to assess whether the procedure was more widely used in Italy than north of the Alps.

Sweating

As we have seen, visible sweat as well as *perspiratio insensibilis,* invisible evaporation through the pores of the skin, counted among the most important excretions in the medicine of the Renaissance period. In the healthy person, sweat served to evacuate the non-assimilated leftovers of the third concoction, which took place in the individual body parts. When a person was ill, sweat freed the body of liquid and volatile morbid matter. As the ancient Hippocratics had already observed, it was a good sign when, during acute illness, a sweat broke out on the so-called "critical" days of a disease, thereby freeing the body of morbid matter and ending the fever.[546] Consequently, physicians were well advised to stimulate excretion via the skin if a harmful, pathological humor inside the body was stirring up trouble, as with fevers and very much in the case of pestilential fevers.[547] Of course they he had to ensure, as with bloodletting, that the flow of perspiration did not weaken the patient too much.[548] There were different ways to open the pores and increase perspiration. One could use warm compresses or warm lavations, rub the skin with a warm, rough linen cloth or

---

542 Falloppia, De cauteriis (1570), fol. 71v.
543 Cod. 11240, fol. 36v.
544 E.g. Trincavella, Consilia (1587), col. 22, col. 197 and col. 263,
545 Biblioteca comunale Aurelio Saffi, Forlì, Fondo antico, Ms. 94, fol. 5v, fol. 80r, fol. 81r, fol. 83r-v, fol. 99r-v, and fol. 106v.
546 Cod. 11210, fol. 63r.
547 Ibid., fol. 62v.
548 Ibid., fol. 63r.

have the patient lie in a previously warmed bed; one could wrap the patients in warm cloths and/or put warm bricks at their feet.[549] One could also rub warm ointments on the skin and thus not only widen the pores but heat up the humors themselves.[550] Sometimes physicians even ordered the patient's hair be cut so that the harmful vapors could escape better,[551] or they prescribed sweat-inducing medications, so-called *sudorifica*.

Requiring more preparation and work were the widespread steam baths and sudatories. We will be returning to these when we discuss bathhouses, but according to Handsch, they could also be set up in the patient's house. One had to put the sick person on a ladder over a bathtub that was filled with hot stones and then pour water over the stones. "Hot" and "moist" herbs could be decocted in this water beforehand. The patient's body and the bathtub were to be wrapped in linens, while only the head was to be left exposed, covered merely with a hat, so that the vital force ("virtus vitalis") would not be weakened due to the excessive heat and the flow of perspiration.[552]

Thermal Springs and Healing Waters

Another important means to cleanse not only the outside but also the inside of the body was bathing in the waters or drinking the water from a spring that was known for its curative virtues. In this sense, Handsch's friend Mitis, for example praised the thermal springs in Teplitz, saying, "The water washes away all the harmful humors of the sick and suffering body".[553] Visiting thermal springs and drinking healing water became increasingly popular in the late Middle Ages and the Renaissance, first in Italy and soon also north of the Alps.

Different thermal springs were distinguished from one another on the basis of the kind of water they had and what each was indicated for. As Handsch's detailed notes make clear, it was expected of the learned physician that he understand which water or spring was suitable and proven for which illness, just as he was to prescribe specific medications for specific ailments. Salty or nitrous springs were said to be good for arthritis, palsy or paralysis, asthma and dropsy.[554] Sulfurous water softened and warmed the nerves and also helped with skin complaints of all

---

549   Ibid., foll. 62v-63r.
550   Ibid., fol. 63v.
551   Cod. 11205, fol. 584v.
552   Cod. 11210, fol. 62r-v.
553   Cit. in Guth, Idyll (1930), p. 163.
554   Cod. 11210, fol. 61v.

kinds, indurations of the spleen and liver, podagra and uterine complaints.[555] Ferrous water could be used for the stomach and the spleen. Handsch also listed thermal springs that were "aluminosae" – presumably containing alum – pitchy or tarry ("bituminosae"), ore-bearing or cupriferous ("aereae", "cupreae") or which contained gold, as well as their respective indications.[556]

The area around Padua was famous for its thermal springs. Handsch's teacher Falloppia devoted large parts of a lecture series to the chymical composition of the various waters and to their beneficial effects in specific diseases.[557] Of the healing baths in Tyrol, the Heiligenkreuz bath near Hall was thought to be beneficial for swellings in the abdominal area or legs, or as a treatment for emaciation. The water in Sellrain was recommended as a treatment for uterine illnesses in particular, especially if the uterus was "contaminated" ("inquinata") as when there was white discharge. The water of the nearby Teffelsbad, on the other hand, had astringent properties according to Handsch and could be recommended as a treatment for hemorrhoids, wounds, and ulcers.[558]

As Handsch took from a consultation letter written by Johann Neefe, it was always important to bear the patient's strength in mind and not overburden him. Accordingly, baths lasting four to five hours were generally sufficient. As for drinking water in the baths, Handsch had already learned in Padua[559] that the amount imbibed should be gradually increased until an upper limit was reached that was still well tolerated and "the water, without causing complaints, had made the person produce five, six, or seven stools".[560]

Handsch later accompanied Ferdinand II, Philippine, and other members of the court to the healing baths in Karlsbad twice, once in 1571 and again in 1574.[561] The princely couple bathed for hours in the thermal springs there and underwent lengthy ablutions. Not only this, they also drank incrementally higher quantities of the water. Even Philippine, in the course of her six-week stay, drank as many as eight seidels a day– approximately four liters[562] – and she also took purgatives.

---

555 Ibid.
556 Ibid.
557 Falloppia, De medicatis aquis (1564).
558 Cod. 11183, fol. 459r.
559 Cod. 11205, fol. 568v.
560 Cod. 11204, foll. 14r-15r: "Ex Naevii regimine"; similarly Trincavella recommended that a noble patient of his – he did not give the name – gradually increase his daily intake (Trincavella, Consilia (1587), coll. 710–11).
561 Cod. 11204, foll. 1r-16v and foll. 28r-30v; Oberrauch, Medizin (2012), pp. 365-368; Stolberg, Krankheitsgeschehen (2021).
562 Cod. 11205, fol. 256v.

Handsch documented the purifying effects: her plentiful urine, her bowel movements numbering as many as seventeen per day, her perspiration, and at the end the painful rashes on her arms that resembled erysipelas.[563] In 1574, Ferdinand began treatment in Karlsbad and then went on to Pürglitz, where he drank water from the thermal springs of Lucca. Here, we see indications of the beginnings of a trade in mineral or healing water, because the water was brought to Bohemia from Italy.[564] He increased the quantity from six pounds or nine cups per day to twelve, then eighteen cups, and went on to a maximum of twenty cups a day.[565] The water produced the desired effect, in Handsch's words: "He made much sweat, stool, and water" ("multum sudavit, cacavit et minxit"). Ferdinand felt better, even if by the end he complained that the water was attacking his stomach.[566]

Dietetics: Eating, Way of Life, Emotions, and Sexuality

Another important pillar of medical treatment was dietetics, the branch of knowledge concerned with the maintenance of health through diet and way of life. Significant attention was devoted to it in contemporary medical literature. In the course of the early modern period, there was a flood of publications on dietetic questions. This literature has garnered considerable attention in recent historical research. Valuable overviews have been given by Sandra Cavallo and Tessa Storey, David Gentilcore, Heikki Mikkeli, and Andrew Wear.[567]

The wealth of extant printed dietetic guidebooks can mislead us, however, into overestimating the significance of dietetics in the lives of ordinary people. While the sheer number of publications concerning health that were brought out in the sixteenth and seventeenth centuries as well as the numerous editions of bestsellers like Alvise Cornaro's *De vita sobria*[568] do allow us to conclude that the printers and publishers had put their finger on a profitable market, the degree to which these works were actually read is another matter. The copies of health guidebooks that have survived show few signs of wear or use, suggesting that many readers tended to search for rather specific information on specific illnesses or pertaining to specific questions, and left large portions of these publications

---

563 Cod. 11204, foll. 1r-4v.
564 Ibid., fol. 29r.
565 Ibid.
566 Ibid.
567 Mikkeli, Hygiene (1999); Wear, Knowledge (2000), pp. 154–209; Cavallo/Storey, Healthy living (2014); Gentilcore, Food (2006).
568 Cornaro, Discorsi (1627).

unread.⁵⁶⁹ We must certainly not assume without further investigation that the dietetic directives were applied in practice. It is possible that such books or booklets gave many readers a sense of security, a trust that illnesses were preventable and controllable should this become necessary down the road.

The interest in dietetic advice appears to have been significantly greater when someone fell ill, especially among the upper classes. After all, dietetics was not only supposed to ward off disease in healthy times; since antiquity, it had been an important component of therapy. Much like the various evacuant and strengthening remedies, dietetics was to support nature in her battle against the disease. Handsch even gave an account of an old patient with jaundice who was dissatisfied with his previous physician because this physician had not given him any dietetic advice.⁵⁷⁰

In both the prevention and treatment of disease, early modern dietetics was based in large part on the ancient teaching of the *res non naturales*. Some authors, with Hippocrates as a model, distinguished five external influences which came from a person's way of life, acted on the body, and could give rise to diseases: eating, drinking, sleeping, movement, and sexuality.⁵⁷¹ Most sixteenth-century writers of health guidebooks and consultation letters for individual patients drew on the traditional Galenic six-point scheme, however. Here, eating and drinking were conflated and three further aspects were added: the air, the passions, and excretions over which were largely beyond control, however.

Most people were simply at the mercy of the local air and its influence. Very few were able to move somewhere else for health reasons. At most, one could avoid leaving the house if the air seemed especially hazardous or insalubrious, for example during a plague or in the damp, cold winter months. Or one could try to clean the air with fire or with aromatic substances and to condition the air within the living quarters depending on a person's disease and *complexio*. If someone had a hot and dry illness, for example, one could sprinkle liquids on the floor and lay out wet flowers.⁵⁷²

When it came to the affects of the mind, the passions or emotions, the mantra was again moderation. Anger, in particular, had to be held in check while positive emotions like temperate joy, especially through pleasant conversation or beautiful music, would promote health. This kind of advice could be seen as an attempt to promote the process of civilization, encouraging people to tame their emotions for their own good if not of that of others. But it remains highly

---

569 Stolberg, Negotiating (2004); Richards, Useful books (2012).
570 Cod. 11205, fol. 574r: "Non placet M. Jacobus [Camenicenus, M.S.] ei, quia non praescripsit diaetam".
571 Mikkeli, Hygiene (1999), p. 57 and pp. 71f.
572 Cod. 11210, fol. 43v.

questionable whether people in the sixteenth century actually worked harder to control their emotions for health reasons. In the letters the sick and their families wrote to distant physicians asking them for epistolary advice based on a detail account of their disease, it is only from the eighteenth century onwards that I have found personal testimonies which show that people indeed worked to keep their feelings from others, for example when affronted or after losing a game and feeling disappointed. And tellingly the reason they mentioned this was not to underline their ability to control their emotions for the purpose of promoting health but quite the contrary: they believed that the suppressed emotion had had a lasting harmful effect on their health.[573]

More human control was possible when it came to sleep, exercise and rest. Moderate movement was considered healthy. But, of course, one was not to overdo it, because here too, as Hippocrates had written, every "too much" was harmful.[574] Sleep had to be long enough to allow sufficient time for concoction, but not so long that the subsequent excretion would be hindered. As a rule, this was seven to eight hours.[575] Sleep position could have a beneficial or detrimental effect on the concoction processes during the nighttime. It was best, Handsch learned, to fall asleep while lying on one's right side, so that food could easily enter the stomach, and then to roll over to the left side so as to encourage the subsequent concoction in the liver.[576] It was dangerous, however, to sleep on one's back, which could cause nightmares, apoplexy, paralysis, and other problems because the intestines in this position pressed on the vena cava.[577]

The medical literature was more ambivalent about sleep during the day. As Handsch learned, Hippocrates and Aëtius of Amida, proclaimed it harmful unless one had slept poorly or not at all the previous night or if the senses were weary.[578] This was because the brain filled with too much fluid during daytime sleep, which caused heaviness of the head ("gravedines capitis") and made the head susceptible to "cold" illnesses.[579] It was better therefore to go for a walk after eating and relax the mind.[580] Handsch explicitly advised the old, jaundiced man mentioned above against napping.[581]

---

573 Stolberg, Emotions (2019).
574 Cod. 11210, fol. 50v.
575 Ibid., fol. 52v.
576 Ibid.
577 Ibid., fol. 53r.
578 Ibid., fol. 52r.
579 Ibid., fol. 52v.
580 Ibid., fol. 52r, "animi aliqua laxamenta adhibenda"; the work of Aëtius of Amida (Aëtius, Libri XVI (1535)) was widely read and quoted in the sixteenth century.
581 Cod. 11205, fol. 574r.

The possibilities of active self-regulation were greatest with respect to nutrition and diet. In the health guidebooks as well as in the consultation letters to individual patients, this topic was often given by far the greatest amount of consideration. The greatest challenge here was adapting the diet to the patient's temperament, age, sex, individual constitution, and way of life.[582] The predominant primary qualities of the food had to be appropriate. For one patient, a strong wine might have a strengthening effect, while for another it might be contraindicated because, in the case of a fever for example, it might increase the pathological heat. Eating habits also had to be taken into consideration. Foods the person commonly ate were preferable; if food that was out of the ordinary was given, it had to be introduced slowly and carefully.[583] Favorite foods were also to be preferred if possible. Handsch noted that foods the patient ate with desire ("cum voluptate") were more readily accepted and concocted by the stomach.[584] One was furthermore not to eat an unruly assortment of foods and it was important to choose the right time to eat. It was healthy to eat at the same times of day, when one's appetite was keen and after one had had some exercise and the previous meal had left the stomach.[585] On the other hand, if a patient suffered from a fever attack and another illness involving paroxysms, it was better to wait until the attack had passed.[586] Following the change of the seasons, it was better to eat warming and drying foods in the wet and cold winter, while in the spring, a more meat-rich diet was good. According to Hippocrates, a rich diet was always indicated in the winter and spring because the inner warmth was strong and concentrated and sleep was long. In the summer, one needed to eat less and to drink more, and cold dishes made sense. In the fall, more food was once again indicated and it was best if it were dry.[587]

The *regimens* physicians recommended for specific diseases in printed guidebooks and in their handwritten letter consultations for upper-class patients could be very detailed. They sometimes listed dozens if not hundreds of foods that were to be preferred or avoided. In the retrospective view, the minutiae of these dietetic directives can be interpreted as an expression of the efforts made by physicians to exhaustively medicalize everyday life in times of both sickness and health, to subject it to the dictates of medical expertise. At the same time, this was a platform for physicians to prove their abilities through meticulous instructions, to

---

582 Cod. 11210, foll. 44v-45r.
583 Ibid., fol. 45r.
584 Ibid.
585 Ibid.
586 Ibid., fol. 45v.
587 Ibid., foll. 44v-45r.

show how they were able to tailor their prescriptions to their patients' individual constitutions.

Turning to the dietetic advice noted down by Handsch – advice either he or other physicians in his professional environment gave to patients in day-to-day practice – we find that it was far from excessive. It was limited to a few points which the patients and their relatives could retain after having merely listened to the physician, and it concerned nutrition above all. Handsch and his colleagues mainly advised against foods that were "difficult to digest", food that was cool and therefore increased mucus production, as well as foods that caused winds. In the case of fevers, they recommended that one avoid wine and other excessively "heating" foods and beverages. Accordingly, Handsch ordered some patients not to eat fish.[588] And indeed one female patient confirmed that after eating fish she felt "heavy in the stomach".[589] Handsch noted down the basic rule: "Fish is forbidden when there is a fever". Some people even came down with a fever after eating fish or suffered a relapse afterwards.[590] Handsch also advised against peas, cabbage, old beer, and other flatulent foods and knew that he was in the company of many a good physician in doing so.[591] He recommended, on the other hand "light fare" such as egg drop soup or chicken[592] and, very frequently, toasted bread.[593] Still today, zwieback or rusks are considered by many people to be particularly "digestible" and appropriate in the case of a fever. A brief comparison with Benedetto Vittore's treatment of his patients in Bologna in the 1540s yields a very similar result: Vittore often recommended some dietetic restrictions but usually his advice was very simple and limited to eating bread soup ("panatella"), broth or some mashed food and to drinking no or only little and watery wine.[594]

Within the *res non naturales*, the excretions were assigned a special status in the context of the Galenic six-point scheme. If excretion was disrupted, it was considered a crucial cause of illness. But excretion could only be indirectly influenced, and only to a limited extent insofar as one controlled the other *res non naturales* so as to promote health. This meant moderate exercise, spending time in warm places, and consuming food and drink that stimulated excretion (or inhibited it). There is a striking contrast between the prominent position of the excretions in theoretical discussions of the *res non naturales* and their

---

[588] Cod. 11205, fol. 519v.
[589] Ibid., fol. 514v.
[590] Ibid., fol. 396v.
[591] Ibid., fol. 396v, fol. 401v, fol. 514v and 574v.
[592] Ibid., fol. 562v.
[593] E.g. ibid., fol. 519v.
[594] Biblioteca comunale Aurelio Saffi, Forlì, Fondo antico, Ms. 94.

marginal position in dietetic instructions or *regimina* for specific patients, even when the latter, following the widespread practice, dealt with all six *res non naturales* in turn.

There was one excretion, however, that in and of itself was largely subject to the human will and human control, namely the excretion of seed. Insofar as it was included in sexuality, this excretion was one of the five points in the Hippocratic five-point scheme. It was not assumed that one could have complete control over this excretion, as nocturnal emission was of course a known phenomenon. Handsch himself experienced it physically and patients described it as well.[595] Furthermore, involuntary, uncontrolled genital discharge of the kind that we would today attribute to an infection, was taken then to be *gonorrhoea* in a literal sense, that is a "semen flux". However, as opposed to the excretion of feces and urine, which could at best be delayed somewhat, or menstrual bleeding, which was not at all subject to the woman's will, the discharge of semen was seen to be largely subject to the deliberate decision of the individual.

Although semen was considered a kind of excrement, it was one that was especially useful and valuable. According to Avicenna it was formed from the best, most delicate parts of the blood and, with man as with woman, was rich in *spiritus,* though more so with man.[596] It could even be used to treat illnesses. Handsch heard from Gallo that a sick patient called Adrianus had been given male seed to drink by an old healing woman, and Handsch added that this advice was also found in the works of medical authors.[597] He even believed he had found an indication in the Hippocratic Epidemics that semen could cure dysentery. Handsch read here that the slightly oily, temperate seed alleviated the acridity of the humors and combatted intestinal ulcers in the person who received it. He concluded that Hippocrates must have permitted anal intercourse.[598]

Far more than with other excretions, however, an excessive excretion of this valuable substance was fraught with danger in the perspective of this time, be it through marital intercourse, "unchastity", or masturbation. As Handsch took from his reading, the loss of seed weakened the senses and the body as a whole, accelerated aging, and damaged the eyes and head, the nerves, the joints, the chest, the kidneys, and the loins.[599] In the consilia of Bartolomeo Montagnana, he read that excessive coitus was often the reason for an obstruction

---

595 Cod. 11183, fol. 142v; ibid., fol. 258v; Cod. 11205, foll. 172r-179r, copy of a letter from Christoph von Hassenstein.
596 Cod. 11210, fol. 9v.
597 Cod. 11207, fol. 43r.
598 Ibid., fol. 87r, "exercere venerem posticam".
599 Cod. 11210, fol. 66v.

of the liver.⁶⁰⁰ In Padua, he experienced how Trincavella traced the complaints of a young man to a weakness of the stomach that had arisen from "too much Venus".⁶⁰¹ Handsch himself attributed the bladder ulcers of a male patient to "too much coitus".⁶⁰² Laypeople as well were convinced and shared their subjective, bodily experience that the body was weakened following a loss of semen. An ailing Bohemian nobleman from the Prague court, for example, did not dare to have intercourse with a woman although he was forty and in the prime of his life, for fear that it would be detrimental to his health.⁶⁰³

Particularly at risk were aging and old people whose vital heat was already diminished. Thus, Lehner advised a patient who was complaining of impotence to avoid the pleasures of Venus entirely, given his age. It was more harmful, he claimed, to lose an ounce of semen than a *seidel* or a pound of blood.⁶⁰⁴ Handsch recalled Lehner's comment about an old tutor who could still have been alive in Lehner's opinion "had he not taken a young wife".⁶⁰⁵ And the severe colic of a certain Dr Andreas – he was presumably in the service of the Archduke at Ambras – was traced in part to his young wife, because too much coitus weakened the liver.⁶⁰⁶ In a book on the history of Bohemia, Handsch found an anecdote about the very old Emperor Maximilian to whom King Wenzel offered his young daughter in marriage. The emperor retorted that there was no better way to kill a man honestly than to give him a young woman as his wife.⁶⁰⁷

Regardless of age, frequent intercourse, it was believed, could also lead to a pathological loss of semen that was independent of sexual activity. Bellocati explained to his students that too much coitus weakened the seminal vessels and their capacity to hold the semen. The result was a pathological efflux of semen, a *gonorrhoea*.⁶⁰⁸ This was particularly true of masturbation, whose harmful effects on the genitals were thrown into relief by sixteenth- and seventeenth-century authors.⁶⁰⁹ The French physician Louis Saporta, for example, attributed the *gonorrhoea* of a young man not to a profusion of semen, but rather considered it the result of a weakness and flaccidity of the seminal vessels, which the

---

600 Cod. 11205, fol. 219v.
601 Cod. 11238, foll. 109v-110r.
602 Cod. 11205, fol. 230r.
603 Ibid., fol. 102r.
604 Ibid., fol. 256v.
605 Ibid., fol. 256v and fol. 266v.
606 Cod. 11183, fol. 313v.
607 Cod. 11205, fol. 257r.
608 Cod. 11238, fol. 131r and 133r.
609 Da Castro, Universa mulierum medicina (1662), p. 97; Ettmüller, Opera (1685), p. 422. Timaeus von Güldenklee, Responsa (1668), pp. 191–193.

young man had brought upon himself in part by "frequently pulling back the foreskin followed by seminal discharge".[610]

If, however, the semen was inappropriately held back and remained in the body for a long time, this too was perilous according to widespread conviction. Withheld semen – this Handsch learned from the Hippocratic aphorisms and from Avicenna – became highly noxious, indeed poisonous.[611] Particularly imperiled were virgins, nuns, and widows, but men too had to reckon with grave consequences for their health if they lived too abstemiously. The seminal substance that in its natural condition was especially pure and valuable was for that very reason particularly inclined to decompose and to release very harmful, in fact poisonous substances if it built up in the body. Just before her (unexpected) death, Gallo advised the chronically ill Baroness of Hungerkasten, whose complaints were numerous, to lie with her husband.[612] As Handsch noted, even sexual dreams ("insomnia Veneris"), which, according to Handsch, women certainly had as well, could have grave consequences. While, for men, the semen left the body, the dreaming woman's seed only passed into the uterus. Because no conception took place, the seed could easily spoil and give rise to the most severe illnesses ("maximos morbos").[613]

The dangers posed by withheld, corruptible semen constituted an important reason why physicians recommended marriage, especially to women. Moreover, coitus warmed the blood and encouraged the evacuation of spoiled blood via the uterus, that is, via menstruation.[614] For these reasons, Gallo told a sick virgin, for example, that a husband would be a "good cure" for her cough, hardened splenic tumor, and disrupted menstruation.[615] Handsch himself gave this advice to an unmarried young woman in Trento. He also added that a clergyman whose name he did not mention and who also worked as a physician had given this advice to women.[616] The idea was common among laypeople as well. The abovementioned Dr Andreas in Ambras thought that his unmarried sister, with her heavy feet, languidness, shortness of breath, pain in her loins, and insufficient menstrual bleeding, had little hope of recovery if she did not marry soon.[617] According to Handsch,

---

610 Sächsische Landes- und Universitätsbibliothek Dresden, Ms. C337, "Consilia praestantissimorum aliquot in Gallia medicorum", foll. 292v-294v: "Pro quodam adolescente gonorrhoea laborante, ex mastupratione et praematuro veneris usu."
611 Cod. 11205, fol. 165r; Cod. 11207, fol. 37v.
612 Cod. 11183, fol. 22*, added slip of paper.
613 Cod. 11210, fol. 9v.
614 Cod. 11207, fol. 209r.
615 Ibid., fol. 83r.
616 Ibid.
617 Cod. 11183, fol. 388v.

a monk had said to a woman, "All of your illness is that you have no desire for men", and it appeared that she agreed.[618] The understanding sketched out here was also presumably at the root of a comment made by an archducal chancery clerk, who said his wife, plagued as she was by pain and a white discharge, lay like a tree trunk ("tanquam truncum") during coitus; this indicated lacking desire and thus an insufficient emission of her accumulated seed.[619]

The idea, then, was to find the proper balance. As long as one did not overdo it, coitus was healthy for body and spirit – this Handsch gleaned from his reading. It relieved the body, strengthened the appetite, alleviated mental upset, and was useful for sad and melancholy people, epileptics, and people with phlegmatic illnesses.[620] As physicians knew from their reading, the notion that coitus helped those suffering from melancholy in particular had already found expression in the work of Galen.[621] Thus Gallo could only agree with an old woman who urged those suffering from melancholy to have intercourse frequently. He himself had actually given this advice before.[622] Gallo explicitly advised the young, unmarried Archduke Ferdinand to have intercourse because he attributed his unusual complaints – which some considered to have possibly been inflicted by witchcraft, while others saw them as the result of melancholy – to withheld seed.[623] Handsch, however, was not prepared to believe this. Even a nun, he felt, would know how to help herself in this situation, and certainly a young prince would.[624]

Handsch also carefully observed the effects the discharge of semen had on his own body. When, over the course of two days, he observed that his pulse was irregular – there were short interruptions and sudden quick beats – he wondered if this could be the result of withheld semen, even though, he added, he had masturbated earlier.[625] When he was suffering acutely from a bladder stone, it appears he hoped he might ease the egress of the stone in this way. After a previous *manuductio* – this was the term that he commonly used for

---

617 Cod. 11183, fol. 388v.
618 Cod. 11205, fol. 211r.
619 Cod. 11183, fol. 460r.
620 Cod. 11210, fol. 66v; at another point, however, he explained that as a general rule epileptics should be forbidden to have sexual intercourse because it weakened the nerves (Cod. 11240, fol. 88r).
621 Cod. 11207, fol. 43r, referring to Galen's commentary on the Hippocratic *Aphorisms* (book 5, ch. 5).
622 Ibid.
623 Cod. 11204, fol. 37r.
624 Cod. 11207, fol. 37v.
625 Cod. 11205, fol. 218r.

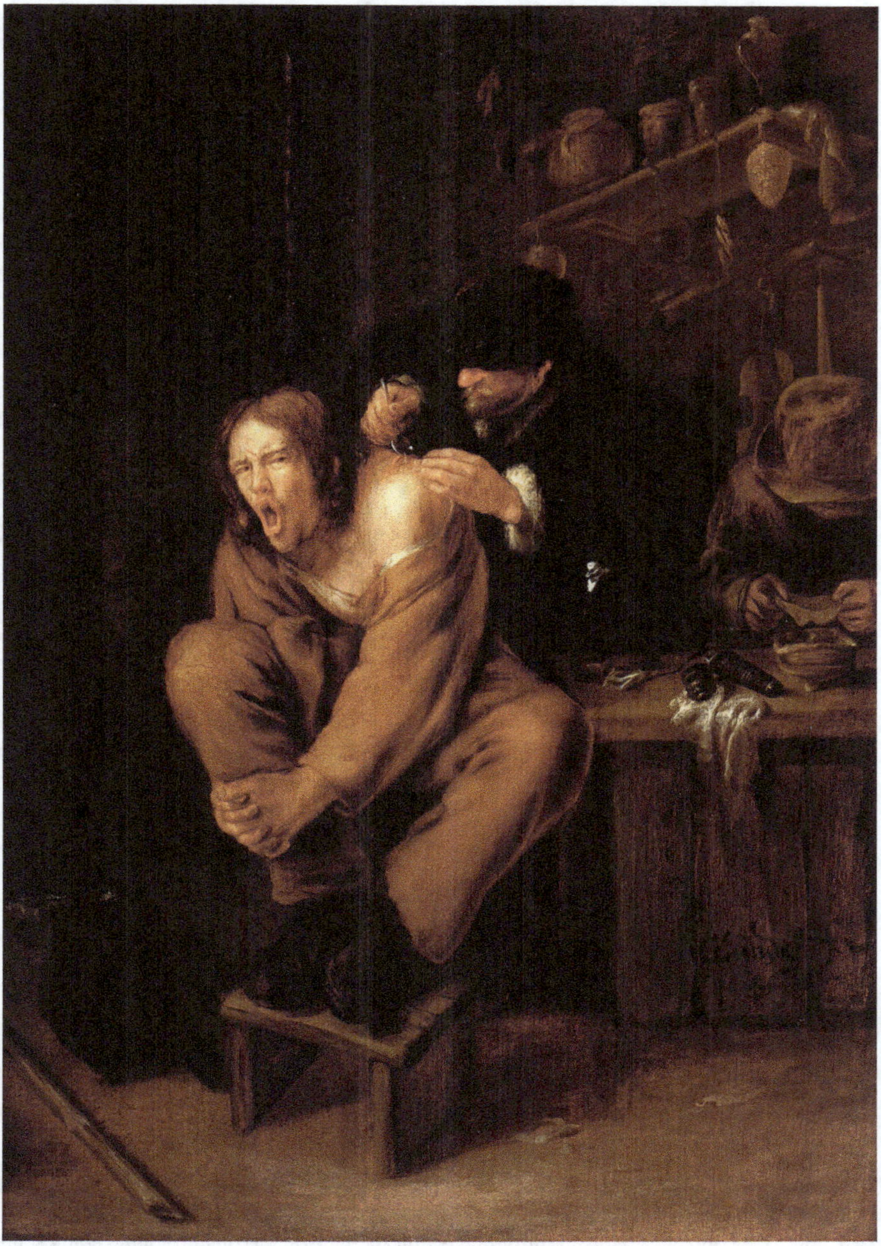

Fig. 7: Painful surgical treatment, oil painting by Gerrit Lundens, 1649, Wellcome Collection, London.

masturbation – earlier in the day, he "forced" a second ejaculation in the evening.[626] As his stone disease progressed, however, he eventually decided that he would forgo a *manuductio* after his midday nap and after his evening meal.[627] He experienced that the *spermatizatio* also had a weakening effect; after having masturbated upon going to bed, he was "weak and exhausted", and it surprised him that he nevertheless had sexual dreams.[628]

Surgery

Surgery was an important branch of medicine and had been firmly established in the medical literature since the Middle Ages.[629] In the sixteenth century, its significance in scholarly medicine grew further, in part thanks to the growing field of anatomy, which was predominantly practiced by surgically experienced physicians. Regarding the status of surgery in medical practice, however, there were great differences within Europe, as we have seen in Part I. In Italy, surgery was broadly recognized. It was taught at universities, sometimes by doctors of medicine such as Gabrielle Falloppia, who also had extensive practical experience in surgery. In German-speaking areas by contrast, surgery was considered the domain of the barber-surgeons (cf. Fig. 7). who were trained as craftsmen and who guarded their guild's privileges, making it difficult for non-members, including the *doctores medicinae*, to gain a foothold in the field.

In the understanding of the time and certainly in the German-speaking areas, surgeons were in charge of "external", manual treatments – terms like "chirurgia" or "Chirurgie" come from the Greek words for "hand" and "work". This included not only the treatment of wounds and fractures but also minor interventions such as bloodletting, cupping, and giving enemas or clysters, along with the treatment of tumors, skin rashes, and ulcers. The medical doctors for their part staked out their territory: the administering of medications for internal use. When it came to the few major, high-risk surgeries that were possible in the circumstances – mainly cutting stones, operating on hernias, and couching – these were primarily the realm of specialized itinerant surgeons.[630]

---

626 Cod. 11183, fol. 434v, "iterum modo cogens quasi".
627 Ibid., fol. 459v.
628 Cod. 11205, fol. 80v, "cum ad introitum lectum spermatizavi, postea in somno etiam somniavi venera, quamvis ad primam spermatizationem iam debilis et exhaustus spermate fui."
629 Pouchelle, Body (1990); McVaugh, Rational surgery (2006).
630 Jütte, Ärzte (1991), pp. 20–23.

As Handsch's notes show, the lines between the surgeon's and the physician's area of activity were ultimately blurred in everyday medical practice north of the Alps, as in other parts of Europe. For one thing, many barber-surgeons did not limit themselves to surgical procedures but practiced medicine as a whole, and they often administered medicines intended for internal use.[631] Even high-ranking rulers sometimes preferred the help of a barber-surgeon to tend to their internal diseases, and Handsch, too, occasionally sought their treatment. Not only this, but doctors of medicine indeed explored surgical matters and surgical cases at length. North of the Alps, they took up the surgical knife only as an exception but if they wanted to present themselves to their patients as competent experts who could deal with any case, they had to at least know how surgical diseases were diagnosed and treated, and they had to be able to give the barber-surgeons instructions if necessary, and to supervise them. In serious cases, especially with high-ranking patients and their staff, learned doctors and barber-surgeons sometimes even cooperated. For example, Mattioli worked with "the barber-surgeons" when he treated the abdominal injury of a certain Virgilius, who was apparently in the service of the Archduke. The man was very unwell. Stool came out of his wound and Mattioli thought that his subdued cough, his difficulty breathing, and occasional expectoration of blood indicated the injury of a lung.[632]

Handsch's notes about medical practice include dozens of entries about surgical cases. Sometimes he only briefly described cases which his teachers, mentors, and colleagues had apparently treated in his presence, for example, the treatment of a fractured shin by Ulrich Lehner[633] or Tremenus's visit to a young man with a head wound.[634] Many of Handsch's entries, however, are very specific and are concerned with craftsmanship and detailed technical knowledge. For example, Lehner taught him how to keep ulcers from closing over prematurely by inserting gentian root. The root swelled, thus dilating the opening.[635] If an ulcer healed prematurely, it was feared that the morbid matter, which until then had been evacuated via the ulcer, would accumulate inside the body.[636] Handsch could thank Mattioli for his recipes for various remedies, which he used on surgi-

---

631 See Staatsbibliothek Berlin, Hdschr. 442, *Arzneybuch* of the bathmaster Hanns Triefseysen.
632 Cod. 11207, fol. 161r-v
633 Cod. 11247, fol. 27v.
634 Cod. 11226, fol. 175v.
635 Cod. 11183, fol. 39v.
636 Cod. 11205, fol. 521v.

cal cases, for example the recipe for a poultice against burns.[637] He also took note of different forms of dressings, which he saw others use, such as a crossed linen bandage slung around the wrist and tied for finger injuries.[638]

But above all, Handsch learned from the craftsmanship of the barber-surgeons, even when he was an experienced physician. These were the professionals who were so violently criticized for their alleged incompetence and ignorance by Paracelsus, Johannes Lange, and other contemporary authors. Handsch's most important source of knowledge for surgical matters was the archducal court surgeon Hildebrand. Hildebrand showed him, for example, where to place the incision when treating an empyema, that is an accumulation of pus in the ribcage.[639] Handsch also noted down multiple times how Hildebrand proceeded in the examination and treatment of severe injuries and deep ulcers. For example, he wrote a detailed account of how Hildebrand and the barber Melchior Störl, working together, treated a young man in Ötting who, in a state of inebriation, had incurred serious head injuries and wounds on his back and arm. With their instruments, they did a thorough examination of his head injuries until the man fainted from pain, or rather seized. They brought him to again by having him smell vinegar and put a spoon in his mouth, apparently so he could clench his teeth without hurting himself. The following day, Hildebrand probed the skull again, using one of his instruments. He discovered a place where the skull was fractured and moved a bone fragment that had been pushed inward back into its proper position. The patient recovered.[640] It was also Hildebrand who examined the ulcerating tumor on the upper abdomen of the terminally ill Anna Welser with a silver pin to determine how far it extended inward.[641]

As a court surgeon, Hildebrand was quite a prominent figure compared to the majority of ordinary barber-surgeons. But Handsch also conversed with a barber about bleeding control during a leg amputation. From him, Handsch learned that he would not cauterize the surface of the wound, as was widely practiced at the time, but would instead fold a wet bladder over it, likely meaning the application of a poultice.[642] Handsch also found it worthwhile to note down what another barber told him about stonecutting: in the case of a bladder stone, he did not insert his finger in the anus to feel the stone in the bladder, but instead

---

637 Cod. 11183, fol. 164r.
638 Ibid., fol. 165r.
639 Ibid., fol. 468v.
640 Ibid., fol. 354r-v; Handsch did not explicitly mention that he could witness the operation but his detailed description leaves little doubt that he did.
641 Ibid., fol. 430r-v.
642 Ibid., fol. 22v.

found the stone with a probe, made his incision, and lifted the stone out with pliers.[643] Handsch further described how a barber in Ambras carefully inspected a chest wound that a guard had inflicted on a tailor, and concluded that the weapon had not penetrated to the inside of the chest and that the patient was not "weydwund", was not fatally wounded in other words.[644]

Handsch took notes for one of the standard surgical procedures of the time in particular detail, the creation of a fontanella, an artificial ulcer that was kept open to allow for the continuous drainage of morbid matter. It seems he had the opportunity to watch a barber do it. The barber applied a small, round plaster, about four fingerwidths back from the edge of the tibia, so as not to risk hurting any nerves and tendons. The plaster had a small opening in the middle, into which the barber put a paste of Spanish flies and then applied a dressing. He then let the paste act upon the skin for ten hours or more. When a blister had formed, he cut it off with scissors, put in elder pith ("medulla sambuci") and lead into the open wound and again dressed the area. The next morning, he removed the elder pith, which had already taken up quite a bit of liquid. In the evening, he filled the now larger opening again with the same paste. This procedure was repeated for several days. When, finally, the scab fell off and an ulcer had formed, he put a small hollow silver sphere about the size of a hazelnut into the opening to keep it open.[645]

From the barber-surgeons, Handsch also learned about medications they used successfully in the treatment of external complaints and injuries. One of them applied a "white ointment" ("unguentum album") on a bruise which a clerk had incurred over his eye. This was a standard remedy. At this opportunity Handsch also learned that it could be used for *decubitus* or pressure sores ("ad excoriationem a iactura") as well.[646] And Handsch furthermore accepted the critique of a barber who pointed out a mistake to him. Handsch had applied the *unguentum album* to the wound of a little girl who had fallen. In his notes on the case he added "error" and includes the barber's question, "What is the white ointment to do, when [the wound] is open."[647]

Sometimes, Handsch even found it worthwhile to write down the experiences and knowledge of medical laypeople in surgical matters. For example, a woman

---

643 Ibid., fol. 211r.
644 Ibid., fol. 372v; Handsch did not indicate the reason why the guard injured the man.
645 Cod. 11207, fol. 216r-v; in another entry (Cod. 11183, fol. 131v), he also noted the recipe for the etching stone, the *lapis corrosivus*, which the surgeon Cunradus used on von Wartenberg's wife to create an ulcer (fontanel).
646 Cod. 11183, fol. 40v.
647 Ibid., fol. 165r.

called the Bögnerin told him that her husband would put a small piece of cloth with glue ("glutine") on his finger after he had cut himself and then the wound would heal.[648] He also had a baker show him the truss he put on for his hernia, which the baker said he had incurred from carrying heavy things. Handsch described its form and design in great detail and even made a small drawing of it.[649] And he took seriously what a stonecutter told him about the treatment of gangrene. The stonecutter's mother suffered from the "cold burn" and the barber-surgeons had already talked about amputation. But the stonecutter applied a remedy made of alum, frankincense, and myrrh and his mother recovered.[650] Even when one of Handsch's landlords recommended placing a still warm, black-plumed hen with its rump cut off over the operation wound after a hand amputation, he took this seriously enough to write it down without commentary.[651]

Several times Handsch sought out and found the opportunity to watch experienced surgeons doing major, invasive procedures and examining and treating serious injuries. He gave a thorough description, for example, of the surgery on a forty-five-year-old servant ("famulus"). The man had had an intestinal hernia for seven years and it had become larger and larger. The surgery took half an hour. First of all, everyone present bent their knees and prayed to God. Then the surgeon placed three incisions and removed the testicle – which was common practice in such cases. The patient fainted. When he regained consciousness, the surgeon asked him a few questions and cauterized the area with a red-hot iron. Handsch quoted the patient saying that this was what hurt him the most. But he had not wanted to get drunk – apparently, this was how some people dealt with the pain of the operation. He had only consumed some spiced wine. Following the procedure, he had to stay in bed for five weeks, but he survived the surgery and the hernia was gone.

Handsch also witnessed the surgical removal of a hernia or hydrocele with a six-year-old boy. The procedure took less than half an hour. The boy was tied head down to a board or beam which was placed at an angle, likely so the intestines would recede as far as possible into the abdomen through their own weight. The boy cried pitifully from the pain. After the operation, he had the cold sweat of fear on his face but was able to walk on his own feet to go to bed.[652] It is likely that Handsch was also present when a surgeon operated on his 13-year-old half-brother Johannes, successfully removing an almost chicken-egg sized bladder

---

648 Ibid., fol. 211r
649 Cod. 11205, fol. 126v
650 Cod. 11183, fol. 2v.
651 Ibid., fol. 297r.
652 Cod. 11204, fol. 16r

stone within a quarter of an hour.⁶⁵³ He only had somebody else's account, however, of the leg amputation a barber performed on an older man in Prague's Angel's Garden. The barber had promised that three blows of the hatchet would be enough – he apparently did not use a saw. In the end, he took almost thirty blows, tormenting the man like a torturer. He was at least able to stanch the blood without using a cautering iron. He only "pinched the veins with wire". The man died three days later.⁶⁵⁴

It has been widely assumed in historical research that learned physicians north of the Alps, generally did not perform surgical interventions themselves. As a student, Handsch made a point of writing down Galen's admonition that a physician was never to perform surgery but must instead only prescribe it, just as the emperor did not fight at the front of his army with a sword but gave the army orders.⁶⁵⁵ Once again, however, a more differentiated picture emerges when we look at everyday medical practice more closely. When it came to minor surgery, Handsch certainly did occasionally take up the knife. He sometimes even gave clysters, though this was typically a task for the barber-surgeons. He learned at this opportunity that it was not the easiest task. Importantly, he found that the person administering the clyster or an assistant had to make sure that the clyster did not slip back out of the anus from the pressure. It had happened to him. Perhaps it was better, he reflected, to wrap the tip of the clyster syringe with fine leather, which he had seen done in Trento. This way, the syringe did not slip out of the anus as easily.⁶⁵⁶ He furthermore mentioned – repeatedly, and without further explanation – surgical cases that he treated himself, for example the case of a certain Hans Reutter, who had been bitten by a dog.⁶⁵⁷

Handsch's training in Italy may have caused him to be particularly open toward surgery but he shared this Italian experience with many other physicians from north of the Alps. There we find indications that other learned physicians, too, who treated surgical cases and even performed surgical procedures personally. For example, Handsch wrote that his colleague Willenbroch had "cauterized the area". Willenbroch was treating a man who had mistakenly taken a big gulp of corrosive sublimate thinking it was wine. In time, a bulge had formed in his upper abdomen, which was hard to the touch like a drum. The area was first opened with a caustic agent ("ruptorium") and then with a lancet. A silver canula was inserted

---

653 Cod. 11183, fol. 211r.
654 Cod. 11205, fol. 492v.
655 Cod. 11231, fol. Ir, with a reference to Galen's commentary on the sixth book of Hippocratic *Epidemics*.
656 Cod. 11205, fol. 147v, "ego clysterizavi".
657 Cod. 11183, fol. 369r.

and it was said that close to forty pounds of blood and pus were passed in the course of a month.[658]

Already in the sixteenth century, several physicians north of the Alps even possessed extensive surgical knowledge and skill. In most cases, they likely owed their expertise to having trained as surgical craftsmen or having studied in Italy. Volcher Coiter, for example, who had earned his doctorate in Bologna, spent more than ten years in Italy, and in 1569 he was appointed the municipal physician and surgeon of Nuremberg.[659] As early as 1560, Steffan Holtman had been employed as a "medical and surgical doctor" with the express condition that he be "willing and ready to let himself be put to use as a surgeon".[660] And even the municipal physician of Fulda, Burkhard Schönfeld, who is not known to have undergone special surgical training or to have studied in Italy, wrote in 1597 about "instrumentis meis chyrurgicis", and so it appears that he at least had his own set of surgical instruments.

---

658 Ibid., fol. 412v, "urebat ipsum hic locus"; in the individual case, such wording always leaves open the possibility that the doctor in question merely gave the order for such an operation, however.
659 Groß/Steinmetzer, Strategien (2005), p. 280.
660 Wolfangel, Ayrer (1957), pp. 60–62, edition of the contract.

Diseases

Renaissance physicians' approach to the illnesses of individual patients centered on the effort to pinpoint the pathological changes inside the body and their causes. In most cases, this meant identifying the particular morbid matter. Fighting and eliminating it, the physicians sought to attack the disease at its roots and ideally eradicate it. It was therefore not essential that the illness be assigned a particular disease name, something which is widely considered the goal or primary task of medical diagnosis today. In his practice journal, Hiob Finzel tellingly was content to sketch the suspected pathogenesis, for instance "raw matter" ("cruditas"), "obstruction of the veins with heat from the liver", or "burnt and putrefied humors". According to Handsch's notes as well, disease names played only a modest role when he and the physicians around him communicated their diagnosis to the patients and their families.

This does not mean that such disease names did not exist. Quite to the contrary, the physicians of the sixteenth century could avail themselves of a wide spectrum of terms, some of which had historical roots tracing back to antiquity. Disease names like *epilepsia, apoplexia* (stroke), *paralysis, catarrhus, asthma,*[1] *phthisis* (consumption), *syncope* (loss of consciousness), *hydrops* (dropsy), *cancer, icteritia/ icterus* (jaundice), *scorbutus* (scurvy), *lepra* (leprosy), *podagra* (gout), *tertiana* (tertian fever), and *quartana* (quartan fever) were well-established in medical literature and practice. In addition, there were names for diseases that were new – or at least perceived as such – like *morbus gallicus* (the French disease) and *sudor anglicus* (English sweat).

Certain disease terms, such as *cancer, scorbutus,* and *lepra* did not immediately indicate the characteristic appearance of these conditions, even to the learned physicians of the day, with their solid knowledge of Latin and often also Greek. In most cases, however, disease names pointed to the external appearance, as with *icterus, hydrops, phthisis,* and *paralysis,* or to a characteristic cardinal symptom, as with *podagra* (literally foot pain), and *febris tertiana*.

---

[1] At the time, "asthma" was used for difficult breathing in general and for sudden attacks of dyspnea, in particular. Handsch quoted the account of a young pharmacist, for example, with "sudden asthma" ("asthma repentinum") who felt pressure in his throat as if he were about to suffocate and was close to collapsing due to a sudden attack in the marketplace: "Es kümpt mir oben ynn die Kele und druckt mich gleich als solte ich bald ersticken"; "heut auf dem Marckt kam es mich gehlig an, benam mir den Athem und gleich wie ich solt umbfallen" (Cod. 11205, fol. 524a r and loose slip of paper without pagination); on early modern "asthma", see also Demaitre, Straws (2002) and Jackson, Asthma (2009), pp. 10–53.

Open Access. © 2022 Michael Stolberg, published by De Gruyter. This work is licensed under the Creative Commons Attribution-NonCommercial-NoDerivatives 4.0 International License.
https://doi.org/10.1515/9783110733549-010

Across different times and cultures, commonly used disease terms share two features which are crucial also for our historical understanding. First, disease terms are far more than mere names. Virtually without exception, they are linked to a concrete idea about the nature and the causes of the patient's complaint and the underlying pathological changes in the body. They stand for a whole concept, for more or less complex models that explain the illness and point to the suitable treatment, helping to literally come to terms with it.

The second commonality has to do with the organizing function of language. Diseases like *cancer* or *tertian fever* are not naturally-given entities. They are abstractions. Patients presenting with somewhat similar but rarely perfectly identical complaints, sensations, physical changes, or abnormal behaviors are matched to a particular disease term and in this way distinguished from patients with other clinical pictures that are subsumed under other terms. As we see clearly when comparing different cultures or time periods, including our own, this act of abstraction and subsumption can follow different criteria and can result in different attributions and categorizations. The spectrum extends all the way to so-called culture-bound syndromes, that is clinical pictures that can only be observed in their specific form in certain cultures and/or sociocultural contexts, such as the South American *nervios,* the Punjabi "sinking heart", or the "liver crisis" ("crise de foie"), which is still known in France today.[2]

The forming and differentiation of disease terms by way of abstraction from individual cases has far-reaching epistemological implications and very concrete practical ramifications. Disease terms reflect an underlying understanding that above and beyond individual cases of illness there are disease entities that can be distinguished from one another, more or less the same way we distinguish different species of plants or animals. In the eighteenth century, there were even attempts to create comprehensive, systematic nosologies which classified diseases on the model of botany.[3] As to diagnostic and therapeutic practice, the use of abstract disease terms implies that different people can suffer from the "same" illness. The diagnosis and treatment of one patient can therefore be based on the experience a physician has gained with others who suffered from the "same" disease.

In medical theory, we call this an "ontological" understanding of disease. It defines disease as a separate entity. It is closely linked to the notion of disease as something that is foreign to the body, that befalls it from the outside. In Renaissance medicine, such an ontological notion of disease was in perfect harmony

---

[2] Simons/Hughes, Culture-bound syndromes (1985); Helman, Culture, pp. 130–132.
[3] Boissier de Sauvages, Nosologia (1773).

with the ruling idea that most diseases were caused by morbid matter that was foreign to the body. In medical theory, such an "ontological" approach is commonly contrasted with a "physiological" understanding. With the latter, disease is conceptualized only as a gradual divergence from an ideal state of health. A prime example here is the interpretation of illness as the expression and consequence of an *intemperies* in the body, a gradual deviation from an ideal balance of the four primary qualities that is specific to each individual body.[4]

A systematic investigation of Renaissance disease concepts based on a comprehensive overview of theoretical writings and sources that describe everyday practice is yet to be accomplished. There are, however, numerous indications that an ontological understanding of disease as sketched out above gained considerable significance in learned medicine since the late fifteenth century. One such indication is that "specifics", whose effects could be explained not in terms of a particular mixture of qualities but with respect to their hidden powers or their "total substance", garnered increasing attention in learned medical practice. An "ontological" understanding of disease also comes to the fore in the way in the physicians' notebooks and practice journals: frequently they collected their observations about various patients who were suffering from the "same" disease under the same heading. Handsch, for his part, repeatedly supplemented his entries on individual patients with references to other, similar cases in an attempt to arrive at generalizing conclusions. For the subsequent time period, collections of *curationes* and *observationes* document and illustrate this striking shift. The titles of late medieval *consilia* frequently followed the pattern "consilium pro N.N.", referring to a particular patient who was seeking advice. The printed collections of *curationes* and *observationes*, by contrast, that began to appear in growing numbers from the mid-sixteenth century onwards put an increasing emphasis, in the titles of individual case histories already, on the disease term, of which the particular case history was an example. And printed collections of *consilia* now began to take the same approach, naming just the respective disease term – "epilepsia", "hydrops", "suppressio mensium", and so forth – in the heading, with no additional information on the individual patient.

Taking this one step further, there was an increasing tendency to organize printed collections of *consilia, curationes* and *observationes* according to diseases and their location in the body. In 1587, the Venetian edition of *consilia*

---

[4] Since only one but sometimes also two of the four natural humors or of the four primary qualities could predominate, Galenist medicine distinguished eight basic types of imbalance (in terms of qualities that were in excess: hot, hot and dry, cold, cold and moist, dry, dry and cold, moist and hot and moist).

and *collegia* of Vettore Trincavella and some of his Paduan colleagues advertised itself as "per locos communes digesta", that is organized by headings or key words. Beginning with "headache" ("cephalalgia"), it sorted the cases according to the classic scheme from head to foot, "a capite ad calcem", and it concluded with the generalized diseases.[5] A few years later, Theodor Zwinger praised the accomplishments which Johann Schenck von Gräfenberg had achieved for the *medica respublica* in his multi-volume *Observationes medicae rarae, novae, admirabiles, et monstrosae*, which was organized by body region and featured an index. According to Zwinger, von Gräfenberg had made accessible to the reader "per locos communes digesta" the various *historiae* and *curationes* that were otherwise only found spread out, scattered and remote, among the works of numerous other authors.[6] If a manuscript or a printed collection strung together the *curationes* or *observationes* on different diseases in a motley fashion, an index often made it possible at least to identify all entries that pertained to a particular disease.

The underlying assumption of trans-individual disease entities was bolstered by the linguistic habits of laypeople. They too used different names for different, more or less characteristic disease patterns. In his notebooks, Handsch quoted a whole host of such vernacular terms. Some, like "Zipperlein" and "Schlagfluss", corresponded for the most part to analogous terms the physicians used, here "podagra" and "apoplexia". Others, like "das Grüne" ["the green"], "das Kalde" ["the cold"] or "Nabelverstürzung" ["umbilical dislocation"], had no direct equivalent in medical terminology. They therefore prove all the more that laypeople, too, tended to define and distinguish different disease patterns, just as they made distinctions between plants and other natural things and gave them different names.

In the following, I will present in more detail some of the most important and widely diagnosed diseases, to which the physicians referred with specific disease terms and which they distinguished from one another. I will discuss, in particular, fevers, consumption, gout, bladder and kidney stones, cancer, dropsy, falling sickness, apoplexy, melancholy, and the French disease; further along, in the section on diseases of women, I will also address suppressed menstruation and suffocation of the womb at greater length, the two most commonly diagnosed female disorders at the time. This list of diseases represents only a small portion of the wide spectrum of diseases that were discussed in contemporary textbooks and presented in printed collections of medical case histories. However, if we look at Handsch's notes on the practice of his Paduan professors and his notes

---

5 Trincavella, Consilia (1587).
6 Dedicatory epistle 19 August 1584, in: Schenck von Grafenberg, Observationum, vol. 2, (1599).

on the patients whom he and his colleagues treated in Prague and Innsbruck, as well as at Finzel's practice journal (though he made limited use of specific disease terms), along with other sources that describe everyday practice, what we find is that in everyday medical practice a large number, indeed (due to the prevalence of fever diseases) probably even the overwhelming majority of patients, were diagnosed with one of the diseases I will discuss. Looking at these widely diagnosed diseases, I will also illustrate, in general, how physicians interpreted the different diseases in their daily work and which diagnostic and therapeutic practices they turned to in dealing with them.

In this way, I also hope to advance a field that has received remarkably little attention in medico-historical research. As Adrian Wilson lamented more than two decades ago, "the history of medical practice is often written without reference to the disease-categories by which past practitioners apprehended the illnesses of their patients."[7] Or as Christopher Lawrence put it: "How the various medical groupings of the Renaissance created and employed disease concepts in their differing social contexts remains largely unexplored."[8] Very little has changed since. With respect to medieval explanatory models for individual diseases, we can now draw on Luke Demaitre's extensive study, which is based on an analysis of fifteen medieval works on medical *practica*.[9] It is also valuable for this study because it helps in identifying long-term continuities amidst innovations. With respect to the early modern period, however, the current state of the art remains very unsatisfactory.[10]

When disease terms appear in early modern sources, and they do so not only in medical texts but also in non-medical contexts, for example in (auto-)biographical, literary, and historical texts, their meaning and the explanatory concepts associated with them may generally only be grasped through a reading of contemporary sources. Otherwise, we risk gross misinterpretation. It is particularly great with terms that are common but have a different meaning today. When, for example, biographies of famous early modern figures equate a source term like "apoplexia" with "stroke" or "cerebral insult" (while in many cases, acute heart disease would be the correct interpretation), or if, in German, "Gichter" or "Vergicht" (convulsions in infants) are misunderstood as "Gicht" (gout) or podagra, then this is no longer sound historical scholarship. It is considered

---

[7] Wilson, History (2000), p. 271.
[8] Lawrence, Democratic (1992), p. 18.
[9] Demaitre, Medieval medicine (2013); see also Demaitre, Straws (2002); on the importance of the genre of *practicae* in the sixteenth century see Wear, Explorations (1985).
[10] Brief outlines of some commonly diagnosed diseases can be found in Evans/Real, Maladies (2017).

questionable, and rightly so, when a historians working on early modern astrological practice, for example, believe they can do without some basic knowledge at least of the ways horoscopes and nativities were constructed and interpreted at the time. The same, one would think, should be true of historical research into diseases and their diagnosis and treatment. Ideally – though this is admittedly setting the bar very high – we would get to the point where we would arrive at the same diagnostic and therapeutic conclusions as the physicians of that time when reading a case history from the period.

Fevers

Fevers were ubiquitous in the medical practice of sixteenth-century physicians. Back in his days as a student in Padua, Handsch noted that while a physician had to know how to heal all diseases, fevers were the most important. After all, he wrote, it was seldom that a person died a natural death ("mori naturaliter") without having a fever. Countless entries in his notebooks are dedicated to patients suffering from fevers and to fevers in general, and he repeatedly documented his own fevers as well.[11]

As is suggested by the plural forms that were commonly used at the time such as "variae febres",[12] "fever" (Latin: "febris") meant more than an elevated body temperature as we understand it today. A "fever" was not a symptom but a disease. More precisely, it was the umbrella term for a series of different diseases with different symptoms and/or causes. An elevated, indeed excessive body heat accompanied many fevers. But fevers could also go hand in hand with coldness. This was manifest in the chills and shivers that were particularly seen with severe fevers. According to Handsch, the population at large even tended to use the term "das Kalte" ("the cold") for "fever".[13] Under the heading "contra febres", he noted a recipe for the "Kalde", which he had from a nobleman, namely a pinch of gunpowder in warm, old beer.[14] Gallo advised Handsch, in fact, to be more explicit than simply diagnosing "a fever" when the urine of a patient was brought to him, because people would understand this to mean "cold" ("frigus"). It was better to specify, for example to say that the patient had a "steady", "inner", or "heating" fever.[15]

---

11 E.g. Cod. 11205, fol. 307 and fol. 397v.
12 E.g. ibid., fol. 304r.
13 Cod. 11207, fol. 154r.
14 Cod. 11183, fol. 241r.
15 Cod. 11207, fol. 198r.

Fevers were very widely discussed in the contemporary medical literature due to their preeminent significance in medical practice, but also due to the controversial theories about the nature of fevers and their frequently observed periodicity. Virtually every major medical author of the time discussed the subject in some detail.[16]

For the entire sixteenth century, the central authority on fevers was Avicenna, whose *Canon medicinae* covered the entire spectrum of fevers in detail.[17] As Handsch's student notes indicate, the relevant sections of the *Canon* were essential reading.[18] With the work of medical humanists Galen's writings acquired a more prominent place in this debate. Handsch made extensive excerpts from Galen's treatise on fevers, *De differentiis febrium*.[19] However, the explanations of the nature and classification of fevers formulated by Galen here and in other works did not offer a comprehensive and coherent theory. To authors of the sixteenth century, they quite often seemed contradictory. In the middle of the sixteenth century, Jean Fernel presented a doctrine of fevers that was more coherent and compelling and found a wide readership. While based on Galen, it also diverged from his teachings in several essential points.[20]

The central theoretical challenge was the difficult question of the relationship between febrile heat and natural vital heat. The doctrine of "implanted" *calor innatus* deemed this special natural vital heat to have faculties well beyond heat as a primary quality. It also relied on a particular substrate, the *humidum radicale*, which provided its nourishment but was eventually used up, causing the vital heat to expire. As we have seen, Avicenna in an oft-quoted definition, which Handsch noted down a number of times, traced fevers to a *calor extraneus*, to a particular "foreign" or "extrinsic" heat that was different from the natural vital heat or *calor innatus* in the body. It was ignited in the heart and spread throughout the body with the vital spirits, the *spiritus vitales*.[21] The term *calor febrilis*, too, which was widely used in the sixteenth century, did not simply refer to a rise in body temperature but to a different kind of heat that

---

16 For an analysis of the complex early modern debates on fever theories and their natural-philosophical context see Lonie, Fever pathology (1981); on the medieval understanding of fevers see Demaitre, Medieval medicine (2013); cf. also Stöhsel, Fieberlehre (1923).
17 Avicenna, Canon (1595), vol. 2, pp. 1–81 (book 4, fen 1).
18 Cod. 11240, fol. 28r: "Leguntur Paduae [. . .] Prima fen quarti, de omnibus febribus."
19 Cod. 11239, foll. 80r-90r.
20 On Fernel's new ideas see Fernel, Universa medicina (1542); Roger, Jean Fernel (1960).
21 Avicenna, Canon (1595), vol. 2, p. 1: "Febris est calor extraneus accensus in corde et procedens ab eo mediantibus spiritibus et sanguine per arterias et venas in totum corpus"; the definition Handsch learnt as a student learnt was "calor extraneus accensus in corde" (Cod. 11240, fol. 3v and fol. 94r).

was distinct from natural heat. Explaining fever at the sickbed, Trincavella like Handsch maintained that the natural vital heat was transformed into a fiery heat.[22] The *calor febrilis* was attributed above all to processes of putrefaction in the body. Handsch learned from Trincavella that "putrid heat" ("calor putredinalis"), which was produced by putrefaction in the body, made its way to the heart and was the cause of fever.[23]

Going by the typical clinical picture, medical literature divided fevers into three basic categories: the simple one-day fevers or *febres ephemerae* (also often *ephimerae*), the chronic hectic fevers or *febres hecticae* (derived from the Greek word ἕλκειν for "to pull" or "to draw out"), which were also called *febres ethicae* at the time,[24] as well as a wide spectrum of humoral or putrid fevers, of *febres humorales* or *febres putridae*, which were connected to a specific morbid matter.[25]

This three-part distinction simultaneously indicated the site of the pathological process within the body. With the *ephemera*, solely the vital spirits were seized by the unnatural, foreign heat and they could quickly free themselves from it, mainly through perspiration via the pores. Thus, *ephemera* epitomized a fever that would take its course quickly and was relatively harmless. An *ephemera* which Handsch experienced himself began in the evening after he had returned from a journey in the hot sun; his limbs felt weak. In bed at night he shivered a little and broke out in a sweat. The next day it was all over.[26] Because of the quick and generally harmless course they took, the *ephemerae* were only of marginal significance in medical practice. They hardly feature in Handsch's notes. In thousands of consultations, Finzel made the diagnosis only twice, tellingly for noble patients who often sought his counsel.[27] Handsch's teacher Fracanzano bemoaned that university lectures on pyretology sometimes did not even include *febris ephemera* at all,[28] even though a simple one-day-fever could develop into a much more severe fever.[29] In the worst case, an apparent *ephemera* proved to be the beginning of a fatal pestilential fever, as Handsch read in Michele

---

22 Cod. 11238, fol. 98r; Cod. 11207, fol. 226v.
23 Cod. 11238, fol. 110v.
24 E.g. Cod. 11006, fol. 106v; Cod. 11200, fol. 144v; Cod. 11207, fol. 62r and fol. 167r.
25 The "burning fever" ("causon"), which still held an important place in medieval medicine (Demaitre, Medieval medicine (2013), pp. 43–44), plays no role in my sixteenth-century sources. Terms like "febris ardens" suggest that such fevers were, by then, considered only as a particularly hot subtypes.
26 Cod. 11205, fol. 217r, "ephimera mea".
27 These were Georg Albrecht von Witzleben (1568) and the wife of Konrad von Iphofen (1572).
28 Cod. 11240, fol. 31r; Fracanzano was referring specifically to his predecessors in Padua.
29 Ibid.

Savonarola.³⁰ Strictly speaking, the fever in such cases was not truly an *ephemera*, however. When it was, patients, because they recovered so promptly, did not usually have the time or a compelling reason to seek medical advice.

With hectic fever by contrast, that is *febris hectica* or *febris ethica*, the unnatural, foreign heat took hold of the substance of the heart and with time that of other organs as well. In Handsch's notes as well as in Hiob Finzel's practice journal, patients suffering from a *febris hectica* played a very minor role, with most entries having to do with cases where physicians had only perceived the danger of a hectic fever developing and where they thought the feverish heat would consume the heart and other *solida* in the body over time.³¹ This danger seemed real primarily when fevers were sustained and resistant to treatment.³² Typically, patients would become emaciated and complain of inner heat. In the case of Emperor Ferdinand I (1503–1564), the physicians' diagnosis of a *dispositio hectica* was based on a triad of catarrh, light fever, and progressive weight loss. In the end, after having been ill for ten months, he was no more than a skeleton and was unable to stand.³³ Physicians in Handsch's professional environment also feared that the Polish queen Catharina was suffering from a hectic fever due to her weight loss and her sensation of heat at night.³⁴ Physicians considered the young Giulio Gallo to be particularly at risk because he was naturally gracile.³⁵ When older patients lost significant amounts of weight, like the seventy-year-old wife of Mattioli, physicians sometimes suspected a *hectica senilis*.³⁶ In everyday medical practice, however, hectic fever demanded the physicians' attention mostly because of its close relation to *phthisis*, that is consumption, where in addition to fever there were symptoms like coughing, hemoptysis, and other pathological changes of the lungs and respiratory tract. We will be returning to this point later.

As opposed to these two types of fevers, the large and heterogeneous group of *febres humorales*, or, as Handsch generally termed them, *febres putridae*, had paramount significance in everyday medical practice and in the contemporary debates about fevers. Unlike the *febris ephemera* and the *febris hectica*,³⁷ they

---

30 Cod. 11207, fol. 115r.
31 Cod. 11238, fol. 120v; Cod. 11205, fol. 259r.
32 Cod. 11207, fol. 191v.
33 Cod. 11183, fol. 196v.
34 Cod. 11207, fol. 167r; presumably, the entry referred to Katharina von Österreich (1533–1573), the wife of King Sigismund II. August of Poland.
35 Cod. 11238, fol. 137r; see also Cod. 11183, fol. 284r, on the heightened risks of people with a hot, biliary *complexio* and a "loose" body (corpus "rarum").
36 Cod. 11205, fol. 272r; similarly ibid., fol. 233r, on one of Gallo's patients with "ethica senilis".
37 Cod. 11240, fol. 6v, "non est praesentia materiae".

were caused by morbid matter. *Febres humorales* or *putridae* arose when humors in the body decayed, spoiled, or rotted. Hot yellow bile and moist phlegm in particular tended to do so, and sometimes both spoiled together.[38] Some patients even believed they could feel the effects and the movement of the febrile matter in their bodies. The fever of the elderly Lord of Meseritz seemed to be abating and he was sweating profusely when suddenly he had a stabbing pain in both knees and he felt how the matter, as it were, painfully descended into both legs and went all the way to the soles of his feet, which the sick man nevertheless preferred to the fever heat.[39]

Aside from the experience of the typical heat of fever, what was behind the association with warmth and moisture was evidently the everyday observation that moist and wet foods and liquids spoiled and rotted particularly quickly in warm temperatures. Physicians were convinced that bad or spoiled food – Handsch mentioned the consumption of fish and mushrooms in particular[40]– led to fevers. The same was true of external influences that engendered a heating of the body. Excessive physical exercise, being out in the sun or even sleeping in the sun,[41] and intense or frequent anger were considered the primary external causes of fevers.[42]

In the interpretation of fevers, but also of other phenomena, the notion of spoiling and rotting was associated with images of obstruction, of stagnancy in the flow of the natural humors within the body. If the natural flow of the humors was impeded, the humors would spoil and rot. The clearest water became murky if it stood long enough. Fever came from stagnancy and spoiling, Handsch noted succinctly.[43] In this sense, the physician could say to the fever patient, "Your blood is obstructed and impeded".[44] Handsch learned early on from Trincavella that such obstructions arose when there was a surfeit of humors or when the matter or humors were too thick or viscous.[45] Decreased menstruation, too, could promote putrefaction and thus produce fevers,[46] as could an insufficient flow of the lochia, which explained puerperal fevers.[47] In such cases, the recommended course of action was to encourage an evacuation of the uterus, for example by

---

38 Cod. 11238, fol. 106r and fol. 116r.
39 Cod. 11207, fol. 227r.
40 Cod. 11205, fol. 396v; Cod. 11207, fol. 35r.
41 Cod. 11205, fol. 398v.
42 Cod. 11238, fol. 71r, fol. 106r and fol. 108r; Cod. 11210, fol. 173v.
43 Cod. 11205, fol. 226v.
44 Ibid., fol. 406v: "Das Blut das ist ym verstopfft und verhindert."
45 Cod. 11238, fol. 98r.
46 Ibid., fol. 71r, Comes de Monte on the *febris interpollata* of the mistress of a young nobleman.
47 Ibid., fol. 99r.

rubbing the legs shortly before menstruation was expected, thus directing the flow of the humors downward.⁴⁸

In some cases, the disease progressed evenly, without ups and downs. Here one spoke of a *febris continua*, a sustained and continuous fever or of a *synochus*. Handsch himself once fell ill with a *febris continua*.⁴⁹ In many cases, however, physicians believed they could discern a recurring intensification or worsening in the form of febrile attacks. The most important forms of such intermittent fevers ("febres interpollatae") were named in accordance with the respective periodicity of the febrile attacks and were at the same time connected with ideas about the cause and nature of the particular morbid matter. Depending on which humor spoiled and decayed, different rhythms could be observed. The medical literature distinguished a multitude of different fever types by the kind of periodicity and the nature of the morbid matter. In medical practice, however, only a few types were frequently diagnosed.

With *tertiana*, or tertian fever, the febrile attacks happened every second day. The term came from the established way of counting: if the patient had an attack on one day, the next day his fever would be calm, but on the third ("tertius") day, there would be a new febrile attack. In Tyrol, according to Handsch, intermittent fevers were thus also called "the evil good", because a good day was followed by a bad one.⁵⁰ As a rule, tertian fevers were traced to preternatural yellow bile. *Quartana* (from "quartus", fourth), or quartan fever, was associated with preternatural black bile and the attacks recurred every third day.⁵¹ The term "double tertian" ("tertiana duplex") designated a yellow-bilious fever from which the patient suffered an attack every day rather than every second day.⁵² The triple quartan fever ("quartana triplex") was likewise characterized by daily febrile attacks, but

---

48 Ibid., foll. 71r-72r.
49 Cod. 11183, fol. 403v.
50 Cod. 11206, fol. 162v, "das böse Gutt".
51 Drembach, De atra bile ([1548]), conclusio XII. In modern medicine, "tertian" and "quartan" are still commonly used terms for the two principal forms of malaria caused by two different subtypes of *plasmodium*. They are characterized by fever paroxysms that recur every second and third day respectively. Tertian fevers in this sense were, according to current knowledge, also widespread in Europe in earlier centuries. Some areas, such as the Maremma in Italy, were then notorious for the "swamp fever", which was attributed to the "mala aria", i.e. the bad, unhealthy air that reigned there. We do not know how many of the cases diagnosed as *tertiana* and *quartana* in the sixteenth century would still be diagnosed as such today. Practice records, such as those of Handsch, suggest that, with fevers, physicians usually expected and tried to determine some kind of periodicity, a cyclical recurrence of the fever attacks.
52 Cod. 11205, fol. 586r; for concrete cases see Cod. 11205, fol. 401r; Cod. 11207, fol. 35r; Cod. 11238, fol. 121v.

here the attacks were traced to preternatural black bile.[53] Handsch's mentor Gallo came down with this type.[54] In the case of the double quartan fever ("quartana duplex") two days with febrile attacks were followed by one quiet, paroxysm-free day; the physician could explain this to the patient with his fingers as counting aids if necessary.[55] *Febris quotidiana,* or quotidian fever, was also characterized by daily attacks of shivers and fever, but it was attributed to spoiled phlegm or blood.[56]

In the sixteenth century, the periodicity of the regularly recurring febrile attacks was not (or was no longer) primarily explained with naturally given rhythmical patterns but rather with a regular mobilization of the respective morbid matter.[57] While the morbid humors during sustained fevers, the theory ran, remained mixed with the blood, they accumulated outside the veins with the intermittent fevers. From there they found their way back into the vessels at regular intervals, and into the heart or the muscles, making them stiff, as Handsch learned in Padua.[58] As a result the different fever types could also transform into others. A simple quartan fever could develop into a triple quartan if the same morbid matter was mobilized at different times in different places.[59] If several humors were involved, hybrid forms could result.

For physicians, the central significance of putrefied humors and processes of decay for the development of most fevers also explained the frequent coincidence of fever and worm infestation. According to the widely-accepted doctrine of spontaneous generation, worms, like fevers, developed from putrefaction. Trincavella and Handsch, visited a nineteen-year-old patient, for example, in whose stool they found worms. Trincavella concluded that the young man had accumulated large quantities of raw, mucous matter in his stomach from which the worms had developed.[60]

As a rule, the stronger the putrefaction, the greater the danger. Fracanzano, Trincavella, and other physicians often called highly malignant fevers "pestilential" without referring to "pestilence" ("pestis"), or plague, in the proper sense.[61] True pestilential fever ("febris pestilens") was considered a disease of its

---

[53] Cod. 11238, fol. 105r.
[54] Cod. 11205, fol. 162v and fol. 598r.
[55] Ibid., fol. 598r.
[56] Cod. 11240, fol. 4r; cf. Cod. 11238, fol. 140r.
[57] Cod. 11183, fol. 471v, on the notion of a *materia fixa*.
[58] Cod. 11240, fol. 4r.
[59] Cod. 11238, fol. 105r.
[60] Ibid., fol. 74r-v; the doctrine of the so-called "spontaneous generation", i.e. of the emergence of (lower) animals from putrefaction, was still widely accepted at the time, although Handsch as a student also noted the doubts that Aristotle had already expressed (ibid., fol. 74v).
[61] Cod. 11238, fol. 106r and fol. 123r; Cod. 11207, fol. 12.

own and distinguished from other fevers. Like consumption ("phthisis", "tabes"), scabies, and certain eye infections, it counted among the contagious diseases and it developed from a contagion of the air ("ex contagione aeris").[62] As Handsch learned from his Paduan professors, however, the manifestation of the plague in the body was not fundamentally different from that of a malignant putrid fever. With both, there was a pronounced putrefaction of the humors. In fevers that developed from a "contagion of the air" the putrefaction was just still more pronounced. Thus, both were to be treated in a similar manner.[63] Furthermore, as experience taught, malignant fevers too and not only the plague in a stricter sense occurred more frequently at certain times and in certain places. They too, as Handsch wrote, had "something epidemic" ("quoddam epidemicum")[64] or even proved contagious. He experienced this in his own family. When his father along with many others in his father's house and in all of Leipa fell ill with fever, he concluded that this intermittent fever ("febris interpollata") was sometimes epidemically contagious ("epidemica contagiosa").[65]

Diagnosing a fever as such was generally a simple matter. Even when the fever patient was subjectively complaining of coldness or was shivering[66] so much that the teeth were chattering,[67] the palpable fever heat that was present in serious cases often left no room for doubt. Here, relatives would say, "He's got heat".[68] And the question Handsch wanted to ask, especially with children, was "does he have heat?" because heat in most cases pointed to a fever.[69] To feel for the feverish heat, the physician could place his hand on the patient's forehead or feel the hands. Archduke Ferdinand II was in the habit of holding out his hands for his physician to feel.[70] As Handsch knew from his own experience,[71] fever patients also often had no appetite, complained about headaches and thirst, felt exhausted and weak and slept badly. With some fevers, red patches appeared on the skin,[72] so-called "Todtensprenkel" ("death speckles")

---

62 Cod. 11239, fol. 19r.
63 Cod. 11238, fol. 96r.
64 Cod. 11207, fol. 200r.
65 Ibid., fol. 210v.
66 Cod. 11183, fol. 406v, "tamen interius dixit se frigere".
67 Cod. 11207, fol. 203r, "das yr die Zene klapperen".
68 Ibid., fol. 71v, "Er hat Hiz".
69 Ibid., fol. 198r.
70 Cod. 11206, fol. 171v.
71 Cod. 11238, fol. 133v, "mea febris 5 dierum"; Cod. 11183, fol. 408v.
72 Cod. 11183, fol. 418v.

or *petechiae*.[73] Other fevers were characterized by severe diarrhea or vomiting, as Handsch experienced himself several times.[74]

Uroscopy was routinely used to diagnose fevers, with the urine typically indicating inner heat by its strong yellow or reddish color, which Handsch also observed with himself.[75] The change in color was considered to be so characteristic that one could simply refer to the "feverish color" ("color febrilis") of the urine[76] or conversely to urine that was not "feverishly colored" ("febriliter colorata").[77] Unfortunately, uroscopy was not very reliable for diagnosing fevers, as leading authorities of the time emphasized. A seemingly feverish, dark color that verged on red might also point to a simple heating of the kidneys, causing the same changes in the urine that passed on its way out of the body.[78] On the other hand, medical experience taught that the urine of a patient suffering from quartan fever often looked like that of a healthy person.[79] And, as Handsch learned from Gallo, the same was true right at the beginning of particularly malignant fevers. Here, healthy-looking urine was even considered to be a bad sign; it showed that the "poison" ("venenum") was in the heart rather than in the veins, where it would reveal itself by causing coarse and cloudy urine.[80]

According to Handsch's notes, uroscopy was particularly valuable when the urine was examined daily over a number of days so that the development of the fever and the underlying morbid matter within the body could be traced. Hardly visible, miniscule particles, the so-called *atomi*, and turbidity indicated that nature was about to concoct and excrete the morbid matter. Coarser particles, cloudy or discolored urine and sediment indicated that nature's efforts were increasingly successful.[81]

Like uroscopy, hematoscopy could show the presence of febrile heat in the body: the blood in the bloodletting bowl was black from the heat.[82] With sustained fevers, where the heat was constant, the physician could therefore predict that the patient's blood would be black as pitch when he or she was bled.[83]

---

73 Ibid., fol. 24r.
74 Ibid., fol. 418v; Cod. 11238, fol. 136r, on Giulio Gallo's fever, with added references to two other fever patients with vomiting.
75 Cod. 11205, fol. 398r.
76 Cod. 11183, fol. 74r.
77 Ibid., fol. 80v.
78 Cod. 11207, fol. 98v.
79 Cod. 11240, fol. 147r, with a reference to Giovanni Arcolani's "De febribus" (fifteenth cent.).
80 Cod. 11207, fol. 17r.
81 Cod. 11238, fol. 96v-100r, notes on patient visits with Tremenus and Trincavella.
82 Cod. 11183, fol. 453r.
83 Cod. 11205, fol. 406v.

Sometimes, the morbid matter that was mixed in with the blood even became visible as a pus-like substance that rose to the surface of the black, clotted blood after it had stood for some time.[84]

In the case of pulse diagnosis, fevers were even the central area of application. With numerous cases, Handsch noted a "feverish pulse", a *pulsus febrilis*, or the lack of one.[85] When the skin rash of a Turkish woman disappeared, he was able to recognize from the pulse (and the heat) that she had not yet overcome the fever.[86] In his notes, he indicated only vaguely the specific pulse qualities that characterized a *pulsus febrilis*. He was essentially content with its designation as "rapid" ("velox"), "very rapid" ("velocissimus") or "accelerated" ("celerius") and, when the fever heat abated or temporarily declined or "slowed" ("tardius").[87]

An examination of the tongue could provide additional insights. Looking at the tongue has long been an integral part of physical examination, with tongue checks widely and routinely performed still today, even if its diagnostic validity has been called into question in recent medical literature. In Handsch's time, physicians believed that they could determine the kind of morbid matter and whether it was excessively heated from a fever by examining the coating of the tongue. His professors back in Padua had shown him what was entailed.[88] With some fever patients, they observed a brown or even black-coated tongue.[89] Sometimes they also touched the tongue with their finger.[90] According to Fracanzano, a very dry and rough tongue signaled that the fever was literally burning inside the body.[91]

The treatment of fevers could take place at several levels. Especially at the beginning of treatment, the physician could seek to cool the *calor febrilis* before giving other medications which might even aggravate the foreign fever heat.[92] In Rhazes, Handsch found an early example of a comparative clinical observation: while travelling, a master and his servant fell ill with a very hot fever. The master was given cold water to drink and survived, while the servant did not receive any water and died.[93] And presumably it was the cooling effect of whey

---

84 Cod. 11238, fol. 71r.
85 E.g. Cod. 11183, fol. 74v, fol. 163r, fol. 282v, fol. 295r, fol. 373r and fol. 414v.
86 Ibid., fol. 373v.
87 Cod. 11205, fol. 320r and fol. 453v; Cod. 11238, fol. 119r and fol. 122v.
88 Cod. 11238, fol. 119v; Cod. 11240, fol. 151r: "In hospitale aspexit linguam febricitanti".
89 Cod. 11207, fol. 17r; Cod. 11183, fol. 418v.
90 Cod. 11207, fol. 17r.
91 Cod. 11238, fol. 118r.
92 Cod. 11183, fol. 64v, on Lehner who first "formam febrilem sc[ilicet] calorem restringuit"; see also Cod. 11207, fol. 180v.
93 Cod. 11240, 148v; Cod. 11238, fol. 4r.

that prompted physicians in England – this according to a report by a febrile fellow student of Handsch from England – to recommend whey as a suitable beverage for fever patients.[94]

For a lasting success of the cure, however, it was crucial that the spoiled, foul morbid matter be drained from the body, thus possibly preventing further febrile attacks which came from its periodic mobilization. Here, the physician was not to be deceived by an apparent recovery. Even if the febrile heat abated, the putrid matter ("materia putrida") that caused the fever might still be found in the vessels, as Handsch learned from Lehner.[95] With dysentery ("dysenteria"), it was therefore important not to combat the diarrhea all too aggressively, because a pestilential fever could arise from retained malignant matter.[96]

Indicated above all were purgatives, a first line of treatment in Padua,[97] and bloodletting.[98] Gallo swore by emetics as well, because corrupted matter, which fed the fever, accumulated in the fever patient's stomach.[99] Once the body and the blood were roughly cleansed in this way, the physician had to attempt to dissolve the obstructions that were thought to always play a significant role with fevers.[100] Handsch noted down a basic rule: "Treating fevers means opening obstructions".[101] In medical experience, blockages in the organs could be dissolved with sour substances, especially vinegar, which simultaneously combatted putrefaction.[102] In Handsch's assessment, a drink with vinegar and aromatic substances was essential in helping a patient who suffered from tertian fever.[103] Further, the physician had to ensure that the foreign febrile heat in the body was not increased by external influences. Handsch was astonished when Mattioli administered his heat-generating quintessence to a fever patient who was already complaining of great heat in the heart region. Probably, Handsch thought, Mattioli wanted to make it look as if he were doing something to fight the disease. Even good doctors made mistakes sometimes, he commented drily.[104] One of the important questions concerning the diet of fever patients was therefore

---

94 Cod. 11238, fol. 128r.
95 Cod. 11183, fol. 74r.
96 Ibid., fol. 221v.
97 Cod. 11240, fol. 87r.
98 Cod. 11205, fol. 226v.
99 Ibid., fol. 154v.
100 Ibid., fol. 226v.
101 Cod. 11183, fol. 410v: "Curare febres est obstructiones aperire."
102 Cod. 11205, fol. 226v; Cod. 11207, fol. 17r and fol. 60v.
103 Cod. 11205, fol. 226v.
104 Cod. 11207, fol. 204v.

whether they were allowed to drink wine, and if so how much. Not only in southern Europe but north of the Alps as well, wine was a common, everyday drink and doctors and laypeople alike considered it to have a generally fortifying effect. It was thought, however, to heat the body, albeit to different degrees depending on the type of wine. And so it was necessary to be cautious.

With acute fevers, many doctors relied more than with other diseases on the healing powers of nature, of the body itself. Often these effects could be clearly discerned in the person's profuse perspiration, which was generally thought to introduce and accompany the abatement of a febrile attack or a fever as such and to signify the successful excretion of the febrile matter via the skin. Some patients spoke of multiple shirts which they had to change within a short period of time.[105] As an explanation and a way to remind sick people to be patient, Handsch wrote down the comparison, "The blood cleans itself little by little", and it was like with rising yeast, because "when the blood makes to ferment, it pools together, creating a heap in the body, and so the hands, feet, and skin remain cold." Once fermentation started, "the heat arrives and finally the yeasts go away, which is the sweat."[106] For this reason, fever patients were also discouraged from going out into the fresh air, because cold air constricted the pores and thus hindered the evacuation of morbid matter. Thus, it makes sense why a doctor gave a febrile boy this warning: "Don't go outdoors, keep yourself warm".[107] When Handsch had a fever, his colleague Tremenus gave him the same advice.[108] And indeed, Handsch had observed the insalubrious effects of fresh air not only with patients, but with himself as well.[109] Even compresses could seem dangerous for this reason. When Andrea Gallo recommended the use of compresses to treat the febrile Giulio Alessandrini, Gallo's son objected. He considered it more important for the *calor* – he obviously meant the *calor febrilis* – to evaporate unimpeded.[110]

Experience taught that urination was another important means of evacuating febrile matter. Thus, if the urine changed significantly, seemed cloudy or had a thick, brick-red sediment reminiscent of blood, this was often a good sign in the opinion of doctors. It indicated that nature of her own power was mobilizing and evacuating the morbid matter. Handsch even derived a general rule from the observation he made many times that the urine of fever patients changed significantly

---

105 Ibid., fol. 226v.
106 Cod. 11205, fol. 202v.
107 Ibid., fol. 398r.
108 Ibid., fol. 193r.
109 Ibid.
110 Ibid., fol. 307v.

when they began to recover: if the urine of patients with a sustained fever was spoiled, this was always a good sign.[111]

With acute fevers, physicians could also draw on the ancient notion of "critical days". According to this concept, acute diseases changed for the better or for the worse on certain days in the course of the disease; in Greek, the words for "crisis" and "decision" have the same root. In fevers, special significance was assigned to the fourth, the seventh, and the fourteenth day of illness, calculated from when the person first fell ill. With acute or malignant fevers – this Handsch learned early on from Ulrich Lehner – a "critical", that is "decisive", evacuation of the morbid matter was essential – with sweat, vomiting, defecation, urination, or another form of excretion.[112] Accompanying his Paduan professors, Handsch saw fever patients whose disease began to recede, on the fourteenth day for example, when a large quantity of urine was excreted.[113] And he experienced how Trincavella used this knowledge of the critical days to predict the recovery of a fever patient on the fourteenth day after the beginning of the illness.[114] When he gave a patient a purgative or a "solutivum" on the fourteenth day of illness and the man died several days later, Handsch upbraided himself ("meum erratum"). It had been wrong to give such a remedy on a "critical day"; he should have waited for nature to do her part.[115]

When a "critical" evacuation indicated the successful work of nature, some doctors even chose to administer hardly any medication at all. Trincavella in Padua, for example, gave little or no medication when there were signs that the illness was taking a favorable course. As Handsch surmised, probably correctly, this was "because he does not want to hinder the work of nature". Only when he saw the visible signs of successful concoction in the urine did Trincavella administer diuretics so as to aid the evacuation of the matter that was manifestly ready to be excreted.[116] In Prague, by contrast, the physicians often administered diuretics even if "raw" urine showed that the morbid matter was far from being perfectly concocted.[117] This was wrong in Handsch's view and in his notes he criticized Mattioli's treatment of fever patients with uncharacteristic vehemence: Mattioli had overburdened the febrile *chartarius* Matthias with numerous medications, whereas Handsch thought it correct to give only few remedies

---

111 Cod. 11206, fol. 35r.
112 Ibid., fol. 318r.
113 Cod. 11238, fol. 98r.
114 Ibid., fol. 106r.
115 Cod. 11183, foll. 48v-50v.
116 Cod. 11238, foll. 97v-98r; Cod. 11183, fol. 119r.
117 Cod. 11183, fol. 119r.

and "to allow nature to do something". As Handsch saw it, the fever only got worse under Mattioli's treatment.[118]

With chronic fevers, above all quartan fever, doctors by their own admission could often no more than hope that nature would eventually overcome the fever. Here their therapeutic capabilities usually reached their limits. Handsch called the quartan fever a "scandalon".[119] Some chronic fevers lasted sixteen weeks or even half a year or longer.[120] As Handsch wrote, Augustus, Elector of Saxony, much like Emperor Maximilian, suffered from a fever for a whole year. His physician did not come away with praise.[121] All physicians could do in such cases was to ask for patience in those suffering a fever. According to Handsch's notes, physicians could say to patients, "You must endure the fever" or, "The fever's rage needs to become exhausted". And they could remind them that even great kings, lords, and princes with their *doctores* had to "endure the fever" because "it must not be obstructed".[122] Fracanzano explained to a patient suffering from an intermittent fever, "I cannot do anything for you; you have to let its rage come to an end".[123] Here physicians could generally count on the patient's understanding. Laypeople were familiar with the idea that diseases followed particular temporal patterns. The wife of a paperhanger, for example, complained that "it was expelled from him too soon" when, after the apparently successful treatment of his fever, her husband suffered from colic, vomited, and had two convulsive seizures.[124]

Some physicians even went a step further. In his detailed study on the history of the doctrine of the healing power of nature, Max Neuburger shone a light on the ideas Gómez Pereira outlined in his *Margarita Antoniana,* identifying them as an important, innovative alternative to traditional fever theory.[125] According to Neuburger, Pereira was the first to proclaim that fevers could have favorable, salubrious effects. Handsch's notes, however, show that this conception did not originate with Pereira. It was known in Italy and Bohemia, and possibly elsewhere, as early as the mid-sixteenth century, and by all indications had much older origins. In Handsch's conviction, fevers could help fight off

---

118 Ibid., fol. 119r-v, "aliquid etiam permittere naturae".
119 Cod. 11206, fol. 104v; see also ibid., fol. 105r: "Hydrops et quartana medicis sunt scandala plana".
120 Cod. 11207, fol. 210r.
121 Cod. 11206, fol. 104v: "Nullam laudem medicus reportat."
122 Cod. 11205, fol. 202v.
123 Cod. 11238, fol. 135r.
124 Cod. 11183, fol. 454r.
125 Neuburger, Lehre (1926), p. 35, on part 2, ch. 5 of Pereira's Werk.

other serious illnesses in children in particular, because they led to an evacuation of spoiled morbid matter. In the case of a ten-year-old boy with quotidian fever attacks, he soon stopped giving any medication. He explained that it was not a dangerous disease, and with "fevers in young people, children, more serious accidental diseases go away; and it is not good to expel it soon; the blood cleanses itself and brings out yeasts like a young wine."[126] Laypeople, too, sometimes considered fevers to be salubrious. A Bohemian chancery clerk, for example, commented on the fevers of two stable boys, saying that "swine fevers" ("febres maiales") were not dangerous but indeed "healthy".[127] According to Handsch, there was even a saying about quartan fever in Italy: "The four-day fever kills the old and heals the young".[128]

Gabrielle Falloppia found empirical evidence of the potential salubrious effect of quartan fever in a man who had been condemned to death and sent to Pisa to be anatomized. When Falloppia gave him a fatal dose of opium while he was in the midst of an acute febrile attack, the fever conquered the poison, as Falloppia told his students. The man survived. But the next day, when he had no fever paroxysm, he was again given the same dose and he died, just as anyone else would.[129] Still today, it is commonly believed by laypeople and medical professionals alike that it is best (within limits) to let the fever take its course instead of turning immediately to antipyretic medication. Yet, as we have seen, there is a crucial difference: in the Renaissance, the healing effect of fevers was seen not in their elevation of body temperature but in the fact that they stimulated nature to evacuate the harmful matter from the body.

The ideas sketched out above regarding the key role played by an often putrid, corrupted, indeed poisonous febrile matter that had to be concocted and expelled by the body provide the background, in turn, for another conviction that is still widely held by laypeople today, namely that fever patients should fast or at least make do with light, easily digestible foods: zwieback or rusks, or as was my own rather unpleasant childhood experience, gruel. Still today, one of the most well-known medical adages goes, "Feed a cold, starve a fever".[130] In his notes, Handsch repeatedly emphasized the therapeutic effects of fasting

---

126 Cod. 11205, fol. 303v, "gehens sonst grosserer zufellige Kranckheit hinweg, ist auch nicht gutt, das man es bald vertreibe, das Blutt reinigt sich, und wirfft gleich wie eyn junger Weyn Hefen auff."
127 Cod. 11183, fol. 361v.
128 Cod. 11206, fol. 104v: "La febre quartana le vecchie mazza, le iuovene sana"; Cod. 11207, fol. 86v.
129 Cod. 11225, fol. 36r.
130 Cf. Helman, Feed (1978).

during an acute fever and he named numerous patients who ate little or nothing during their fever and recovered quickly.[131] Girolamo Gallo, for example (he was likely the brother of Handsch's patron Andrea Gallo), a notary in Trento, gave his feverish son nothing to eat except a little bread soup (*panatella*) in the evening. The son only suffered two attacks before he was healthy again.[132] The reasons for the therapeutic effect of fasting during fevers were obvious to physicians at the time. In their view, what was crucial for healing was the concoction and excretion of the febrile matter by the inner nature of the body and her tool, the vital heat. If the patient abstained from food, the vital heat could concentrate entirely on its fight against the morbid matter.[133] Only when the fever began to abate was it advisable to increase food intake so that the weakened body could regain strength.[134]

Consumption

Consumption, or, in the medical terminology of the time, "phthisis" or "phthysis", was a frequently diagnosed and feared disease. In Handsch's notes, it had a preeminent place.[135] Of the cases he documented with fatal outcomes, it was the deadliest by far. This stands in striking contradiction to the printed collections of medical case histories or *observationes,* where it only plays a marginal role. This is undoubtedly the result of the choices made by the authors or compilers of these collections. Because treatment in most cases ultimately met with failure, consumption offered neither the opportunity to illustrate the most suitable therapeutic approach to readers nor did it allow the authors to advertise their outstanding therapeutic skills.

Retrospectively, the early modern term "consumption" is often more or less equated with the modern diagnosis of "pulmonary tuberculosis". This is rather problematic. The bacterial pathogens were not yet known and some patients who were diagnosed as "consumptive" at the time may have, in today's assessment, died from pulmonary carcinoma, severe emphysema, or another disease.

---

131 Cod. 11238, fol. 139v.
132 Ibid.
133 Cod. 11205, fol. 397v, "quia natura semper agens ita aget in materiam morbificam"; Cod. 11238, fol. 139v, "natura tum tantum est intenta circa materiam".
134 Cod. 11238, fol. 137v.
135 In addition to the cases mentioned here, Handsch documented further cases of patients he himself or the physicians around him suspected of suffering from consumption in Cod. 11183, fol. 344r.

However, early modern consumption doubtlessly ranks among those diseases where the possibility of a plausible retrospective diagnosis – though rejected on principle by some historians – cannot be categorically and sweepingly denied.[136] How much and in what way such a retrospective diagnosis serves historical insight – or whether it might stand in the way of it – is a different question, of course.[137]

The clinical picture that was associated with the diagnosis of *phthisis* or consumption in the Renaissance is very similar to modern "pulmonary tuberculosis" and at the same time, in its combination of symptoms, it is very specific. Based on the dissection of deceased "consumptive" patients, small lumps and growths in the lungs were described, along with other post-mortem findings that still today are considered distinctive for pulmonary tuberculosis.[138] In the body of Emperor Ferdinand I, for example, who passed away in 1564 after having been ill for ten months, a hardened, dried-out pulmonary lobe was found that had become attached to the spine.[139]

According to the medical judgment of the day, the most important signs of consumption were a chronic, often agonizing cough with profuse tenacious and malodorous sputum as well as a feeling of heat in the body and night sweats. As the disease progressed, the sputum typically became bloody and there could even be massive bleeding. Emaciation and hair loss set in,[140] and, toward the end, increased respiratory distress to the point where patients feared asphyxiation.[141]

In his notes, Handsch documented a whole host of cases of consumption. Many of the patients were relatively young. A young, thin patient called Wenzel Crispin, for example, spat up blood and had a persistent cough. He became

---

136 Demaitre, Medieval medicine (2013), p. 44, has come to a similiar conclusion.
137 On retrospective diagnosis, in general, see Rath, Moderne Diagnosen (1956); Leven, Krankheiten (1998); Stolberg, Möglichkeiten (2012); Stolberg/Walter, Martin Luthers viele Krankheiten (2018).
138 Colombo, Re medica (1559), p. 265.
139 Cod. 11183, fol. 196v; in addition, several ounces of "sand" were found in the kidneys, suggesting that they were affected as well. Afterwards, the body was treated with myrrhe, storax and similar substances that had a pleasant smell, presumably to help preserve the corpse (ibid.).
140 Ibid., fol. 264r; the Hippocratic aphorisms already ranked alopecia among the typical symptoms of consumption. According to Brasavola alopecia could have different causes but in the case of consumption it indicated the approaching death. Just as the trees lost their leaves in fall, the hair fell off the head, when the *humidum radicale* dried up (Brasavola, In octo libros (1541), p. 775).
141 Some patients reported other, less typical symptoms which, as the physicians were well aware, could also indicate a concomitant second disease. Young "Resch phtysicus", for example, had swollen arms and legs but according to Handsch he also drank a lot, was a "magnus potator".

emaciated, bedridden, and gasped for breath. He could only speak tremulously and finally, after months of illness, he died.[142] At the Ambras court, Handsch and Willenbroch treated a Turkish girl who was only fifteen or sixteen years old. She developed a chronic cough and finally began to expectorate "greenish", slimy, almost pussy sputum and sometimes bloody matter as well. She died within less than a year.[143] An older female patient had been suffering from a cough for two years when Handsch saw her. She was emaciated and complained of night sweats, slimy and sometimes bloody sputum, as well as hair loss, and she became bedridden in the end. Handsch predicted that she would soon die. To his surprise, he saw her in town a few weeks later, but not long after this he heard that she was doing poorly again.[144]

Consumption was considered contagious and "hereditary" in the broad definition of the time – broad in the sense that one could, for example, "inherit" scabies from someone by wearing his or her clothes. A colleague of Handsch, with whom Handsch treated the ailing Johann von Wartenberg, said that he preferred to attend someone who was suffering from the plague rather than a consumptive patient. He held that just stepping on the sputum of someone suffering from consumption with bare feet was enough to become infected ("inficitur").[145] It was believed that the disease could be passed on through contact with a sick person or his or her sputum, and from parents to children. With consumptive adolescents in particular, Handsch accordingly made note of the death of a parent or sibling from consumption or hectic fever which was often associated with it, for example the mother of Wenzel Crispin and the brother of the wife of Korzaur.[146] His notes suggest that the fear of contagion and inheritance was also widespread among laypeople. The Lord of Peyersberg, for example, feared that his son, who was about sixteen years old, had consumption because the boy's mother had died of the disease.[147]

Consumption also numbered among those diseases that were long connected to particular professions. Handsch supplemented his excerpts of Pietro d'Abano's *De venenis* with a note in the margin saying that some metal workers became consumptive, and in another entry he named specific cases.[148]

---

[142] Cod. 11183, fol. 473v.
[143] Ibid., fol. 368v.
[144] Ibid., fol. 264r.
[145] Ibid., fol. 239v.
[146] Ibid., fol. 81r and fol. 473v.
[147] Ibid., fol. 405v.
[148] Cod. 11240, fol. 75r; Cod. 11205, fol. 237v.

According to the dominant teachings, what was central to the pathological process within the lungs was a sharp biting morbid matter that, like with other forms of a *catarrhus*, ran down into the lungs. The seriously ill wife of Blasius even believed she could physically perceive its movement inside her body. In her back she could "feel in the night how it ran down cold". In the margin, Handsch commented: "Note: a manifest sign of catarrh".[149] The hotter, more acrid or bilious the matter, the greater the danger for life and limb, because it was all the more able to eat away at the pulmonary vessels and cause a bloody cough. On the other hand, as Bellocati in Padua recounted from his own clinical experience, a case of consumption that was mucous and moist could go on for twenty or thirty years.[150] To some degree, Handsch believed he could confirm these findings from his own physical experience. When he once had a head cold ("coryza"), his left nostril, through which the morbid matter was draining, was as if raw inside. The matter itself tasted salty. His conclusion from this was that the same thing must happen in the lungs. When a salty catarrh drained into the lungs, the lungs too would become raw inside and an ulcer would form. The sputum would become bloody and consumption would ensue.[151] In another entry, he concluded that a salty catarrh, since it could even eat into the hard substance of the teeth – cavities at the time were linked to catarrh – was all the more able to corrode the soft lungs.[152]

Some consumptive patients seemed to be rotting from the inside out. They perpetually expectorated ill-colored, fetid, and purulent sputum, the odor emanating from their mouths was nauseating.[153] The *foetor* coming from the wife of an archducal chancery clerk, who sometimes also spat up blood, was likened to that of feces by the court surgeon Hildebrand.[154] Apparently, this stench was even considered a decisive diagnostic sign among laypeople. Rejecting a physician's diagnosis of consumption, an ailing patient said, "If my lungs were foul, I would stink from the throat."[155]

If the foul, corrupted matter accumulated in a cavity, a so-called empyema would result, that is a local collection of pus in the lungs. This could be a preliminary stage of consumption if an ulcerous decay set in over time, or it could be an accompanying symptom of consumption if, for some time, the matter had

---

149 Cod. 11205, fol. 509v: "Nota manifestum signum catarri".
150 Cod. 11240, fol. 91r.
151 Cod. 11205, fol. 119v.
152 Ibid., fol. 243v: "Meum de phtysi".
153 E.g. Cod. 11183, fol. 264r; Cod. 11205, fol. 165r.
154 Cod. 11183, fol. 484v.
155 Cod. 11207, fol. 75v.

no access to the respiratory tract and thus could not be coughed up. In living persons, empyemas could only be diagnosed with certainty when they formed near the ribcage and were visible from the outside. In these cases, they could be opened surgically if necessary by making an incision in the skin.[156] As Giovanni Battista da Monte explained in a *consultatio,* an empyema generally resolved itself at some point insofar as it burst and its matter was evacuated through the air passages or the skin, or it was excreted with the urine or stool. The girl who was the subject of his consultation had been ill for four years and was severely emaciated. Her stinking sputum pointed to excretion via the airways, but on top of that, an accumulation of matter could be seen externally on her left side. While Da Monte did not expressly declare the girl consumptive, he was obviously thinking in this direction. He feared a fatal outcome and warned of the danger of contagion. Everyone who helped her, he stressed, especially children and relatives, must not have a conversation near her, meaning in all likelihood that they must not stay longer than absolutely necessary.[157]

Consumption was diagnosed primarily based on the appearance of the sputum. Typically, consumptive sputum was plentiful, more or less strongly discolored, and at times malodorous. To determine if the sputum was purulent, the patient could be asked to spit into a water-filled vessel – more precisely, Handsch indicated a glazed clay vessel.[158] If there was pus in the sputum, it would sink to the bottom. Handsch described how he himself and his colleagues actually asked patients to collect their sputum in water-filled containers.[159] The physicians in Handsch's professional environment also gleaned from the Hippocratic *Aphorisms* that the sputum could be thrown on glowing embers: purulent sputum would give off an unpleasant smell.[160] When Mattioli suggested this at the bedside, Handsch was critical, thinking it dangerous due to the possibility of contagion.[161] Another time, however, when he was treating a patient he suspected of being consumptive, he advised her to do precisely this and then asked her maid if it stank.[162]

Bloody sputum was seen as especially characteristic for consumption, as Handsch had already learned from Fracanzano in Padua. Fracanzano made a point of asking patients about it. With one severely emaciated patient who was complaining of tightness in the chest and a coarse voice, Fracanzano initially

---

156 Cf. also Cod. 11183, fol. 468v.
157 Da Monte, Consultationum (1554), pp. 272–73.
158 Cod. 11183, fol. 405v, "vas terreum vitreatum".
159 Ibid.; Cod. 11207, fol. 75v.
160 Brasavola, In octo libros (1541), pp. 775–76, on book 5, aph. 11.
161 Cod. 11207, fol. 75v, "quia phtysis contagiosa est."
162 Cod. 11205, fol. 537v.

wondered if he was dealing with a case of *asthma*. But the following day, having seen the man's somewhat bloody sputum, he committed to the diagnosis of *phthisis*.[163] In later years with his own patients, Handsch paid close attention to this sign.[164]

In the medical thinking of the time, *phthisis* or consumption was closely connected to hectic fever, to *febris hectica*. The two diseases often co-occurred and both pointed in their names to emaciation, to a dwindling or consumption of body mass, but they referred to two different pathological processes. At the center of the contemporary understanding of consumption was an ulceration and putrefactive decay in the lungs, caused, as a rule, by a more or less specific and contagious morbid matter. Hectic fever, by contrast, was by definition not associated with morbid matter.

For physicians, there were great challenges involved in treating consumption. With good reason, Handsch named consumption first among the incurable diseases whose treatment he did not want to take on: the physician could at most prolong the life of the consumptive patient but he could never free him or her of the disease.[165] This was also for "mechanical" reasons: once ulceration had occurred, it was impossible to heal it because the lungs were in constant movement.[166] When the wife of Korzaur coughed up blood for the first time – this was considered to be a clear indication of ulceration – all of the physicians immediately lost hope, according to Handsch. He continued to visit her in the following weeks, but then he, too, "left" her ("reliqui ipsam"). Less than two weeks later, she was dead.[167]

If there was a chance at all of recovering from consumption, it was at the outset of the disease. Physicians could thus blame the patient for not seeking their advice sooner and thereby hold them responsible for the failure of the treatment. Along these lines, a physician explained to the consumptive Lord of Tetschen that he had "hesitated too long; if I had seen you earlier, I would have liked to help you."[168]

Given its nature, consumption was therefore a disease which demanded for the most part that physicians be content with a "cura palleativa", as Handsch's relayed the term derived from the Latin "pallium" for "cloak"; it was a term

---

[163] Cod. 11183, fol. 121r.
[164] Ibid., fol. 264r.
[165] Cod. 11240, fol. 42r: "Incurabiles morbos non suscipere, ut est phtisis, apoplexia, asthma in senibus, hydrops inveterata, oculorum vicia, bene possunt prolongari vita et praeservari homo ab illis sed non liberari."
[166] Cod. 11205, fol. 237v; similarly already in his Paduan years Cod. 11240, fol. 29v.
[167] Cod. 11183, fol. 82v.
[168] Cod. 11205, fol. 165v; the physician was probably Andrea Gallo.

which had come increasingly into use since the late Middle Ages.[169] As we have seen, if a radical, curative treatment – one that got to the root of the disease – was no longer possible, all that remained to do was "cloak" the symptoms and attempt to slow down the progress of the disease.

Thus, to the extent that Handsch documented the medical treatment of individual consumptive patients, he primarily indicated remedies that served to alleviate the symptoms. According to his notes, physicians gave white sugar, rose sugar (*zuccarum rosatum*), and other remedies that were meant to ease expectoration ("facilentia sputum").[170] This was presumably also the goal of a *mixtura pectoralis*, which Johannes Willenbroch ordered be taken by the consumptive Turkish girl at Ambras three times daily with the help of a "wooden spoon".[171] When a significant amount of blood was being coughed up, the physician could attempt to direct the flow of blood away from the lungs by way of bloodletting. Handsch assumed that this was the intention of an unnamed physician who ordered bloodletting on five occasions for an approximately 29-year-old male patient whose severe cough was producing blood, as Handsch learned from the patient's account.[172] However, bloodletting came with the risk of weakening the consumptive even further.

Unlike with most other diseases, Handsch rarely mentioned tried and tested recipes and specifics to combat consumption. Mattioli, he noted, praised a recipe against consumption that came from Valescus of Taranta (c. 1500) and with which he had accomplished "miracles" ("miracula").[173] The archduchess Helena (1543–1574) allegedly found fox lung very helpful in fighting her cough and above all her consumption. At the command of the prince, two foxes were caught and killed and their lungs were prepared by the apothecary. Nevertheless, she died at the young age of thirty-one.[174]

Gout and Podagra

Podagra or, in vernacular German "Zipperlein", was among the most frequently diagnosed chronic diseases in the sixteenth century. The Greek root word "pod" indicates its primary location, the foot. "Agra" and "agrios" refer to hunting,

---

[169] Cod. 11240, fol. 36r; see above and Stolberg, Cura palliativa (2007).
[170] Cod. 11205, fol. 477v; Cod. 11207, fol. 75v and Cod. 11205, fol. 107v; Cod. 11206, fol. 75r, "facilientia sputum".
[171] Cod. 11183, fol. 368v.
[172] Cod. 11205, 512v.
[173] Ibid., fol. 510r.
[174] Cod. 11183, fol. 344r.

trapping or, maybe most relevant in this context, getting wild. Handsch gave "dolor pedis", "foot pain", as the Latin translation.[175] The term referred in most cases to a specific clinical picture that was very similar to what we still today call "gout". The disease had been known since antiquity and was described and discussed at length in ancient medical literature.[176] The typical, characteristic symptom of *podagra* was (and still is today) a paroxysm of pain in the metatarso-phalangeal joint at the basis of the big toe. Patients described the pain as very intense and sharp. Some screamed with pain[177] or were terrified of just being touched on the affected area. Handsch described how some patients with *podagra* remained in their beds for several days or ventured no further than the privy because merely putting their foot on the floor was already too painful. Sometimes the ankles, other joints of the feet, or the knee were affected,[178] or the hand joints. In these cases, the disease could more precisely be called "gonagra" for knee pain, "chiragra" for hand pain and so forth. These conditions, which sometimes occurred simultaneously with foot pain,[179] were all considered to be manifestations of *podagra*, however. In other words, the term "podagra" did not only refer to the actual pain in the foot but also described a disease entity, a clinical picture which could manifest in different locations in the body. In his notes, Handsch occasionally also used terms such as "arthritis" and "artetica" for joint complaints. But special disease names for clinical pictures similar to what we call rheumatoid arthritis today were hardly in use at the time, not even among learned physicians. Presumably patients who would today be considered rheumatics or arthritics were then counted in with *podagra* patients.

Another typical and common symptom of *podagra*, though it was not always observed, were hardened bumps ("nodi podagrici") beneath the skin in the area of the painful joints.[180] Modern medicine explains them as local collections of urate crystals. Handsch had heard from a canon that if you opened them, a whitish, gypsum-like substance came out.[181] Falloppia called these bumps "tophi", a term which is still in use today and comes from the Greek word for "tuff". In Ferrara, he told his students, had removed a number of these tophi from a man with *podagra* and then cut them open to examine them.[182]

---

175 Cod. 9666, fol. 42r.
176 Porter/Rousseau, Gout (1988), pp. 13–20.
177 Cod. 11205, fol. 127r.
178 E.g. Cod. 11207, fol. 191v, on the "genugra" of the sick wife of a private tutor.
179 Concrete cases in Cod. 11183, fol. 189r; Cod. 11238, fol. 140r; Cod. 11207, fol. 197r.
180 Cod. 11205, fol. 252v, on the "nodi podagrici" around the finger joints.
181 Cod. 11238, fol. 142v, "extrusit proprie gypsum".
182 Cod. 11225, fol. 28v, notes on Falloppia's lectures on tumors "praeter naturam".

In the dominant understanding of the human body and its diseases, these bumps or tophi and what was generally localized pain in a single joint left little room for doubt about the nature and genesis of the disease. The disease was caused by a mobile morbid matter, which preferably settled in that location, a "humor praeter naturam", or "materia peccans", as Jean Fernel and Girolamo Capivaccia called it. Occasionally, Handsch referred to it as a "materia podagrica", while Johann Willenbroch called it a "gifftige verterbte Feuchtickeit" ("poisonous spoiled humor").[183] This substance was described as somewhat slimy, perhaps borrowing from the experience of the slightly mucilaginous, chalky water that produced visible deposits in thermal baths.[184] The morbid matter formed deposits in the area of the affected joint, causing the typical, intense pain, and it frequently presented itself to the observing eye, when it formed tophi.

Podagra was therefore an important subform of a "flux". A "flux" was mobile morbid matter in motion that accumulated in a certain location in the body. Handsch made a note of the Italian word for "podagra" – "la gotta" – derived from the Latin "gutta" for "drop". This image of dripping morbid matter is still preserved today in the term "gout" and we find the same in various other European languages: in Spanish and Portuguese with "gota", in French with "goutte". As long as it had not solidified, this liquid and thus mobile morbid matter could move on to a different location. Thus, in the perception of patients and physicians, *podagra*, too, had the potential to shift from one location to another, from one joint to another.[185] With this in mind, one female lay healer from Zittau cautioned of the danger of *podagra* even in a patient who had no joint complaints at all: "His chest is unclean with fluxes; if the fluxes gain the upper hand, we'll have to worry that they go to his back, arms and legs, and they could ultimately give him podagra".[186]

As with most fluxes, the morbid matter responsible for *podagra* was ultimately traced to an insufficient concoction of the food, caused by the inadequate heat or strength of the concocting parts, above all by their inability to cope with unsuitable, excessive food.[187] It was a humanist topos that the rich and powerful, whose lives abounded in the pleasures of eating and drinking,

---

183 Cod. 11183, fol. 325v; epistolary *consilium* by Girolamo Capivaccia for an unnamed nobleman from Salzburg, Padua 1575, in: Scholz, Consiliorum (1611), pp. 191–200.
184 Cod. 11205, 242v.
185 Cod. 11183, fol. 128r.
186 Cod. 11205, fol. 550r: "Er hat eyn unreyne Brust, von Flüssen, auch so die Flüsse uberhandt solten nemen, ist zubesorgen, es komme ym ynn den Recken, Arm, und Beyn, undmöcht er entlich das Podagra uberkomen."
187 Epistolary *consilium* by Girolamo Capivaccia for an unnamed nobleman from Salzburg, Padua 1575 in: Scholz, Consilia (1611), pp. 191–200.

were the most frequent victims of the disease. They paid for their flouting of the rules of moderate, healthy living with the almost unbearable pain of *podagra*.[188]

As with catarrh, physicians located the origin of the gouty flux in the head for the most part. It was there that the rising vapors and fumes cooled down, liquefied, and flowed downward into the joints. Looking at these ideas, we may better understand why Jean Fernel and other physicians at the time claimed that gout was closely related to *sciatica*. This was because – as Handsch had already learned as a student – the morbid matter responsible for *podagra* flowed down from the brain predominantly along the spine. If the ligaments in the hip area blocked the morbid matter as it moved down to the legs, then this would cause the characteristic pain that radiated down into the upper legs.[189]

According to Handsch's notes, an important predisposing factor in gout was a weakness or limpness of the ducts, ligaments, sinews, or "nerves" – the terms were often not strictly distinguished from one another at the time – in the area of the affected joint. This made it easier for the morbid matter to accumulate there.[190] Matthaeus Collinus, himself a victim of *podagra,* told his wife not to consume vinegar because it was an enemy of the "nerves".[191] There is no mention in Handsch's notes of the consumption of red meat, which today is considered as an important source of excessive levels of uric acid and thus in the genesis of gout. Physicians did, however, caution against thick, strong ("crassus") red wine, recommending instead white wine or mead, as did Mattioli in the case of Ulrich Lehner.[192]

Older people were considered to be particularly susceptible. Most of them, Handsch wrote, would have a *dispositio podagrica* or a weakness in the legs which led them to have complaints there when fluxes flowed downward in the body.[193] As the Hippocratic *Aphorisms* taught, women were much less susceptible to the disease because of their monthly cleansing. If women did show the signs of *podagra,* this could therefore indicate that their menstruation was obstructed.[194] *Podagra* was furthermore a disease that both physicians and laypeople considered to be hereditary.[195] As a young physician in Prague, Handsch made a note that one sufferer of podagra produces another sufferer of podagra.[196]

---

[188] Porter/Rousseau, Gout (1998), pp. 28–33.
[189] Cod. 11240, fol. 132r.
[190] Cod. 11207, fol. 47r.
[191] Cod. 11205, fol. 307r.
[192] Cod. 11207, fol. 102v.
[193] Cod. 11205, fol. 434r.
[194] Ibid., fol. 410r.
[195] Ibid., fol. 293v.
[196] Cod. 11207, fol. 57r.

For the most part, the medical prevention and treatment of *podagra* followed in a very direct and logical manner from the ideas that have been presented here. The aim was to curb the production of the phlegmy matter from which the morbid matter specific to *podagra* was created. To this end, *digestiva* were used. They strengthened the stomach and its inner heat and thus improved the concoction of food in the stomach, preventing the production and accumulation of raw, mucous matter.[197] Morbid matter that had already built up in the body was – as always – to be voided by means of suitable remedies, for example powerful purgatives or a diuretic like terebinth.[198] One man suffering from *podagra* was even given guaiac wood by Mattioli, which was mostly used to treat the French disease. Presumably Mattioli hoped to evacuate the morbid matter with the sweat.[199]

Going sometimes into considerable detail, physicians also impressed upon their patients the necessity of a thorough cleansing of the body so as to rid it of the morbid matter. This is shown in an epistolary consultation by the Zwickau physician Stefan Wild, which Handsch transcribed, presumably for future use with his own patients. Wild explained to the man that he had to "always keep the body quite clean" so that the fluxes did not accumulate again. If he had been bled regularly in the spring and fall, he should continue to do so and if necessary he should have cupping done as well. In addition, he prescribed powders that kept the "body lithe, supple, and clean [. . .] without purging too much", and which strengthened the stomach, as well as "morsels" or *morsuli*, which strengthened the head, stomach and the veins.[200]

In addition came the external treatment. Bloodletting could be done on the side opposite the affected side. Following the principle of *revulsio,* this aimed at drawing the morbid matter, to the extent that it was still mobile, out of the depths of the afflicted joint and the surrounding area.[201] But above all, an effort was made through ablutions and the application of ointments or compresses to alleviate the complaints and to strengthen the limb with its "nerves" and ligaments so as to slow down the further influx of morbid matter. Many kinds of

---

197 Cod. 11205, fol. 242v.
198 Cod. 11207, fol. 83v, fol. 197r and fol. 184v.
199 Ibid., fol. 39r.
200 Cod. 11183, fol. 305v-313r, cit. foll. 310v-311r, "alles Geeders".
201 Cod. 11207, fol. 22r, on Mattioli's explanation of the difference in comparison with erysipelas, in which a *revulsio* was not called for, because the morbific matter accumulated right underneath the skin; Cod. 11205, fol. 306r-v, on Handsch's treatment of the podagric wife of Collinus, which was flawed, as he came to realize; Cod. 11207, fol. 158r, on Ulrich Lehner, who treated his own *podagra* "contra regulas et praecepta communia", when he ordered bloodletting from the affected foot.

remedies were used here, for example pike fat or herbal decoctions.[202] According to Handsch, Ulrich Lehner reaped great praise for his *oleum generosum*, with which he had successfully combatted the pain of sciatica and *podagra*.[203] Presumably intended for local application, Handsch prescribed opium mixed with egg yolk to Collinus's wife, who was suffering from *podagra*. When it brought no relief, an opium poultice was made for her.[204] Gallo requested that his legs be fanned when he suffered from the pain of *podagra*.[205]

There were dangers involved in the local treatment of *podagra,* similar to those which loomed when an ulcer healed too soon. *Podagra* might be very painful, but it was also said that *podagra* patients tended to live a long life. This could easily be explained from a humoral-pathological perspective. With *podagra,* the morbid matter accumulated far away from the vital parts or organs. To a certain extent, this process could be likened to excretion, and the formation of tophi was indeed quite close to excretion. It made sense that the urine of *podagra* patients had a good, healthy color and consistency, as opposed to the dark coloration seen with pestilential diseases, where the morbid matter permeated the entire body and its blood,[206] and as opposed to stone disease, where the body evacuated the morbid matter through the kidneys and bladder. As we will be seeing in more detail, gout and stone disease were otherwise seen as closely related.

For the physician treating cases of *podagra,* this meant that he had to proceed with caution. If he impeded the further influx of morbid matter to the affected joint or mobilized the morbid matter in the affected body part without creating another excretory pathway, then the harmful matter could move to the vital organs, potentially with fatal consequences.

Handsch's Paduan professors had already told cautionary tales. Antonio Fracanzano, for example, had the story of a Venetian patrician who was freed of his *podagra* by a lay healer by means of strengthening and astringent remedies that were applied externally. But because nature was not able to direct the morbid matter to the joint as she was wont to do, she sent it to the area of the pharynx. The man developed tightness of the throat ("angina") and died of suffocation in the fifth year.[207] In another similar case, a lay healer promised to heal a nobleman suffering from *podagra*. He gave him a remedy and indeed the

---

202 Cod. 11183, fol. 45v.
203 Cod. 11200, fol. 198r; the composition is not known.
204 Cod. 11205, foll. 305v-306r.
205 Cod. 11207, fol. 8r.
206 Ibid., fol. 186r-v, "lindt und rein [. . .] one sonderlich [zu] purgiren".
207 Cod. 11238, fol. 128v.

podagra came to an end. Five months later, however, the sick man suffocated because the morbid matter, or so was the assumption, could no longer flow to its habitual place.[208] Learned physicians tended to blame the *empirici* for making such potentially fatal errors when treating *podagra*. Handsch also experienced, however, how his first medical teacher Ulrich Lehner washed the feet of a *podagra* patient with a decoction and how the patient then developed an inflammation and narrowing of the throat ("angina") and lockjaw ("tetanus"). He conjectured that the external treatment had strengthened the feet so that they no longer absorbed the morbid matter, whereupon nature sent it somewhere else.

This is all to say that it was important not to strengthen the affected limb too much or make it contract too much, and not to interrupt the influx of the morbid matter too abruptly. Handsch thus preferred to simply wash the area with salt water rather than externally apply alum and other more astringent remedies.[209] Gallo even rebuked Lehner (who suffered from *podagra*) for washing his feet and thus loosening the "nerves" and widening the passageways. He himself – as mentioned, Gallo, too, suffered from *podagra* – had not washed his feet in ten years. Lehner, however, who evidently suffered from stiff joints as well, thought that the "nerves" became suppler through washing.[210]

It was furthermore important to cleanse the body with purgatives before carrying out topical treatment, just as it was important to continue giving remedies afterwards on a regular basis that would prevent a renewed accumulation of morbid matter.[211] For similar reasons, Gallo asserted that one must not be content with administering gentle purgatives because of the risk of merely moving the morbid matter from the joint and mobilizing it without successfully driving it out. Rather, it was necessary to administer powerful purgatives that effectively evacuated the matter, just as he had done in Vienna with a *podagra* patient. After taking them, the man passed sixteen stools. According to Gallo, the treatment did him good and he was able to walk again without a cane.[212]

As an addition or an alternative to these treatment approaches that targeted the cause of the disease, numerous other remedies were used or at least recommended which were considered effective against *podagra* based on experience, without clear knowledge of the causal connections. Gallo, following Arnaldo de Villanova, swore by the beneficial effects of cilantro. He said he had administered

---

208 Cod. 11251, fol. 13r.
209 Cod. 11205, fol. 246r.
210 Cod. 11207, fol. 47r.
211 Cod. 11205, fol. 276r; Cod. 11238, foll. 128v-129r.
212 Cod. 11207, fol. 197r; Gallo gave nitrate, among others.

close to one hundred pounds of it in his lifetime.[213] Thaddeus Hagecius of Hajek (1525–1600) told Handsch of the excellent effects of mullein oil.[214]

As so often, Handsch also noted down what he heard from patients and other laypeople about treatment practices of ordinary folks. He learned that in the population at large, numerous remedies were being used to fight gout.[215] Some of these were herbal remedies to be ingested or externally applied, for example a mixture of cloves, saffron, sage, cream, and other ingredients. This was administered by an old woman in Italy and was said to be so effective that it made fools of the physicians.[216] A noble patient in Prague owed his knowledge of the beneficial effects of juniper to a farmer.[217] Another informant told Handsch of a sufferer of *podagra* who was helped by a distillate made from the blossoms or roots of mullein.[218] The private tutor who worked for the Lords of Berka swore by warm brandy, which was also taken by another acquaintance of Handsch as a remedy for his sciatica.[219] The recommendation to drink donkey milk[220] was among the more unusual suggestions, but in lay experience, such remedies had proven effective. Further treatments of this kind included the external application of ants, which were presumably thought to help draw the morbid matter out of the joint and into the skin.[221] From the Count of Helfenstein, Handsch received the advice that a compress with warmed frogspawn could help in the case of hot *podagra*.[222] And an archducal servant recommended as a proven remedy ("pro certum compertum") a bath in a tub filled with dung water, a recommendation that calls forth associations with approaches that were later also followed by some physicians and became known as *Dreckapotheke* ("filth pharmacy"). Going by the principle of similarity or sympathy, the fecal water was presumably thought to pull the impure morbid matter to the outside.[223]

---

213 Ibid., fol. 42v.
214 Cod. 11205, fol. 127r; Handsch indicated his source only as "M. Thaddeus" in Prague.
215 "The women recommended so many remedies" ("tot remedia consuluerunt mulieres"), Handsch wrote about the podagric wife of Collinus (Cod. 11205, fol. 306v); see also Cod. 11183, fol. 45v, on various proven remedies that Handsch learnt from a gem polisher.
216 Cod. 11251, fol. 85v.
217 Cod. 11251, fol. 111r.
218 Cod. 11205, fol. 127.
219 Cod. 11183, fol. 248v.
220 Cod. 11251, fol. 38v.
221 Cod. 11205, fol. 263r.
222 Cod. 11251, fol. 157v.
223 Cod. 11251, fol. 117r; on the "Dreckapotheke" see Paullini, Heylsame Dreck-Apotheke (1696); one patient also told Handsch that he had been advised to use donkey dung against his jaundice and Handsch recorded this recommendation in his collection of proven remedies (Cod. 11205, fol. 575r).

Because *podagra* generally came in episodes, physicians doubtlessly experienced how patients recovered under their care insofar as the paroxysms began to occur less frequently, at least for some time. As Handsch's notes suggest, however, a permanent cure could only be hoped for exceptionally. Along with falling sickness, dropsy, and leprosy, *podagra* was one of the four "main diseases" that perpetually pushed medical care to its limits. With *podagra,* as Handsch learned from his reading of Manardi, there was no better remedy than patience.[224] As Daniel Schuster has shown, physicians met this challenge in part by attributing something positive to the disease. It was certainly true, on the one hand, that *podagra* was an "unbidden", indeed an "evil guest" whose bed patients made by indulging in food and drink. At the same time, it tended to afflict the rich and powerful and thus was attended by an element of distinction.[225] Not least of all, then, *podagra* could serve the self-fashioning of humanist scholars.[226]

Stone Disease

Attempting to assess the prevalence of certain diseases in the sixteenth century based on modern diagnostic criteria, such as "pulmonary tuberculosis" or "cardiovascular" disease, is highly problematic. Most diagnoses that stood at the center of learned medicine in the Renaissance do not easily translate into modern medical terminology. Diseases were defined and distinguished from each other based on very different physiological and pathological concepts. Some diseases, as we know them today, are characterized by such unique signs and symptoms, however, that the diagnostic criteria then were basically the same as those today. In this case, a plausible retrospective diagnosis is often possible. A prime example are kidney- and bladder-stones. The sufferers not only felt the painful colics. When we read premodern accounts of people who saw the stones they excreted with their urine and felt them with their fingers there can be no reasonable doubt about the diagnosis.

Even when the bodily manifestations of a disease – as defined by modern medicine – are very characteristic, we can assess its prevalence in previous centuries only very roughly at best. How often a disease is mentioned in physicians' notebooks and correspondence or in medical publications cannot be taken for a reliable reflection of its incidence or prevalence. The attention received by a

---

[224] Cod. 11206, fol. 127v.
[225] Schuster, Festung (2021).
[226] Storchová, Tempting girl (2016).

certain disease was strongly influenced by its severity and the degree to which explaining, diagnosing, and treating it gave rise to controversy. In certain cases, however, the attention paid to a disease that we still know today was so great and the frequency in which it appears in the sources seems so disproportionate, in the light of modern epidemiological data, that one cannot help but get the impression that it was more widespread then than it is today.

Two diseases stand out in this respect in the Renaissance: podagra or gout and kidney- and bladder-stones. Accounts of stone disease are virtually ubiquitous in sixteenth-century sources and even a conspicuous number of famous figures are known to have been stricken with stones; Martin Luther, Philipp Melanchthon, Erasmus of Rotterdam, and Handsch's employer Archduke Ferdinand are just a few names among many others.[227] We can only speculate about the reasons but by all appearances kidney- and bladder-stones were considerably more common at the time.

Kidney and bladder stones played an important role also in Handsch's notes. Again and again, he documented cases of stones and noted down diagnostic signs and successful treatments. Later in life, he also documented his own suffering from stones, describing the severe stone colics that afflicted him along with the stones he excreted.[228] The characteristic symptom was an intense, agonizing pain in his loins when the stone entered the ureter, sometimes accompanied by nausea, cold sweat, and vomiting. Archduke Ferdinand, too, suffered badly and would come to tears from the pain.[229] Some sufferers compared the pain of excreting a stone to that of childbirth.[230] The colics could last for days and the pain could radiate into the legs and testicles, as Handsch knew from his own harrowing experience.[231] When the stone entered the bladder, the colics abated. Handsch quoted the Archduke as saying, "Now I felt that the stone fell into the bladder; now the hardship is over, the pain has abated, and the apprehension has passed".[232] The subsequent excretion of the stone via the urethra was typically accompanied by a sharp or stabbing pain.[233]

---

[227] Handsch mentioned Melanchthon and Erasmus explicitly (Cod. 11183, fol. 57v and fol. 239v); on Archduke Ferdinand's stones see Cod. 11204 and Stolberg, Krankheitsgeschehen (2021).
[228] Cod. 11183, fol. 425v, documents first indications in December 1570.
[229] Cod. 11204, fol 53v and fol. 54v.
[230] Cod. 11205, fol. 138r.
[231] Cod. 11204, fol. 45v and fol. 63r; Cod. 11183, foll. 436v-437v.
[232] Cod. 11204, fol. 44r: "Itzund hab ich gefhület das das Steinle in die Blasen gefallen ist, nue hats kein Not, der Weetagen hat nachgelassen, und die Bangickeit ist vergangen."
[233] Cod. 11183, fol. 438r.

Sometimes, as Handsch also experienced personally, the stone did not enter the urethra but instead obstructed the bladder exit. The risk of this happening was greater with smaller stones, as Handsch learned from Gallo, who had told him of a horse whose bladder contained three fist-sized stones that apparently did not interrupt the flow of urine.[234] Archduke Ferdinand experienced various times that bladder stones obstructed the flow of urine. He was making water "with difficulty" he said at that point.[235] Once he was unable to make water for twenty-four hours.[236] The same misfortune happened to Handsch when he was travelling in the vicinity of Innsbruck. He was in severe pain until a catheter ("syringa") – presumably he sought the help of a surgeon – allowed ample urine to flow out and he was immediately relieved.[237] According to Mattioli's detailed account, sick "Bohuslaus" too – this was possibly Bohuslav Felix von Hassenstein (1517–1583) – had to be helped with a catheter while he was travelling in Burgundy. The situation was so dire that a stone cutter had already been called.[238]

Handsch's descriptions of the pain suffered by small children with bladder stones are particularly dramatic; he observed this not least of all with his little half-brother Johannes. Here, he did not describe the ureteric colic that is typical of adults, but the stones did block the bladder exit so that the urine could only exit one drop at a time.[239] The excretion of the bladder stones via the urethra could be very painful. The nine-year-old son of a nobleman, for instance, had to make water often and when he did the pain was so sharp that, as Handsch had been told, he paced the room from the pain he was in.[240] Handsch's half-brother Johannes, too, writhed in pain at times like these, and sometimes screamed or even crawled under the bench and pressed so hard against his belly that the skin turned dark – presumably from bruises.[241] Sometimes he also rubbed his shanks so much that they became very red.[242] Other boys always had their hand in the groin area.[243] The boys – and this was true of Johannes as well – often wet their beds at night.[244] About a nine-year-old boy it was said that he would always

---

234 Cod. 11207, fol. 120v.
235 Cod. 11204, fol. 64r.
236 Ibid., fol. 67v.
237 Cod. 11183, fol. 470r.
238 Ibid., foll. 133r-177v, esp. foll. 141r-142r.
239 Cod. 11205, fol. 105r.
240 Ibid., fol. 258r.
241 Cod. 11295, fol. 105.
242 Cod. 11205, fol. 472r.
243 Cod. 11183, fol. 211r.
244 Ibid., fol. 211r.

urinate with difficulty, and often, and also into the bed. He had been suffering from stones several times a year for four years. If at some point he no longer wetted the bed, Handsch added, this would be a sign of healing.[245]

Stones could often easily be diagnosed by the sufferers themselves and by those around them. Not only were the complaints frequently severe and characteristic. Sooner or later, most patients found stones or sand in their chamber pots. Thus, going by the sandy urine and the vomiting of a sixteen-year-old boy, "the women", according to Handsch's account, concluded that he had stone disease.[246] In another case, Handsch was sent sand that had been passed with the urine wrapped in a piece of paper.[247] A further characteristic sign when the condition was acute was bloody or at least reddish or brownish urine. One chaplain likened his bloody urine to spoiled blood from bloodletting, and he said that little stones came out after his urine.[248] If the urine was left to stand for some time, reddish or even sandy sediment would often collect at the bottom.[249] In other cases there was no sediment or bloody coloration, but the matter responsible for the formation of sand or stones manifested in a milky, whey-like cloudiness of the urine.[250]

If sandy matter in the urine was not accompanied by greater complaints, this did signal the danger of stone disease, yet one could hope in such cases that the morbid matter would be passed as tiny particles before larger concretions formed. According to Handsch, when the urine flask was swirled and sand could be seen, one could say to patients that without this sand, they would have stones.[251] Indeed, Handsch and the physicians he worked with quite often found sandy matter in the urine of sick people who did not complain of stones.[252] As Handsch remarked under the heading "Aphorismus Hipp[ocratis] falsus", these observations disproved the Hippocratic teaching according to which sand in the urine allowed one to conclude that the patient had bladder stones.[253] Considering the common observation that sand stuck to the sides of chamber pots and matulas

---

245 Cod. 11205, fol. 262v.
246 Cod. 11183, fol. 279v.
247 Ibid., fol. 122v.
248 Ibid., fol. 278r; similarly ibid., fol. 276v.
249 Cod. 11205, fol. 107r and fol. 124r.
250 Ibid., fol. 105r and fol. 262v.
251 Cod. 11206, fol. 168r.
252 Cod. 11207, fol. 151v, fol. 160v and fol. 214r, "ego saepius vidi"; ibid., fol. 54v; here Gallo also was referring to sand in the urine of the Archduke, however, who eventually did suffer from stones.
253 Ibid., fol. 149v.

when they were in use over a longer period of time, it could even be presumed that sand was passed very frequently with the urine and was sometimes only too fine to be visible to the naked eye.[254]

Difficulties arose occasionally in distinguishing the painful excretion of stones from what was called "colics" ("colicae") at the time. Colics were understood as spasmodic intestinal pain, which both physicians and patients ascribed mainly to winds in the bowels. As a matter of fact, the term "colic" as we use it today – usually referring to the pain when kidney or gallstones are expelled – comes from the Greek word "kolon" for "bowel". In retrospect we can assume that "colics" were sometimes triggered by gallstones as well, which physicians of the period knew primarily from post-mortems.[255] As a student, Handsch learned that (intestinal) colics first were more to the front of the belly and then moved towards the back and were stronger after eating. With kidney stones, by contrast – this Handsch took from his reading Guainerio – the pain remained in the same place.[256] Urine that was brown and bloody could also point to an ulcer in the efferent urinary tract, but in this case the typical paroxysms of pain were absent.[257]

In the medical understanding of the time, the formation of stones corresponded in large part to the genesis of other diseases that could be traced to "fluxes", that is to local accumulations of morbid matter. Along these lines, Giovanni Battista da Monte explained that stones had the same nature as other *fluxiones*. As opposed to other fluxes, however, they solidified as concretions due to the influence of intense heat.[258] Da Monte assumed that the disease originated with the four natural humors, and most frequently, a mixture of bile and phlegm occurred.[259] However, for Handsch and the physicians in his professional environment, kidney and bladder stones could not be traced to natural phlegm but rather to an unnatural, thick, viscous, sticky, mucous matter which accumulated in the stomach whenever food was insufficiently concocted. The urine of the lithiatic Lady of Wartenberg was white and thick with mucus.[260] When the raw, mucous matter entered the kidneys and was greatly heated there, it hardened like

---

254 Ibid., fol. 214r.
255 Benivieni, De abditis (1994), p. 153; Solenander, Consilorum (1609), p. 493, on a stone in the gall-bladder of Duke Wilhelm von Cleve of the size of a chestnut.
256 Cod. 11240, fol. 145r.
257 Cod. 11205, fol. 138r.
258 Da Monte, Consultationum (1554), pp. 422f.
259 Ibid., p. 423.
260 Cod. 11240, foll. 130v-131r.

clay that was made into bricks.²⁶¹ The same matter could also be deposited in other, cooler places in the body and cause complaints there without hardening.

On this basis, Handsch offered the patients and their families a detailed account of how the stones were generated in the body. When a man delivered the urine of Valten Eberspach's wife, Handsch told him that her stone disease was caused by the fact that "her loins" were "phlegmy". This phlegmy matter, he continued, "causes her complaints in the loins, and the same phlegm can at times go into the kidneys, which are hot and narrow, so that it is as if loam went into the oven where it can be turned into stone. The same matter can also go into the uterus and fill its ducts with phlegm, so that the menses will not happen regularly; this makes vapors rise into the head, making her feel strange, as well as toward the heart, giving her complaints there."²⁶²

Going into greater length still, he explained the disease to the sick wife of the captain of Reichstadt: "You have a weak stomach that does not digest the food well and so produces a lot of phlegm. The phlegm collects every day from food and drink and is the source and root of all your complaints. Depending on where the phlegm from the stomach goes, that is how you will feel. Sometimes it goes down on the left side, into the spleen, where it causes pressure or stings, or you will feel it in your left side. Sometimes it goes down into the right side, into the liver, then you will feel it in your right side. Sometimes it goes to the back or loins, where you will feel it. In sum, wherever the phlegm goes, you will feel it, but the root and stem are in the stomach. Sometimes the phlegm goes into the kidneys and becomes a stone; it is like putting dung or loam in the oven to make a brick. Sometimes it goes down to the uterus and soils or obstructs it so that your period does not go as it should and is not fully accomplished."²⁶³

---

261 Cod. 11183, fol. 283v, "pituita crassa, tenax et glutinosa"; Cod. 11183, fol. 150r; Mattioli attributed the stones of sick Bohuslaus to "pituosis excrementis"; see also Cod. 11205, fol. 105r, on a "materia pituitosa" as "calculi fomes".
262 Cod. 11205, fol. 207v, "davon empfindet sie ynn Lennden ein Beschwernus, und derselbige Schleym kompt bisweilen ynn die Nieren, und die syndt hitzig und eng, ist gleich, wie Leym ynn Backofen keme, es mag der Stein deraus werden. Es mag auch dieselbig Materi ynn die Mutter [Gebärmutter, M.S.] komen, und verschleympt die Genge der Mutter, das die *menses* nicht recht gehen, und raucht davon eyn Dampff yn Kopff, das yr seltzam wirt, und gegen dem Herzen, das yr beschwerlich ist umb das Herzgrübel."
263 Cod. 11205, foll. 195v-196r: "Yr habt ein schwachen, blöden Magen, der verdeuet die Speis nit wol, derhalben macht er vil Schleym, der Schleym samlet sich teglich aus Essen und Trincken, und ist eyn Ursprung und Wurzel aller euer Kranckheit, denn nachdem sich der Schleym aus dem Magen hin und wider legt, also fület aber [oder, M.S.] empfindet yr euch. Bisweilen sinckt er auff die linke Seyten ynn Milz, da druckt, aber [oder, M.S.] sticht, aber [oder, M.S.] fulet es yr ynn der lincken Seyten, Bisweilen syncktt er ynn die rechten Seyten, ynn

This account of the formation of stones also explained why stone disease and *podagra* were so closely related, as emphasized by Da Monte in a letter of consultation written for Cardinal Pietro Bembo.[264] Both diseases could be traced to a mucous matter that was produced when food was insufficiently concocted in the stomach. In the case of *podagra*, this matter accumulated in and around individual joints, while with stones, it made its way to the kidneys. It was not surprising then that both, as experience taught, could occur at the same time, or successively or in alternation in the same patient. Stones accompanied "Queen Podagra", as Antonio Guainerio had written.[265] Handsch personally knew quite a number of people who were tormented not only by *podagra* but also by stones, one of whom was Ulrich Lehner.[266] Handsch's mentor Gallo told a patient that he could free him of his stone, but warned him that the familiar *podagra* would return.[267] Handsch explained the disease of the daughter of the Lord of Gendorf by saying to those present, "All those who accumulate much phlegm usually have sand or stone".[268] Using more chemical terms, Gallo likewise told those near him at the sickbed that stones came from matter that was mucous and, he added, salty. In the kidneys, a nitrous quality ("nitrositas") developed from this.[269]

An important predisposing element for stone disease was – just as with *podagra* – a weak or overtaxed stomach lacking sufficient heat for concoction.[270] As a possible cause for his own urinary retention, which ultimately had to be remedied with a catheter, Handsch named his indulgence in cold wine, which would have cooled the stomach.[271] It also appears that Handsch gave credence to several patients when they claimed their stones had been encouraged by

---

die Leber; da fulet yr es ynn der rechten Seyten. Bisweilen legt er sich ynn den Rucken, aber [oder, M.S.] Lennden, und da fulet yr es, ynn summa, wo er sich hin legt der Schleym, da fulet yrs, aber die Wurzel und der Stock ist ym Magen. Bisweilen legt sich der Schleym ynn die Nieren, so wird ein Stein daraus, und ist gleich wenn man Kot aber Leim [oder Lehm, M.S.] ynn Backofen thutt, so wird ein Zigel daraus. Bisweilen sinckt er hinab ynn die Mutter, unnd verunreiniget aber [oder, M.S.] verstopfft sie also, das euer Zeit nicht rechtschaffen und volkomen gehen [sic!]."

264 Da Monte, Consultationum (1554), p. 436. In today's medicine, a similar correlation is described: When there is an elevated level of uric acid, which is responsible for gout in the modern understanding, there is also a high incidence of kidney and bladder stones made from urate.
265 Cod. 11207, fol. 104r and fol. 212r.
266 Ibid., fol. 212r, lists several patients that confirmed Guainerio's observation; Handsch mentions further patients in Cod. 11205, fol. 224v and Cod. 11183, fol. 44v.
267 Cod. 11207, fol. 24v.
268 Cod. 11205, fol. 293v.
269 Cod. 11207, fol. 120r.
270 Cod. 11205, fol. 230v.
271 Cod. 11183, fol. 470r, on the successful treatment of Ferenberger and his stones.

their consumption of barley beer.[272] Even the resolution he expressed in this context – he was no longer going to engage in a *manuductio* after eating – seems to point in this direction: the act came with the danger of drawing the vital heat needed for concoction away from the stomach.[273] Eating foods that were hard to digest also overburdened the stomach. Handsch traced the stones of a castellan to his excessive enjoyment of mushrooms, for example.[274] On principle, cheese and milk products were off limits for those suffering from stone disease.[275]

As with *podagra*, physicians and laypeople alike believed there was also a hereditary element in stone disease. After his father died of a stone, a patient was all the more fearful of stone disease in himself when he found sandy sediment in his urine.[276] Handsch explained that if the father had gout, and perhaps stones as well, then "usually the children will have a stone as well and are phlegmy".[277]

When patients suffered acutely from stones, physicians – but also the *empiricus* in Leipa[278] – had patients lie for an extended period of time in a bathtub filled with water infused with herbs, presumably in the hope that the external heat would widen the urinary passages.[279] According to Handsch, a widespread household remedy was to apply a small satchel with hot oats.[280] In addition, there were various medications. Handsch heard of a monk in Bologna who had allegedly passed more than a thousand stones and had not been able to pass water for four days. He then rubbed scorpion oil into his chest and member and it helped.[281] In Handsch's experience, administering the sweet *manus Christi* to children who were feeling pain during urination had proven beneficial.[282] To alleviate the pain, physicians used strong analgesics like philonium.[283]

---

[272] Cod. 11205, fol. 186r.
[273] Cod. 11183, fol. 459v.
[274] Cod. 11207, fol. 24v.
[275] Ibid., fol. 113r.
[276] Ibid., fol. 160v.
[277] Cod. 11205, fol. 293v.
[278] Ibid., fol. 409r; Handsch even recorded the plants which the *empiricus* recommended adding, among them oats, chamomille, mugwort and juniper berries, which first had to be boiled in water.
[279] Ibid., fol. 111r and fol. 112r.
[280] Ibid., fol. 558v; Cod. 11204, fol. 70v, on a female Bohemian empiric, who successfully used such little bags.
[281] Cod. 11251, fol. 42r.
[282] Cod. 11205, fol. 263r and fol. 285r.
[283] Ibid., fol. 111r.

If the stone obstructed the flow of urine from the bladder, a catheter could bring instant relief – it is still the means of choice in situations like these today.[284] If the stone had already entered the urethra and the patient was a boy, one could attempt to suck it out with the mouth. This was done by a lay healer on the little son of a tailor who suffered from stones.[285] Gallo knew of a woman in Trento who inserted her finger with its long fingernail into the anus of a person experiencing urinary retention and broke the stone; what must be meant here is that she did this by applying pressure to the bladder or urethra.[286]

In the long-term prevention and treatment of kidney and bladder stones, the most essential tools in physicians' toolkits were diuretics like terebinth.[287] Before they were administered, however, the body had to be cleansed to the greatest degree possible of phlegmy morbid matter, for example with expectorants, laxatives, and clysters. Were this not done, the phlegm would be voided with the urine and would aggravate the complaints.[288] Some patients also sought healing in spas and by drinking the waters from thermal springs, as was increasingly popular in the upper classes. Hans Reiter, for example, plagued as he was by stones and bloody urine along with signs of paralysis in his legs, went to Karlsbad, but without success. The following spring, he visited Partenkirchen, but his condition only worsened.[289]

In addition, medications that were believed to have a more or less specific effect on stones could be given, although the lines between such specifics and purgatives were sometimes blurred. Leonhard Fuchs recommended among other things St. Benedict's herb,[290] while Mattioli praised the effects of heather.[291] Erasmus von Rotterdam, following the advice of Wilhelm Copus, alleviated his complaints with a decoction of licorice.[292] Others thought horseradish could serve to break up stones.[293] Some physicians also developed special mixtures of drugs. One physician gave Ebersbach's wife, who was tormented by severe stone colics, his own "stone breaking drink" ("haustum saxifragium"),[294] and Handsch himself sometimes gave patients a "powder to fight the stone".[295]

---

284 Cod. 11183, fol. 470r.
285 Cod. 11205, fol. 105r; similarly ibid., fol. 409v.
286 Cod. 11207, fol. 103r.
287 Cod. 11183, fol. 470r.
288 Cod. 11207, fol. 120r-v; this was Gallo's advice.
289 Cod. 11183, fol. 433r.
290 Cod. 11207, fol. 83r.
291 Ibid., fol. 121v.
292 Cod. 11183, fol. 239v.
293 Cod. 11205, fol. 495r.
294 Ibid., fol. 111r.
295 Cod. 11207, fol. 205v.

Among laypeople, various plant- and animal-derived substances were considered to have a beneficial effect. One old woman praised blackthorn blossoms in warm beer, which had allegedly healed her husband. They also tried it on Handsch's half-brother Johannes but it was to little avail.[296] A servant of Heinrich Hirschberger told Handsch about his own father who successfully treated himself with a powder of roasted rose hips.[297] Handsch had also heard of the use of pigeon dung as a treatment for stones.[298] And evidently following the principle of treating like with like, Handsch's stepmother recommended pike teeth.[299] This principle of *similia similibus,* adopted centuries later by homeopathy, also apparently justified the use of other remedies against stones. The brother of one of Handsch's landladies, following the advice of a farmer, took a remedy that contained pulverized snail shells, among other things.[300] Another person reported the good effects of (presumably grated) peach pits, that he said made him pass quite a number of little stones.[301] And a mother had her little boy, who suffered from recurrent stones and pain in his limbs, drink the crushed bladder stones; he was freed from his stone disease until he became a grown man.[302]

Physicians sometimes reported the success of a treatment, yet often the complaints kept coming back. Even an eminent medical authority like Johann Neefe recommended to Ebersbach's wife that she continue with her "home remedies" in spite of the fact that he had a powder against stones in his repertoire.[303] If nothing helped and especially if stones continued to block the bladder exit, making urination impossible, sometimes only lithotomy remained as a last resort. Cutting stones, the surgical removal of the bladder stones, was performed, as a rule, by an experienced surgeon. But physicians were involved insofar as some patients and their families expected helpful advice. They wanted to know, as the mother of a nine-year-old boy who suffered from stones put it, "Whether I should have him cut".[304] It was a difficult decision. The operation was very painful and, because of the risk of great blood loss, dangerous. Not only that; it was still possible that new stones would form after a successful operation.

---

296 Cod. 11205, fol. 472v.
297 Cod. 11183, fol. 108r.
298 Cod. 11251, fol. 115r.
299 Cod. 11205, fol. 113r.
300 Cod. 11251, fol. 115r.
301 Cod. 11183, fol. 108r.
302 Cod. 11205, fol. 242v.
303 Ibid., fol. 409v.
304 Ibid., fol. 262v.

In retrospect, we can only speculate about the success rate of these surgeries. Unlike with hernia operations – which, granted, were often only undertaken when the bowel was incarcerated – there is considerable evidence in contemporary sources that favorable outcomes were not infrequent in stone cutting. Gallo even once had a boy "cut" despite the resistance of the other physicians – and with success.[305] Handsch's half-brother Johannes, too, was ultimately operated on at the age of thirteen. The procedure lasted fifteen minutes and the surgeon found a stone that was almost as large as a chicken egg. Johannes recovered completely, Handsch added.[306]

Cancer

Cancer is widely perceived regarded as a disease of modernity. Already in the Renaissance period, however, cancer was feared like few other diseases. People knew of the terrible pain, the bodily decay, the stench, the months of excruciating suffering that often preceded the fatal outcome.[307] In the medical literature, cancer was traditionally attributed to some "cancerous" morbid matter which accumulated in a certain location or organ. This cancerous matter was thought to be similar to black bile but acrid, caustic, or even poisonous. An excessively heated liver was considered a prime cause of the disease because it burned the humors and this gave them a biting sharpness. An obstruction of the natural excretions, above all of menstruation, could play a role as well. If the matter accumulated in one place in the body, a tumor formed which in the best circumstances would remain where it was, though it could still disrupt the flow of humors or press against neighboring organs. In many cases, however, the acrid cancerous matter became more aggressive over time. It began to eat away at the surrounding area. The flesh would rot and decay and when the matter reached the skin it would break into ulcers. Foul-smelling fluids, blood, and sometimes small particles of flesh would be evacuated. Moreover, it was believed that the cancerous matter often "infected" the blood and humors over time. Like poison or a contagium, just the smallest quantities could affect the whole body and destroy it over time.[308]

---

305 Ibid., fol. 263r.
306 Cod. 11183, fol. 211r.
307 Kaartinen, Pray (2012); Stolberg, Metaphors (2014).
308 Overviews in Wolff, Lehre (1929); Rather, Genesis (1978); detailed late medieval account in Montagnana, De herpete (1589), foll. 54r-85v.

Apparently physicians diagnosed and treated cancer patients relatively rarely in their practice. If cancer plays only a marginal role in sixteenth-century collections of medical case histories this could again be explained by the fact that cancer hardly ever allowed the author of the case history to highlight his outstanding diagnostic acumen or therapeutic skills. In most cases, the treatment failed and the physician could only seek to palliate. Even Handsch, in his extensive personal notes, mentioned cancer only here and there, however, and among the thousands of cases Hiob Finzel documented in his practice journal there are only two patients he diagnosed with cancer.[309] Yet this must not be mistaken as evidence that cancer, as we know it, was rare. Life expectancy was significantly lower than today, due in large part to the high infant and child mortality, but if a person survived childhood in the Renaissance, he or she had good prospects of reaching the age of sixty or even seventy and of falling ill with cancer.

There are other reasons, why Renaissance physicians rarely diagnosed and treated cancer. To start with, in many cases, the physicians quite simply would not have recognized the cancer as such. Cancer, as they knew it, revealed itself almost exclusively as a subcutaneous tumor that could be seen from the outside, as an ulcer of the skin or of a mucous membrane or as cancerous fluid that oozed forth from the bodily orifices. Galen had already emphasized that a *cancer occultus* could deploy its destructive powers also hidden inside the body. Thus, the physician could voice his suspicion that there was an "inner cancer" or at least an "inner tumor" of the stomach or liver.[310] During the patient's lifetime, cancerous tumors and ulcers inside the body were generally impossible to recognize, however. Only an autopsy might later reveal such a *cancer internus*.[311] As a result presumably many a patient who would today be considered as suffering from cancer was diagnosed at the time with diseases like consumption, hectic fever, or dropsy.

It seems quite likely, for example, that old Anna Welser died of cancer if we read Handsch's extensive account of her final disease in the light of today's medical ideas. She had a tumor in the area around her stomach ("tumor in stomacho") and eventually a red apostema formed next to her stomach, which, on the advice of a physician and a barber, was made to burst. A large amount of pus issued forth. According to Handsch's description, the stench was so awful that the physicians could hardly stand to stay in the room. With time, the ulcer developed into gangrene, into "cold fire", and blackened on the inside. When

---

309 Ratsbibliothek Zwickau, Ms. QQQQ1, Ms. QQQQ1a and Ms. QQQQ1b.
310 Cod. 11206, fol. 16v.
311 Ibid.

Hildebrand wanted to test for depth, his silver probe disappeared almost entirely into the body. In the end, ingested food exited the body via the ulcer. The old woman became weaker and weaker until she could hardly breathe and she passed away.[312]

Because cancer was almost exclusively diagnosed when it manifested on the outside, physicians north of the Alps were also less likely to treat patients for professional reasons. Ulcers like other diseases (or manifestations of disease) of the skin were commonly taken to belong primarily in the domain of barber-surgeons. Treating such external complaints was their prerogative. Thus it was the court surgeon Hildebrand who showed Handsch a case of "cancer of the mouth" ("cancrum oris") which had visibly distended the patient's upper jaw and had caused an ugly discoloration inside the mouth.[313] Hildebrand also allowed him to touch the large, knotty and hardened goiter of a poor woman which had grown in the past months and in his opinion was cancerous. He gave her a simple external remedy that was to halt the influx of matter and soften the induration.[314]

The Renaissance understanding and experience of cancer as a disease that manifested itself primarily on the body's surface had another major consequence which is often overlooked in historical research: cancer was diagnosed primarily in women. According to modern medicine, most kinds of cancer that commonly occur with both sexes worldwide affect inner organs such as the lungs, colon, stomach, and liver. They show on the outside only as a general physical deterioration or, at most, through symptoms like blood in the sputum or stool. Only skin cancer is visible on the surface of the skin but it is not as common. This explains why the majority of cases of cancer that were diagnosed in the early modern period involved women with uterine or breast cancer. These two common kinds of cancer could be perceived directly with the senses. With breast cancer, the growing tumor could often be felt under the skin, and as the disease progressed, it evolved into a festering ulcer. The decay of a cancerous uterus was not visible from the outside but the frequent excretion of a foul, stinking discharge was all the more a telltale sign.

From a contemporary point of view, the predominance of cancer in women was not surprising. It confirmed the widespread idea that women were by their very nature impure and continually accumulated waste matter in their bodies. They required a "monthly cleansing" to shed this matter. A woman who missed her periods could not free herself from the accumulated waste matter, which therefore built up in her body. It collected in and around the uterus above all,

---

312 Cod. 11183, foll. 430r-431r.
313 Ibid., fol. 286v.
314 Ibid., fol. 383r.

which served its natural excretion, and in the breasts, which for their part were closely connected to the uterus. When the menstrual flow was obstructed, the waste matter could easily harden into a tumor in the uterus or in the breasts and ultimately degenerate into aggressive, acrid cancerous matter that would eat its way into the surrounding area and the skin or mucous membrane. For this reason, it was not surprising that women fell victim to cancer especially during and after menopause.[315]

Although treating the cancerous growths and ulcers was primarily the surgeon's task, physicians could still hope to make a difference when patients consulted them. They could seek to fight the production of the sharp, burnt cancerous matter with medicines that cooled the liver, or by diverting the flux of cancerous matter away from the ulcer. They were well aware, however, that they could usually only hope to slow down the process but not achieve a cure. Presumably it was the painful awareness that their treatment was of little avail in most cases together with their reluctance to scare patients which made physicians avoid the diagnosis of cancer, even if the condition was advanced. The wife of a royal judge, for example, had a hardened growth in her left breast and blood issued from it. Yet Handsch did not even note down a suspicion of breast cancer.[316] Another patient who had been mostly bedridden for months, was plagued by nocturnal pain in the umbilical area; she experienced coarse, impure discharge from her uterus, was emaciated, and her feet were beginning to swell. She died two months later. In retrospect, it seems very likely that she was suffering from uterine cancer. Handsch, however, only wrote that her uterus was "contaminated" ("inquinata").[317]

Dropsy

People suffering from dropsy, or *hydrops* (from the Greek word *hydor* for water) similarly posed a great challenge to physicians. The prognosis was commonly poor. As in cases of consumption, quartan fever and *apoplexia,* the physicians were often powerless. Patients' lives could, at most, be prolonged but the disease itself usually could not be cured.[318] "Hydrops et quartana sunt scandala plana", Handsch reminded himself repeatedly.[319] He decided not to accept any patients with dropsy of long standing because it was incurable in his experience. Some

---

[315] See the chapter on disordered menstruation.
[316] Cod. 11183, fol. 241v.
[317] Ibid., fol. 208v.
[318] Cod. 11240, fol. 42r.
[319] Cod. 11183, fol. 9v.

physicians did claim they had successful therapies for dropsy. Mattioli boasted that he had cured close to twenty dropsical patients, but Handsch tellingly added "if we may dare to believe it".[320]

Patients and their relatives feared the disease and anxiously asked at times whether there were signs of dropsy.[321] As in the case of cancer, this fear may have been the reason why physicians, even when they were faced with a greatly swollen abdomen and/or extremities, often chose not to give the diagnosis of dropsy but at most hinted at the possible danger. Katharina von Loxan, for example, had already developed swollen feet, a distended belly and complained about shortness of breath when Mattioli told her that she would develop dropsy in half a year if she did not undergo appropriate treatment.[322]

As students in Padua learned in Falloppia's anatomy classes,[323] three basic forms of dropsy could be distinguished: *anasarca,* in which the entire body and especially the extremities became bloated with water; *ascites* (from the Greek *askos* for "water bag"), which meant an accumulation of water in the abdomen; and *tympanites,* in which the abdomen was distended by excess gas.[324]

The typical symptoms of the different forms of dropsy or edema were relatively easy to identify. With general dropsy, *anasarca,* the feet in particular but also the face and the rest of the body became swollen. If one pressed with a finger on the swollen body part, the resulting dent remained visible for some time.[325] The swelling had increased, a patient who had been sick with dropsy for four years, reported, and when somebody pressed his feet a dimple remained.[326] To this day, this "pitting" is considered as a characteristic sign for dropsy. A dimple also remained in the swollen feet of a seriously ill accountant but in this case Handsch was not sure it indicated dropsy since the abdomen and the scrotum were not distended in the typical manner ("more hydropis").[327]

Ascites and *tympanites* manifested themselves in a massively swollen and often tense abdomen. When the sick person moved or one briefly compressed the belly with the hands from both sides, a noise as from water in a water bottle was typically heard with *ascites.* By contrast, if one knocked against the tympanitic

---

320 Ibid., fol. 333v.
321 E.g. Ibid., foll. 79v-80r; since the patient did not have typical symptoms of the disease, Handsch thought that perhaps an *empiricus* had arrived at this diagnosis.
322 Ibid., fol. 429v.
323 Cod. 11210, fol. 144v.
324 Cod. 11207, fol. 65v.
325 Cod. 11183, fol. 443r.
326 Cod. 11205, fol. 265v.
327 Cod. 11207, fol. 108r; the man died nevertheless.

abdomen with the hand, it sounded like a drum; "tympanum", in Latin, means "drum". The different forms of dropsy often coexisted. A sixteen-year-old *hydropicus* in the *Bruderhaus* in Innsbruck, for example, had swollen legs in which a dimple remained for some time after pressing a finger into them. A slap of the hand on the belly produced a sound. And when a physician pushed the belly from both sides, a gurgling was heard.[328]

Advanced dropsy was a dramatic sight. A dropsical man called Fröhlich, for example, had swollen legs and a distended abdomen. His fingernails had become blue and he suffered from severe shortness of breath. Shortly before he died, the only way he could sleep was to sit in a chair.[329] According to Gallo, it was a very bad sign when dropsical patients developed a cough – again this conclusion would be shared by doctors today – because it would indicate that the lungs were filling with water.[330] In other cases, the abdominal veins protruded visibly. Handsch observed this with a dropsical boy. A further possible symptom was blood welling up in the mouth.[331]

Physicians today attribute the typical signs of dropsy, that is massive water retention in the abdomen, the extremities and sometimes even in the face or lungs, primarily with chronic heart or kidney failure, or cirrhosis of the liver. The physicians of the sixteenth century traced the origins of dropsy to the liver almost exclusively. From his reading of Galen, Handsch learned that dropsy was associated with a weak liver.[332] In sixteenth-century medical practice, physicians and laypeople alike ascribed dropsy more precisely to an obstruction or induration of the liver, as Handsch's notes tell us.[333] Palpation and autopsy findings confirmed this assumption in some cases. As a student in Padua, Handsch saw a feverish boy, for example, who was beginning to develop dropsy and according to Trincavella had a "weak liver" ("imbecillitas hepatis"). Palpation revealed a "tensed" liver of uneven consistency, with harder and softer parts.[334]

The connection between the liver and dropsy was grounded in the notion that the liver generated the blood from chyme. If the liver was weakened, indurated, or

---

[328] Cod. 11183, fol. 443r; the physician whom Handsch mentioned as "Dr. Achilles" was probably Achilles Jelmin.
[329] Cod. 11183, fol. 448v.
[330] Cod. 11207, fol. 70r.
[331] Cod. 11183, fol. 43r; protruding veins on the abdominal wall together with massive bleeding from the esophageal veins are considered an important sign of liver cirrhosis today, which, in turn, is a leading cause of ascites.
[332] Ibid., fol. 43r.
[333] Cod. 11006, fol. 85v; Cod. 11183, fol. 289.
[334] Cod. 11238, foll. 98v-99r.

too cold,[335] it created imperfect, watery blood. Thus, Handsch explained to a miller that the liver was the blood's workshop. Half of his liver, however, had hardened and did not produce good blood.[336] The assumption of watery blood also furnished the explanation for the watery urine that physicians considered a characteristic sign of dropsy,[337] and it underpinned their advice that great restraint was to be shown when letting the blood of dropsical patients: it would make the blood even more watery.[338]

Handsch further noted the possibility that the kidneys might not be doing their work as they should. In the healthy body, they attracted watery fluid from the liver and the rest of the body in what was understood as an active process. If the kidneys' power of attraction was too weak, the fluid remained in the body and what followed was dropsy.[339]

In medieval medicine, dropsy had sometimes also been traced to the spleen.[340] Handsch mentioned this interpretation in connection with an old court physician from Kaaden. An old woman healer had palpated the area of the spleen and declared that his spleen was obstructed and indurated, and that dropsy was developing. It seems that the court physician believed in the healer's diagnosis because he had himself treated by her; it was said that she had cured many dropsical people before him.[341]

Physicians relied on a wide selection of primarily remedies when treating dropsy. Purgatives and remedies that were said to have a diuretic effect were particularly important. Falloppia told his students about a physician from Modena who was very successful with his prescriptions of spurge (*euphorbia*), which worked very well to void the "waters". According to Falloppia, the remedy burned in the throat, however. He preferred cassia, which also drained the water well, without burning in the throat.[342] In several entries, Handsch also noted down the

---

335 E.g. a young dropsical postmaster, whom Gallo treated, was believed to suffer only from an *intemperies frigida* of the liver and was cured (Cod. 11205, fol. 266r).
336 Cod. 11205, fol. 203r; Handsch used the term "pistor", which, at the time, could refer to a miller but sometimes also to a baker.
337 However, Handsch also noted exceptions to this rule (Cod. 11238, fol. 127v).
338 Cod. 11207, fol. 213v; Handsch was surprised that Gallo ordered bloodletting in the case of a patient whose arms were already swollen but presumably Gallo hoped to promote the movement of the blood and to resolve obstructions by this means.
339 Ibid., fol. 121r.
340 Demaitre, Medieval medicine, p. 277.
341 Cod. 11205, foll. 220v-221r.
342 Cod. 11251, foll. 29v-30r; similarly Cod. 11210, fol. 144v.

prescription of iris and white swallow-wort (*vincetoxicum*), praising its good results.[343] Handsch learned from Gallo that late medieval authors like Gordonius and Nicolaus Florentinus, as well as the author of *Antidotarium Nicolai* had written about curing dropsy with iris. Some used only the juice, while others also administered the roots, mixed with sugar and raw egg.[344] White swallow-wort was also recommended by Mattioli in his commentary on Dioscorides, where he described it as a remedy that dispelled dropsy "marvelously".[345] Based on Amatus Lusitanus, peach blossoms were prescribed as well.[346] Bellocati told of a dropsical patient he treated with nothing but cucumber juice.[347] Mattioli celebrated the successes he had with an oil of garden rue,[348] while Gallo lauded the efficacy of celery juice.[349] Willenbroch treated dropsy with a remedy containing alder buckthorn, or he used antimony.[350]

One could also try to void the excessive water with sudorific remedies.[351] And it was possible to reduce water intake. Gallo advised a patient not always to take a drink when he got thirsty.[352] From a *germanus* in Padua – presumably a fellow student – Handsch heard the story of a dropsical man who purportedly recovered after he had remained tied to a board for eight days without food or drink.[353]

In extreme cases, one could also try to void the water with surgical interventions. As we have seen, Falloppia gave his anatomy students a detailed description of the procedure of paracentesis, a small incision made in the abdominal wall to drain water, but warned of the danger.[354] In his later notes, Handsch did not once mention a case in which he or the physicians in his professional environment recommended this procedure.

---

343 Cod. 11183, fol. 124v, fol. 193v and 443r.
344 Cod. 11207, fol. 70v and fol. 160r; based on his own experience, Gallo preferred the root of *palma Christi*, however, which, he argued, burnt less when it was swallowed (ibid.).
345 Mattioli, New Kreutterbuch (1563), fol. 337r.
346 Cod. 11205, fol. 137v.
347 Cod. 11106, fol. 150v.
348 Cod. 11207, fol. 26v.
349 Ibid., fol. 61r.
350 Cod. 11204, fol. 46r.
351 Cod. 11207, fol. 65v; allegedly Gallo successfully cured a patient with swollen arms and legs this way.
352 Ibid., fol. 52r.
353 Cod. 11240, fol. 144v.
354 See the chapter on surgery in Part I.

Lay healers combatted dropsy with plant-based remedies such as rhubarb,[355] radish decoctions,[356] and wormwood oil, which Philippine Welser in one instance sent to an impoverished dropsical man.[357] But they also used remedies of what later came to be called "Dreckapotheke" or "filth pharmacy". An acquaintance of Handsch treated his swollen legs externally with dried sheep dung that had been brought to a boil in milk. He had learned about this from a lay healer who treated the swollen bellies of children in this way.[358] The sick court physician from Kaaden mentioned above was told by the woman healer he was consulting to soak a piece of cloth in his own urine every day and apply it. The "oils" from the urine would soften his clogged and hardened spleen and open the ducts. The man followed her advice but used the urine of a healthy young boy instead of his own. He believed that his spleen was healed after eight days but was still feeling weak.[359]

Falling Sickness

Today, epilepsy is generally considered a chronic, cerebral disorder characterized by seizures; it is not particularly rare[360] and in the majority of cases begins before the age of twenty. In the sixteenth century, *epilepsia* or the "falling sickness"[361] commonly manifested in very dramatic ways and was of great concern to physicians. It is one of the most frequently mentioned complaints in Handsch's notebooks. More than with any other disease, Handsch used emotionally charged words such as "horribilis" or in German "greulich" ("dreadful") and "scheuzlich" ("awful") when describing seizures he witnessed personally.[362]

Early modern physicians defined the term "epilepsy" very broadly, and in the following I will use the term as it was used at the time and forgo quotation marks. There was a triad of symptoms that was considered typical, even pathognomonic for epilepsy: a sudden attack of massive convulsions, temporary loss of consciousness, and foaming at the mouth. And so, when Handsch was called

---

355 Cod. 11183, fol. 45r, on the wife of a patient.
356 Cod. 11251, fol. 46v, on an *empiricus*.
357 Cod. 11183, fol. 366v.
358 Ibid., fol. 43r.
359 Cod. 11205, fol. 221r.
360 Today the prevalence is estimated to be in the area of 0,5 to 1 % of the general population.
361 Historical overview in Temkin, Falling sickness (1971); Handsch referred to the disease as "fallende Sucht" in German (e.g. Cod. 11207, fol. 169r).
362 Cod. 11183, fol. 423r, fol. 442r and fol. 443r; Cod. 11205, foll. 118v-119r.

because someone had had a convulsive attack, one of his routine questions for the relatives was whether the person had foamed at the mouth before or after the seizure.[363]

Various kinds of convulsions and even repeated fainting were also sometimes interpreted as epilepsy, however, or at least as indications of it. What physicians often saw – and this is reflected in Handsch's notes – were "epilepsies" in the form of massive convulsions in infants. These were also known as "mater puerorum".[364] Today, we would suspect febrile convulsions in many of these cases. Handsch relayed what the mother of an infant had said: "When it came over him, it bent his hands and made him froth at the mouth; he was pale as death, entirely still, and if he had not vomited green and yellow, I would have thought he had died."[365] Physicians of this time furthermore considered as epileptic the twitches and cramps they saw with the dying just before their death. This confirmed and amplified, in turn, the perception of epilepsy as a highly dangerous, often fatal disease.[366] Handsch even declared St. Vitus Dance to be a kind of epilepsy. He had seen beggars jump around and then lie on the ground as if dead.[367] He also recognized a connection to pathological *melancholia*, by which he must have meant melancholics who suffered episodes of insanity or mania.[368]

In their daily lives and in their social environment, the general population, and with them the physicians, were confronted with epileptic seizures in this broader sense quite frequently. Handsch's stepmother told him about a beggar who had entered their house and then collapsed on the floor in the parlor. He was "shaken cruelly and was seized a good long while".[369] Handsch also suspected that a beggar boy had just had an epileptic seizure when he saw him

---

363 See also Da Monte, Consultationum (1554), p. 63; Handsch recorded relevant descriptions among others in Cod. 11183, fol. 95v, fol. 123v, fol. 193r, fol. 260r, fol. 418v, fol. 423r, fol. 430 and fol. 442r.
364 Cod. 11205, fol. 227v; Cod. 11207, fol. 169r.
365 Cod. 11205, fol. 565v: "Wenn es yn ankam, so krummet es ym die Hende und *spuma* vor dem Maul, bleich wie todt, gar still [. . .] und wenn er sich nicht gebrochen hett geel und grün, so denckt sie, er were gestorben"; the child was Thomas Mitis' little son.
366 E.g. Cod. 11183, fol. 289v, on the death of a patient who first had cramps and signs of paralysis in her arms and legs and, in the end, died after an epileptic fit; Cod. 11205, fol. 227v, on a child who, according to the mother's account, rolled its eyes during the fits and had foam in front of its mouth, laughed again but died soon after; Cod. 11238, fol. 140v, on Bellocati's story of a patient with tertian fever who had five fits within an hour and who died the following day.
367 Cod. 11205, fol. 2r.
368 Ibid., fol. 402v.
369 Ibid., fol. 430r, "grausam geschüttelt, unnd eyn gutte Weil gehalten".

lying as if dead next to a fire in a square. Upon closer inspection, he discovered that the boy had foam at the mouth and that his arms were still trembling a little.[370]

The causes of epilepsy had already been described in the Hippocratic writings. The famous treatise on the "sacred disease" attributed the disease to an obstructed flow of phlegm from the brain.[371] In the Middle Ages and in the Renaissance, this conception remained alive and was developed further.[372] Leading authorities such as Jean Fernel and Giovanni Battista da Monte explained that superfluous thick phlegm in the brain blocked the brain's ventricles (which were considered the primary seat of brain function) or the openings or ducts through which the animal spirits, the spirits of the soul, flowed from the ventricles to the body. As opposed to apoplexy, this was not a complete but a partial blockage, however. The animal spirits then struggled against the resistance in a disorderly commotion, thus causing the erratic movements and massive convulsions. In the case of a boy who always moved slowly after a seizure and also appeared quite simple-minded, Handsch, thinking along these lines, ascribed the epilepsy to accumulated phlegm.[373] The hard clenching of the teeth was also considered typical. Today, epileptic seizures continue to be feared for the serious bite injuries to the tongue that may result. Lay people and physicians attempted to counter this risk by putting a wooden spoon, a piece of wood wrapped in cloth, or a wax candle between the seizing person's teeth if they had a chance.[374]

By the middle of the sixteenth century, the restricted movement of the animal spirits, caused by a phlegmy obstruction, was no longer the only explanation. According to Jean Fernel, abscesses or diseased meninges could also cause epilepsies, as could be shown by opening the skulls of deceased epileptics.[375] Physicians further thought that epilepsy could be caused by poisonous vapors or by a "bad" ("mala") "poisonous" ("venenosa") quality that rose from the lower regions of the body to the brain. The source could be retained menstrual blood in the uterus, for example; in one case, it even was believed to stem from an injured fingertip.[376] According to Da Monte, this poisonous quality that spread through the body was

---

370 Ibid., fol. 505v.
371 Temkin, Falling sickness (1971).
372 Eadie/Bladin, A disease once sacred (2001).
373 Cod. 11205, fol. 119r.
374 Cod. 11183, fol. 380v, fol. 406r and fol. 415r; in ibid., fol. 237r, Handsch also mentioned a special, purpose-made silver spoon with holes which, in Handsch's view, risked damaging the teeth, however.
375 Fernel, Universa medicina (1644), p. 495.
376 Da Monte, Consultationum (1554), p. 64 and p. 97; Fernel, Universa medicina (1644), p. 495.

called an *aura*.³⁷⁷ In this case, the actual cause of epilepsy was not located in the brain but in the lower body regions.³⁷⁸ Physicians spoke of epilepsy "per consensum" or "per sympathiam"³⁷⁹ or simply of "stomach epilepsy" ("epilepsia stomachica"). When an archducal chaplain's arms and legs suddenly began to tremble violently, Handsch noticed his yellow eyes and identified the cause as acrid bilious vapors that had risen to the brain.³⁸⁰ After inspecting a sick man's urine, his colleague Willenbroch suspected viscous bile which had become "sharp" from heat and which would, when it then rises as vapor, stung and bit the meninges.³⁸¹

As Handsch learned from his mentor Gallo, epilepsy in infants usually did not arise from an excess of phlegm in the brain but from a weak brain or harmful vapors. Da Monte held that living or necrotic worms in the body, which were a particularly frequent occurrence in the first years of life, could also release vapors and cause seizures.³⁸² When the little daughter of the archducal court surgeon Hildebrand suffered a seizure, during which her eyes were half closed and her legs and arms flailed about, Willenbroch accordingly gave her a remedy for worms.³⁸³ Handsch's teacher Gallo liked to use rhubarb syrup as an excellent remedy for worms and epilepsy,³⁸⁴ and Handsch also noted down the recipe for a "powder for epilepsy and worms".³⁸⁵

Physicians identified various predisposing and promoting factors, among them weakened, slackened nerves. Handsch wrote down as a "general rule" ("regula generalis") that baths were harmful to epileptics, and that epileptics must be forbidden from having sexual intercourse because it weakened the nerves.³⁸⁶ When, in an epistolary consultation, Gallo told an epileptic not to ingest vinegar, among other things, Handsch assumed this was because vinegar was bad for the nerves.³⁸⁷ Strong emotions were thought to constitute an important direct trigger for epileptic seizures,³⁸⁸ in particular intense anger, which set the phlegmy matter in the brain in motion, which then clogged the openings

---

377 Da Monte, Consultationum (1554), pp. 63–64; the term "aura" is used today to describe the the strange subjective sensations which some epileptics report at the approach of a fit.
378 Fernel, Universa medicina (1644), p. 495.
379 Da Monte, Consultationum (1554), p. 97.
380 Cod. 11183, foll. 345v-346r.
381 Cod. 11206, fol. 37v.
382 Da Monte, Consultationum (1554), p. 97.
383 Cod. 11183, fol. 409r.
384 Ibid., fol. 244r.
385 Cod. 11206, fol. 29r.
386 Cod. 11240, fol. 88r.
387 Cod. 11205, fol. 310v.
388 Da Monte, Consultationum (1554), p. 66.

of the cerebral ventricles.[389] Wine as well was considered dangerous.[390] Experience taught that the drinking habits of mothers and wet nurses could promote the development of seizures. In Leipa, Handsch observed that the infants of mothers who indulged in wine tended to suffer from epilepsy.[391] Another observation, which he made more than once, was that epileptic seizures tended to occur after a bout of colic.[392]

For the treatment of epilepsy, physicians used medicines against worms and a wide selection of herbal remedies, including hellebore and peony, the classic epilepsy remedy.[393] More than once Handsch also mentioned the external use of rue or peony root on the feet or buttocks.[394] In the eyes of some physicians, the severity of the disease and the dramatic symptoms called for the use of mineral preparations such as antimony or saltpeter.[395] Additionally, they used specifics, including various animal-derived remedies.[396] In a small book, Handsch found a reference to a *novum experimentum,* which described the bones of the green lizard as very useful in the treatment of epilepsy.[397]

Some means and methods, last but not least, relied on magic. In the works of Antonio Guainerio, which continued to find frequent mention in the sixteenth century, Handsch read that amulets and healing charms ("carmina") were recommended for epilepsy.[398] And he also wrote down a number of practices used for epilepsy by laypeople. Handsch learned from one of his landladies that it helped to cut off some hair, singe it in a flame and hold it to the nose of the person who was having a seizure.[399] Handsch was also shown a special "hand band" for epilepsy that was made from hair and small balls.[400] An acquaintance told him

---

389 Cod. 11205, fol. 149r.
390 Ibid., fol. 310v.
391 Ibid., fol. 311r, "vinosae"; see also Cod. 11207, fol. 58r, on wet nurses; it is impossible, in retrospect, to assess the degree to which convulsions of the infants of mothers and wet nurses who were heavy drinkers were due to the toxic effects of alcohol or indeed withdrawal symptoms.
392 Cod. 11183, fol. 320r, on the court painter in Ambras, Teuffel; on Tyrol, in general, ibid., fol. 321r and fol. 296v, "in hac regione fieri solet".
393 For a detailed examination of the treatment of epilepsy in children recommended by contemporary writings on the diseases of children see Manzke, Remedia (2008), pp. 71–89.
394 E.g. Cod. 11206, fol. 28v; Cod. 11210, fol. 138r, on the root of peony.
395 Cod. 11205, fol. 132v and fol. 133r; Cod. 11207, fol. 83v, on nitrate pills.
396 Schattner, Bewältigungsverhalten (2012), p. 58.
397 Cod. 11240, fol. 149r.
398 Cod. 11106, fol. 185v; magical rituals, charms and similiar means continued to be commonly used against epilepsy for a long time to come (Schattner, Bewältigungsverhalten (2012), p. 61).
399 Cod. 11183, fol. 321r.
400 Cod. 11205, fol. 171v.

about a noble lady who had been given a male and a female skull, which she had someone gild. To prevent epileptic seizures, women had to drink from the female and men from the male skull.[401] In the opinion of the people ("vulgi opinione"), wrote Handsch, epileptics would be healed if they drank the blood of a freshly beheaded person, served by the hangman. However, his stepmother, he noted, had told him about somebody for whom this had done nothing.[402]

Apoplexy and Paralysis

Apoplexy – *apoplexia* in Latin, and "Schlag" ("stroke") or "die Handt Gottes" ("the hand of God") in German[403] – was the byword for sudden death in Handsch's day. Still today, Germans speak figuratively of people who seem "as if struck" ("vom Schlag gerührt")[404] or "hit" ("getroffen"). Handsch wrote down a whole host of these cases in his notebooks. He knew about some of them through stories that had been told to him: Cardinal Bernardo Cles of Trento died of *apoplexia* when he was preparing a banquet.[405] In Prague, a thirty-five-year-old Jesuit died just four hours after climbing up the hill to the Prague Castle.[406] Other cases Handsch experienced first-hand or in his immediate circles. For example, Ulrich Lehner was called to see a man who was suddenly unable to speak or write one morning and was foaming at the mouth. He died a day later wheezing.[407] And Handsch was with Lehner the night Lehner himself succumbed to *apoplexia*.[408]

To physicians and laypeople alike, a feeling of dizziness was an important warning sign of *apoplexia*.[409] Some patients also first showed spasms, for instance a young woman in Ambras, who succumbed to *apoplexia*.[410] Handsch thought

---

401 Ibid., fol. 307v, "contra epilepsiam".
402 Ibid., fol. 469r; on this widespread belief see also Schild, Blut (2007); the practice is documented, e.g., for late seventeenth-century Nürnberg, where the blood of the executed was collected in a vessel and given to the poor epileptics (Schattner, Bewältigungsverhalten (2012), p. 56).
403 Cod. 11183, fol. 348v.
404 In Latin, Handsch used the expression "tactus apoplexia" (ibid., fol. 142r).
405 Cod. 11205, fol. 237v.
406 Cod. 11183, fol. 123r.
407 Cod. 11205, fol. 236v.
408 Cod. 11183, fol. 433v.
409 Ibid., fol. 460v; Cod. 11207, fol. 194v, on a patient with vertigo, who felt as if he were about to be seized by an *apoplexia*. Handsch used the term "Vergicht" which like the similar German term "Gichter" translates into "cramps" or "convulsions".
410 Cod. 11183, fol. 466r.

that lavender was a good preventive, or mustard, which could be chewed.[411] It was also said that the Saxon Elector had saved an old man with the smoke of amber when he was about to go into a state similar to *apoplexia*.[412]

Apoplexia had in common with the modern concept of "apoplexy" or "stroke" that it was not always fatal. Here laypeople spoke of a "Stuck vom Schlag", a "piece of stroke".[413] The consequences were sometimes limited to different degrees of paralysis, often hemiplegia, which is still considered a typical consequence of a stroke today. Patients were unable to move arms and legs on the affected side or dragged one leg,[414] and the mouth was twisted to one side.[415] Signs of paralysis were thus an important warning for the risk of *apoplexia*. After a mild case of *apoplexia*, some patients lived on for many years. However, as Handsch experienced various times, there was always a risk that a second, fatal attack of *apoplexia* would follow, sometimes within hours or days.[416]

In its central elements, the medical explanation of *apoplexia* was similar to that of *epilepsia*. As Handsch learned in Falloppia's anatomy classes, there were two kinds of excretions found in the brain: The vaporous, smoky excretions escaped through the cranial sutures. The thicker, more viscous and phlegmy kind, by contrast, could only be emptied via the larger ducts that led away from the skull. If this drainage was obstructed, there was a risk of an *apoplexia*.[417] Handsch wrote later that he usually told people to try and remember their dreams if they were worried about having a stroke. If they could not remember, this was a sign that their *virtus imaginativa* was beginning to become cloudy from the presence of phlegmy substances ("materiae pituitosae"), which were usually responsible for *apoplexia*. If, on the contrary, they could remember their dreams well, it was an indication of open, unobstructed ventricles.[418] As Handsch mentioned in another entry, the risk of *apoplexia* and *epilepsia* was particularly great in the springtime because the peccant humors were mobilized.[419] Physicians and laypeople alike also perceived a hereditary element. Handsch wrote about patients who feared *apoplexia* in part because their parents or siblings had died of it.[420] He concurred

---

411 Cod. 11205, fol. 122r.
412 Cod. 11251, fol. 38v.
413 Cod. 11183, fol. 433v.
414 Cod. 11183, fol. 142r.
415 Ibid., fol. 245r.
416 Ibid., fol. 50v, fol. 399v and fol. 433v; Cod. 11205, fol. 127v.
417 Cod. 11210, fol. 24r.
418 Cod. 11205, fol. 302v.
419 Cod. 11207, fol. 182r.
420 Cod. 11183, fol. 348v.

with this assessment and offered an anatomical explanation: just as people differed in their outward appearance, some people had a greater risk from birth because their ventricles were narrow and could become obstructed more easily.[421]

This explanatory framework related *apoplexia* closely to *epilepsia*. With both diseases, patients lost consciousness, though with *epilepsia* this was only temporary. Physicians observed that, like the *epileptici*, the *apoplectici* often foamed at the mouth. With *epilepsia*, the phlegm did not obstruct the ducts from the skull as completely as it did with *apoplexia*. As Handsch observed in the case of the court painter Teuffel, it was thus possible that patients first suffered epileptic seizures and finally – here he apparently suspected a complete obstruction – succumbed to fatal *apoplexia*.[422] Physicians and laypeople considered strong emotions, especially rage, to be significant triggers for both diseases.[423] It was said of King Matthias, for example, who died unexpectedly at the age of forty-seven, that he suffered a fatal stroke while eating due to an intense rage ("ex magna ira").[424]

Especially among laypeople, the interpretation of *apoplexia* as a disease of the brain was only one of two interpretations, and the second one was possibly more prevalent, but here the sources are sparse. It was reflected in the synonymous use of the term *Schlagfluss*, which was widespread among German-speaking laypeople, and remained so until the very recent past. Just as with *apoplexia*, the typical characteristic of a *Schlagfluss* was the sudden, dramatic manifestation of the disease, the *Schlag* or stroke, which often resulted in death but in this case, as the word *Schlagfluss* indicates, the stroke was seen as a subform of a *Fluss* or flux.[425] Morbid matter flowed to the heart which thereby became the locus of the deadly process. It thus made sense when, as Handsch wrote, an archducal chancery clerk who had serious chest complaints feared that an *apoplexi*a "ex catarrho" might be attacking him, that is a stroke caused by morbid matter which was flowing downward. He had started to "feel strange, tight, and narrow in the chest as if he had to die, and his left arm had become heavy."[426]

In learned medicine, the distinction between apoplexia as a disease of the brain and as a disease of the heart was not always clear either. Nobody died from

---

421 Cod. 11206, fol. 126r.
422 Cod. 11183, fol. 411v.
423 Cod. 11205, fol. 149r, on the belief of the "vulgares"; Cod. 11183, fol. 51r, on the irascible ("iracundus") Eduard Seidelhuber, who became hemiplegic and later died.
424 Cod. 11193, fol. 474v; as Handsch added, a similar story was narrated about King Wenzel of Bohemia.
425 In Cod. 11205, fol. 272r, Handsch also recorded as an *error vulgi* the belief that in *apoplexia* a drop of blood fell from the brain into the heart.
426 Cod. 11183, fol. 450v.

paralysis alone, Handsch thought; in addition, there had to be something like *apoplexia* "which suffocates the heart".[427] And concerning some *apoplectici*, he wrote of death by "suffocation", presumably because of their death rattle.[428] Physicians also shared the lay opinion that corpulent people were particularly at risk. This made sense, because, as Gallo explained to Handsch after reading Rhazes, with both congenital and acquired obesity ("obesitas"), the veins were narrow and could become blocked easily. For this reason, fat people ("pingues") fell victim to paralysis and *apoplexia* more easily.[429] From his reading of Haly Abbas, Handsch further learned that a *plethora*, a surplus of blood in the body and the veins, would lead to paralysis and *apoplexia*. A perpetually sweaty face was an important sign.[430]

The dual nature of the "stroke" as a disease of the brain, on the one hand, and of the heart and vessels on the other is crucial for a correct interpretation of premodern sources. When these sources mention people who died of a "stroke", "apoplexy" or "Schlagfluss", we ultimately cannot know whether what occurred was cerebral insult in the modern understanding, or whether the heart might have been the main site of the disease, as in a myocardial infarction, for example. The "pressura", "angustia pectoris"[431] and the "heaviness" of the left arm of which the above-mentioned chancery clerk complained would certainly make any physician today suspect *angina pectoris* and the risk of a myocardial infarction. Therefore, if historians describe the death of a historic figure based on the historical diagnosis of a stroke, *Schlagfluss* or *apoplexia* without marking these terms as historical, that is to say when they essentially consider the death – as happens regularly in history writing – to have resulted from apoplexy in the modern sense, they risk making a gross misjudgment. All we know with some certainty is that the person died a sudden death – and, depending on the case, the cause for it could have been a number of things. Sometimes only, supplementary information about previous episodes of paralysis or complaints in the chest area suggests one interpretation rather than another.

---

427 Cod. 11205, fol. 270v.
428 Ibid., fol. 236v and fol. 237v, on cardinal Bernardo Cles.
429 Ibid., fol. 268v; as Handsch remarked in another entry, however, skinny people could also suffer an *apoplexia* (Cod. 11183, fol. 449: "Macilenti etiam apoplectici"); see also Stolberg, "Abhorreas pinguedinem" (2012).
430 Cod. 11205, fol. 268v.
431 Cod. 11183, fol. 450v.

Melancholy and Madness

"Melancholy" – "melancholia" in Latin – has received much attention in studies in the history of the Renaissance, including from literary scholars and art historians.[432] The ambiguity of the term "melancholia" as well as the adjective "melancholicus" has also led to a fair share of misunderstandings, however. Three interrelated levels of meaning for "melancholia" and "melancholicus" must be distinguished. Derived from the Greek words for "black" and "bile", "melancholia" first of all denoted one of the body's four natural humors, black bile. It was described as cold and dry and having a tough consistency. Its primary seat in the body was the spleen, whose size, according to Falloppia, varied depending on the amount of black bile that had accumulated in it.[433]

If black bile predominated in someone's body, this person had a melancholy temperament, in short, was a "melancholicus". The person typically exhibited certain "melancholy" character traits and physical characteristics, without being sick. In the tradition of the Middle Ages, these included having dark skin and dark hair, a tendency to solitude and a certain sadness, miserliness, and a good, "tenacious" memory. In the Renaissance, under the influence of Neoplatonism, the "melancholic" temperament underwent a radical re-evaluation. Marsilio Ficino and various later authors elaborated on a passage from the pseudo-Aristotelian *Problemata*, according to which the *melancholici* – Ficino counted himself among them – possessed outstanding mental faculties.[434]

In its third level of meaning, "melancholia" was a disease term. The difference between this usage and the melancholic temperament has often been overlooked in historical research and indeed there were areas of overlap. In the Renaissance period, some cases of the disease "melancholia" continued to be ascribed to an excessive, pathological, and ultimately morbid dominance of the natural black bile. Like most other diseases, however, "melancholy" in the sixteenth century was generally attributed not to an imbalance of the humors but ascribed to a particular morbid matter – in this case black, or more specifically black and burnt matter. It could develop when natural black bile was exces-

---

432 The classical study is Klibansky, Panofsky and Saxl, Saturn und Melancholie (1992); see also Steiger, Melancholie (1996); Sullivan, Beyond melancholy (2016); overviews of the long-term developments in Fischer-Homberger, Hypochondrie (1970) and Jackson, Melancholia (1986).
433 Cod. 11210, fol. 2r.
434 Ficino, De triplici vita (1978); Wittstock, Melancholia translata (2011).

sively heated and vapors rose from it,⁴³⁵ but also from yellow bile and even blood, when were burnt in the body. Thus, Jakob Horst attributed the *melancholia hypochondriaca* of one his patients to her hot liver which was burning the warm blood.⁴³⁶ Jakob Horst and Johannes Neefe also ascribed the melancholy of Caspar von Rechenberg to his melancholy, burnt blood, and a malignant humor, from which harmful vapors rose up to the head, weakening the brain and causing Caspar's sadness, fearfulness, and faintheartedness.⁴³⁷ With another patient, Horst identified an obstruction of the spleen caused by an excess of a melancholy humor, whose inner cause he located again in the heated liver that burnt the blood, thus creating melancholy blood. Added to this were the external causes of worry and sorrow following the death of his wife.⁴³⁸

Physicians often also used the term "atra bilis" instead of "melancholia" to refer to the acrid, caustic, dark, burnt blood or black or yellow bile that caused the disease "melancholia". It was described as very similar to or indeed identical with the morbid matter which caused ulcers, cancer, and other skin alterations – which also explains the connection that was made, somewhat surprisingly at first glance, between melancholy and scurvy. Scurvy, in the early modern sense of the word, was characterized by ulcers of the gums and skin. In the case of the patient last mentioned, Horst could thus diagnose both *hypochondria melancholica* and scurvy, or at least a certain predisposition for it.⁴³⁹

The lines between *melancholia* and *mania,* or fury, which medieval authors still sought to distinguish to some degree,⁴⁴⁰ became further blurred in the early modern period. "Melancholia" essentially became a generic term for different manifestations of "insanity" or "madness", covering symptoms from violent fury to abject, unprovoked sadness and all the way to great fearfulness.

Lycanthropy, or werewolf delusion, was considered a major variant of pathological melancholia. In Prague, Handsch saw a farmer who, perhaps because he was impoverished, had hidden in the straw in the fields. He was discovered during a search for a disappeared boy. The farmer claimed that he was a wolf and was in the habit of eating children. He was taken to the hospital and treated

---

435 See Drembach, De atra bile ([1548]), Aii: "Quandoque in homine ita aßatus adustusque deprehendatur [melancholicus humor], ut eum inde morbum efficiat, qui etiam absque febre mentem infestet, timorem et moestitiam pariat."
436 Staats- und Universitätsbibliothek Göttingen, Ms Meibom 146, pp. 186–188, letter to Ascha von Mohrenfeld, undated, in German.
437 Ibid., pp. 222–228, letter to Caspar von Rechenberg, February 1569.
438 Ibid., pp. 160–167, letter to Melchior Richardus, the prefect of the treasury of Duke Julius of Braunschweig-Wolfenbüttel, 10 May 1585, in German.
439 Ibid.
440 Demaitre, Medieval medicine (2013), pp. 135–138.

with bloodletting until he fainted.[441] In milder cases, lycanthropy sufferers inclined toward solitude and showed a special affinity for cemeteries and corpses. As to bodily symptoms, the disease was associated above all with ulcers on the legs, which were interpreted as consequences of the acrid, burnt black and bilious matter.[442]

The three semantic levels of "melancholy" and their interconnections are also reflected in Handsch's notes. Handsch and the physicians in his professional environment considered various patients to have a "melancholy" *complexio*.[443] According to Gallo, a dark reddened face in particular pointed in this direction.[444] With some patients, the physicians suspected a mixed choleric-melancholic *complexio*: both yellow and black bile predominated in this case.[445] In the case of an archducal secretary, this was indicated by his black beard, reddened face, and hulking body.[446]

Black bile could sometimes be seen with the naked eye in the patient's blood or excretions. Again and again, Handsch described the *melancholia* he observed as blackish matter in the blood from bloodletting[447] or in the stool, including sometimes his own.[448] A layman like Archduke Ferdinand, too, could arrive at the conclusion that his stool was "melancholy"; Handsch described it as "blackish gray, dark".[449] However, physicians agreed that what they saw in most cases was preternatural, thickened, and, above all, burnt black bile.[450] Trincavella in Padua ascribed the strong induration of a woman's spleen to a "materia crassa, melancholica".[451] In the case of the later Emperor Maximilian II, Trincavella concluded that he had a hot, dry temperament and generated a lot of blood, which, due to "burning" ("ex exustione"), tended toward melancholy, as could be seen in his excrements and on his skin.[452] A hot, dry temperament indicated the dominance of hot yellow, not cold black bile. When diagnosing the Trento bookseller Hieronymus, Handsch suspected that a hot liver was generating

---

441 Cod. 11226, fol. 79v.
442 Stolberg, Lykanthropie (2001); Metzger, Wolfsmenschen (2011).
443 E.g. Cod. 11183, fol. 113r; Cod. 11205, fol. 324r.
444 Cod. 11207, fol. 29r; Gallo contradicted Handsch here who had assumed a sanguinic temperament, persumably because of the redness.
445 Cod. 11205, fol. 324r-v.
446 Ibid., fol. 482v.
447 Cod. 11206, fol. 34r; Cod. 11204, 34r.
448 Cod. 11183, fol. 165r and fol. 200r-v.
449 Cod. 11204, fol. 34r.
450 Cod. 11205, fol. 124v.
451 Cod. 11238, fol. 89r.
452 Cod. 11207, fol. IIr.

burnt, "melancholy" blood.[453] As mentioned above, acrid, burnt "melancholy" humors were also seen as an important cause of ulcers, cancer, and scurvy. Presumably because of the distinctive skin symptoms, some physicians even saw burnt, melancholy matter as a cause of the French disease.[454]

In Handsch's notes and in other contemporary sources that describe everyday practice, "melancholia" and the "melancholici" referred primarily to a quite clearly defined disease then that was caused by burnt, or otherwise unnatural "melancholic" matter and came in several subforms, each with characteristic symptoms. Handsch documented a whole host of cases of *melancholia*, and some of his entries were unusually elaborate and detailed. *Mania* by contrast, figures only marginally in Handsch's notes, usually in connection with *melancholia*, in expressions like "maniaci melancholici".[455] Handsch and the physicians in his professional environment counted *insani* and *maniaci*, that is people with marked delusions and "mad" or violent behavior among the *melancholici* just as they did patients whose main complaints were sadness, despondency, and fearfulness.

The symptoms of insane or raging *melancholici* were sometimes very dramatic, recalling the psychotic episodes of schizophrenics as described by psychiatry today.[456] A twenty-five-year old melancholy cantor, for example, believed that he was God and had created the mountains around Innsbruck. He tore off his clothes and rubbed himself with excrement. He wanted to hug the physicians and sometimes he sang. When Mattioli beat him with a switch, he fell silent. Later, he cried a lot and was finally taken home as someone who had taken leave of his senses ("amens").[457] A young melancholy woman did not speak with anyone for an entire year, not even with her relatives. Once, she hit her head against the wall and cursed without any apparent reason.[458] Coming from a woman and in a society strongly shaped by religion, cursing would have been considered a possible symptom of madness much more so than today. Some *melancholici* thought they were princes. For example, an insane ("insana") young woman who had been chained at home objected when someone addressed her, saying, "How dare you use an informal tone with me?" She tore up her clothes, lay naked, sometimes

---

453 Cod. 11238, fol. 138v.
454 Ibid., fol. 98v.
455 Cod. 11207, fol. 5v; Cod. 11226, fol. 75v, marginal note on Willenbroch's treatment of a *maniacus*.
456 In some cases, the descriptions suggest, from a modern point of view, an alcohol-induced delirium, e.g., in the case of a certain Fassbinder, who came home drunk and developed such frenzy that he had to be tied to his bed. He cursed and did not seem to recognize anyone but fully recovered within a few days (Cod. 11183, fol. 426v).
457 Ibid., fol. 389v.
458 Ibid., fol. 59v.

laughed, sometimes cursed. She temporarily improved but during a relapse, she beat the boys and girls she saw in the street.[459] Handsch added to his entry that a young man in Prague had stolen a sword from the workshop of a swordsmith and had run raging across the square with it. Only with difficulty could he be taken to the dungeon.[460]

Melancholia when suffered by women in childbed could sometimes be a heavy burden for them and for the people around them. Modern medicine knows similar phenomena by the name of postpartum depression or psychosis.[461] Handsch experienced the dramatic manifestation of the disease first hand with the wife of Caspar von Mühlstein. The birth had gone well. Seven hours after her water broke, she gave birth to a child. However, on the fourth day after the delivery, she became delirious. She believed people wanted to kill her. After the wife of the court surgeon Hildebrand gave her different remedies, her mind cleared up but that improvement did not last. People prayed for her wellbeing at church. She continued to have delirious thoughts, saying among other things: "My husband is gone, my child too, and I will follow soon myself." Intermittently, she was more lucid. Her child was given to another woman and a small dog was found to suckle from the sick woman and thus free her of the superfluous milk. Her lochia became less bloody. She seemed to be slowly doing better, but six weeks after she gave birth she still had delusions. She said strange things, wanted to interpret the Old and the New Testament and at one point threw herself down in front of Willenbroch, praying to him as if he were Christ. Come the new moon, things got worse. She began yelling again, hid under benches, and made a move to hang herself, and the physicians saw all this as a sign that her *melancholia* was returning. Willenbroch prescribed opiates and antimony, but to no avail. When he finally gave up, Handsch took over treatment and prescribed clysters, sleep-inducing medication, and other remedies. She was beginning to get better. She only cried sometimes. Eventually her husband informed him that her monthly period had stopped. She was indeed pregnant again, and the delusions stopped.[462]

In a similar case in 1563, Handsch was in charge of treatment from the beginning. Delivery and the passing of the afterbirth were uneventful. But one week later, the woman came down with a fever, headaches, a rash on her chest, and became delirious. She believed she was close to dying, asked for a candle to be lit, and said goodbye to her children. In the days that followed, it continued to seem as if she had lost her mind. But she only complained about a "dropped uvula"

---

[459] Cod. 11205, fol. 415r.
[460] Ibid., fol. 415r.
[461] On the more recent history see Marland, Dangerous motherhood (2004).
[462] Cod. 11183, foll. 461v-465r.

("uvula lapsa"), had much "catarrh" in her throat and was hardly able to speak. Several days later, the women gave her a sitz bath for an hour and washed her head. They said this had to be done fourteen days after the birth. Finally, Handsch ordered bloodletting from the *vena saphena* on the leg. He knew from Mattioli that this promised to be beneficial because it restored menstruation – presumably by drawing the blood downwards. The patient became lucid again, though sometimes she sat pensively and laughed. Another woman who had just given birth and then became sick with melancholy recovered but then fell ill again during her next pregnancy and hurt a maid with a knife.[463]

The clinical pictures of other *melancholici* were less dramatic. Some only laughed without cause.[464] Or, in the estimation of those close to them, they had "confused fantasies",[465] said peculiar things and told strange stories,[466] for example about the devil,[467] or spoke, like a *scholasticus melancholicus*, incessantly and partly in Latin, about all kinds of things.[468] About a noble *melancholicus*, Handsch wrote, "He talks like a madman and yet sometimes goes for a stroll in the alleys, knows the people, sometimes acts friendly, eats well". The man complained that there were many "who berate him and knock against the bed at night".[469]

While such cases involving varying degrees of insanity come up comparatively frequently in Handsch's notes, he made fewer notes about manifestations of *melancholia* that were characterized mainly by deep sadness or despondency, a condition that would thus be closer to "depression" in today's understanding. About the *melancholia* of Jan von Wartenberg, he noted, "It sometimes came over him like a swoon, making him sad and scared without reason."[470] Jan soon felt better. The *melancholia* of another nobleman called Wenzel was more serious. He proved to be reasonable and respectful with the physicians. But he was always sad ("tristis") and Lehner was concerned that he might hang himself.[471] With other patients as well, prolonged sorrow and fearfulness[472] or their hiding away

---

[463] Ibid., fol. 470r.
[464] Ibid., fol. 59v.
[465] Cod. 11205, fol. 262r.
[466] Ibid., fol. 238r; Cod. 11240, fol. 37v.
[467] Cod. 11183, fol. 176r.
[468] Cod. 11205, fol. 235v.
[469] Ibid., fol. 224v.
[470] Cod. 11183, fol. 239v.
[471] Cod. 11205, fol. 237v and Cod. 11240, fol. 37r; he died soon after but it is unclear whether he actually killed himself.
[472] Cod. 11205, fol. 501r, on the wife of Oswald Kamm.

under the roof[473] indicated *melancholia*. In the case of Archduke Ferdinand II, Handsch restricted himself to more subtle remarks. The Archduke was plagued by stones, but, as Handsch noted down in July of 1570, "there was also a symptom of melancholy, apprehension [. . .] because he felt something that he did not want to tell." The physicians watched over him all night. Whether the Archduke had possibly hinted at delusional ideas or even suicidal thoughts remains unclear.[474] Several weeks later – his stone complaints were ongoing – Ferdinand called for the physicians before daybreak and again complained about "apprehension".[475]

A widely diagnosed, milder variety of *melancholia* was *melancholia hypochondriaca*. In the course of the early modern period, the concept of *hypochondria* would develop from it, becoming increasingly disconnected from its original, primarily somatic associations and developing into the term for an exaggerated fear of disease as we still know it today. The term "hypochondria" referred to the area in the body where the disease was believed to originate, that is the upper abdomen. The term is composed of the Greek words for "under" ("hypo") and "cartilage" ("chondros") – referring to the costal cartilage. The established explanation of the disease "hypochondria" was that pathogenic vapors rose from the abdomen to the heart, lungs, and brain. They compromised the functions of those organs and led to associated symptoms. Sometimes physicians also used the expression *melancholia myrachalis*, which was derived from the Arabic words for "abdomen" or "upper abdomen".[476]

With regard to the treatment of insane *melancholici*, numerous stories circulated in the medical literature about lunatics who were supposedly cured by cleverly exerting an influence on their *ratio* or by deliberately provoking powerful affects. From Lehner, Handsch heard a story about a *melancholica* for whom a visit by a make-believe hangman was arranged. The visit gave her such a fright that she was cured.[477] Yet, the medical treatment of both the insane and the deeply sad *melancholici*, as documented in Handsch's notebooks, reflects the predominant medical view of *melancholia* as a physical disease. Various drugs were used, including remedies such as *terra sigillata*, that is Armenian clay, which was believed

---

[473] Cod. 11183, fol. 23r.
[474] Cod. 11204, fol. 42v, "et aderat quoque symptoma melancholicum, die bangickeit, nam dicebat sibi quid esse quod nemini vellet dicere."
[475] Ibid., fol. 44r; for a more detailed account see Stolberg, Krankheitsgeschehen (2021).
[476] Cod. 11226, fol. 75v, student notes on a lecture by Trincavella.
[477] Cod. 11205, fol. 235v.

to be effective against a range of poisons.⁴⁷⁸ In addition, physicians resorted to surgical procedures. They prescribed copious bloodletting, if necessary until the patient lost consciousness, apparently to empty the black-bilious, burnt blood and see it replaced by newly generated, healthy blood. As Handsch observed, Gallo also frequently relied on the beneficial effects of cauterization with a red-hot iron, which Rhazes had recommended for such cases. The above-mentioned disconsolate, melancholy Wenzel, for example, was cauterized on the top of his head.⁴⁷⁹

The French Disease

In the late fifteenth century, a disastrous new epidemic spread across Europe in only a few years: *morbus gallicus,* or the "French disease".⁴⁸⁰ As opposed to the plague, the disease was not immediately lethal but it often had a protracted progression over many years and brought great suffering. People from all ranks, including the highest circles of society were affected One of its most famous early victims was the humanist Ulrich von Hutten.⁴⁸¹ And in a remarkably plainspoken manner, the physicians of Martin Luther considered the possibility that his complaints derived from an affliction of *morbus gallicus*.⁴⁸² Handsch, for his part, knew of various prominent patients who suffered from the disease: one of his acquaintances told him that the Duke of Saxony and several young noblemen at his court had been treated for the French disease.⁴⁸³ And he learned from Mattioli that his own employer, Archduke Ferdinand II, had suffered from it when he was young,⁴⁸⁴ as did Karl and Hans Georg Welser, two close relatives of Ferdinand's wife Philippine.⁴⁸⁵

From the perspective of modern medicine, early modern *morbus gallicus* had much in common with today's syphilis. It was very likely caused by a bacterium that would have been at least very similar to *treponema pallidum,* the recognized cause of syphilis. Most of the symptoms that were linked to a diagnosis of *morbus*

---

478 Cod. 11183, fol. 237v; Cod. 11207, fol. 27v.
479 Cod. 11240, foll. 36v-37r.
480 Overviews in Bloch, Ursprung (1901/1911); Leven, Geschichte (1997), pp. 36–38 and pp. 53–60; Arrizabalaga/French/Henderson, Great pox (1997); Stein, Negotiating (2009), esp. pp. 23–66.
481 Hutten, Artzney (1519).
482 Stolberg/Walter, Martin Luthers viele Krankheiten (2018).
483 Cod. 11207, fol. 222v.
484 Cod. 11204, fol. 37v.
485 Cod. 11183, fol. 202v and fol. 413v.

gallicus then – ranging from skin alterations and hair loss to tumors, intense headaches and tinnitus – are considered symptoms of the different stages of syphilis. Paleopathological examinations have shown changes in the bones like those typical for syphilis.[486] And just as syphilis, *morbus gallicus* was transmitted primarily through sexual contact, as contemporaries soon realized. Even the term "syphilis" as a name for *morbus gallicus* was coined as early as the sixteenth century by Girolamo Fracastoro,[487] though medical writers initially used it only to a very limited extent; in Handsch's extensive notes, it occurs only peripherally.[488]

For our historical understanding of the experience of *morbus gallicus* and of how people dealt with it in the early modern period, equating it with the modern-day "syphilis" is not really helpful, however, and in some respects misleading. For one thing, the historical images and ideas connected with *morbus gallicus* emerged in a very different context and were shaped by it. This context was the doctrine of the significance of different types of more or less specific morbid matter as the key to understanding the vast majority of diseases. Moreover, the typical clinical picture of *morbus gallicus,* which we find documented in numerous contemporary descriptions, in case histories, and in the personal testimonies of patients, only partially overlaps with that associated with syphilis today, especially with regard to the extent and the intensity of the pathological changes. The common perception of syphilis as a venereal disease that affects above all the genitals – without an awareness of the many pathological changes that may occur inside the body when it goes untreated – does not come close to doing justice to the perception and the experience of *morbus gallicus* in the sixteenth century. To avoid such anachronistic misunderstandings, I will therefore continue to use the term "morbus gallicus" along with the term "French disease", which corresponds to the term "Franzosenkrankheit" as commonly used in German at the time.

Already in Handsch's time, the characteristic symptom of *morbus gallicus,* especially at the outset of the disease, was an ulcer on the glans penis, under

---

[486] Walker et alii, Evidence (2015).
[487] Fracastoro, Syphilis (1530).
[488] According to the old catalogue of the Austrian National Library in Vienna, Handsch made excerpts from a treatise by Da Monte's *De lue syphilido* in Cod. 11126, foll. 146r-148v; in the microfilm of this manuscript these pages are missing, however. The user is informed that the sequence of pages in the film corresponds to the original. Unfortunately, I could not consult the orginal due to the bad condition of the manuscript but presumably the pages have gone lost. According to the frontispiece, Da Monte's *Methodus* (1553) included a "De syphillidos lue tractatus" but the passage itself has the title "Lectiones de morbo gallico" (ibid., foll. 14r-32v).

the foreskin, often accompanied by swelling in the groin area.[489] In addition, *gonorrhea* was considered a frequent early symptom.[490] Today, this is considered a distinct, sexually transmitted disease that is caused by a specific bacterial pathogen. At the time, however, "gonorrhea", from the Greek words for "semen" and "flux" referred generally to a pathological flux of what was believed to be seminal fluid. Handsch claimed that the vernacular expression for it was "kalde Seyche" ("cold piss"), presumably derived from the German word "seichen", meaning to pass water.[491] As such, *gonorrhea* could also occur in women. Handsch suspected *gonorrhea*, a voiding of female *sperma*, for example when the wife of Collinus told him about the whitish liquid that sometimes flowed from her vagina the morning after she had had intercourse with her husband. What made it likely in Handsch's view that this was her own semen was her description: she sometimes felt lust during coitus and then felt weakened afterward.[492] To distinguish a literal *gonorrhea* from purulent discharge – which we would assume it to have been in many cases – was not always easy. And so Handsch wrote about a male patient who said that he did not know whether the "filth" that was issuing from him was "nature", that is spermatic fluid, or perhaps pus.[493] What he considered a "flux of semen" even reeked in the case of a Polish patient.[494]

According to medical doctrine, the main causes of *gonorrhea* were, first of all, a pathologically changed, all too watery, liquid, or excessively heated seminal fluid – qualities which promoted its expulsion. Secondly, there was a weakening of the *facultas retentrix* or a relaxation and widening of the seminal vessels.[495] The latter explained the occurrence of *gonorrhea* following frequent coitus which would cause a slackening of the seminal vessels. This is how Handsch in Padua made sense of the *gonorrhea* suffered by a certain Balthasar. He resolved that when dealing with similar cases, he would ask whether the *gonorrhea* had happened after intercourse.[496] Counseling another young man on his *gonorrhea*, he recommended that the man avoid coitus and lustful thoughts and advised him to stay away from spicy, salty, and sour food, as well as from garlic and strong wine, all of which were believed to promote sexual desire and/or the emission of semen.[497]

---

489 E.g. Cod. 11183, fol. 203r; Cod. 11247, fol. 33r.
490 Cod. 11205, fol. 580v, referring to various patients who initially had *gonorrhea* but then developed the French disease.
491 Cod. 11240, fol. 98r; similarly: Cod. 11238, fol. 134v.
492 Cod. 11205, fol. 248v.
493 Ibid., fol. 507r.
494 Cod. 11183, fol. 285v.
495 Cod. 11238, fol. 130v.
496 Ibid., fol. 131r.
497 Cod. 11205, fol. 581r.

Experience taught, however, that *gonorrhea* primarily occurred after intercourse with "unclean" women and easily developed into the French disease or accompanied it.[498] Handsch's friend Giulio Gallo, for instance, had a bout of *gonorrhea* "post venerem", as indicated by the spotting on his shirt and his painful urination. Some weeks later, a rash ("scabies") developed on his thighs and he experienced swelling in the groin area.[499] Handsch observed a similar development with other patients whose pathological "seminal flux" was ultimately joined or followed by the symptoms of *morbus gallicus*.[500] Handsch also learned that Archduke Ferdinand II not only had been treated for the French disease as a young man but had also suffered from *gonorrhea* for six months.[501] Some physicians simply spoke of a *gonorrhea gallica*.[502]

The clinical picture of fully developed *morbus gallicus* was dramatic and often readily recognizable by anyone looking at the sufferer. The affected body parts usually included not only the genitalia but also the skin, the mucous membranes, and not least of all the bones. In women, in whom the genital changes tended to be less obvious, these latter symptoms were often predominant.

On the skin of the face and the body, the disease manifested in countless red spots ("maculae") or purulent pustules ("pustulae").[503] They could become quite large, and their surface, like the skin in general, was often described as crusted-over or flaking and white.[504] In the late fifteenth and sixteenth centuries, these skin alterations seem to have been more dramatic and striking than in later times.[505] The physicians here also talked about a "French scab" or "scabies gallica",[506] which could affect the face and hands, or even the entire body.[507] Judging by his colleague Tremenus's ugly, flaking rash, Handsch was quite certain, for example, that Tremenus, although he denied it, had contracted *morbus gallicus*, and Handsch was all the more certain as Tremenus "confessed" that he used to have an ulcer on his penis. Not only this but he was always, as Handsch observed, in the company of a "whore" ("scorta").[508] Simply seeing the pustules in the face of a man who was

---

498 Cod. 11126, fol. 127v.
499 Cod. 11238, fol. 134r.
500 Ibid., fol. 134r-v.
501 Cod. 11204, fol. 49r.
502 Cod. 11183, fol. 434r, on a sick man in Karlsbad.
503 E.g. Ibid., fol. 435v, on the red *maculae* of a young "Pfenningmeister" (presumably the archducal treasurer); Cod. 11207, fol. 163v.
504 Cod. 11183, fol. 117r.
505 See also Leven, Geschichte (1997), p. 55, note.
506 Cod. 11183, fol. 203r.
507 Ibid.
508 Ibid., fol. 431r.

bringing in a flask of his urine – which, he claimed, came from another patient – Gallo was equally certain. So, seemingly only from his examination of the urine, he was able to determine quite exactly the age of the patient in question – that of the messenger – along with the symptoms, that is the known, typical accompanying symptoms of *morbus gallicus* and the man confirmed everything.[509] The palms of the hand were sometimes affected, too. A young man, who apparently worked with a barber and, according to Handsch also consorted with a whore, even developed ulcers there.[510]

In the experience of physicians, only leprosy, if anything, could cause similar skin changes. The physicians in Handsch's professional environment were in fact not always certain whether a patient was sick with *morbus gallicus* or *elephantiasis*, a common synonym for leprosy at the time.[511] With lepers, however, they expected to find halitosis.[512] Further signs that were typical of *morbus gallicus* could readily allay the remaining doubts physicians had – and there were plenty of signs. As Handsch learned early on as a student of Fracanzano,[513] these signs did not necessarily appear all at once, but many of them occurred almost exclusively with *morbus gallicus*.

One typical sign was the pustules and venereal wart-like proliferations in the area of the anus which some patients developed, or "warts in the cranny of the arse", as Handsch referred to them.[514] They itched and wept and sometimes patients found it painful just to sit down.[515] When they suspected a case of *morbus gallicus*, Lehner, Handsch himself and other physicians he knew asked explicitly about them.[516] Another very characteristic skin change that manifested with many patients over the years were the so-called *gummositates* or *gummata*. These were indurated nodules or lumps in the skin. Handsch observed such *gummositates* in a number of patients. They could by very painful, and they could ulcerate and open.[517] Answering Handsch's question, one woman said they "[sting] as if there is pus inside". She had *gummositates* on her forehead

---

509 Cod. 11207, fol. 182v.
510 Cod. 11183, fol. 435v.
511 Cod. 11205, fol. 267v.
512 Ibid., on Gallo's diagnosis of *morbus gallicus* in a young man with swollen legs and hands, pustules, and hair loss.
513 Cod. 11226, fol. 127v.
514 Cod. 11183, fol. 124v; Handsch listed a series of patients here; he named further patients ibid., fol. 77v, fol. 435v and in Cod. 11207, fol. 152r.
515 Ibid., fol. 117r, on a certain Thomas "ex hospitali", and fol. 118r, on the "incisor" Johannes (possibly one of the artisans who made the woodcuts for Mattioli's famous herbal).
516 Cod. 11207, fol. 152r; Cod. 11183, fol. 117r.
517 Cod. 11183, fol. 72v and fol. 252v.

and four more, the size of acorns, on her back.⁵¹⁸ Sometimes the mucosa of the tongue and throat was affected as well.⁵¹⁹ It was therefore necessary for a physician to ask specifically about ulcerations in the throat when suspecting *morbus gallicus*.⁵²⁰

A further typical symptom was seen in the partial loss of head hair, eyebrows, and beard. In the worst cases, only vestiges remained.⁵²¹ This too the physician had to include in his list of questions when *morbus gallicus* was suspected and when hair loss was not already clearly visible.⁵²² However, as Handsch learned from Mattioli, not all patients experienced hair loss, and it was something that could also occur with leprosy.⁵²³

Many sufferers also complained of severe headaches, especially in the evenings and at night. In one entry, Handsch listed a whole host of male patients and one maid from Padua who suffered from strong headaches due to *morbus gallicus*.⁵²⁴ The pain was caused by the disease attacking the skull bone, Handsch explained to one patient.⁵²⁵ With some patients, the headaches coincided with *gummositates* or other indurated tumors of the head.⁵²⁶ In the case of the dean Paulus in Reichstadt, the entire nasal bone had crumbled from ulceration, which also changed his voice. He spoke "in a hollow tone", as if his nose were stuffed, thought Handsch.⁵²⁷ The pains that *morbus gallicus* patients complained of very often included "rheumatic pains" in the limbs and joints, and this was a further symptom explicitly inquired about by physicians and even one apothecary.⁵²⁸

Handsch furthermore encountered many people with suspected cases of *morbus gallicus* who complained of *tinnitus,* a ringing or whistling in the ears. One of them said that he could hardly speak anymore because of it.⁵²⁹ According to

---

518 Ibid, fol. 117* r-v.
519 Cod. 11207, fol. 152r and fol. 212r; Cod. 11183, fol. 203r.
520 Cod. 11238, fol. 130r.
521 Cod. 11183, fol. 118r, fol. 252v and fol. 399v, massive loss of beard; Cod. 11205, fol. 267v and 323r; Cod. 11238, fol. 238r; Cod. 11207, fol. 154v and Cod. 11183, fol. 203r, loss of eyebrows.
522 Cod. 11238, fol. 130r: "Nota inquirenda de morbo gallico".
523 Cod. 11207, fol. 154v; Mattioli had previously discussed the differences between *morbus gallicus* and *elephantiasis* (Mattioli, Morbi gallici (1535)).
524 Cod. 11205, fol. 323r; Cod. 11183, fol. 27v; Cod. 11238, fol. 4v, on the case of a soldier with severe headpain due to the French disease.
525 Cod. 11205, fol. 323r.
526 Cod. 11238, fol. 98r.
527 Cod. 11205, fol. 415v (cit.) and fol. 471r.
528 Cod. 11183, fol. 72v (pharmacist), fol. 87v, fol. 252v and fol. 285v.
529 Cod. 11207, fol. 169r and fol. 171r, on a servant of Holzer's, the merchant Martinus and on the strong young relative of captain.

Fracanzano, epilepsy, vertigo, and insomnia counted among other possible consequences of *morbus gallicus* if the morbid matter accumulated in the head.[530]

The writings of the classical authorities offered no information about the nature and the causes of *morbus gallicus*. However, the paramount significance of the new disease in contemporary society and therefore in medical practice led to a wealth of treatises and it soon entered the university syllabus as well. Now students of medicine received a thorough schooling in the nature, causes, symptoms, and treatment of the disease. When Handsch studied in Padua, he saw many cases with Fracanzano and Falloppia.[531] In Padua, Handsch also produced notes from Antonio Fracanzano's lecture titled *De morbo gallico*.[532] These notes provide a good overview of the understanding of the disease at the time.

Fracanzano explained to his students that *morbus gallicus* was a new disease and that there were a number of different ideas concerning its emergence. He went on to say that he concurred with Niccolò Leoniceno,[533] who thought that Portuguese sailors had brought the disease with them from "India" – meaning the Caribbean – to Spain and Italy, or that it had its starting point in their intercourse with a leprous whore ("leproso scorzo"). At any rate, the army of the French king Charles VIII, which was moving through Italy at the time, had spread the disease quickly after that.

Fracanzano had no doubt that the disease was transmissible and in this he was of the same mind as the overwhelming majority of contemporary medical authors. He explained to his students that the disease was always transmitted by a *contagium*, a special kind of morbid matter that, when it entered another body, produced a more or less identical clinical picture.[534] Trincavella similarly held that the disease was as widespread in "India" as smallpox was in Europe, which it had invaded "per contagium".[535]

Fracanzano sketched out the different routes of transmission, which were similarly explained in numerous other treatises on *morbus gallicus*. In their daily practice, Handsch and the physicians in his professional environment also described these routes of transmission when explaining the infection to

---

530 Cod. 11226, foll. 125v-126r.
531 Cod. 11238, foll. 89v-91r.
532 Cod. 11226, foll. 123r-140v, "Tractatus de morbo gallico, dictatus ab Excell. D. Antonio Frankenzano, Padua, Anno 1552 in Februario." Probably this was a private lecture but Handsch does not explicitly specify that it was. From Francanzano's later years in Bologna student notes on a lecture on the French disease are extant in print (Francanzano, De morbo gallico (1564); see also Fracanzano, De morbo gallico fragmenta (1574)).
533 On Leoniceno see Mugnai Carrara, Profilo (1979).
534 Cod. 11226, fol.125: "Semper per contagium fit."
535 Cod. 11238, fol. 98v.

patients. There was soon a consensus that the most significant route of transmission by far was coitus, as the typical, early genital symptoms suggested. In the cases encountered by Handsch and his mentors in their practice, there was often little cause for doubt in this respect. As mentioned, some patients declared or it was known about them that they consorted with "whores"[536] or saw prostitutes ("meretrices") regularly, like the unmarried merchant Fabianus.[537] Others at least admitted that they had had a thing with a woman[538] or, like a certain Florian, they were known to be "libidinosus". Florian's physician bluntly told him "You caught something from careless women".[539] In the case of a patient who suffered from *gonorrhea*, which Handsch thought was caused by *morbus gallicus*, Handsch concluded without much ado that he had gotten the disease from an "impure woman" ("impura muliere").[540]

Some patients swore it was impossible for them to have contracted the disease from coitus, as they had had "nothing to do with any woman for two years."[541] And in Fracastoro's writings, Handsch read that some people suffered from the French disease without having been infected.[542] Fracanzano, however, urged his students to be skeptical here: one should give little credence to those who claimed that the disease was not passed on through a contagion, citing as proof monks who lived strictly by the rules and nevertheless suffered from *morbus gallicus*. If one cared to look more closely, one would see that they knew very well how to look after their needs in secret.[543]

Some authors thought it was possible that the disease could be transmitted by drinking from the same cup or sleeping in the same bed as someone infected with the disease.[544] For this reason, the physician Wolfgang Reichert urged his son Zeno, who was about sixteen years of age, not to – as was common at the time – share his bed with a fellow student, whom Reichert suspected of being ill with *morbus gallicus*. For those sleeping in the same bed, no disease was more dangerous and more contagious, he said.[545]

---

536 Cod. 11183, fol. 435v.
537 Ibid., fol. 176v.
538 Ibid., fol. 117v, "se cum mulierem rem habuisse"; Cod. 11205, fol. 580v, "fassus est [. . .] concubuisse".
539 Cod. 11205, fol. 239v.
540 Cod. 11205, fol. 507r.
541 Ibid., fol. 204r; similarly Cod. 11207, fol. 137r.
542 Cod. 11205, fol. 204r.
543 Cod. 11226, fol. 125v.
544 Renner, Handtbüchlein (1557), fol. A IVr.
545 Ludwig, Vater und Sohn (1999), pp. 104–106, 22 July 1522.

There had furthermore been a long-established explanation in Handsch's time for those cases in which the disease manifested and showed its true face only years after a possible or suspected sexual infection. Here the physicians were building on the ancient doctrine of a "seed of disease".[546] They were assuming that the *contagium* in the form of a *seminarium,* a collection of seeds, was able remain inactive in the body for a long time as plant seeds hid in the ground. Only when nature initiated a "critical", "climacteric" movement ("motum criticum clymactericum"), as it did at regular intervals as the years went by, would the blood and the *seminarium* of the *morbus gallicus* be mobilized and the blood "infected." Gallo compared this to a small amount of red paint added to milk. Only when stirred did the entire liquid become red.[547] This allowed physicians to explain how the disease could break out long after "suspicious" contact – and after years of marriage – without having to allege infidelity. For example, when a tailor's wife who had been married for six years fell ill with the French disease, Handsch had no doubt that she had been "infected" ("infecta") by her husband. He wrote that the husband had undergone treatment with guaiac before his wedding but had not made a complete recovery.[548]

The notion of a seed of disease that could sometimes lie dormant for years further helped explain *morbus gallicus* in children. Some children clearly got infected by a wet nurse who had the French disease. Others, however, developed the symptoms only years after they were born. With the court surgeon Hildebrand, Handsch saw a girl with *morbus gallicus* who had pustules on her lips, head, anus, and vulva.[549] Gallo believed that children like her had received the morbid matter from the father's seed but the seed of the disease had sprouted only years later.[550] The girl's father had himself suffered from the disease.[551] Amatus Lusitanus published an especially striking case history in his *curationes,* to which Handsch referred in his notes. He wrote of a man who fell ill with *morbus gallicus* and was treated, seemingly with success. He no longer had symptoms. Ten years later, he married a "highly chaste" woman who gave birth to two healthy children within the following five years. In the seventh year of their marriage, however, she had another child, a boy who was infected ("infectum") with "scabies gallica". The woman had hitherto been healthy, but before this delivery, she had developed small ulcerations in the region of the labia.

---

546 Nutton, Reception (1990).
547 Cod. 11183, fol. 204r.
548 Ibid., fol. 177* r.
549 Ibid., fol. 457v.
550 Cod. 11205, fol. 204r; Handsch does not even allude to the possibility of sexual abuse.
551 Cod. 11183, fol. 457v.

Following the birth, she was unwell; something was not right with her breasts and she had to give the child to a wet nurse. The wet nurse subsequently also developed a *scabies gallica*. She infected her husband and two neighbors' children, whom she nursed. The mothers of those children were also infected by the *contagium*. In this way, the disease spread within a short time from the husband to eight other people. Amatus concluded that the husband had evidently carried an old hidden seed of the disease,[552] though he would certainly have been aware of the alternative explanation, namely that the husband had had an affair.

The exact nature of the morbid matter and the reasons for its specific effects were the subject of lively discussion in theoretical writings.[553] Fracanzano explained to his students that the *contagium* acted by "infecting" the blood. It spread through the blood and arrived at the liver. Handsch later heard a more detailed description from a Jew ("judaeus") who said that it began with an ulcer under the foreskin and then entered the body.[554] According to Fracanzano, the *contagium* acted through its "specific form" ("forma specifica"), which came with specific powers. It led to a severe, dry overheating of the liver. This in turn gave rise to the actual, morbid agent in the body, namely burnt blood, which could be joined by further burnt humors. It was the effects of the burnt blood and possibly other burnt humors that led to the infinite variety of symptoms ("symptomata infinita") and sequelae. Other authors, however, including physicians from Handsch's circles in Prague, ascribed the symptoms to a viscous, phlegmy morbid matter, which manifested as foam that could be seen in the urine. Trincavella believed that with *morbus gallicus* both a thick, mucous, and a burnt black-bilious morbid matter were at work.[555]

When it came to treating patients, the precise nature of the morbid matter was ultimately of peripheral significance, as Handsch's extensive notes on *morbus gallicus* make clear. The crucial point was that the morbid matter could be transmitted and that it could have various, in part very specific effects that were difficult to explain at the level of primary qualities.

To improve the condition of patients and successfully treat the disease, physicians believed that, as with most other diseases, the decisive action to be taken was to rid the body of the morbid matter. Some patients therefore went to one of the popular baths.[556] These were thought to help expel the morbid matter

---

552 Amatus Lusitanus, Curationum (1552), pp. 291–293.
553 Cf. Arrizabalaga/French/Henderson, Great pox (1997).
554 Cod. 11183, fol. 177* r.
555 Cod. 11238, fol. 98v.
556 Cod. 11183, fol. 334r, on a patient with the French disease who seems to have been in the service of Archduke Ferdinand II and like the Archduke went to Karlsbad after having tried a

from the body via the urine and, in the case of thermal springs, via the sweat. However, two specific remedies quickly gained preeminence in the treatment of *morbus gallicus*. One was mercury, which had already been recognized as a remedy for scabies and similar skin symptoms in the Middle Ages, as Handsch knew from his reading of Avicenna and Fracastoro.[557] The other was guaiac or guaiacum – "pox wood"[558] – which had allegedly proven successful in "India", in the treatment of the disease which was very widespread there.[559] The effects of guaiacum and of mercury became manifest in the evacuations they brought forth. Guaiacum was taken as a drink and its most hoped-for effect was the production of copious sweat. Mercury was administered in the form of ointments or unctions to be applied to the skin, or with mercury fumes. With mercury, the morbid matter was voided mainly with profuse salivation. Both methods of applying mercury could also be combined. Mattioli and Neefe did just that. And, as Handsch noted, the fluxes would run even better if one covered the chest.[560] Since the treatment had to mobilize the morbid matter before it could be evacuated, the patient's condition could initially worsen. Increasing numbers of pustules might develop, as Handsch experienced with the sick Memminger. When the blood had become increasingly purified ("purificatus") however, things started to improve.[561] In addition, mercury and guaiacum were believed to have a specific effect against the morbid matter. Gallo even compared guaiacum as a remedy for the French disease with bezoars, which were considered a universal antidote against many morbid poisons.[562]

Handsch dedicated many entries in his notebooks to the treatment of *morbus gallicus*, repeatedly describing every last detail of the procedures. At first glance, this might seem surprising because after all, the disease was principally characterized by external pathological changes and these, at least north of the Alps, were the domain of barber-surgeons. The workings of the morbid matter and the disease process as such were, however, located within the body – the domain of the learned physicians. Many of the agonizing symptoms, too, made themselves felt inside the body, ranging from rheumatic pains to paralyses to

---

treatment with guaiacum; ibid., fol. 434r, on a man whom the physicians diagnosed as suffering from *gonorrhea gallica* and an ulcer in the bladder.
557 Cod. 11207, fol. 144r; cf. Avicenna, Canon (1595), vol. 2, p. 248 (book 4, fen 7, tr. 3); see also Arrizabalaga/French/Henderson, Great pox (1997), p. 240.
558 Cod. 11183, fol. 428v.
559 Cod. 11238, fol. 98v; for a detailed account of the common ways of treating the French disease see Stein, Negotiating (2009), pp. 147–170.
560 Cod. 11183, fol. 180v.
561 Cod. 11207, fol. 136v.
562 Ibid.

ringing in the ears and headaches. When mercury unctions were used, it was almost inevitable for the practitioner to touch the patient, and learned physicians preferred to leave such manual tasks to the lesser educated healers. A guaiacum concoction, by contrast, could be ingested like any other medication. Along with the less drastic side effects of mercury, this would have been an important reason why *empirici* most often treated the French disease with mercury unctions, as Handsch found, while the *doctores* used guaiacum.[563]

Whether mercury or guaiacum was chosen, it was important to prepare the body with purgatives, as Manardi had already recommended.[564] The body first roughly had to be cleared of morbid matter and other waste matter. Otherwise, excessive amounts of morbid matter threatened to reach and affect the skin when guaiacum or mercury was given.[565] Some patients first underwent bloodletting, likely for the same reason. However, if obvious skin symptoms had already begun to show, this procedure also came with a risk. The skin changes indicated that at least some amount of the morbid matter had already been pushed out to the skin and a bloodletting could draw the matter back inside the body.[566]

Treatment with highly toxic mercury was a great strain on the body and not harmless for the practitioner either. Handsch mentioned remarkably often the involvement of "Jewish" healers in these activities – there was a significant Jewish community in Prague.[567] He repeatedly took the opportunity to observe them and other non-academic healers when they were performing mercury therapy. In addition, patients who had undergone mercury treatment told him about their experience with the procedure.[568]

Mercury unctions were the less complicated method. People said that the patient had to "lie in the unction".[569] A mercury-containing ointment was applied to the naked body and this process of rubbing ointment on the skin was commonly repeated twice or three times.[570] Handsch learned from healers, like the Jew Esaias, how they made the bluish ointment with mercury. It was mixed with butter, pork fat, and various kinds of plant matter and then heated.[571]

---

[563] Cod. 11240, fol. 36r.
[564] Cod. 11106, fol. 127r.
[565] Cod. 11183, fol. 72v.
[566] Cod. 111207, fol. 13r.
[567] Albrecht, Prag (2012), p. 1649 and p. 1659.
[568] See also Uhlig, Suche (1938), p. 334, on the interrogation of an itininerant "Jewish" healer who boasted of his successful treatment of patients with the French disease.
[569] Cod. 11205, fol. 244r; similarly, Cod. 11183, fol. 177r.
[570] Cod. 11183, fol. 177* r.
[571] Ibid., fol. 177r-v.

Esaias applied an amount about the size of a hazelnut on each extremity, including the neck and the lumbar region.[572] Like some other healers he used a spatula for this.[573] Others got their patients to spread the ointment with their own hands, as far as they could reach. In the case of one French-diseased patient, Esaias used his own hands only when rubbing the ointment on the man's back, gluteal fold, and genitalia.[574] Even a nobleman like Bernardus Hoddeiovinus was simply given the amount of mercury ointment necessary for three unctions by a Jewish healer.[575] Handsch took the opportunity to note down that the *empirici* chose to not use their own hands to rub the ointment on their patients, instead telling them to do it themselves. They knew that the mercury, if it entered their own body, would eventually cause shaking in their hands. Other entries of course show that not everyone observed this rule. "The hands of the *empirici* tremble because of the frequent unctions", wrote Handsch in his notes about the treatment of Florianus, whom the barber, using his hands, had rubbed with ointment at the oven.[576] Handsch personally knew a *judaeus* named Moises who suffered this effect.[577]

After the unction had been applied, patients were told to run a sweat either at the oven or in a warm bed.[578] The unctions were repeated until the effects of the mercury began to show, with the entire treatment lasting several weeks.[579]

Mercury fumigations were more complicated. When Handsch once administered the treatment himself, he was bitterly rebuked by the patient's brother because the flow of saliva did not initially manifest as expected. In the brother's view, Handsch had no business performing a treatment that he knew nothing about.[580] Handsch wrote down how different practitioners proceeded, among them Mattioli,[581] a barber, and an old man who had done these fumigations on occasion. For the fumigation, patients had to undress and sit in a tub or basin ("tina", "labrum") or another large vessel that could be closed off with wooden

---

572 Ibid., fol. 177r-v.
573 Ibid., fol. 177v.
574 Ibid., fol. 117*.
575 Cod. 11205, fol. 323v.
576 Ibid., fol. 244r, "empiricis propter crebras unctiones tremunt manus."
577 Ibid., fol. 323v; in another entry, Handsch mentioned the trembling hands of a goldsmith (ibid., fol. 134r); at the time, goldsmiths routinely worked with mercury.
578 Ibid., fol. 244r-v.
579 E.g. ibid., fol. 244v, "3 Wochen ist er ynne gelegen".
580 Cod. 11183, fol. 254r.
581 Ibid., foll. 211v-212v.

rings or similar means[582] or could at least be shrouded with linen or blankets in such a way that hardly any fumes escaped.[583] A bowl with embers was placed inside the vessel and sprinkled with a small amount of "French powder",[584] that is cinnabar[585] or another mercury-containing substance, which was sometimes combined with frankincense, styrax, myrrh, and similar aromatic plants.[586] According to Mattioli, two ounces of cinnabar were sufficient for fumigation, while four to five were needed for an unction.[587]

Some historians have assumed that the aim of the fumigation method was to have patients inhale the mercury fumes.[588] Handsch's notes show that this was precisely what practitioners, at least in the Prague of his day, generally took a more nuanced approach. He wrote about a patient who was fumigated for about an eighth of an hour with his head outside and then for an equal amount of time with his head exposed to the smoke, when, we may assume, the release of mercury fumes was already decreasing.[589] Other practitioners kept the patient's head outside the fumigated space for the entire time[590] or they gave the patients a *strophiolus*, apparently a kind of straw or breathing tube, through which they could breathe fresh outside air.[591] But even with respect to this latter solution, Handsch had his misgivings because some mercury fumes would still enter the mouth if the patient opened it.[592]

The individual sessions did not last long. The barber Ludwig was even content with the duration of a *Pater noster*.[593] But one sitting was not enough. Ludwig carried them out every other day,[594] and an old lay healer even repeated the procedure twice a day. In general, as Handsch's notes on different patients tell us, the cure entailed five to seven sittings and went on for about a fortnight.[595]

---

582 Ibid., fol. 201v and fol. 212v.
583 Ibid., fol. 203r and fol. 253r.
584 Ibid., fol. 202r.
585 Ibid., fol. 202r and fol. 253r; Cod. 11238, fol. 132v.
586 Cod. 11183, fol. 201v.
587 Ibid., fol. 202r.
588 Stein, Negotiating (2009), p. 154; Stein supports her argument with an engraving by J. Harrewijns (reproduced ibid., p. 155) but it seems to me that the engraving shows the heating of the patient's bed in order to promote sweating rather than fumigation with mercury.
589 Cod. 11183, fol. 202r.
590 Ibid., fol. 253r.
591 Ibid., fol. 203r and fol. 253r.
592 Cod. 11238, fol. 132v.
593 Cod. 11183, fol. 203r.
594 Ibid., fol. 203r.
595 Ibid., foll. 201v-202r and fol. 253r.

Sometimes practitioners locked their patients up in a room for this period,[596] perhaps to keep cold outside air from entering, which could close the pores and thus hinder the flow of sweat. An Italian mason told Handsch that he was locked up in a chamber whose doors and windows were hung with cloths for three days.[597]

It usually took a couple of days for treatment with mercury to produce results, and this was true of both fumigation and the unctions. Then the desired effects became manifest – from today's perspective, these were the symptoms of massive acute mercury poisoning. It was an ordeal for the patients. For days, they expelled such large amounts of saliva and phlegm that some of them could hardly sleep.[598] One patient's wife communicated that "It went out of him like brimstone", and when he was able to go to sleep for a little while, the liquid ran down on him and into his armpits.[599] The gums and tongue became painfully swollen and often ulceration occurred in the mouth.[600] It was not uncommon for the teeth to loosen.[601] Some patients could no longer eat solid food, only broth, which they had to drink with a straw.[602] Handsch had even heard of several patients who had supposedly died of the treatment because they were unable to eat or drink anything due to a swollen, closed-up throat.[603]

Handsch repeatedly described the patients who had undergone this treatment as pale and weak.[604] Some suffered serious and lasting harm. The court surgeon Hildebrand was visited by a young woman who had been treated with mercury fumigation for *morbus gallicus* and now had a tremor in her head and limbs.[605] Another common side effect was hair loss, including facial hair.[606] In this respect, the consequences of the treatment were similar to a recognized symptom of the French disease. In the physicians' experience, the hair at least grew back fairly well given some time, though not as handsomely as before.[607]

---

596 Cod. 11205, fol. 244v.
597 Ibid., fol. 501v.
598 Cod. 11183, fol. 117* r and fol. 202r.
599 Ibid., fol. 202r.
600 Ibid., fol. 202v.
601 Ibid., fol. 202v.
602 Ibid., fol. 117* and fol. 202r; Cod. 11205, fol. 244v; Cod. 11238, foll. 132v-133r.
603 Cod. 11183, fol. 177*.
604 Cod. 11183, fol. 117*.
605 Ibid., fol. 399r.
606 Ibid., fol. 203r, continued on fol. 202*r; Handsch added, however, that her husband had also hit her on the head.
607 Ibid., fol. 202*v and fol. 177*.

Some sufferers reported a marked improvement following the cure. The pustules abated or disappeared altogether,[608] ulcers healed, swelling went down.[609] Some patients – among them Hoddeiovinus[610] – believed themselves completely healed, whereas others retained pustules, ulcers, or other skin symptoms which showed that the disease was still doing mischief in their bodies.[611] Some patients continued to complain of pain in their extremities and joints.[612] Handsch wrote, referring to his reading of Fracastoro, that once the bones were affected, a complete cure was no longer possible.[613]

Although the treatment with guaiacum was less complicated and safer its duration alone was a strain. Sometimes physicians did not allow their patient to leave the house for weeks.[614] In Augsburg and other German cities, "wood" or "pox" houses were set up for the treatment of people with the French disease.[615] The remedy was administered as a wood decoction which patients had to imbibe every day over the course of several weeks.[616] The recommended amounts to be used in the remedy varied somewhat. Gallo added two pounds of the wood to sixteen pounds of water, while Mattioli added the same amount to twenty-seven pounds of water. Da Monte added one pound to fourteen pounds of water of chicory.[617] As Handsch observed when Gallo and Mattioli treated the sick Memminger, the patient had to take the remedy twice a day, early in the morning and in the third hour of the afternoon. Afterward, he had to be in bed or in the warm parlor where he would sweat, wipe off the sweat with warmed cloths, and change his clothing and cloths. He was not allowed to eat much: to begin with, he could have chicken and chicken broth with bread only every other day, adding biscuit and raisins from the eighth day on. We may assume that the physicians wanted to give nature and the inner heat a chance to focus entirely on fighting the morbid matter. The hungry patient was allowed to eat a little more after a while, but he was counselled to keep restraining himself even after he had completed the treatment.[618]

---

608 Ibid., fol. 117* r.
609 Ibid., fol. 203r.
610 Cod. 11205, fol. 323v.
611 Cod. 11183, fol. 202*v.
612 Ibid., fol. 254v.
613 Ibid., fol. 212r.
614 Cod. 11207, fol. 137v.
615 Stein, Negotiating (2009), p. 91.
616 Cod. 11238, fol. 265v.
617 Cod. 11207, fol. 137r; in her sources for Augsburg, Stein (Stein, Negotiating (2009), p. 149) has found lower concentrations, with two pounds of guaiacum on seven liters of water.
618 Cod. 11207, foll. 136v-138r.

Thus, even the so-called wood treatment demanded quite a lot from patients. When Mattioli, for example, treated a man called Schrenk over a period of forty days, he allowed the sick man to eat no meat, only toasted bread without salt.[619] Handsch as well underwent a wood cure at some point – whether it was for *morbus gallicus* remains unclear – and during that time he very much longed for beer.[620]

After the treatment, some patients believed they were much better or even considered themselves healed. Others, however, were bitterly disappointed. The skin symptoms experienced by Schrenck, for example, abated only temporarily. Before long, he showed Handsch repulsive pustules on his head.[621] One patient, whom the physicians had convinced he should repeat the wood cure even though he did not show the respective skin symptoms, went so far as to complain, "I felt much healthier before than [I do] now, because I lay in the wood."[622]

In retrospect, it might seem surprising that so many sufferers agreed to undergo treatment with mercury or guaiacum, considering the unpleasant effects that accompanied and followed the procedure as well as the uncertainty of its success. However, the disease not only produced massive symptoms and could be transferred to one's wife and children, it was also highly stigmatizing. Tellingly, Handsch sometimes used phrases such as "he confessed to me" ("confessus est mihi")[623] and "he admitted" ("fassus est"), when writing about patients who told him about the signs of a suspected *morbus gallicus*. Of course, one aspect was that, with men, the physicians commonly associated the disease with moral wrongdoing, with "lasciviousness", and coitus before or outside marriage, possibly even with a prostitute. Yet the suspicion that the sufferer of *morbus gallicus* had had intercourse with "impure" women was not everything. In addition, the body of the sufferer was clearly dominated by impurity, and impurity at the time was highly charged both morally and culturally, as we can see in the disparaging view – even the condemnation – of "impure" professions. Worse still, the massive skin changes that could hardly be concealed, especially when they occurred in the face, were not only deemed repulsive but to pose a very real, physical threat for fellow human beings. The lesions signaled nature's efforts to rid the body of impure matter, and the contagious matter voided in this way was a threat to others. The dean Paulus, for example, experienced how

---

619 Cod. 11183, fol. 324r.
620 Ibid., fol. 218v.
621 Ibid., fol. 324v; however, according to Handsch, the patient had not followed the dietetic recommendations of his doctors.
622 Cod. 11207, fol. 222r.
623 Cod. 11183, fol. 177r and fol. 431r.

no one wanted to have a drink with him anymore because of the visible, massive affliction of his nose.[624] In the case of the Ambras head chef Martinus, all it took was losing some mobility in his arms and a rumor circulating that he had been treated for *morbus gallicus* and his life took a tragic turn. Handsch did not believe it was *morbus gallicus*. He could not find any rash and instead suspected a partial paralysis of the arm. Old Anna Welser, however, was unwilling to tolerate the man at Ambras Castle any longer. Saddened ("tristis"), he took his leave and went to Innsbruck.[625]

In light of this, physicians were well advised, especially when working with high-ranking patients, to err on the side of caution when dealing with a potential diagnosis of *morbus gallicus*. When examining the thirteen-year-old daughter of the Lady of Berka, Mattioli nevertheless voiced his suspicion, because it seemed obvious. After all, the girl was losing eyebrows and the hair on her head; she had red pustules and later a "mangy" rash on her body. Still, her mother did not want to hear of it. She held that her daughter had no inner complaints, and perhaps it all came from water or the cold. Handsch wrote that, "perhaps for the lady's sake" Gallo had then offered that he suspected leprosy. Mattioli stood by his opinion, making the rather valid point that a diagnosis of leprosy would not be any better.[626] In the case of a young relative of an army captain, Gallo did not specifically name the disease but simply proceeded with the common wood cure.[627] Of course, laypeople knew that mercury and guaiacum were primarily used in the treatment of the French disease, which explains why Archduke Ferdinand took offence when the physicians treated his sixteen-year-old son with guaiacum the wood cure (*decoctum ligni*).[628]

Patients themselves, especially if they were of higher standing, tried to keep their guaiacum cure secret, which was not always easy considering that the treatment took several weeks. In the case of a teacher who was likely working for the Prague court, Handsch was firm in his opinion that the man's position did not allow for the possibility of others seeing him ("manifeste") drink the guaiacum decoction. Mattioli therefore prepared the remedy at home and allowed the patient to leave his house.[629] Discussing another case, Handsch warned that, for patients who had other diseases, simply mentioning the possibility of doing a wood

---

624 Cod. 11205, fol. 415v.
625 Cod. 11183, fol. 399v.
626 Cod. 11207, fol. 154v.
627 Ibid., fol. 170r.
628 Cod. 11205, fol. 299v.
629 Cod. 11207, fol. 212r.

cure was enough to raise their hackles. "Lying in the wood" was invariably associated with the French disease.[630]

Considering the often severe side effects and other consequences of a mercury treatment and of – though less pronounced – a treatment with guaiacum, and considering the difficulty of keeping the lengthy treatments a secret, it is not surprising that both physicians and patients sought alternatives. They placed their hopes on less taxing remedies that were said to possess specific powers for treating *morbus gallicus*. According to Mattioli, the Italian physicians reported positive experiences with administering antimony not only for other diseases but for the French disease as well.[631] Other physicians allegedly had patients send in their urine, whereupon they would add saffron to it and instruct the patients to drink it but Handsch admittedly only learned this by hearsay.[632] He did hear from Gallo directly, however, that sea holly worked well to treat the ulcers caused by *morbus gallicus*. Mattioli administered it with guaiacum.[633] Lay healers, too, treated *morbus gallicus* with tried and tested medicinal herbs. A barber told Handsch that a certain woman had treated him when he had fallen sick with *morbus gallicus* in his youth. She had cured the serious skin changes in his face and on his entire body with masterwort in white wine, and then performed cupping.[634]

Toothaches

Dentistry was not yet a specialized discipline of medicine in the sixteenth century and the number of treatable dental complaints was limited. The central concerns were caries, loose, crumbling, and rotting teeth, and the resulting pain in and around the tooth. Only a major paleopathological study would be able to definitively determine whether tooth decay was less widespread than it is today. On the one hand, dietary habits were different at the time and people ate much less sugary food. On the other hand, we must not assume that people's dental hygiene was as rigorous and regular as it is today. Handsch thought it worthwhile to dedicate an entire entry in one of his notebooks to dental hygiene, writing that one should "wash" one's teeth every day.[635]

---

630 Ibid., fol. 110r.
631 Cod. 11183, fol. 241r.
632 Cod. 11125, fol. 34v.
633 Cod. 11207, fol. 155r.
634 Cod. 11251, fol. 110v.
635 Cod. 11183, fol. 479r.

There is no doubt that toothaches were widespread and that they had an important presence in people's everyday life. Some people were lucky: Michel de Montaigne wrote, "I have always had excellent teeth, and only now is old age beginning to threaten them. [. . .] Now, a tooth has fallen out, without causing pain, all by itself; the natural end of its time had come."[636] But early modern testimonies and medical reports tell us of countless people who suffered from harrowing toothaches. It seems that hardly anyone was spared. Martin Luther complained about fierce toothaches[637] and even someone like Friedrich von der Pfalz had to stay in his room all day because of the toothache, as he wrote in one of his brief journal entries.[638] In addition, the pain often persisted for a long time, due to the limited possibilities of treatment. Handsch's notebooks, too, contain dozens of entries on the subject of toothaches. He himself had suffered from agonizing toothaches at a young age,[639] as did his mentor Mattioli[640] and many of the patients Handsch mentioned, both low- and high-ranking.[641]

It is often assumed that toothaches were the domain of barber surgeons and itinerant tooth pullers in the early modern period. Handsch's numerous entries and contemporary letter consultations show that patients also sought the advice of a learned physician when they suffered from a toothache. This is not really surprising. As with so many other complaints, physicians and laypeople alike ultimately attributed caries and tooth decay to "fluxes". In the case of toothaches, the pernicious matter at work was acrid, and corrosive, and accumulated in and around the teeth.[642] For anatomical reasons, fluxes from the upper area of the

---

636 Montaigne, Essais (1953), p. 377.
637 Luther, Werke (1934), p. 549, Nr. 1686.
638 Friedrich IV., Tagebuch (1880), p. 216.
639 Cod. 11205, 232v, on the toothache he suffered during the night when he stayed with Collinus.
640 Cod. 11183, 173v; Cod. 11207, fol. 55r.
641 Cod. 11183, fol. 61v, on sick Gendorf; ibid., fol. 366v, on Georg Welser; ibid., fol. 383r, on Katharina von Loxan, who had her socalled "Augenzahn" ("eye tooth") pulled out from our maxilla, which tended to cause secretions from the eye ("gern darnach flüßig"), as Handsch added; Cod. 11205, fol. 120r, on the tailor Kritzel, who suffered, at the same time, from nasal secretions and tinnitus; Cod. 11207, fol. 208r, on "domina nostra" (possibly referring to Anna of Bohemia and Hungary, the wife of emperor Ferdinand I – the entry is in a notebook from Handsch's time with Gallo); Cod. 11238, fol. 131, on Handsch's "patrona" (probably referring to his landlady in Padua); ibid., on a librarian in Trento (probably a certain Hieronymus whom Handsch mentioned repeatedly); ibid., fol. 143r, on a certain Fabricius; Cod. 11251, fol. 115v, on one of his landladies.
642 Universitätsbibliothek Erlangen, Trew, Montagnanus Nr. 4, letter from Camillo Franchini to Joachim Camerarius II., Bologna, 28 November 1565, on a flux to the teeth and to the ears, which plagued Philipp Camerarius; see also Fernel, Consiliorum (1644), pp. 254f.

skull were considered the principal source of toothaches and loose teeth. This was the very place that was suspected to be the origin of "catarrhs" in general, which sometimes drained from the nose, but often settled in the lower respiratory tract, in the joints, or other places in the body, where they caused pain and other disease symptoms.[643] Thinking along these lines, an archducal chancery scribe believed his loose tooth and the surrounding sore flesh to be "ex catarrho". Using gold wire, a lay healer affixed the tooth to the neighboring, more firmly anchored teeth.[644] Another patient complained of "a flux in the teeth" and said, "I have a piercing pain in half my head".[645] Handsch quoted his landlady, who suffered from a toothache, as saying, "gushes and fluxes are coming in".[646] In his dramatic story of a nun who was about forty years of age, Claudius Deodatus described how, one year previously, she "was attacked by a wild, unusual head flux" and since then "suffered and had to endure a miserable, painful flux onto the teeth of her right jaw, along with an unbearable, unforgiving toothache".[647]

In lay culture, there was also the idea of a "tooth worm", a small animal that literally ate the tooth from the inside. Treatment accordingly aimed at luring the worm out of hiding and killing it.[648] An acquaintance told Handsch about a "very certain remedy" ("pro certissimo remedio") for the tooth worm. One had to roast the berries of the *alkekengi* (*physalis*), mince them, mix them with wax, put the mixture on glowing embers and let the smoke rise into one's mouth.[649] We may assume that, following the principle of similitude, the powdered earthworms that Thomas Erastus recommended for a noble patient's toothache also aimed at the tooth worm; the old physicians, he claimed, had praised it highly.[650] The notion of the tooth worm may also have been based in the belief

---

643 Along the same lines, Ernestus Henricus wrote to the Bamberg physician Sigismund Schnitzer, for example, that fluid matter from the head had settled on the teeth and on the throat of their patient (Hornung, Cista 1626, pp. 366–7 (www.aerztebriefe.de/id/00000584, S. Reiher); see also the undated *consilium* by Johannes Crato von Krafftheim for a *nobilis matrona* in Scholz, Consiliorum (1592), pp. 219f. (translated from the German original).
644 Cod. 11183, fol. 364r.
645 Cod. 11207, fol. 203r.
646 Cod. 11251, fol. 115v.
647 Undated letter from Claudius Deodatus to Wilhelm Fabry (c. 1615), in German, in Fabricius, Wund-Artzney (1652), pp. 397–399, cit. p. 397.
648 Cf. Hubmann, Zahnwurm (2008).
649 Cod. 11183, fol. 266r.
650 Undated letter from Thomas Erastus to Graf Georg Ernst von Henneberg-Schleusingen (www.aerztebriefe.de/id/00004335, T. Walter).

that one could sometimes see a small "worm" at the root tip when a tooth was pulled. To some extent this accorded with the physicians' belief that the immediate cause of the pain was located in the dental nerve.[651] At a time when Handsch suffered from a severe toothache, he was able to look in the mirror and see a hole in the side of the tooth. And when he drank cold water, he felt the pain right away, which, he noted, corresponded with the Hippocratic aphorism that cold was hostile to bones and teeth.[652]

In the majority of cases, physicians ultimately attributed toothaches to a morbid matter that accumulated in and around the tooth; therefore, they could try to redirect the morbid humor the way they did with other fluxes and catarrhs. Handsch knew of a girl at the Ambras court who applied ranunculus to her wrist, apparently to cause an irritation of the skin; her toothache disappeared within half an hour.[653] In the same vein, Count Heinrich of Mansfeld wrote that a "flux" had fallen into his tooth and that he had to have cupping done to alleviate it.[654] Thomas Erastus advised a count who suffered from ear- and toothaches to have someone "create a blister" in the appropriate place, that is to use powerful skin irritants to cause the morbid matter to collect in the skin and to leave the body when the blister opened.[655] Johannes Crato recommended to one of his female patients that she have cupping done on both her arm and her shoulder blades, and to have plasters applied to her ears that would create blisters. He explained to her that in itself pulling teeth did not bring about healing, but it was beneficial because it allowed the morbid matter to drain. For the same reason, he held, the removal of a tooth could sometimes alleviate headaches.[656]

In addition, physicians used different analgesics that were said to be effective for toothaches. Some physicians praised brandy,[657] and laypeople too fended off their toothaches with "strong waters".[658] Handsch had good experiences with

---

651 Cod. 11205, fol. 232v.
652 Ibid., fol. 231r and fol. 239r.
653 Cod. 11183, fol. 397r; however, the resulting painful blister on the wrist had to be treated by a barber surgeon afterwards.
654 Staatsbibliothek Berlin, Ms. boruss. fol. 687, fol. 176r-177r, letter to Leonhard Thurneisser, Schraplau, 12 May 1581.
655 Letter from Thomas Erastus to Georg Ernst Graf von Henneberg-Schleusigen, 24 July 1573 (www.aerztebriefe.de/id/00004340, T. Walter).
656 Undated *consilium* by Johannes Crato von Krafftheim for a *nobilis matrona* in Scholz, Consiliorum (1592), pp. 219f. (translated from the German original).
657 Cod. 11251, fol. 31r.
658 Letter from Anna Leszczyńska to Leonhard Thurneisser, 20 January 1582, ed. in Wotschke, Blasius (1925), p. 24 (www.aerztebriefe.de/id/00016021, U. Schlegelmilch).

brandy when he had a toothache.[659] Toothaches tended to get worse, however, when he drank a lot of wine.[660] Handsch further praised the pain-relieving effect of salt. He rubbed it on the tooth and gums or rinsed the tooth with salt dissolved in warm vinegar. Reading Galen and Aëtius of Amida, he learned that salt helped with gout because it strengthened the nerves and muscles, and he suspected a similar effect on the dental nerve.[661] The contemporary collections of "proven" *experimenta* and secrets proposed many more remedies.[662] The court surgeon Hildebrand recommended garlic, which Amatus Lusitanus had praised as well.[663] Handsch heard from a barber that the pepper-like Spanish chamomile (pyrethrum) helped with toothaches.[664] One of Handsch's landladies treated her toothache successfully by putting a little red coral in the hole.[665] Some people even rinsed their mouths with human or horse urine.[666] Archduke Ferdinand II was said to have paid 200 kroner to a Venetian lay healer to obtain the recipe for a secret against toothache (and further remedies).[667] For much less money, people could buy a "tooth powder" from merchants. Handsch purchased a small bag of it in Prague for three kreutzers. He examined it and decided that it consisted of alum and a root that had been ground up. He acknowledged that the astringent effect of alum was indeed beneficial.[668]

For severe and prolonged toothaches, opium was the drug of choice. It was used locally or internally. Handsch laid about six grains of opium on the tooth of his servant Bartholomäus and instructed him not to let them move from the tooth and not to swallow his saliva. However, this was exactly what Bartholomäus did. He slept through the night, and the next morning Handsch found him in bed, lying as if stunned.[669] To a maid Handsch gave an opium pill for oral use. She complained about its bitter taste but after half an hour her pain was gone.[670]

---

659 Cod. 11207, fol. 208r.
660 Cod. 11205, fol. 247v.
661 Ibid., fol. 232v and fol. 255r.
662 E.g. Stocker, Empirica (1601), pp. 49–52.
663 Cod. 11251, fol. 113v.
664 Cod. 11183, fol. 371r.
665 Cod. 11251, fol. 115v.
666 Cod. 11205, fol. 292v, on a maid servant and on the Frau von Wartenberg in Leipa.
667 Cod. 11251, fol. 142r; Handsch was to translate the prescription from Italian into German.
668 Cod. 11205, fol. 254v; one of Handsch's acquaintances, a painter in Trento, confirmed the beneficial effects of alum (Cod. 11228, fol. 143r).
669 Cod. 11183, fol. 370v.
670 Cod. 11205, fol. 239v; he added in the margins that they had a stronger effect in another case.

Mattioli tried a number of remedies in vain and finally also reached for opium.[671] In the case of the emperor's wife, Anne of Bohemia and Hungary, not even opium pills brought relief. Handsch assumed that opium in this form did not reach the dental nerve and suggested dissolving it in red wine first.[672]

A toothache could also be addressed with magical, sympathetic healing methods. In Handsch's collection of tried and proven *experimenta*, we find the recommendation that one attach the tooth of a deceased person to the painful tooth. This would soon cause the affected tooth to fall out. Of course, one had to ensure that no healthy teeth were touched by the dead person's tooth by accident.[673]

If the pain did not go away or if the decay of a tooth was advanced, usually the final resort was a manual, surgical treatment. A clergyman in Saalfeld, for example, lamented to the famous physician Caspar Ratzenberger in Weimar that the "Devil" had taken four of his upper teeth and three more were loose already. He went on to explain that his vocation required him to give many speeches. He asked Ratzenberger to prescribe him a remedy to stabilize the teeth ("ad stabiliendos eos") and have it prepared right then and there in Weimar.[674] Handsch noted down that one patient got a barber to cauterize the inside of a hollow tooth with *aqua fortis* (nitric acid) or mercury water.[675] A gatekeeper, named Martin, told him from his own experience that one had to make a nail red hot and lay it in vinegar and then touch the painful tooth with it.[676] When the court surgeon Hildebrand had a toothache, he daubed *aqua fortis* on the surrounding swollen gums and then cut the flesh off. He claimed that the pain was gone the next day.[677] In a later entry, Handsch also noted down the use of nitric acid to destroy the afflicted crown of a tooth, leaving only the root, which would then be covered by the gums.[678]

In many cases, the tooth ultimately had to be pulled because the pain persisted or the tooth was crumbling. It seems that most people had to undergo this ordeal several times during their lifetime. Somebody like Alexander Bösch would have been no exception. As he wrote in his memoirs, toothaches had

---

671 Cod. 11207, fol. 54r.
672 Ibid., fol. 208r.
673 Cod. 11200, fol. 20v; in the notes of his mentor Gallo, Handsch found instructions for another ritual "Contra dolorem dentium" (Cod. 11207, fol. 83v).
674 Letter from Philipp Caesar to Caspar Ratzenberger, 19 April 1582. (www.aerztebriefe.de/id/00023288, U. Schlegelmilch).
675 Cod. 11183, fol. 296v.
676 Ibid., fol. 382r.
677 Ibid., fol. 410r.
678 Ibid., fol. 457r.

plagued him badly and often, before and after he switched to a pastorate in Hemberg, and he needed to have many teeth pulled.[679] Colin Jones's claim that people in the early modern period showed their teeth much less when smiling to hide their inevitable gaps certainly seems plausible in this light.[680]

Tooth extraction was commonly done by local barber-surgeons or itinerant "tooth pullers" who went from county fair to county fair noisily hawking their services (Fig. 8). As an example for the use of the Latin word for "to yell" or "to shout", "clamare", Handsch wrote, "[they] immediately take to yelling like tooth pullers". His phrasing here does not indicate whether the tooth pullers might also have called out or yelled at the moment they pulled a tooth to drown out their patient's shriek of pain.[681] The travelling surgeons did not have a good reputation but some of them knew their trade. A tooth puller from Wendlingen who was a trained surgeon and came to the Michaelmas market in Augsburg even gained the respect of the otherwise highly exacting and critical Augsburg medical college. They found that anyone could see that he was masterful at pulling teeth.[682]

Barber-surgeons and tooth pullers had special instruments, but using them well required strength and skill. Besides a number of different pliers, they mainly used the so-called pelican. The tool was set down on healthy neighboring teeth to loosen and more easily pull the diseased tooth using leverage.[683] Obviously, one had to be careful not to accidentally damage a healthy tooth in the process.[684] Handsch was not spared the painful first-hand experience of having a tooth pulled. It was a difficult and exhausting procedure. First, the barber cut off the gums around the affected tooth, using a scalpel. Then he pulled at length on the tooth with forceps. While Handsch cried out in pain ("cum magno meo clamore"), the barber struggled, but to no avail. Finally, the barber let off and Handsch was given a bandage around his head. A second and certainly no less painful attempt also failed. The barber gave up and sent Handsch to another, older barber, who got the job done. Handsch summarized, "the pain during the extraction is great", and afterwards he continued to experience pain in the right side of his head

---

679 Bösch, Liber familiarium (2001), pp. 91–93.
680 Jones, Smile revolution (2014).
681 Cod. 9671, fol. 51r.
682 Letter to the authorities in Augsburg, 22 November 1597 (www.aerztebriefe.de/id/00003579, S. Herde).
683 Hoffmann-Axthelm, Geschichte der Zahnheilkunde (1973), pp. 132–165, with illustrations of various instruments used to pull teeth and to perform other interventions on the teeth at the time.
684 Cod. 11183, fol. 297r.

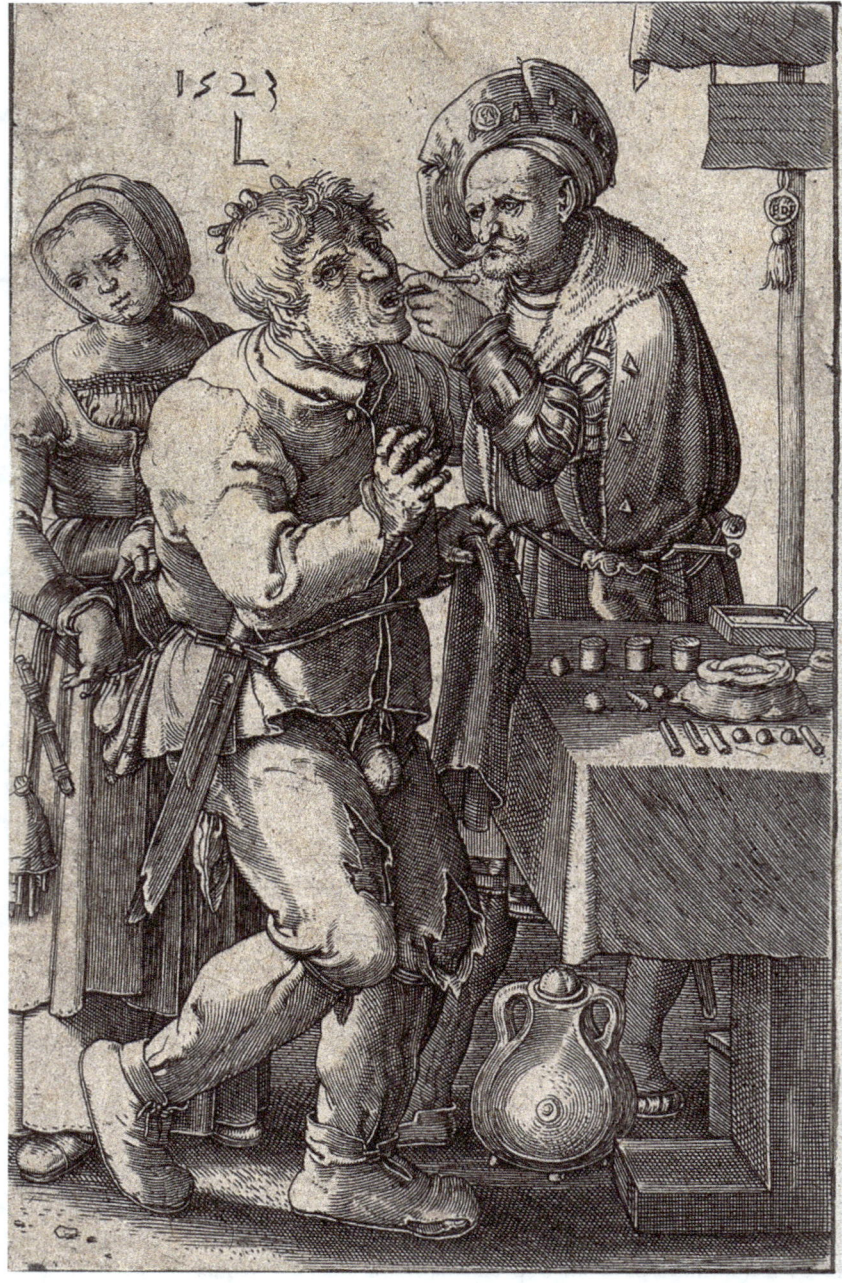

Fig. 8: Lukas van Leiden, Dentist, 1523, Wellcome Collection, London.

and in the gums.[685] From the seventeenth century, an account about a slightly drunk barber has survived who pulled a young man's molar with such great force that he dislocated his lower jaw. The young man was no longer able to open his mouth and thus suffered permanent damage.[686]

The art of tooth filling appears not to have been widespread at the time. The Ulm municipal physician Johannes Stocker, who died in 1513, described the procedure early in the sixteenth century.[687] Though this is earliest known account of this kind, it is unlikely that he invented the technique. The fact that a barber was able to show it to Handsch in a *Liber experimentorum*,[688] suggests that Stocker for his part could draw on an established surgical tradition. According to this *Liber experimentorum*, when treating a hollow tooth, first the inside had to be cauterized with a hot golden pen until the root was dead. Following this, amalgam ("amalgama"), a compound of mercury, vitriol, and other substances of the kind used by goldsmiths, had to be inserted into the hollow tooth. There, the mass would become hard as rock and stay in the tooth. Handsch related that when a tooth of Archduke Ferdinand was repaired, the much more expensive pure gold leaf was used, resulting in a gold filling.[689] When Handsch was very much tormented by his toothache, he wondered if he should fill the hollow with "auripellem" – presumably referring to thin layers of gold.[690]

---

685 Cod. 11205, fol. 291v-292r; afterwards, the old barber surgeon also told him the story of a man, whose bleeding after the tooth extraction could not even be stopped by means of cauterization and who died in the end (ibid.). In retrospect, this was quite possibly an early account of the dangers of tooth extraction in a patient with hemophilia.
686 Expert opinion of the Medical Faculty in Tübingen, 8 May 1655 (www.aerztebriefe.de/id/00012413, A. Döll/T. Walter).
687 Hoffmann-Axthelm, Geschichte der Zahnheilkunde (1973), pp. 151–152, with a photographic reproduction of the recipe found in a manuscript from 1528, Stadtarchiv Ulm, Handschrift Xlyffer, foll. 75v-76r; cf. Stocker, Empirica (1601).
688 Cod. 11183, foll. 296v-297r.
689 Ibid., fol. 297r.
690 Cod. 11205, fol. 232v.

Pediatrics

For a long time, medical historians assumed that infants and children were only rarely treated by physicians in the early modern period. Supposedly, families accepted their children's diseases as God-given and were possibly even somewhat relieved when a child died, given the large numbers of children families tended to have. It was furthermore thought that if people sought medical help at all rather than simply being content with home remedies, it was to midwives that they turned. More recent studies have shown, however, that physicians in the seventeenth and eighteenth centuries certainly did treat a substantial number of children.[691] A look at sixteenth- sources makes clear that this was far from a new development. Handsch's notes as well as Ulrich Lehner's and Hiob Finzel's practice journals along with the occasional case history found in published collections of *observationes* show that already in the Renaissance, physicians addressed the diseases of children, and did so on more than just a theoretical level: they were consulted quite often when children and even infants were sick.

While children frequently came down with diseases that were also diagnosed in adults, yet there were some diseases that could be observed mostly or almost exclusively in children. It was furthermore deemed necessary to consider the particularities of the child's body when choosing a treatment, especially when selecting and dosing medications. The treatment of childhood diseases therefore required a certain degree of specialized knowledge. And so it was with good reason that the diseases of children and their treatment occupied an important place in the medical textbooks of the time. The authors were able to rely on classical and medieval predecessors. One prominent author who had addressed childhood diseases in detail was Rhazes, whose *Liber ad Almansorem* was considered core literature of practical medicine in the sixteenth century.[692] The late fifteenth century also saw the first autonomous treatises on childhood diseases written by Western physicians.[693]

Interest in pediatrics grew in the course of the sixteenth century.[694] Students of medicine at the Upper Italian universities learned about childhood

---

[691] Newton, Sick child (2012); Ritzmann, Sorgenkinder (2008).
[692] Rhazes, Treatment of small children (2015).
[693] Sudhoff, Erstlinge (1925); Mauch, Libellus (1937).
[694] Austrius, De infantium (1540); Phaer, Regiment of life (1545); Vittori, De aegritudinibus infantium (1557); Ferrarius, De arte medica (1577); overviews in Manzke, Remedia (2008) and Schäfer, Regimina (2008); on the later developments, see Ritzmann, Sorgenkinder (2008).

diseases in lectures[695] and were introduced to the treatment of sick and injured child patients. Cases of child patients are found time and again in the printed *consilia* written by Paduan professors who discussed their diagnoses and treatments in front of the gathered student body during *collegia*.[696] Student notes from Ferrara document that Antonio Musa Brasavola and Lucas Ricardus visited various sick children with their students, including a child ill with dysentery, a girl with right-sided paralysis, one who had worms and epilepsy, one with a "scabious" rash on her head, and another who had fallen and hit his head.[697] Infants of the highest social circles, such as Johanna (1547–1578), the daughter of the later emperor Ferdinand I, sometimes even received medical treatment in the early days after their birth.[698]

Handsch and his colleagues from Prague and Innsbruck, too, frequently treated sick children and youths. In Prague, Handsch was occasionally called to attend to sick students at Collinus's private school in the Angelus Garden, likely in part because he had been employed there in the past. Some of these children and youths suffered from typical childhood diseases like measles and the much-feared smallpox.[699] At one point, Handsch treated five boys who had fallen ill with the measles.[700] They recovered quickly but with other children he observed a swelling of the abdomen and legs following the measles.[701] Febrile diseases in general were common during childhood. As Handsch witnessed at Gallo's home, physicians treated their feverish children with very mild remedies like sweet cooked plums that helped with bowel movements and were nutritious at the same time, or with infants, they limited themselves rubbing them with rose ointment.[702]

Abdominal complaints were widespread, especially among the very youngest, first and foremost the so-called "Reißen" or "jerking pain". People said about children who cried a lot that they had "a jerking pain in the belly". Handsch and Gallo attributed these complaints at this young age not to worms but to winds from milk or porridge.[703] "He has intestinal winds", one could say

---

695 Mercuriale, De morbis puerorum (1583).
696 E.g. Da Monte, Consultationum (1554), pp. 96–102 and 146–156, what seems to have been an oral communication about two girls with epilepsy viz. headaches.
697 Biblioteca Ariostea, Ferrara, Ms Antonelli 531, Curationes Antonii Musae Brasavoli.
698 Cod. 11205, fol. 168v and fol. 201r.
699 Cod. 11183, fol. 421v, mentioning numerous children who suffered from these diseases; cf. Leven, Geschichte (1997), p. 46.
700 Cod. 11183, fol. 404v.
701 Ibid., fol. 422v.
702 Cod. 11205, fol. 236r.
703 Cod. 11207, fol. 6v.

in such cases, according to Handsch.[704] The eight-month-old boy of a man called Schmidt, for example, was calm most of the time and slept well, but every night at nine o'clock he began to cry and thrash around.[705] Conveying the experience of mothers, Handsch wrote that kale, too, could cause children to howl with pain. One could hear it rumbling in their bellies and their mouths trembled. Handsch added in the margin that Gallo recommended breastfeeding children instead of giving them porridge, and that was how Gallo's wife had done it with their own children. It appears that in Bohemia mothers often breastfed their children for a long time, as we can surmise from Handsch's note that women wanted to know early if they were pregnant again so they would have time to wean their children. As Handsch's stepmother told him herself, she breastfed his half-sister Sabina for eighteen months.[706] A woman from the highest circles of society even waited two years before she weaned her son. She stayed away from him for three days before she saw him again, and she put bitter gentian powder on her breasts so as to spoil breastfeeding for the child.[707] As we know today, breastfeeding significantly decreases the probability of getting pregnant and presumably women at the time were well aware of this effect and often welcomed it.

Further, physicians often dealt with worm infestation in children – and certainly not only in Prague.[708] Mattioli passed on the experience of an old physician who held that, just as the uterus was involved in most diseases of women, worms played a part in most childhood diseases.[709] Physicians took worms very seriously and thought they could sometimes have fatal consequences. They believed they observed that epilepsy in particular was often accompanied by worms and then sometimes resulted in death.[710] Handsch and his colleagues furthermore thought they had discovered an important diagnostic sign: they observed that children

---

704 Cod. 11205, fol. 213v.
705 Cod. 11207, fol. 6v.
706 Cod. 11205, fol. 118v; Sabina was born in 1545, about ten years before Handsch took these notes.
707 Ibid., fol. 563v.
708 Cod. 11183, fol. 351v.
709 Cod. 11206, fol. 99r: "In omnibus morbis puerorum concurrunt vermes, mulierum uterus"; similarly ibid., fol. 161v, "In omnibus morbis mulierum matrix habet suam partem, et in puerorum morbis vermes."
710 Cod. 11183, fol. 413r, on the death of Scheur's infant. The child suffered from worms and epilepsy. Garlic juice, lemon juice and numerous other remedies were to no avail. The child died.

who had worms in their bellies rubbed their noses. They assumed that foul vapors rose from the worms and reached the sensitive noses of the children.[711]

Epilepsia or *mater puerorum*, to which Handsch usually referred with the German "Vergicht", but which was also known by the names "Gichter", "Fraisen", "Fräsel", and "Fressel", was a disease that was widely diagnosed in children at the time. The convulsive fits that typically occurred when children had a fever, were also considered *epilepsia,* as we have seen. However, some physicians here preferred the term *convulsiones*.[712] *Epilepsia* in children was feared.[713] Handsch thought epilepsy was "terrifying" to behold. He had apparently witnessed seizures with his nephew, the son of his sister Catharina. The nephew had writhed and "flailed" ("aufgeworfen") so much that the bench cracked.[714] Another boy whom Handsch saw got well again but later presented with slowed movements and great "stupidity" ("stupiditas").[715]

Children with symptoms we would probably attribute to the heart or lungs today were likewise diagnosed by ordinary people as victims of *Vergicht* or *Fräsel*. One such child was the three-year-old child of a man called Miltelius, who coughed violently, struggled for air, and had blue lips.[716] From his observations of different patients, Handsch even concluded that the blue color was an indication of epilepsy. He had seen this blue coloration with an infant in Prague, for example, who died of *mater puerorum* in a bath.[717]

Handsch very frequently mentioned sick infants and small children from his own family and the families with whom he roomed. His entries include what he learned from their mothers, for example that a child who cried and kicked his or her legs likely had a belly ache,[718] or that infants who were still nursed got abdominal cramps when the mother was pregnant again and – a common occurrence – developed an appetite for sauerkraut, vinegar, and other sour things.[719]

There were a number of childhood diseases that were of special interest to Handsch. For instance, he made several entries about *Mitesser* (blackheads) or "comedones" (from Latin "comedere", "to eat" or "to share food") in children, equating them with worms under the skin and thus taking up an idea that was

---

711 Ibid., fol. 391r, on the daughter of Frau von Wels; Cod. 11207, fol. 25v.
712 Cod. 11183, fol. 287v, referring to Dr. "Achilles", i.e., presumably to Achilles Jelmin.
713 See also Manzke, Remedia (2008), pp. 67f.
714 Cod. 11205, fol. 119r.
715 Ibid.
716 Cod. 11183, fol. 463v.
717 Ibid.
718 Ibid., fol. 296v.
719 Ibid., fol. 297r.

widespread among the populace. Whenever infants lost weight, he wrote, one had to suspect such subcutaneous *comedones*.[720] One of his landladies suspected *comedones*, when her four-week-old infant seemed to be losing weight. *Comedones* were usually hidden from view, wrote Handsch, and the heads only came up when the child was given a bath and thoroughly smeared with honey. He evidently thought that the worms were attracted by the sweet food. The thing to do next was to rub them off with toasted bread. He added that, in Bohemia, a knife was used for this purpose as well.[721]

On the whole, Handsch and his colleagues were confronted with a broad spectrum of diseases in children, ranging from fairly harmless or at least quickly passing complaints to prolonged and even terminal diseases. Sometimes they also saw surgical cases in a broader sense, injuries that is or pathological changes of the skin or the mucous membranes. The boy of a man called Schindler had gotten slaked lime in his eyes, which consequently became painful and swollen.[722] Another had painful pustules in his mouth and throat.[723] A four-year-old girl suffered from a fistula in her upper abdomen, which exuded light-colored liquid.[724] The body and head of the fifteen-week-old daughter of Handsch's landlord Nicolaus was covered in ulcers.[725] Gallo and Mattioli found a large tumor on the neck of another child and could not agree whether to cauterize it or to fight it with liquefying remedies.[726] A girl who was also treated by both physicians suffered from a lacrimal fistula.[727] A disease that was common among children and youths was scabies. The treatment could be very painful: when a ten-year-old girl was suffering from a scabies rash on her head and face, the surgeon Hildebrand recommended putting a cap coated with pitch on her head and using it to pull out the hair; he claimed that the seat of the malady was in the hair follicles.[728]

Parents might seek the advice of a physician or apothecary when their children were sick, but not only then. No longer able to bear his children's crying at night, an acquaintance of Handsch went to an apothecary and got a soporific,

---

[720] Ibid., fol. 323v, "semper suspicare de vermibus subcutaneis. Mittesser."
[721] Ibid., fol. 287v.
[722] Cod. 11207, fol. 24r.
[723] Ibid.
[724] Cod. 11183, fol. 429v.
[725] Cod. 11205, fol. 221v.
[726] Cod. 11207, fol. 26v.
[727] Ibid., fol. 31v.
[728] Cod. 11183, fol. 451v.

which made his children sleep calmly.[729] As Handsch reported during his time in Prague, several apothecaries there regularly prepared soporifics whose ingredients included mandrake and henbane, and they were given to crying infants on a nightly basis. The consequences were devastating, Handsch remarked: the natural vital heat was destroyed, its nature tainted, and the children were pale and shaky. The apothecary Balthasar knew of an infant who had been given opium frequently and had become unable to go to sleep without it. A woman had even told him about a boy who had died of opium.[730]

Physicians who worked with children needed to take their constitution into account when choosing a treatment.[731] In his *Antidotariolus*, a collection of recipes from different sources, Handsch wrote down various remedies to be used specifically with infants and children.[732] Among them were various recipes, for example one from Andrea Gallo, for coughing in children in general but also specifically for a three-year-old girl whose swollen belly and cough Gallo attributed to her cold spleen,[733] and one from Ulrich Lehner for a three-year-old epileptic boy.[734] Even more so than with adults, the taste of a remedy was an important consideration. When the daughter of Blasius came down with a fever and showed signs of a worm infestation, Gallo was going to give her cassia with *hiera picra* but Handsch objected on account of the "repulsive" taste.[735]

Physicians experienced time and again that they were helpless in the face of the diseases of children. The belly and face of a poor, apparently older feverish boy, for example, became distended and he ultimately died.[736] During his time in Innsbruck, Handsch gave a haunting description of how the infant of the Welsers died – this was likely the little daughter of Hans Georg, a brother of Philippine and Rebecca Welser.[737] Her body was hot. She had not slept for several nights but kept nursing from the wet nurse. It was advised that the wet nurse drink goat's milk to counter the acridity associated with the milk and stool. But in the night the nurse had some "fright" and developed pustules on her lips and a pain in her

---

729 Cod. 11205, fol. 2v; presumably this was the same Blasius whom Handsch called a "coterraneus" in another entry and who was thus probably from Leipa.
730 Ibid., fol. 137v.
731 Manzke, Remedia (2008), pp. 227–234.
732 Cod. 11200, fol. 140r.
733 Ibid., fol. 1v and fol. 215r.
734 Ibid., fol. 214v.
735 Cod. 11207, fol. 42r.
736 Cod. 11183, fol. 421v.
737 Cf. Hirn, Ferdinand II. (1887), pp. 359–60, on the death of a three-month-old daughter of the couple.

loins. After that, old Anna Welser did not let her nurse the child anymore. Instead, the child was fed goat's milk with a wooden spoon and, when the new nurse was long in coming, boiled water that had run through sweet *conserva rosarum*. The new wet nurse arrived in the evening, but close to midnight Handsch and the apothecary were called to attend to the infant. The child had stopped moving her arms and legs; she "kreiste", as Handsch put it, that is she evidently suffered convulsions. Breathing stopped and her eyes glazed over. She died within the hour.[738]

---

[738] Cod. 11183, fol. 401r.

Diseases of Women

The diseases suffered by women had been explored at length in ancient and medieval medical writings.[739] Yet, in the learned medicine of the sixteenth century, an unparalleled interest in women's diseases is observable. Gynecology, as the field would later come to be called, became a distinct subject area, even a subdiscipline of male-dominated medicine.

There were three interrelated developments that essentially propelled this interest in diseases of women in the sixteenth century. For one thing, there was the renewed appreciation of Hippocrates as the second central authority next to Galen. Such appreciation stemmed not least of all from the medical humanists' "rediscovery" of the Hippocratic writings, including those on diseases of women.[740] Second, physicians were coming to understand that successfully treating sick women could be a boon to their medical practice. Having the trust of women could open doors, especially among the upper-classes, and give a physician access to their families and relatives (Fig. 9). Third, a conviction took hold among learned physicians that the bodies of women and men were fundamentally different, calling for different medical treatment.

This last point requires explanation. In a book that attracted much attention a couple of decades ago, Thomas Laqueur claimed that early modern learned medicine until far into the eighteenth century adhered to a "one-sex-model".[741] He held that, following a model of analogy that had already been formulated by Galen, learned medicine described the genitals of women and men as identical. The stronger vital heat of men simply drove their genitals to the outside, while with women they remained inside the abdominal cavity. The ovaries thus corresponded to the testes, the uterus to the scrotum, and the vagina to the male member. Laqueur's thesis – and this is why I have to go into some detail – received a considerable response and continues to be quoted approvingly. At the time it was proposed, the thesis fit perfectly with a then fairly new current that understood "sex" primarily as "gender", that is as a cultural category. There were also anatomical illustrations that seemed to offer a powerful confirmation of Laqueur's thesis insofar as they depicted the female genitalia as very similar to the male.

---

739 For surveys of medieval gynecology see Green, Women's medical practice (1989); Green, Making women's medicine masculine (2008); on the famous "Trotula" see also Spitzner, Salernitanische Gynäkologie (1921).
740 King, Hippocrates' woman (1998); Bourbon, Jean Liébault (2010).
741 Laqueur, Making sex (1990).

However, criticism of Laqueur's thesis was not long in waiting and, today, it must be considered to be definitively disproven.[742] Even in the old medical writings, such as in Hippocrates, there are passages in which the anatomical differences between the sexes were emphasized.[743] An analysis of numerous medical texts from the sixteenth and seventeenth centuries fails a fortiori to offer proof of the dominance of a "one-sex-model". On the contrary, it shows that the vast majority of medical writers were convinced of a fundamental anatomical difference between man and woman. Authors emphasized that the uterus and the scrotum had very little in common and that the "testes" ("testiculi") in men and women likewise were of different size and nature.[744] Galen's model of analogy was of course known by physicians in the Renaissance; Handsch's teacher Fracanzano also introduced his students to it.[745] At the same time, reading the notes Handsch took in the anatomy lectures of Fracanzano and Falloppia in Padua, it becomes clear that it is quite impossible to claim the dominance of a "one-sex model" in early modern learned medicine, not in university teaching either. The female "testiculi", Handsch noted down, were much smaller than the male ones. They differed from them in their form and construction ("figura et constructione") and did not have a skin either.[746] To this day, the Falloppian tubes carry the name of Handsch's teacher who was the first to describe these structures precisely, underlining how profoundly they differed from the seminal vessels of men.[747]

Looking back, one cannot but arrive at the sobering conclusion that Laqueur "reconstructed" the learned medical discourse of that time without looking at the bulk of the relevant works which were written in Latin, the dominant language of scholarly medicine at the time, except for the few he could access in English translations and that he moreover offered a highly selective reading of those texts he did use.

The learned physicians also made more dedicated efforts than ever in the sixteenth century to showcase the difference between the male and the female bodies apart from the anatomy of the organs of reproduction. This went so far that some assertions of anatomical difference were made which we no longer accept today. Sixteenth-century anatomists found, for example, that not only the pelvis was wider in women compared to men, which allowed them to give

---

742 Park/Nye, Destiny (1991); Stolberg, Woman (2003); King, One-sex body (2013).
743 King, One-sex body (2013).
744 Stolberg, Woman (2003).
745 Cod. 11226, fol. 93v.
746 Cod. 11210, fol. 9v.
747 Falloppia, Observationes (1561), foll. 195v-196v; see also the chapter on anatomy in Part I.

birth more easily, as Handsch learned from Falloppia.[748] They also found the collar-bones in women were straighter and thus contributed to the beauty of the female breast. They were more curved in men, by contrast, which facilitated the throwing of spears and other weapons. In some women, Renaissance anatomists even found a hole in the area of the lower sternum, through which, they believed, vessels passed that took blood from the uterus to the breasts, where it was turned into milk.[749]

Apart from the anatomical differences of the genitals and the skeleton, there was a widespread consensus that the female body, compared to the male, was characterized by its lesser vital heat and thus by a predominance of moist and cold qualities. The boundaries between the sexes were, however, not as clearly defined here as they were when fundamental anatomical differences were described. Some women were considered very hot, while moisture and cold determined the physical constitution of some men so much so that it approached that of women.

If women and men profoundly differed in their build and therefore in their physiology, the obvious implication was that they should be treated differently when they were ill. And, conversely, the many female diseases attributed to the uterus and from which men were correspondingly spared offer a further important proof – ignored by Laqueur – for the supposition of a fundamental difference between the male and the female body. When it came to health, physicians also saw the uterus as responsible for more than local complaints like inflammation, ulcers, and cancer: they regarded it as the source of a wide range of diseases also in the rest of the body due to its central role in women's monthly "cleansing", due to the harmful vapors that could rise from it, and due to its connection with the other organs.

The newly awakened medical interest in diseases of women found reflection in various treatises and other works on the *morbi mulierum* or *morbi muliebres*.[750] One widely read collection of writings on the subject was the *Gynaeceia*. Helen

---

[748] Cod. 11210, fol. 31v; by contrast, Falloppia explained, it was not true that the sagittal suture extended to the root of the nose in women and that women had only 32 teeth against 33 in men (ibid.).
[749] Platter, De corporis (1583), book 3, table II; Stolberg, Woman (2003); on the particular interest in such skeletal differences as evidence for the different nature of women in the Enlightenment see Schiebinger, Skeletons (1986).
[750] Da Monte, Opuscula (1558), vol. 2, pp. 704–785; Marinello, Le medicine (1563); Dunus, Muliebrium morborum (1565); Liébault, Trois livres (1582); Bottoni, De morbis (1585); Mercado, De mulierum (1587); Massaria, Praelectiones (1600); Mercuriale, De morbis (1601); Varanda, De morbis (1620); see also Maclean, Renaissance notion (1987), esp. p. 46.

King has examined its history in great detail.[751] The *Gynaeceia* were first published in 1566 by the Zurich physician Caspar Wolf. In his dedicatory letter to two of his colleagues from Memmingen, he wrote that what had moved him to compile the collection was the discussion he had had with his teacher Conrad Gessner about a female patient. This occasion made him remember manuscripts of works of several different authors who had written about "women's things" ("de gynaeciis").[752] Revised editions by Caspar Bauhin[753] and Israel Spach[754] followed in 1586 and 1597. They added texts by contemporary authors including lectures by the Paduan professors Girolamo Mercuriale and Albertino Bottoni.

As is indicated by this inclusion of contemporary lectures in the *Gynaeceia*, university teaching in the sixteenth century was an important catalyst for the increasingly profound and widespread exploration of diseases of women. We do not know when or where the first lectures specifically devoted to diseases of women or to writings such as the Hippocratic *De morbis mulierum* were held. But we do know that as early as the beginning of the 1550s – that is preceding the first edition of the *Gynaeceia* by a decade – lectures about women's diseases were held in Montpellier and Padua. From Montpellier, notes on a lecture given by Guillaume Rondelet have come down to us.[755] In Padua in the winter of 1551–52, Georg Handsch took extensive notes from a private lecture given by Fracanzano about the *De morbis muliebribus*,[756] and in the decades that followed, the subject of women's diseases was firmly established in the teaching at Padua. It appears that all Paduan professors turned to the subject, as is evidenced by students' notes on lectures by Girolamo Capivaccia[757] and Girolamo Mercuriale,[758] as well as, from 1591, the notes by Hieronymus Besler on a private lecture by Alessandro Massaria's on *De morbis mulierum*.[759]

Soon, a canon of diseases considered as specifically female and connected with the uterus developed in lectures and publications and was discussed regularly. Building on the treatment of female anatomy and physiology, three major

---

751 King, Midwifery (2007).
752 Wolf, Gynaeciorum (1566); the date of the dedicatory epistle is 1564.
753 Bauhin, Gynaeciorum (1586).
754 Spach, Gynaeciorum (1597).
755 Forschungsbibliothek Gotha, Chart. 499, foll. 194–228v; on Rondelet's biography see Dulieu, Rondelet (1966).
756 Cod. 11226, foll. 92r-119r, "privatim incipit", 16 December 1551; in a letter to Mattioli and Willenbroch (Prague, 24 November 1559) Handsch mentioned "libellum" *De morbis muliebribus* by Fracanzano which Ulrich Lehner owned (Cod. 9650, foll. 53v-55v).
757 Forschungsbibliothek Gotha, Chart. 629, fol. 111r-152v, *De uteri affectionibus*.
758 Ibid., foll. 347r-405v, *De morbis muliebribus*.
759 Universitätsbibliothek Erlangen, Ms 981.

parts came to be routinely discussed: First, disordered menstruation, second, the pathological changes to or in the uterus, and third, the pathology of pregnancy, childbirth, and the puerperium.

These three elements can also be found in the detailed notes Handsch prepared from the above-mentioned lecture by Fracanzano in 1551–52. A brief characterization of the fairer, softer, and hairless female body and women's finer hair of the head is followed by a treatment of anatomy, discussing the "testiculi"; the "os uteri", through which the male seed was thought to be led inside and which closed up after conception; and the "collum uteri", the vagina, along with the exterior genitals. Fracanzano then expounded on menstruation and how it could become disordered and described the diseases of the uterus such as "suffocation of the womb" and genital discharge, from which nearly all women were said to suffer to a greater or lesser degree.[760] Concluding his lecture, he turned to questions regarding conception and infertility[761] as well as complaints of pregnancy, including the strange appetite for charcoal, chalk, and such things, which pregnant women sometimes experienced. He discussed the different causes of a miscarriage, dealt with the possible complications during childbirth, and ended with the diseases of childbed.

Disordered Menstruation

Menstruation was a much-discussed topic in the early modern period.[762] Physicians and laypeople agreed that menstruation was of paramount importance for the health and life of women. With female patients, as we can also see in Handsch's notes, the *menses* or *menstrua*, played a major role. When a woman's menstruation was interrupted without her being pregnant, or when the menses were simply less than usual, this was generally considered the principal cause of disease. This view followed directly from the prevailing interpretation of the nature of menstruation: due to her weaker vital heat and her colder temperament, the grown woman concocted her food less well than the man. As a result, she constantly accumulated impure, even spoiled, putrid matter in her body, which had to be emptied every month. Handsch read in Musa Brasavola that some

---

760 Cod. 11226, fol. 107r-v.
761 In this case, Handsch wrote only the headings, leaving space for the notes. Probably he missed these lectures.
762 Vgl. Stolberg, A woman's hell (1999); Stolberg, Monthly malady (2000); Stolberg, Erfahrungen (2004); Stolberg, Menstruation (2005); Hindson, Attitudes (2009); Read, Menstruation (2013); see also, based on vernacular French sources, McClive, Menstruation (2015).

countrywomen did not menstruate and were nevertheless healthy and strong. They dissolved the matter through their movement and physical labor and in this respect resembled female animals, which did not menstruate either (and which transformed some of the matter that was destined for excretion into fur and horns).[763] But for the vast majority of women, menstruation was vital. Da Monte held that, besides conception, the central task of the uterus was to void the excremental matter that women accumulated in their bodies because of their coldness.[764] And Handsch very similarly quoted Trincavella, who wrote that the uterus was made by nature in such a way "that the excrements that are inside the female body due to her sex are cleared out by [the uterus] as if through a cloaca, which is why, as intended by nature, the excrements that are taken there are discharged from it every month."[765] He noted in another entry that, in men, the body was purified sometimes every quarter, sometimes every year through hemorrhoidal bleeding ("mundificatur"), the way it happened through menstruation in women.[766]

Menstrual blood was seen as unclean and harmful, poisonous even, certainly when it was held back in the body past its time.[767] One of the earliest *observationes* in Handsch's student notebooks was about a feverish young woman whose condition did not improve even after she had been given large amounts of purgatives. When Handsch's teacher Comes de Monte was consulted, he identified a "suppressed" menstruation as the crucial cause and prescribed rubbings (likely for her legs, to draw the blood downwards) to encourage the menses.[768] Some diseases were considered a typical result of a disordered, "obstructed", "held-

---

763 Cod. 11205, fol. 165.
764 Da Monte, De uterinis affectibus (1554), fol. 65r. "Uterus est excrementorum sentina", a contemporary reader added to this passage in handwriting (Staatliche Bibliothek Regensburg, Med. 607).
765 Copy of a *consilium* by Trincavella, Cod. 11238, foll. 168–177v, cit. fol. 172v, "uterus enim a natura alioqun confectus est, ut id quod in muliebri corpore ratione sexus excrementosum est, per eum tanquam per cloacam purgaretur, unde naturae instituto singulis mensibus eo delata excrementa excernuntur". Disregarding the numerous passages of this kind which can be found in treatises in Latin, the dominant language of learned medical discourse, Cathy McClive, in her study of menstrual theory in early modern France, has denied that menstruation was widely believed to serve as a means to cleanse the female body of impure matter. She bases this claim on historical studies, which concluded that Hippocrates and Aristoteles both did not "pathologize" menstruation (McClive, Menstruation (2015), p. 109), but the theories and notions of Renaissance physicians (and lay people) frequently were quite different from the ancient ones.
766 Cod. 11240, fol. 94r.
767 Cod. 11207, fol. 10r.
768 Cod. 11238, foll. 71r-72r.

back" menstruation, and one of them was the widely diagnosed "suffocation of the womb", which we will be discussing at greater length. Growths and cancerous tumors of the uterus that resulted from the local accumulation and induration of insufficiently voided excremental matter were likewise feared.[769] Ultimately, nearly any disease could be attributed to insufficient menses and the resulting accumulation of harmful matter, which could settle in different parts of the body and, on top of that, could release vapors. "The woman has an impure uterus and if it is not cleansed we will have to worry that she gets seriously ill with headaches, lumbar pain and infertility", a lay healer from Zittau concluded from the urine of a sick woman.[770]

Women monitored their menstrual cycle meticulously, and, as we can see from Handsch's notebook entries, physicians inquired about it regularly. They would hear from women, for example, that their menses had come at the right time but were not the way they should be ("sed non debito modo", in Handsch's Latin translation), that they were "not right", that the quantity was not sufficient ("non sufficienter", "non debita quantitate", "non in iusta quantitate"), or that they had not come on the expected day, or eight days too early.[771]

Like the blood from bloodletting, menstrual blood could be examined visually and could hold important diagnostic clues. Handsch sometimes asked specifically about its color.[772] The *menstrua* could be pale, "faded as if it had been washed", as one woman said.[773] It had not stained the other side of the chemise, said the wife of Collinus. "Ask women in this way", Handsch then added in the margin, evidently referring to the coloring of the chemise.[774] He learned from a young woman with severe abdominal pain that her *menstruum* by contrast was "blackish, the color of brick, like burned blood", while it had been "good" before her wedding.[775] Unlike with urine and stool, women were apparently not willing to show physicians their *menstruum* collected with a cloth. Handsch thought it noteworthy that he once, in a privy, saw an *anitergium*, which we may interpret as a cloth used to wipe oneself – and on it he also saw some *menstrua*. He described its sticky appearance, like thin, clotted blood-colored snot.[776]

---

769 See the chapter on cancer.
770 Cod. 11205, foll. 549v-550r.
771 Cod. 11183, fol. 10v, fol. 82r, fol. 388v, fol. 402v and fol. 406v; Cod. 11205, fol. 293v; Cod. 11206, fol. 32r.
772 Cod. 11205, fol. 521v.
773 Ibid., fol. 289r.
774 Ibid., fol. 252v.
775 Ibid., fol. 544r.
776 Ibid., fol. 239a v.

Any medical theory of menstruation had to be able to explain why women did not menstruate during pregnancy and, if they breastfed their children, for half a year[777] or, like Handsch's stepmother,[778] even three quarters of a year after giving birth, and nevertheless remained in good health. In his lecture, Fracanzano offered the explanation that the menstrual blood served to feed the fetus during pregnancy and after the birth flowed to the breasts to feed the newborn. But this was only plausible at first glance.[779] Why, of all substances, should impure, excremental, even harmful and poisonous matter serve to feed the child developing in the womb? Handsch read that Avenzoar (Abū Marwān ibn Zuhr, 1094–1162) had already voiced his doubts about this interpretation of Galenic doctrine. He thought that, when Galen had spoken of *menstruum* in this context, he had merely followed common usage but actually meant good, natural blood, which flowed to the uterus.[780]

The necessity of having to explain the interruption of the period during pregnancy and nursing thus was the starting point for an alternative interpretation of menstruation that gained momentum in the scholarly writing of the late sixteenth century. Traces of it are already found in Galen.[781] According to it, the menses served the excretion of pathogenic matter only when the woman was sick. In times of health, menstrual blood was no different from regular, natural blood. During her fertile years, the woman was able to create more blood from her food than her body consumed. During pregnancy, this good, pure blood served to feed the fetus. When she was not pregnant, it had to be excreted only to avoid a *plethora*, a superabundance of blood in the body that could threaten to burst the vessels. The blood became thick and viscous, began to flow more slowly and there was a danger that it could come to a halt completely.[782]

This explanatory model, however, had much less of an impact on medical practice, on the interpretation of women's diseases, and especially on the bodily experience of affected women than one might suspect. The uterus continued to be seen to play a central role in the excretion of impure substances. A reduced or entirely "obstructed" menstruation was still feared as a primary cause of disease, and the *menstruum* often remained linked with images of impurity and spoiled

---

777 Ibid., fol. 239a v, on the wife of a certain Nikolaus, who neverless did not have any noticeable complaints except for some occasional discomfort in the umbilical area.
778 Ibid., fol. 437r. When menstruation resumed, the mother-in-law reported, she immediately got pregnant again.
779 Cod. 11226, fol. 92v.
780 Cod. 11240, fol. 143r: "Ex Avenzoar".
781 Galen, De venae sectione adversus Erasistratum, in idem, Opera (1822), vol. XI, pp. 147–378.
782 Liébault, Infirmitez (1582), p. 329 and pp. 337–341.

matter.[783] In Handsch's time, physicians almost inevitably interpreted menstruation as a discharge of impure, excremental matter.

If menstruation was reduced, had become irregular or stopped entirely, it thus became a most pressing matter to promote it. By rubbing the legs vigorously, as recommended by Comes de Monte, or by letting blood from one of the "women's veins" (*venae saphenae*) or both, as was expected by women,[784] one could try to direct the flow of blood downward to the uterus in the days before the next expected period.[785] There were also several herbs and medications used to facilitate menstruation,[786] and a local intervention was possible as well. One physician from Zittau prescribed a patient whom he was treating with Handsch a pessary with a number of different herbs, to be inserted into her vagina.[787] Handsch himself recommended a remedy to a patient which she was to throw on glowing embers. Once smoke arose, she was to lead it into her vagina by means of a funnel. He explained to the sick woman that the uterus would be heated in this way "and the veins will open".[788]

Given the fundamentally very positive assessment of regular and plentiful menstruation, it was quite unusual for physicians to hear complaints about excessive menses. A rare exception was the wife of Steinberger, who found herself weakened by copious menses that started again while she was still nursing her child.[789]

Not surprisingly then, the natural end of menstruation with age – called *cessatio mensium* in the medicine of the day and what modern medicine termed "menopause" about 200 years ago – had downright negative associations and was seen as a variant of an "impeded", "obstructed", or "withheld" menstruation.[790] After all, there was no plausible reason why an aging woman should no longer need her monthly cleansing. On the contrary, her vital heat, further weakened by her age, was even less able to ensure the concoction of food and, if necessary, of pathogenic substances. And so, Gallo held that a kind of morbid matter that was at least similar to menstrual blood could spoil the uterus, when

---

783 Duden, Geschichte (1987).
784 Cod. 11205, fol. 473r; Handsch owed his knowledge to a bathmaster.
785 Ibid., on Johann Neefe's advice "ut tribus diebus ante periodum mitteret saphenam dextram"; similarly ibid., fol. 627r, copy of a *consilium* by Johann Neefe, recommending bloodletting a day or two before the expected monthly bleeding.
786 Ibid., fol. 489v, on Ulrich Lehner's menstrual powder.
787 Ibid., fol. 457v.
788 Ibid., fol. 490r.
789 Ibid., fol. 189v.
790 Historical overview in Stolberg, Woman's hell (1999).

the menses stopped, and it could badly affect the other organs as well.[791] The increased incidence of breast and uterine cancer as well as other serious diseases during this stage of life seemed to illustrate time and again the fatal consequences of waste matter remaining in the body of the aging woman.

The cessation of the menses was thus framed as a major cause of disease and was associated not only with infertility but also with impurity and filth. This may be one reason why women in Western cultures today tend to perceive and experience menopause more negatively than women in many other parts of the world. It is hard to find writers who could also find some merit in it. Expressing a thought that strike us as quite modern today, Felix Platter tried to see something positive in the cessation of the menses with age, at least with regards to the human race as a whole: divine providence had wisely ordained that the woman was not fertile all her life, because if she were, mankind would multiply so much that the whole earth could not provide enough food.[792]

Only few contemporary authors addressed the cessation of the menses and its effects on the female body at some length. The only fairly detailed description that is known from Handsch's lifetime comes from Giovanni Marinello, written in 1563. The symptoms Marinello names are markedly different from those we connect with menopause today. They echo the contemporary belief that the consequences of menopause resembled in many respects the consequences of a suppressed menstruation at a younger age: "Those women, in whom the menses have ceased or did not start, like those with whom they cease due to age, are always ailing, especially in the body parts that are connected with the uterus or somehow relate to it, such as the stomach and the head. As soon as their menses cease, they experience pain, apostemas, eye complaints, failing eyesight, vomiting, fever, and they desire men more than ever. Their sickly uterus moves up and down the whole time or does other things that are hard to bear. This soon leads to tightness in the chest, a fainting heart, breathlessness, hiccups, and other troublesome symptoms of which the woman sometimes dies. It can also cause an expectoration of blood, hemorrhoids, and, especially in young women, severe nosebleeds and innumerable other complaints, too many to describe here."[793]

---

[791] Cod. 11207, fol. 68v; Francanzano held a different opinion also on this topic. He thought that the ageing body dried up and made menstruation dispensable (Cod. 11126, fol. 94r). It was widely believed, in fact, that the bodily substance dried out with age but, as the frequent catarrhs among the old indicated, fluid, harmful matter could accumulate all the more easily in the spaces between the hardening solids.
[792] Platter, Quaestionum (1625), p. 110.
[793] Marinello, Medicine (1563), fol. 87v.

In Handsch's detailed notes, the complaints that are considered typical of menopause today, especially hot flashes and sweats, are of only marginal importance. But his entry on the aging widow Anna does go to show that laypeople knew the change of life as a phenomenon *sui generis* and gave it a name. Anna lamented to Handsch: "I have a fair share of the women's disease because sometimes a heat shoots through me, from the bottom up to the crown, then soon goes away, and sometimes it is followed by a shiver."[794]

Such sensations of rising heat could also be understood as a symptom of hot vapors that rose from accumulated menstrual blood. This meant that whenever Handsch noted down the remarks women or their relatives made regarding an cessation of the menses, the main question was whether the menstruation had stopped due to age or due to a preternatural and treatable obstruction. It was known of course at what age the menses usually stopped. "A woman has her period until she is fifty years [of age]", said one of Handsch's patients.[795] And a *matrona* at the Ambras court confirmed that women usually had a menses until they were fifty years old, allowing, however, that some had still borne children at this old age.[796] A woman with an "obstructed" menstruation and complaints in the head and upper body accordingly came to the conclusion that it was not because of her age that her menstruation had stopped: this was meant to happen at the age of fifty, but she was only forty.[797]

As opposed to other forms of *retentio mensium,* there was no hope treating *cessatio mensium*. All one could do was to try and compensate for the absent monthly cleansing through the use of other excretory pathways. When an older woman asked Lehner for a remedy that would get her menstruation going again – she thought that it had only been held back for a long time – Lehner said this was not possible because her menstruation had stopped due to her age. When she insisted, Handsch gave her a purging agent and a tonic.[798]

Insofar as menstruation served to void impure, excremental matter, there was an area of overlap with *fluor albus,* or the "whites". Tellingly, the physicians also spoke of a "white menstruation" ("alba menstrua").[799] Fracanzano explained to his students in Padua that nearly all women suffered from this discharge to some

---

794 Cod. 11205, fol. 637v: "Ich hab der Frauen Kranckheit ein gutt Teil, denn bisweilen uberscheust [sic!] mich auch ein Hiz, von unten bis auff die Scheitel hinauf, vergehet bald und bisweilen kompt auch ein Schauer nach der Hitz."
795 Ibid., fol. 434v: "Ein Weib hat yre Zeit bis auff 50 Jahre."
796 Cod. 11206, fol. 36r.
797 Cod. 11205, fol. 326v.
798 Ibid., fol. 346r.
799 Cod. 11183, fol. 460r.

degree.⁸⁰⁰ And so, Handsch later thought he could risk to tell a woman, after examining only her urine, that "the whites" would "at some time affect her strongly".⁸⁰¹ When he saw a sick woman's urine in Prague that was pale and had phlegmy admixtures, he dared to tell her outright that she had white *menstrua*. The woman, who had previously proven to be "headstrong" ("morosus") admitted this immediately and was now willing to take the recommended medicines.⁸⁰² According to Fracanzano's cautioning, physicians should know better than to promise a quick recovery to women who had white discharge. It could persist for years, and many women tried all kinds of treatment in vain.⁸⁰³ The whites were not only an aesthetic issue. Plentiful, frequent *fluor,* like *gonorrhoea,* caused women to fear that they would grow increasingly weak. The consumptive Blasia complained that her "whites" had "returned now", that "it runs below like milk and that weakens me."⁸⁰⁴ Some women complained of concomitant symptoms. An unmarried woman named Maria, for instance, suffered from abdominal cramps and lumbar pain; her feet and breathing were heavy, and she felt languid. Her brother had no hope for her recovery if she did not get married soon.⁸⁰⁵

Suffocation of the Womb

Most premodern diagnostic terms conceptualized symptoms and complaints in ways which, although they differ markedly from those accepted today, are similar to disease entities we still know today. The suffocation of the womb is one of the most striking exceptions. The disease was characterized by a set of symptoms and physical sensations that we are no longer familiar with.

Sometimes early modern physicians used the more general term *passio hysterica,* literally "uterine complaint". The term "hysteria", still familiar today, derives from it. Still in the twentieth century, it signified a disease that physicians and laypeople identified as physical, one that could produce dramatic, even seemingly theatrical symptoms, as extant film footage shows. With the rise of the nerves beginning in the seventeenth century, hysteria came to be framed as a disease of the nerves rather than the uterus, which meant that men, too, could be afflicted by it. In Handsch's time, however, the (largely synonymous) terms "praefocatio" and

---

800 Cod. 11226, fol. 107v.
801 Cod. 11205, fol. 397r.
802 Cod. 11206, fol. 33v.
803 Cod. 11226, fol. 107v.
804 Cod. 11205, fol. 557r.
805 Cod. 11183, fol. 388r.

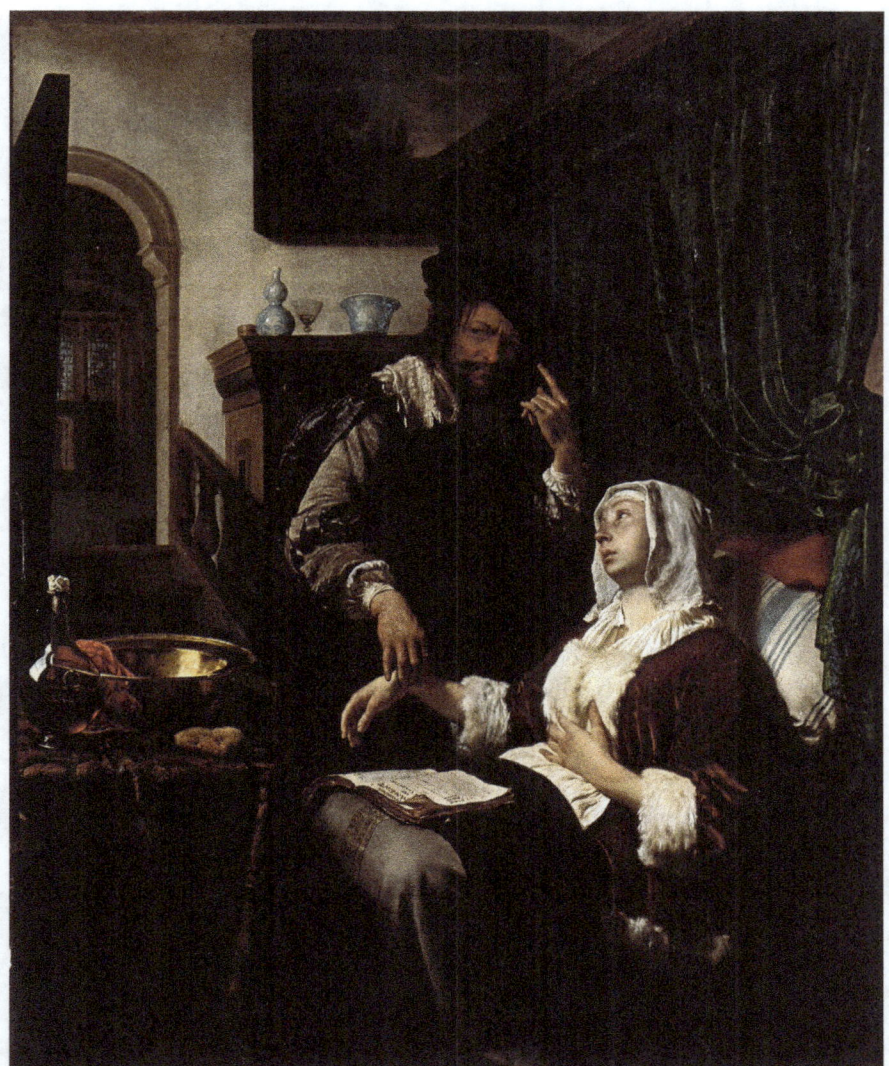

Fig. 9: Unknown painter, after Frans van Mieris (orig. 1657), The doctor's visit, Wellcome Collection, London.

"suffocatio" of the "uterus" or "matrix" were most common. The term was usually rendered as "suffocation of the mother" or "suffocation of the womb" in English.[806]

---

[806] The corresponding German term was "Gebärmuttererstickung".

The term "suffocation" is to be taken quite literally. Affected women complained of difficulty breathing and a strong sense of pressure in the chest. They often even lost their voice and, like the newly widowed wife of Kneysel, as well as a maid in Padua, and one of Handsch's landladies,[807] all they could do was gesture and point to their chests.[808] Some women also developed heart complaints. When the young wife of Heidenreich had a bout of suffocation of the womb, she not only complained of "narrow-chestedness". The blood, Handsch related her account, "shoots up from her thighs; the veins in her left arm sometimes become swollen" and "around the heart, she has a burning sensation".[809] The wife of Handsch's mentor Collinus complained that her heart beat quickly at times. Even her husband had sometimes heard it beating when he lay next to her.[810]

Some women only had one such attack[811] but the attacks could also recur and persist over longer periods, as in the case of Handsch's mistress Philippine Welser.[812] These were often highly dramatic episodes. The descriptions given by physicians overlap to some degree with those of epileptic fits, and sometimes the two diagnoses were noted down side by side.[813] Collinus's wife, for example, fell to the floor in church. She screamed and then fainted and had to be taken to the rectory.[814] An old neighbor of Handsch collapsed in church, and at first was believed dead.[815] Other women, too, came close to fainting during the attack or actually did lose consciousness,[816] or they lay in bed at night as if petrified and their husbands tried in vain to wake them up.[817] One husband described his wife as looking like a dead person during the attack.[818] Relaying the complaints of a peasant woman, Handsch wrote about how she was affected once a month, as if she were swooning and could move neither hands nor feet.

---

807 Cod. 11183, fol. 286r; in this case Handsch only suspected a suffocation of the womb.
808 Cod. 11207, fol. 113v; the Kneyselin still could scream, however, just not talk.
809 Cod. 11183, fol. 379v: "Das Geblüt scheust ir auß den Schenckeln hinauff, die Adern im lincken Arm lauffen ir auff bißweilen"; "umb das Herz aber brennet es sie".
810 Cod. 11205, fol. 248r.
811 In ibid., fol. 508r, Handsch listed four women who only suffered a single attack or at least recovered fully.
812 Stolberg, Krankheitsgeschehen (2021).
813 Cod. 11183, fol. 279r.
814 Cod. 11205, fol. 248r.
815 Ibid., fol. 508r; two days later, she was better again.
816 Ibid., fol. 439r.
817 Cod. 11183, fol. 197v.
818 Cod. 11205, fol. 438r, on the Baroness of Hungerkasten.

The first two years, it had pushed against her heart. But now there was tearing pain around the heart and she felt something beneath her heart, as if a vessel were pulsing. Then she also felt it in all limbs, with a whirling in the hands and feet. Her feet went limp she did not feel one of them in eight days, and as for the legs, the shins were as if broken. She also felt cold in her body and head and was dizzy. It burned when she passed water, and beneath the ribs on her left she felt "how it rises up hot, a vapor in the throat, often making the throat raw and as if swollen, pressing against my heart". She had been advised to have bloodletting done but thought she was too weak and had to die.[819] Anticipating later debates about apparent death, that is about the danger of mistaking unconscious people for dead, some authors even recommended that burial be held off for three days, or until the stench of death brought certainty, when a woman had a severe attack, collapsed, and showed no signs of life. It was claimed that, occasionally, women who seemed dead after an attack had come back to life.[820]

Suffocation of the womb was certainly not a rare condition at the time. Handsch documented a whole series of cases.[821] In the practice journal of Hiob Finzel, *praefocatio matricis* is even by far the most frequent diagnosis of all. During his approximately ten thousand consultations in Weimar, Eisenach, and Zwickau, he made the diagnosis more than a thousand times. This, however, suggests that he understood *praefocatio* as essentially synonymous with *passio hysterica* in the general sense and that he frequently gave the diagnosis even when he merely suspected the cause of a woman's disease to be in the uterus. Physicians widely believed that the uterus was involved at least to some degree in most diseases suffered by women.[822]

Suffocation of the womb and hysteria had been described and discussed by numerous authors since ancient Greece.[823] In an effort to understand the specific nature of the mysterious disease process at work, physicians and laypeople

---

819 Cod. 11205, foll. 476v-477v, "wie es heyß aufgehet, eyn Broden [Dampf, M.S.] ynn Hals, das offt der Halse rohe wirt und wie geschwollen, druckt mich ans Herz."
820 Vietor, De praefocatione (1610), thesis 17; Stupanus, De praefocatione (1612), thesis 11.
821 Cod. 11183, fol. 279r; Cod. 11205, fol. 293r; for further references see the following notes. In English practice journals and case collections from the seventeenth century the diagnosis of a suffocation of the womb is also repeatedly documented (cf. Williams, Hysteria (1990)).
822 Ratsbibliothek Zwickau, Ms. QQQQ1, Ms. QQQQ1a and Ms. QQQQ1b; in about a hundred entries Finzel diagnosed hysterical complaints, however, and sometimes together with a *praefocatio matricis* which suggests that he distinguished the two to some degree; see also Stolberg, A sixteenth-century physician (2019).
823 King, Once upon a text (1993); on the older historiography see Micale, Approaching hysteria (1995).

took recourse to two different explanatory models for the suffocation of the womb.[824] According to an idea that was widespread among laypeople up until the nineteenth century, the uterus literally rose up during an attack, pressing on the diaphragm and the chest. This notion fit in well with the perception of the uterus as an autonomous, even animal-like creature inside the body of the woman, a notion that had already surfaced in Plato. And this interpretation was confirmed time and again by women's accounts. Affected women complained specifically of the bodily sensation of a mass rising up in the abdomen and held that this mass could only be the uterus. In Handsch's notes, too, there are at least echoes of this notion. The daughter of the Lord of Gendorf complained of pain in her left side and claimed that it felt as if there was something like an apple in there.[825] To the wife of a man called Blasius, it seemed one night that something rose up from the area of her uterus and fell down again when she sat up.[826] Her husband described her condition, saying that it sometimes came over her almost like a swoon and, "in the same swoon, it rises up to her heart or below the chest, and it feels to her like swelling that has come up under her heart".[827]

Galen, however, had already called into question the idea that the uterus could actually rise up physically.[828] In the sixteenth century, closer anatomical examination of the female reproductive organs gave rise to further doubts about this explanation. Fracanzano taught his students that the uterus was firmly anchored in place by the vagina.[829] Therefore, it could not rise upward just like that. And yet, in medical practice, the possibility of an *ascensus uteri,* of the literal rising up of the uterus, continued to claim its place. The obvious contradiction was solved by shifting the imagery, by turning the rising of the uterus into a "striving" or extending and expanding upward. For one female patient, Gallo prescribed pills that he had invented himself "against the movement of the uterus" ("contra motum matricis").[830] For treatment during an acute attack, Handsch and his colleagues commonly used unpleasant and pungent substances such as

---

[824] In his notes, Handsch also mentioned a third, Galenic explanation of the *praefocatio* as the result of a poisonous ("venenosa") *intemperies* (Cod. 11126, fol. 101r) but judging from the sources I have seen this – rather paradox – notion did not play any role in sixteenth-century medical practice.
[825] Cod. 11205, fol. 296v.
[826] Ibid., fol. 510v; since Handsch once had also witnessed an attack in the same woman he suspected a "dispositio matricis praefocativa".
[827] Ibid., fol. 544v; "species praefocationis ab utero", Handsch added in the margin.
[828] Galen, De locis affectis. In: idem, Opera, vol. VIII, pp. 428–9.
[829] Cod. 11210, fol. 11r, "ynn derselbigen Omacht steiget es yr zum Herzen aber [oder, M.S.] unter die Brust, und ist yr wie eyn auffgelauffen Geschwulstichen unter dem Herzen".
[830] Cod. 11207, fol. 113v.

castoreum, asa foetida, camphor, or singed partridge or peacock feathers, which they had people hold up to the women's noses.[831] The aim was to drive the uterus downwards with the unpleasant smell. As Neefe put it, this was to ensure that the "mother lies down again" and that the "swoon" leaves the sick woman again.[832] Bitter drinks like absinth in wine could serve this purpose as well. The mother of Handsch's fellow student Daniel Cellarius used this remedy when she felt an attack of suffocation of the womb approaching.[833] Conversely, the smell of fragrant substances could trigger *praefocatio* in sensitive women, pulling the uterus upward. Handsch thus had to admit to himself that it had been wrong to allow a female patient who was vulnerable in this respect to eat oranges.[834]

By contrast, when fragrant substances were brought near the woman's womb this promised to lure the uterus down.[835] In Lehner's collection of *secreta*, Handsch also discovered the advice of applying cups to the genitalia. When he treated the wife of Kneysel it he did not dare suggest this method, however, because of the female bystanders. Gallo, who had prescribed her pills "against the movement of the uterus", also expressed concerns. He did not doubt the efficacy of the cupping but feared that the downward pull on the uterus might be too powerful.[836]

The prevailing explanation for suffocation of the womb in learned medicine was a different one. Once again, the idea of a morbid matter, a *materia peccans*, played a key role. The critical causes of suffocation of the womb here were seen either in menstrual blood or in the female seminal fluid. If they were retained in the body and accumulated in the uterus or in its vicinity, it was assumed that they released a putrid, foul vapor ("vapor putrefactus"), which rose to the upper abdomen and caused a stomachache,[837] to the chest, taking away the breath, and to the heart and brain.[838] Here, the suffocation of the womb became yet another variant of the diseases that resulted from morbid vapors. With this interpretation, the uterus itself could remain in its natural place, firmly attached to

---

831 Cod. 11183, fol. 127r and fol. 286r; Cod. 11205, fol. 248r, on Lehner who made the sick wife of Collinus smell "devil's dirt" ("Teuffels Dreck"), i.e. *asa foetida* as Handsch assumed; Cod. 11205, fol. 449r and fol. 457r, on castoreum and scorched partridge feathers; Cod. 11207, fol. 113v, on castoreum and partridge and peacock feathers. For the same purpose, some authors also recommneded *sternutatoria*, i.e. substances that provoked sneezing (Stupanus, De praefocatione (1612), thesis 13).
832 Cod. 11205, fol. 445r.
833 Cod. 11251, fol. 17v.
834 Cod. 11205, fol. 450r.
835 Ibid., fol. 440r-v; Stupanus, De praefocatione (1612), thesis 13.
836 Cod. 11207, foll. 113v-114r.
837 Thus Lehner, according to Cod. 11006, fol. 35v.
838 Cod. 11210, fol. 11r, quoting Antonio Fracanzano.

the surrounding anatomical structures. At the same time, the rising vapors offered a plausible explanation for the wide range of other symptoms of which the affected women complained, such as dizziness and headaches. Fine vapors could easily rise up all the way to the skullcap, and in adults, the closed cranial sutures hardly allowed them to escape. When Mattioli, suspecting *praefocatio matricis,* asked a patient's husband if his wife's throat and neck became swollen during the attack, he was likely thinking of a distension due to rising vapors.[839]

Such rising vapors also helped explain the various heart complaints. As we have seen, some of the women not only complained of a sense of pressure but also of a burning sensation in and around the heart. Vapors were hot by definition. They could also mingle and interfere with the vital spirits, causing an accelerated or very weak heartbeat, a "fluttering of the heart" ("tremor cordis").[840] As we have seen, the women might even faint. Physicians also used the term a "syncope" in this context, a term that modern medicine still uses in a similar sense, for a brief spell of unconsciousness caused by insufficient blood supply to the brain. Handsch read in Galen that the *vapores* were almost like a poison, and that they were the reason why women stopped breathing and hardly had a palpable pulse.[841]

To give a precise diagnosis and be able to choose the right course of treatment when following this second explanatory model, it was important to determine the nature of the *materia peccans*. First of all, the physician had to decide whether the suffocation of the womb was due to rotten menstrual blood or putrefied seminal fluid. In the case of the Baroness of Hungerkasten, Handsch's notes tell us that the evidence at hand led to the assumption that harmful vapors from spoiled menstrual blood were at the bottom of her *praefocatio* or *strangulatio matricis,* literally her "uterine strangulation".[842] The patient mentioned insufficient menses. In addition, the skin of her hand showed an ugly brownish discoloration and later this happened with her chest. A rule of thumb ("regula") said that most women whose menses did not occur in the necessary fashion either had internal symptoms or showed ugly external changes.[843] The

---

839 Cod. 11183, fol. 197v.
840 Cod. 11205, fol. 495v.
841 Ibid., fol. 439v, with a reference to *De locis affectis*.
842 Ibid., fol. 453v; Handsch owed the term "strangulatio" to Johann Neefe but it was quite commonly used at the time and can be found, for example, already in Brasavola (Brasavola, In octo libros (1541), pp. 829–30).
843 Cod. 11205, fol. 439r.

famous Johann Neefe arrived at the same conclusion, and to a woman he explained the pathological process within her body as follows: "As explained in the included note in Latin, you fainted from the uterus rising, and this is a complaint that women experience quite often. It happens because they do not have their female roses in the right way, or otherwise accumulate a lot of bad humors in the body and in the mother. Bad vapors rise from them, irritate the mother and cause fainting along with difficulty breathing, as if the woman is going to suffocate."[844] In his practice journal, Finzel too noted down various cases of *praefocatio matricis* that resulted from disordered menses.

In some respects, suffocation of the womb thus resembled *melancholia hypochondriaca*. Both diseases were attributed to harmful, poisonous vapors that rose up from the abdomen, and some of the complaints that were considered typical can be found in descriptions of both clinical pictures. The proximity of "hysteria" and "hypochondria" in later times by all indications stemmed from this tradition of explaining the symptoms in terms of rising *vapores*. The difference is that *melancholia hypochondriaca* and later *hypochondria* were diagnosed almost exclusively in men. The reasons are obvious. Given the dominant position of the uterus in their bodies, it was natural to diagnose women with suffocation of the womb or *passio hysterica* when they had complaints that in men indicated vapors that originated from the upper abdomen, the *hypochondrium*.

Reading Handsch's notes and other published case histories of patients who suffered from suffocation of the womb, today's reader will likely be inclined to consider the disease as largely psychosomatic. The symptoms and the legitimacy they acquired thanks to the official medical diagnosis also promised considerable secondary morbid gain, as we would call it today. Over a period of months, the Baroness of Hungerkasten, for instance, called on an impressive number of physicians and at least one lay healer who attended her at her bedside, often even at night.[845] Neefe confirmed her in her conviction that she was suffering from a serious disease, saying that it was truly a disease that was not to be scoffed at.[846] At one point, she hastily drew up her last will.[847] Another

---

844 Ibid., fol. 443r-v, early August 1558: "Wie ich aus beiliegendem lateinischen Zettel vormercke, so ist euch die Omacht von Aufsteigen der Muetter herkommen, und tregt sich solcher Zufall bei Weibespersonen gar offt zu, kompt daher, das sie ire weibliche Rosen nicht zu rechte haben, aber [oder, M.S.] sonst vil boser Feuchtikeit ym Leibe unnd ynn der Muetter samlen, von denen steigen denn böse Dempfe über sich, errhegen die Muetter, und verursachen Omacht, schweren Athem als wollte eyn Weibesperson ersticken."
845 E.g. Cod. 11205, fol. 460v, fol. 462r and fol. 462v.
846 Ibid., fol. 449r.
847 Ibid., fol. 439r.

time she asked for a sacramental candle ("sacram candelam"). With her complaints and her symptoms, she held the attention of the people around her. She declared her disease "amazing" ("mirabilis"),[848] and, according to Handsch, she told her guests at the table that she thought she would die any day. At great length, she described her various and unusual complaints, which in this way served as a mark of distinction, even though they may strike the modern readers as remarkably vague: "Not that it hurts me, but it makes me feel anxious that I'm indeed not healthy; it sometimes goes to my ears and stings me and then it scatters like the wind; and that is in the right side of my head."[849] Handsch further described how, if she believed she was going to faint, she kept everyone around her on their toes, calling and incessantly insisting that people bring her warm cloths and rub her back with them, for example.[850]

Far beyond such aspects of secondary morbid gain, the suffocation of the womb of the early modern period may in retrospect be understood as a physical "idiom of distress", to use a term introduced by researchers in the sociology of health and illness and in cultural anthropology. Especially clinical pictures that – like the suffocation of the womb – are characterized mainly by powerful subjective complaints and occur in larger numbers only at certain historical times and in certain cultures or even only in certain groups and situations, may be understood according to this explanatory approach as a metaphorical expression of suffering or at least of the affected person's discomfort in his or her situation, which they express through physical symptoms: the physical complaints become a medium of communication. This is observed especially in societies and cultures where people have limited recourse to legitimate ways of making their discontent heard verbally. A striking modern example is the illness called *nervios* in South America.[851] When South-American refugees suffering from *nervios* complain of dizziness and fainting, feeling as if the ground beneath their feet is about to give and make them fall, from an outside perspective this may be understood as a metaphorical expression of their uprootedness, their disorientation, their fear of instability.[852] In cases like these, it is not an individual whose personal conflicts become somatized. It is an

---

848 Ibid., fol. 495v.
849 Ibid., foll. 495v-496r: "Nicht das mirs wehe thete, sondern es ist mir bange dabey, das ich nicht frey gesund bin, es kumpt mir bisweilen für die Ohren und sticht mich und darnach zerteilet sich es wie Wynde, unnd dis ist ynn der rechten Seyten des Hauptes."
850 Ibid., fol. 439v.
851 Davis/Whitten, Nerves (1988).
852 On *nervios* see Guarnaccia/ Farias, Social meanings (1988); Davis/ Low, Gender (1989); Low, Culturally interpreted symptoms (1985); Low, Embodied metaphors (1994); the historical origins of the notion of *nervios* in the premodern concept of "nervous diseases" are obvious.

entire collective that "acts out their life circumstances" with their own bodies, as Kaja Finkler put it, drawing on Merleau-Ponty.[853]

We may understand clinical pictures that were specific to certain historical periods in a very similar way, including the "nervous diseases" of the late seventeenth and eighteenth centuries.[854] Of course, this is an interpretation in hindsight, a special form of retrospective diagnosis. Even the underlying concept of somatization is genuinely modern and Western,[855] as it is based on the idea that there exists an independent domain of the "psychological" that acts on the body. In the early modern period, this conception was hardly present. As we have seen, emotions were perceived primarily as physical phenomena. And women suffering from suffocation of the womb evidently experienced their complaints in a very similar way to other conditions that we would interpret as decidedly physical, somatic phenomena today.

For a historical understanding of clinical pictures with which we are no longer familiar today, at least not in the form that they took, it is necessary to bear the above-mentioned reservations in mind, while at the same time understanding that an interpretation of them as "idioms of distress" can offer valuable insights. We know little about the life circumstances of the women whom Handsch and other physicians diagnosed with suffocation of the womb. In light of what we know about the position of women in culture and society at the time, however, the physical symptoms described by women certainly paint a vivid picture. The affected women complained of an intense feeling of constriction and pressure; they became speechless and quite often fainted. They thought their heads would burst from the pain, or they became dizzy. Some felt a burning sensation, a tearing pain, or other complaints in and around the heart, the very place that was recognized at the time as the physical seat of the emotions, not only by physicians. Another aspect of the clinical picture was a predisposition to crying for no apparent reason.[856] The Baroness of Hungerkasten, for her part, unexpectedly burst into tears when she heard religious singing at church.[857]

It is also telling how, in cases of suffocation of the womb, physicians and women paid heightened attention to negative affects as possible triggers. Handsch shed light on the illness of the Baroness of Hungerkasten by writing that she had "burdened herself with many worries that are too heavy for a woman". Giovanni Battista da Monte even named affects as a possible independent cause of

---

[853] Finkler, Universality (1989), p. 174.
[854] For a more detailed account see Stolberg, Experiencing illness (2011), pp. 170–195.
[855] Kleinman/Kleinman, Somatization (1985).
[856] Cod. 11205, fol. 248v.
[857] Ibid., fol. 499v.

suffocation of the womb. In his experience, it sometimes came "ex ipso animi affectu", specifically from the jealousy and anger of wives whose husbands were unfaithful to them.[858] This at the same time indicates suffering that stemmed from society and its norms. While being unfaithful even just once cast doubt on a woman's most important attributes – honor and purity – and could undermine her entire existence, women were expected to accept the unfaithfulness of their husbands without complaint. They were not allowed to become "hysterical" in today's sense of the word, which for its part derives directly from the historical context sketched out here. In his detailed notes about the case of the Baroness of Hungerkasten, Handsch repeatedly brought up negative affects generally but also her suffering due to her husband's unfaithfulness specifically. The patient herself explained that she had become sick "from shock and great insult", precisely because her husband had a lover, as Handsch wrote in his comment.[859] In the society in which she lived, even the noblewoman that she was had to accept without complaint that her husband had a lover, or in her words, a "whore" ("meretrix"). Her husband even told her that, unlike her, his lover had "whimpered in actu coitus".[860]

As this account already suggests, it was with remarkable openness that some of the women brought up their own sexuality and hinted at possible connections to their illness. Their accounts offer rare glimpses into female sexual experience. It was known and accepted at the time that women, too, could have strong sexual desires. Going by the classical Galenic teachings, a woman's feelings of sexual desire even constituted a necessary condition for conception and pregnancy, because only if she felt pleasure did she release her semen. Handsch knew that "naturally" ("naturaliter"), women, too, had to experience pleasure ("delectatio") during coitus, because semen also flowed from the *testiculi* inside their bodies, and this flow caused a tickle ("titillatio").[861] From the viewpoint of a patriarchal society, it was all the more important, then, that female pleasure be fenced in and that female pleasure be enjoyed strictly within the legitimate context of matrimonial intercourse. However, this context quite possibly did not offer women anything near what they wished for. While the wife of Collinus said that she sometimes ("interdum") felt pleasure when her husband lay with her,[862] the

---

858 Da Monte, Consultationum (1554), pp. 539–40.
859 Cod. 11205, fol. 484v.
860 Ibid., fol. 463v, "in actu coitus hett gewinselt".
861 Ibid., fol. 464r.
862 Ibid., fol. 248v.

Baroness of Hungerkasten, plagued by particularly varied and persistent complaints, told her physicians that she felt no desire and pleasure whatsoever during coitus.[863] And Handsch also heard from the wife of Blasius that she did not enjoy herself ("se non delectari") during coitus.[864] In the case of the Lord of Gendorf's daughter, who was about seventeen years old and married to a much older man ("senescenti viro"), the patient herself assumed that the main cause for her lack of enjoyment was the great age difference combined with the sad thoughts this evoked in her. The idea of old men who were unable to fully satisfy the sexual needs of their wives was a topos of the time, and Handsch shared the young woman's opinion.[865]

Conception and Pregnancy

Besides disordered menstruation, which could have various pathological consequences, and suffocation of the womb, which was in part attributed to disordered menstruation and was the principal specifically female disease, conception, pregnancy, birth, and the postpartum period constituted the third large topic area works on diseases of women addressed at the time.

Handsch, in his notebooks, wrote about the question of contraception only peripherally. Once, in conversation, he brought up the Hippocratic story about a woman who leapt down the stairs following coitus to drive out the semen and prevent pregnancy. In response, a teacher told him that he had heard about a woman who held a fragrant substance up to her nose to prevent pregnancy. Making an analogy with suffocation of the womb, Handsch assumed that the uterus, attracted by the fragrance, moved upward, instead of moving downward toward the semen, as was generally thought necessary for conception.[866] He added in another entry that prostitutes did not get pregnant because their uterus was too moist from frequent coitus, implying that they were therefore unable to retain the semen.[867]

Handsch likewise had little to say about the causes and possible treatments of infertility. However, we know from other sources that learned physicians –

---

863 Ibid., 453v, "se nullam delectationem et appetitum habere in coitu"; similarly ibid., fol. 463v and fol. 464r.
864 Ibid., fol. 211r.
865 Ibid., fol. 293r, fol. 295r and fol. 296v; at first, Handsch considered her fits to be epileptic but when he saw her three years later she complained about some weakness and at times suffered from suffocation of the womb.
866 Ibid., fol. 308v: "Quae prohibent impregnationem".
867 Cod. 11240, fol. 2v, citing Hippocrates.

and not only the midwives, as one might think – were certainly asked for advice in this delicate issue. The *consilia* of Jakob Horst provide good insight into how physicians explained and treated infertility. Horst saw the cause mainly in the woman but his recommendations for treatment aimed at both husband and wife. In 1579, for example, he explained to a married couple seeking help that both of them had a natural deficiency, albeit the wife's was much greater than the husband's. The husband, he went on, had a lot of black blood and phlegm and little good blood, and this was exacerbated when his drinking got out of hand. The semen, however, was created from the best blood. Without a doubt, the husband therefore had little good, fertile semen and there was little hope of conceiving even if they had coitus every day. He told the husband to refrain from "matrimonial mingling" for seven days, not to practice it too often thereafter either, and to refrain from excessive drinking.[868] As for the wife, her uterus was burdened and weakened from a lot of moisture, which made it ill-suited for conception and even if it succeeded, the uterus was insufficiently able to retain the "fruit". He therefore recommended remedies to warm and strengthen the uterus, to help void the superfluous moisture from it, and to correct its "bad complexion".[869]

Horst sometimes combined his medical advice to infertile couples with rather concrete instructions on how to behave. For example, in a *consilium* written for an unnamed high-ranking couple, which was labelled "secret", he concluded that the bodies of both spouses were too moist. Due to the moisture, the uterus of the wife was so slack and slippery that it lost the semen. He not only prescribed medications for both to use internally and externally, but also advised the husband to wait until seven days after the wife's menstruation had stopped and then, remembering his fear of God and his duty, to inflame his wife with flattery before setting out to perform the "conjugal act". The greater the "passion" ("fervor"), the better. To counter a premature efflux of semen post coitum, they should use cushions to position the woman with her head lower than her legs, and afterwards she should stay like this and not move. They could repeat this a week later.[870] In the case of Ursula and Melchior Lengen as well, Horst prescribed

---

[868] In another case, he advised the husband to take medicines that would promote concoction ("Dauung") and purge the body (Staats- und Universitätsbibliothek Göttingen, Ms Meibom 146, pp. 400–403, copy of an undated letter, in German).
[869] Staats- und Universitätsbibliothek Göttingen, Ms Meibom 146, pp. 406–411, Liegnitz, 23 February 1579 (copy); in another case, Horst also pointed at the wife's burnt bile as causing a weakness of the womb and infertility, when it was mixed with natural semen, but also diagnosed a cold, corrupted uterus (ibid., pp. 84–98, German *consilium* for Radegunde von Losenstein in Schallaburg, January 1584).
[870] Ibid., pp. 246–250, Iglau, 21 October 1579; the letter is in Latin but addresses the husband personally as "Magnifizenz".

medications to treat the cold and moist uterus that was unable to attract and retain semen, and he also advised the husband to entertain his wife before coitus in such a way that both would engage in the "conjugal act" eagerly, and subsequently the wife should lie still.[871]

The diagnosis of pregnancy was of paramount importance for physicians and other healers.[872] It was known, of course, that menstruation usually ceased during pregnancy; only exceptionally did the menses continue for some time in pregnant women. The absence of menses, however, by no means provided certainty that a woman was pregnant. Like the gradual swelling of the lower abdomen, it was merely one possible indication. Both signs were ambiguous. The "monthly cleansing", which rid the woman every month of the spoiled, putrid blood that collected inside her, could fail to materialize for many reasons; as we have seen, a disordered menstruation was considered one of the principal causes of women's diseases.[873] A growing belly on the other hand was unspecific. One explanation for an increasing abdominal girth, other than pregnancy, was that blood accumulated in and around the uterus when menstruation stopped and caused the lower abdomen to protrude, as with pregnancy. Moreover, with an "obstructed" menstruation the body was observed to rid itself of the accumulating waste matter through vomiting. Thus gestational vomiting, another sign that is considered typical of pregnancy today, became ambiguous as well.

When they were pregnant, women who had given birth before might recognize the subtle changes in their bodies, which experience told them were distinctive. In this sense, Laurent Joubert wrote that he mainly trusted the women who had given birth to many children when they noticed changes in their bellies and breasts. They were experts ("du metier").[874] The typical sign noticed most by women was apparently that their breasts became harder.[875] In his notes, Handsch referred to a discussion about "how to examine the pregnant woman". He thought that one had best feel the mouth of the womb ("os vulvae"). But "the

---

871 Ibid., pp. 266–269, Schweidnitz, 16 October 1579; Horst referred to husband and wife in the third person but the letter was written in German and therefore almost certainly addressed directly to the couple.
872 See Stolberg, Uroscopy (2015), pp. 82–90; Stolberg, Enthüllungen (2020).
873 Stolberg, Erfahrungen (2004).
874 Joubert, Erreurs (1578), p. 281.
875 Cod. 11183, fol. 443r.

women" ("mulieres") had said no, and that you could tell from the breasts.[876] Handsch's sister Apollonia told him that the "puffed-up", plump lips of women also indicated pregnancy.[877] In addition, the medical literature named signs that pointed to a successful conception directly after coitus. When the male semen was retained, that is when it did not flow out, this was seen as an important indication.[878] This was complemented by subjective sensations which suggested that the woman had released her own semen during the act, which played a part in conception, according to Galenic doctrine. To Laurent Joubert we owe an unusually detailed, early, but from today's perspective also somewhat baffling description of how women portrayed their sexual climax: "In this moment, the woman feels a tightening or contraction combined with a small tremble, like a shiver in her depth, in the area of the uterus. It is similar to when we pass water and at the end sometimes feel a little shudder from the contraction of the bladder. The woman also feels a greater cold along her spine than usual."[879]

Women did not usually have the certainty they desired until half-way through their pregnancy, when they could feel the baby move. According to Handsch, one reason why married women wanted to know if they were pregnant again was so that they could start to wean their babies.[880] Moreover, for those who got pregnant unintentionally, an early diagnosis meant that they could find a course of action. Pregnancies out of wedlock were certainly not rare in early modern societies, yet the consequences for women could be grave, and could spell their ruin. They could face dishonoring penalties. Parents or employers might chase them away in disgrace. Life as a married woman and mother of a family was now no longer a possibility for most.[881] If they learned of their pregnancy early enough, women might have a chance to get married in time, or at least they could travel to relatives, where they could hide from view and deliver their child there. Not least of all, they could try to abort their pregnancy by provoking a miscarriage.

By far the most commonly used method to diagnose a pregnancy in its early stages was uroscopy. It also offered the advantage that women did not have to call for the physician or go to him in person, which might not go unnoticed, especially

---

876 Ibid., fol. 23r.
877 Ibid., fol. 243v.
878 Joubert, Erreurs (1578), p. 283.
879 Ibid., p. 283, "a l'instant la fame sant quelque resserremant et contraccion avec petite rigueur, comme frisson au profond, à l'androit de sa matrice: tout ainsi que par fois nous santons a la fin du pisser quelque petite horripilacion, par la contraccion de la vessie. Et mesme du long de l'echine [sic!] la fame sant plus de froid que alheurs."
880 Cod. 11205, fol. 93 and fol. 432v.
881 Labouvie, Andere Umstände (1998).

in smaller communities. It was enough to give one's urine to somebody discreetly, to a maid, a relative, or, in the country, to one of the messengers who regularly took a number of urine flasks from different villagers to a uroscopist.

Numerous entries about uroscopic pregnancy diagnosis can be found in Handsch's notebooks. He himself, he claimed, saw the urine of many women who wanted to know if they were pregnant.[882] Medical treatises on uroscopy described the various "typical" signs that could be found in the urine of pregnant women: a reddish color[883] and minuscule grains, or "atoms", that danced in the liquid like dust particles in oblique sunlight.[884] The latter were, however, not always present, and their absence did not permit one to rule out pregnancy. It was said, by contrast, that almost without fail, the urine of a pregnant woman was cloudy or had a whitish sediment, which indicated a coarse, grainy admixture. When Handsch's sister Anna was pregnant, such cloudy, white sediment was noticeable.[885] The urine of his stepmother as well had a the whitish sediment when she was pregnant.[886]

Medical authors were very much aware that uroscopic pregnancy diagnosis was a rather uncertain affair. They put great emphasis on warning their colleagues not to rely on uroscopy alone, especially when attempting to diagnose a pregnancy. They painted the risk of humiliation if they failed to identify a pregnancy and vice versa of the danger of mistaking a pregnancy for an obstruction of the menses and inadvertently ending it with menstruation-stimulating remedies. Handsch learnt this the hard way when he diagnosed disordered menstruation after examining the urine of a female armor maker. As it turned out, the woman was visibly pregnant and could perfectly feel her baby moving.[887] At the same time, only few physicians doubted that uroscopy could in general be helpful in diagnosing a pregnancy, and even if they did they had good reason not to air their doubts too openly. After all, there were many barbers, barber-surgeons, and lay healers who diagnosed pregnancies from urine, and the population trusted this method. Undoubtedly, women knew from experience that uroscopists could be wrong. But the mistakes of individual uroscopists did not call into question the overall value of uroscopy as a means of diagnosing pregnancy. They only underlined the importance of choosing someone who knew his craft well.

---

882 Cod. 11205, fol. 76v.
883 Paré, Œuvres (1633), p. 687.
884 Cod. 11205, fol. 199v; cf. e.g. Avicenna, Canon (1595), fol. 51v.
885 Cod. 11205, fol. 89v.
886 Ibid.
887 Cod. 11205, fol. 515r.

Occasionally, physicians, women, and relatives also looked to other methods of establishing or ruling out pregnancy. Handsch wrote about the maid of a court official, for example, whose mistress was convinced that she, the maid, was pregnant from a servant. The maid's belly became swollen, yet she denied that she was pregnant. Gallo advised the court official to give the maid a spoonful of fresh honey before she went to bed. If this gave her a bellyache and she sweated, she was pregnant. The maid did have a bad night and sweated – and it turned out that she was indeed pregnant.[888]

During pregnancy the main question was whether bloodletting should be performed or whether, on the contrary, it would be harmful. Considering the widely-recognized importance of the "monthly cleansing" for the woman's health, this question was as central as it was difficult. Some pregnant women asked for bloodletting. Since pregnant women had to do without their habitual "monthly cleansing", it must have seemed obvious to them that they risked accumulating a large quantity of impurities, acrimonies, or other pathogenic matter, from which her body should be freed.[889] On the other hand, the woman might be weakened and the fetus deprived of the nutritious blood it needed to grown. When Handsch was called to a woman who was well advanced in her pregnancy, he was therefore unsure. His teacher Lehner, however, explained to him that the Hippocratic aphorism that advised the greatest reserve in this regard was not to be understood as an absolute prohibition. And indeed, Handsch's notes include the express recommendation of his Paduan professor Fracanzano as well as of Amatus Lusitanus that bloodletting be performed on pregnant women in certain cases. Not least of all, Lehner's own wife was bled once during pregnancy and she subsequently gave birth easily.[890]

Bloodletting furthermore was considered an important preventive against a looming miscarriage or premature birth. The best explanation for a miscarriage often seemed to be that the pregnant woman's body discharged blood or other superfluous humors via the uterus and in a sense washed out the growing baby in the process. Consequently, it made sense to counter this risk by providing an alternative excretory pathway. On other hand, one accepted cause of miscarriage was an insufficient supply of nutrition to the child. In the case of Andrea Gallo's wife. Handsch suggested that one reason for the *abortus* she suffered was that she had frequent nosebleeds during the pregnancy which deprived the child of the necessary nutrition.[891]

---

[888] Cod. 11183, fol. 342r: "De melle ad explorandam impraegnationem".
[889] Ibid., fol. 383v.
[890] Cod. 11205, fol. 10v.
[891] Ibid., fol. 191v.

Birth and Childbed

Obstetrics in the narrower sense of providing assistance at birth was taught increasingly at universities in the sixteenth century. In Padua, Handsch heard Fracanzano discuss at great length the causes of a difficult birth and the best ways of dealing with it. Among the causes on the maternal side, the affects played an important role. The consolation and assistance of female bystanders who had given birth many times themselves was therefore helpful to calm the worried mind. Fear was described as a serious impediment to the birth process. It led to the vital heat becoming concentrated around the heart rather than reaching the uterus, where it was needed to move the birth process along. Similarly, the presence of people who made the delivering woman feel shame caused the blood and vital spirits to flow to body parts other than the uterus. Pain as well could slow down the birth, especially with first-time mothers, as the woman compressed the vital spirits instead of driving it toward the uterus. If a woman was feeling generally weak, this could further add to a difficult birth. A woman who had just overcome an illness did not give birth very easily. Also, the birth canal itself could be constricted or blocked, for example due to inflammation, or from a bladder stone or hardened feces in the adjacent bowels. With very corpulent women, the fat could press on the mouth of the uterus and thus keep it from opening sufficiently.[892]

To make delivery easier, Handsch learnt, physicians were to tell women to lie on their backs and/or stand up, climb stairs or walk. According to Aristotle, it was also conducive to have intercourse in the ninth month because this would tear the "ligaments". Further, baths or at least sponge baths with a moisturizing herbal decoction were said to help relaxation when the time of birth was near. To make expelling the baby easier, the Hippocratic writings recommended that the birthing woman sneeze and exert pressure while she held her breath. It was therefore wrong, Fracanzano explained, that women were told by midwives not to scream. On the contrary, they should scream as much as they could.

One could strengthen birthing mothers by giving them Malvasia wine. And if they fainted, strong smells like that of vinegar would bring them around. If the waters flowed at first but then dried up again, almond oil could be administered. Fracanzano had done that successfully with a relative of his in Vicenza.[893] There were various remedies, which either stimulated or relaxed the uterus as necessary. The woman could also could hold a magnet in her left

---

892 Cod. 11226, fol. 116r.
893 Ibid.

hand or, as was widely practiced, tie an eagle stone (aetites) to her thigh. They would make birthing easier thanks to some *proprietas occulta*.

In other cases, the reasons for difficulties during the birth process were in the child. The unborn child was expected to play an active role. Weak children did not help tear the "ligaments" once the nutrition they were receiving was insufficient. The child might also be too small to free itself. In such cases, the midwives helped out using their nails. On the other hand, it was difficult to push out overly large or malformed children. If the child was in a preternatural position and its hand came out first, for example, the midwife had to put a lot of grease on her arms and attempt to reposition it. This was very dangerous, however, especially if the midwife lacked experience.

Turning to external factors, cold air above all was harmful, according to Fracanzano, as it caused the birth canal to close. For this reason, giving birth in the winter was more difficult. Yet, excessive heat was disadvantageous as well. When women moved too much because they got impatient, the child would not come out with its head first, as intended by nature. And women giving birth should by no means fall asleep, even if they were exhausted from the pain. If a midwife noticed that a birthing mother was asleep, she was to wake the woman up.

As we see from Handsch's notes, students of medicine in Padua as early as 1550 could thus acquire quite a comprehensive and detailed knowledge of obstetrics. It came in large part from the older literature but was also based on knowledge of common practice and, in some cases, on the personal experience of the professor. The future physicians were not very likely to apply their knowledge directly on their own patients. Women who were about to give birth sought advice and help almost exclusively from midwives and other women. Male healers were called in only if necessary, when the mother or the child in the womb had died and a surgical intervention was required. In those cases, usually a barber-surgeon took over. Among the 8,000 consultations recorded by Hiob Finzel, only three had to do with a "difficult birth", two of which were for the same woman in two consecutive years, a woman who belonged to one of the most noble families in the area.[894] What is even more striking is that there is no evidence that he assisted personally with any birth whatsoever. In Handsch notes there is no mention either, anywhere, that he or one of his colleagues were actively involved with a delivery. He was not even present at deliveries that took place in his own family circle. It is possible that Handsch was at a disadvantage here compared to his many married

---

[894] Ratschulbibliothek Zwickau Ms. QQQQ 1b, December 1573 and December 1574 (Frau von Planitz) and January 1574 (the wife of Bartholomaeus Schmid).

colleagues, but there are no sources that indicate that other physicians gave their own wives or daughters obstetric assistance.[895]

And yet, Handsch not only took detailed notes on Fracanzano's lectures. He continued to write notes about obstetrics even after he had finished his studies, giving us valuable insights into the everyday obstetric practice of that time. He must have had his reasons. Probably he wanted to be able to answer questions, give advice to female patients, and if necessary instruct midwives.

Handsch gained this practical knowledge about obstetrical matters almost exclusively from women, especially from those in his own family and sometimes from midwives. He wrote down various remedies, which, in the experience of the women and the midwives, helped with birthing. They were not to be given too early, not before the water had broken.[896] Among his recipes there is one for "linseed oil for delivery".[897] From his mentor Andrea Gallo, Handsch learned that women would drink ordinary oil in the days before giving birth for its "relaxing effects".[898] The countess of Thurn told him that she boiled immature roses in wine around the time of the delivery and drank the decoction. Twice already, she had experienced how this had successfully expelled the child.[899] During a difficult birth, women liked to take a warm bath. Handsch's stepmother and his landlady both helped themselves in this way, and the landlady even delivered in the bathtub.[900] Cold, and especially cold feet, by contrast, were considered unfavorable, perhaps because this was thought to indicate or cause a decreased influx of vital spirits.[901] Handsch also took seriously means that tended to be seen as belonging to magic, even back then. For example, he wrote about the beneficial effect of the so-called "Hasensprincken", a small bone at the knee of a hare, which resembles a kneecap. What counted for him, evidently, were once again the good experiences that women told him about.[902] Handsch also heard that, after giving birth, women drank Malvasia wine mixed with oil.[903]

The women in Handsch's circles also taught him how to care for newborns. He learned from his sister Apollonia how to keep the child's blood loss from the

---

895 The prescription diary of the Dutch physician Cornelis Booth from the first half of the seventeenth century (Universiteitsbiblioteek Utrecht, ms. VII E 49) documents his medical treatment of his two wives and of other female relatives in times of pregnancy.
896 Cod. 11183, fol. 287r.
897 Ibid., fol. 135r, "oleum lini ad partum".
898 Cod. 11205, fol. 143(a)r.
899 Ibid., fol. 166r.
900 Ibid., fol. 119v and foll. 286v-287r.
901 Cod. 11183, fol. 206v.
902 Cod. 11205, fol. 411r.
903 Cod. 11183, fol. 287r.

umbilical cord to a minimum: one had to push the blood in the umbilical cord toward the child, tie the umbilical cord, and cut it off.[904] His little niece Catharina had lost blood unnecessarily because the midwife had not tied off the umbilical cord properly.[905] Handsch noted down that, on the day after delivery, the women gave honey to the newborn to suck on, "so that it cleans itself".[906]

He also learned that midwives had various means at their disposal to waken and strengthen the newborn's vital spirits if necessary. When the wife of Hans Georg Welser at Ambras delivered her daughter after about ten hours of labor, the child seemed almost lifeless. But, as Handsch wrote, the "prudent midwife" ("prudens obstetrix") immediately opened the little girl's mouth and her color soon improved.[907] He wrote about such practices in more detail when Mattioli's wife gave birth. She, too, had a difficult delivery and the child, a son, appeared to be close to dying; he was pale and his body looked white. One of the women present, he learnt, then spat a mouthful of Malvasia wine on the child and went on to sprinkle him repeatedly with warm Malvasia and other wine. In addition, they held various strong smelling, chewed substances such as cinnamon, cloves, and garlic to his nose. The child's color soon improved and he survived.[908] Sometimes, however, all help came too late. According to Handsch's account, the wife of the apothecary Achatius also had a difficult birth. An arm was the first part of the baby's body to leave the uterus. The birthing mother was given an expelling remedy but ultimately the dead child had to be pulled out with force.[909]

When they had given birth, women tended worry that the *membrana secundina,* that is the placenta, might not be expelled completely. Hiob Finzel made notes in his practice journal about three women who had recently given birth – two from the nobility – who sought his advice because they feared that the placenta or parts of it had remained in their abdomens.[910] When Handsch's landlady delivered a son but the placenta would not follow, Mattioli advised a fumigation with leaves of the savin juniper (Juniperus sabina); to everyone's surprise, she then gave birth to a second son – a twin brother.[911] When Gallo's wife was going to deliver, the midwife explained to Handsch that one should keep an onion handy so that it could be held to the nose of the birthing mother after the child

---

904 Ibid., fol. 264r.
905 Cod. 11205, fol. 117v.
906 Cod. 11183, foll. 206v-207r.
907 Ibid., fol. 387r.
908 Cod. 11205, fol. 339v.
909 Cod. 11183, fol. 402r.
910 Ratschulbibliothek Zwickau, Ms. QQQQ 1, Ms. QQQQ 1a and Ms. QQQQ 1b.
911 Cod. 11205, fol. 287r.

was delivered and the placenta was to come next; this would prevent the uterus from moving upward. As in the treatment of suffocation of the womb, the sharp smell of the onion was apparently meant to drive the uterus, and with it the placenta, downward. The same idea presumably was behind the practice of holding strong-smelling camphor to the mother's nose following delivery.[912]

The postpartum period was taken to last (up to) six weeks. The term "Wochenbett", which is still used for the childbed in modern German, derives from the premodern term "Sechswochenbett" or "six-weeks-bed". Accordingly the puerperant woman was referred to as "Sechswocherin", a "six-weeker".[913] Some physicians went for a somewhat shorter time. Willenbroch held that the cleansing via the uterus following birth took about three to four weeks, and according to Fracanzano, the period was around thirty days.[914]

Childbed was widely feared as a time of danger. As the woman had to go without menstruation during her pregnancy, she was especially in need of a cleansing afterwards, to rid herself of all the accumulated waste matter. "A lot of filth issues from women during these days", Handsch noted down.[915] In this sense, the physicians spoke of the "menstrua" of women who had recently given birth.[916] The patients shared the same conviction. Finzel made entries about several female patients who sought his advice on account of their insufficient lochia.[917] The concern that the heating effect of wine might promote fevers was likely behind the idea that women in childbed should not – as was common practice in many regions – drink wine during the first eight or fourteen days after giving birth.[918] If in some cases the "menses" – this term, too, referred to lochia here – were too plentiful, Fracanzano's approach was to redirect them to the breasts using cupping. The administration of astringent remedies, however, had to be monitored carefully so as not to stop the flow.[919]

A number of tried and tested practices were directed at the newborn. According to Handsch, many women wiped the face of the newborn child with

---

912 Ibid., fol. 150v.
913 Cod. 11226, fol. 117r; Cod. 11205, fol. 423v.
914 Cod. 11183, fol. 462r.
915 Cod. 11205, fol. 100v.
916 Ibid., fol. 436v.
917 Ratschulbibliothek Zwickau, Ms. QQQQ 1, Ms. QQQQ 1a and Ms. QQQQ 1b; e.g. the wives of Michael Gebauer ("retentu sanguine post partum", November 1569) and of Balthasar Gebert ("impeditus fluxus post partum", December 1570).
918 Cod. 11183, fol. 355v.
919 Cod. 11226, fol. 117v.

menstrual blood to protect it against birthmarks and other ugly skin changes.[920] In Leipa, Handsch was told that infants often fell ill when their wet nurse was angry and then drank something, because this caused her blood to surge and her milk to change.[921]

Infant nutrition was another important issue. Physicians generally were in favor of infants being nursed by their mothers. Sometimes there were problems, however. Women knew what to do when their breasts began to hurt. When Handsch's sister Anna felt pain in her breasts and thought she was pregnant, her mother said that this kind of pain in the breast was not typical of early pregnancy. Rather, it came from withheld milk. Handsch advised her to drink fennel-infused water, but his stepmother warned him that this would only promote lactation and make matters worse. She thought it was better for Anna to take a bath. She herself had sometimes felt breast pain after giving birth and had successfully treated it with hemlock or by using a cupping glass to suck the milk out.[922] And there were other women who used glasses to pump excessive, pain-causing milk from their breasts.[923] Another method was to get puppies to latch on instead, as in the case of Hans Georg Welser's wife.[924]

There were times, especially if a woman in childbed was ill, when the women and physicians agreed that it would be better to take a break from nursing. Ideally, a wet nurse was on hand to breastfeed the infant. A *proba lactis* could be performed to determine whether milk was sufficiently nutritious: milk taken from the wet nurse's breasts was left to sit in a bowl for a while. If a layer of white "cream" ("Römle") formed on the surface, it meant that the milk was not too watery.[925] If no suitable wet nurse could be found, families made do with almond milk, which the child sucked from a cloth.[926]

---

[920] Cod. 11251, fol. 48v.
[921] Cod. 11183, fol. 240v.
[922] Cod. 11205, foll. 103v-104r.
[923] Ibid., fol. 577v.
[924] Cod. 11183, fol. 387r; see also ibid., fol. 462r.
[925] Ibid., fol. 287r.
[926] Ibid., foll. 206v-207r.

Knowledge from Experience: The Rise of Empiricism

A central foundation of the self-image and self-representation of sixteenth-century physicians continued to be their profound knowledge of the works of both ancient and – increasingly – more recent medical authorities. Even in Padua, Bologna, and Montpellier, where practical training had a particularly prominent place, the curriculum was devoted above all to reading and commenting on the Galenic and Hippocratic texts and on Avicenna's *Canon medicinae*. Numerous later entries in Handsch's notebooks illustrate that physicians in their everyday practice consistently took recourse to these writings when dealing with diagnostic, prognostic, and therapeutic questions, and treated them as the definitive authority when an issue was under dispute. Handsch's notes show that a physician could be expected to know numerous passages by rote, even on very specific issues, and to put them to good use at the sickbed. They prided themselves of their detailed knowledge of the authoritative texts and sought to surpass each other. At one point, Handsch lost a jug of wine because he was not prepared to believe that, according to the Hippocratic aphorisms, melancholy and frenzy tended to occur in the springtime, in spite of the fact that spring was considered an especially healthy time of year.[1]

Beginning in the late fifteenth century, however, the authoritative books were increasingly accompanied by another book: the "book of nature". Empirical approaches acquired greater significance.[2] In the history of science and the history of medicine, the esteem for empirical knowledge that burgeoned during this period has been thoroughly researched and appreciated with respect to anatomy and botany above all. Coming from anatomy, "autopsia", or seeing for oneself, became a central epistemological ideal. In botany, a major reason for relying on empirical knowledge came from the fact that the new, exotic plants from Asia and America and even many plants from central and northern Europa did not find mention in the works of the ancient authorities. Public controversies about who could claim to be the first who discovered or describeed a new anatomical structure or a new plant became a common phenomenon.

By contrast, historians have devoted far less attention to the role of practical medicine in the rise of empirical approaches than it deserves. I would argue that medical practice was at least as important as a major driving force behind this development. Admittedly, in hindsight, unlike with anatomy and botany –

---

[1] Cod. 11207, fol. 181v; cf. book 3, aph. 20, in Hippocrates, Aphorismi (1538), p. 127.
[2] Very useful overview in Wear, Medicine (1995).

Open Access. © 2022 Michael Stolberg, published by De Gruyter. This work is licensed under the Creative Commons Attribution-NonCommercial-NoDerivatives 4.0 International License.
https://doi.org/10.1515/9783110733549-013

and this is certainly the principal reason for the meager historical attention – there were hardly any new discoveries in practical medicine at the time which are today thought to still hold water in medicine.[3] Such a retrospective judgement, however, does not come close to doing justice to the perception of the physicians of the period. They were convinced that, precise empirical observation at the sickbed would lead to important new insights and would help them to gain an ever firmer grasp on the disease process and to treat patients more successfully.[4]

Several developments impelled medicine in general toward the acquisition of knowledge through observation. Front and center here was the transformation of natural history, which took place over a long period of time and which was also largely responsible for advancing this development in botany and anatomy. Beginning in the late Middle Ages, the "particulars", the knowledge of the individual things of nature, their characteristics and faculties as compared to the "universals", increasingly garnered attention.[5]

Although things might seem otherwise at first glance, medical humanism, too, fostered empirical tendencies in its own way. Historians have often largely reduced medical humanism to a philological endeavor, to the point of declaring the philological work of humanism an end in itself. And, more than anything, they have highlighted the humanist disparagement of the (Latin translations of the) works of Arabic authors. This view does not fully do justice to the motives of the medical humanists, however. The reconstruction of the authentic teachings of ancient authors was not an end in itself. Rather, from the point of view of the humanists, the ancient medical works embodied experience that had proven true and valid over centuries of medical practice. Giving new life to the legacy of ancient medicine in its original form was therefore of great practical interest. The aim was to "practise medicine in the manner of the ancient physicians", as Jerome Bylebyl wrote about Giovanni Battista da Monte, and thus to place medicine on a new foundation.[6] Some Hippocratic works especially, above all the *Aphorisms* and the *Epidemics*, presented themselves to the reader as empirical accounts or at least as collections of individual insights that were gained from experience.

---

3 See e.g. the somewhat anachronistic assessment by Oberrauch (Oberrauch, Medizin (2012), p. 362) who claims that there were no substantial developments in sixteenth-century medicine, due above all to the slow progress in anatomy.
4 Stolberg, Empiricism (2013).
5 Park, Observations (2011); see also Premuda, Discepolo (1963); for an overview of the later developments see Ben-Chaim, Experimental philosophy (2004).
6 Bylebyl, School of Padua (1979), p. 341.

And even in Galen, the physicians found case histories here and there. These case histories flagrantly served his self-adulation and were intended to serve as proof of his diagnostic acumen and his superior curative abilities. Nevertheless, they were considered valuable in the sixteenth century, so much so that they were collected and published as a model for modern medical practice.[7]

Furthermore, in medical lay culture experience was valued highly and physicians grew up within this culture, were socialized into it throughout their childhood and youth, before they embarked on their academic studies. Laypeople's use of medicinal herbs and even their trust in healing charms and other magical-sympathetic cures, were founded on experience, on the observation that the sick got better. In early modern vernacular collections of recipes, we regularly find expressions such as "tried and tested" or in Latin "probatum est" at the end of the recipes, sometimes even including the place and time of the successful application.[8]

A last factor, finally, which may well even have contributed decisively to the empirical turn, is more difficult to pin down. Since the fifteenth century, the number of learned physicians began to rise dramatically, and for many of them, medical practice was their principal source of income. And they found that the most important means by far to acquire esteem and authority and attract patients was not bookish learning but successful cures. Physicians made use of numerous remedies whose effects could not be – or could only very indirectly be – traced to the specific mixture of the primary qualities (cold, hot, dry, and wet) and to the secondary qualities derived from these such as "softening" and "purgative". Rather, these remedies were characterized by specific effects on certain complaints and diseases or they at least appeared to be capable of targeting particular humors or types of morbid matter and attracting and voiding them. Such specific faculties could not be explained rationally based on the perception of a dominant cold or wet quality for example. They could only be inferred from the observation of their effects on the patient.

Even Galen, who was very critical of physicians who wanted to base their medicine on experience alone, relied heavily on empirical observation when choosing medications.[9] As Handsch gleaned from his reading of Galen, "Experience is the most reliable judge of the faculties inherent in medications".[10] The

---

[7] Champier, Historiales campi (1532).
[8] E.g. Staatsbibliothek Berlin, Hdschr. 442, recipe book from the late sixteenth century, on an eye ointment that had proven helpful in Austria and Hungary, in 1575.
[9] Debru, Galen (2000), p. 625.
[10] Cod. 11239, fol. 29r: "Experientia est certissima iudicatrix facultatum quae medicamentis insunt."

scholastic physicians of the Middle Ages had accepted this to a degree. Toxic effects, for example, as Handsch learned when reading Pietro d'Abano (1250/ 57–1316), could not always be attributed to a peculiar mixture of primary qualities. Similarly, the successful application of strong antidotes such as St. John's wort (hypericum) and swallowwort (vincetoxicum) could not be explained by the mixture of elementary qualities. It was owed, rather, to their inherent specific faculties or to astral influences.[11]

Empirica, Experimenta, and Secret Remedies

In the sixteenth century, learned medicine widely recognized the significance of specific faculties of many remedies that could only be apprehended by observing the effects on patients. Knowing the characteristic mixture of primary qualities of each medicinal plant remained indispensable but the specific effects on different diseases were widely ascribed to occult (in the literal sense of hidden), supraelemenary powers.[12] A well-known example was peony, which had long been appreciated as an effective remedy for epilepsy, among other things. Some animal-derived substances, too, were believed to have a *proprietas specifica*. Johannes Willenbroch, for example, thought that freshly killed and halved doves, placed on the heads of the mad ("phrenetici"), had a specific effect.[13] In Padua, Handsch experienced how, after a dissection, his fellow students scrambled to get their hands on the fat of the dissected corpse, which was appreciated for its therapeutic effects.[14]

A second essential element was also at work. Physicians often relied on more than the effect of just one medicinal plant. They used formulas, mixtures of different healing plants which they devised themselves or took from the literature or learned from colleagues. Before even setting up their own practice, medical students eagerly noted down the "tried and tested" remedies their professors shared with them. Many of such recipes can be found in Handsch's student notes. The notes taken by one or several students of Antonio Musa Brasavola, who accompanied his (or their) professors on sick visits in Ferrara, mainly recorded the mixtures of drugs they prescribed.[15] As a student in Padua, Johannes Brünsterer assembled

---

11 Cod. 11240, foll. 74r-81r, here fol. 76r and fol. 81r.
12 Richardson, Generation (1985).
13 Cod. 11183, fol. 182v.
14 Cod. 11210, fol. 191v, "scholares raptim abscindebant pinguedinem ad medicationes profuturam."
15 Biblioteca Ariostea, Ferrara, Collezione Antonelli, Ms. 531.

close to fifteen pages with notes on different mixtures of medications under the heading "Empirica quaedam".[16]

The great appreciation physicians had for tried and tested recipes as well as the overarching significance of these recipes in everyday practice is reflected by the extensive collections of *experimenta* which physicians compiled for their personal use. "Experimenta" must not be misunderstood as "experiments" in the present-day sense. At the time, it was the common term for "tried and tested" or "proven" medicines. Even before he started his medical studies, Handsch as an assistant of Ulrich Lehner in Prague began to collect in an *Antidotariolus* formulas which he received from Lehner and other physicians or which he found in books.[17] Included here were secret remedies such as the "electuarium secretum" of a certain Ludovicus, which was to protect against asthma, the "mirabile secretum" of a Mantuan physician named Calderano, and recipes for mixtures of drugs that referred in their names to the physicians or healers who created them, such as an "unguentum magistri Galeacii", a "confectio magistri Fontani", and an "electuarium magistri Antonii". Whole sections of Handsch's notebooks are devoted to the "experimenta et secreta" of a particular physician. As an addition to his notes from his time with Lehner, Handsch would later compile a further substantial volume with *experimenta*.[18] When Handsch was treating patients, he drew from his collection of recipes. Again and again, he turned to the *experimenta* of other physicians, for example to Johann Neefe's laxative syrup.[19] Handsch even used the plague powder of a certain "Dominus Venceslaus" on himself, and, during the great plague epidemic, he left some for his brother and his brother's family, all of whom, it appeared, remained healthy as a result.[20]

Handsch and the physicians he worked with were not shy either about their use of the collection of "empirical" drugs which Benedetto Vittore published in 1551.[21] Mattioli praised Vittore's anti-paralysis pills, among other things.[22] Gallo took Vittore's book with him when he visited a noble patient.[23] Even the remedies of non-academic healers and laypeople earned the attention of the physicians

---

16 Universitätsbibliothek, Erlangen, Ms. 911, foll. 307–322.
17 Cod. 11200: "Antidotariolus. Formulae medicamentorum aliquot. Georgius Handschius Lippensis. Pragae 1549."
18 Cod. 11251: "Experimenta quaedam brevia comparatu facilia vulgaria probata excerpta passim ab authoribus et secretis aliorum medicorum".
19 E.g. Cod. 11183, fol. 275r and fol. 458v.
20 Cod. 11200, fol. 30r and fol. 31r.
21 E.g. Cod. 11183, fol. 314v, on Dr. Merla; ibid., fol. 479r; Cod. 11207, fol. 89v, on Gallo's praise for Vittore's oil against dropsy; cf. Vittore, Medicatio empirica (1551).
22 Cod. 11183, fol. 479r.
23 Cod. 11207, fol. 224r.

if they seemed to prove their worth in practice. One treatment Handsch took note of was administering a decoction of horse manure to combat jaundice.[24] And he heard from an old farmer that a drink made with boiled hazelwort (asarum) would drive away "das Kalte", that is the "cold" fever.[25]

With the help of their *experimenta*, physicians stood a chance of achieving superior curative results, which would make them stand out among their peers, allow them to win the trust of wealthy and noble patients, and perhaps even secure them a position as the personal physician to a prince or king. Handsch praised one of the *secreta* he had noted down, adding that with its help he had "attained glory and money quite a number of times".[26] For good reasons, any self-respecting physician developed his own specific mixtures of drugs and secret remedies. Gallo, for example, had allegedly saved numerous people from the plague with a *secretum*.[27] Tremenus had a *secretum*, which he often applied to the stomach area.[28] According to Handsch, the *unguentum mirabile*, which Mattioli "invented" ("ex inventione [. . .] Mattheoli") quickly healed all fresh wounds.[29] And Mattioli claimed that he had healed many cold fevers with another remedy, which he shared with Handsch "pro secreto".[30]

Physicians who possessed powerful secret remedies could even hope to turn them into an important source of financial profit. Handsch wrote that Lehner was so intent on keeping secret the formula for an electuary he had developed that he had the ingredients produced by three different apothecaries. He asked a lot for the remedy, charging twelve large silver coins for an ounce of it.[31] Others sold the formula for their *secretum* for a steep price. From a certain Hans Kochmüller – he was clearly not a physician – Handsch received the recipe for a remedy against wounds for which Kochmüller's employer, a knight, had allegedly paid eighteen

---

24 Cod. 11183, fol. 381v.
25 Cod. 11205, fol. 413v; on the medicinal use of hazelwort since antiquity see Marzell, Haselwurz (1958).
26 Cod. 11200, fol. 4r.
27 Ibid., fol. 25r; see also the "Experimenta et secreta Doct. Gerhardi Medici Archiducis Ferdinandi", which include a "secretum expertum ad ischiatiken" (ibid., fol. 142v); Cod. 11006, fol. 181r: "Ad gibbum secretum doctoris Petri regii medici". On the rich early modern semantics of the term *secretum*, which could refer to manifold forms of secret knowledge as well as to very concrete instructions on how to make certain medicines and other substances see Eamon, Science (1994) and Eamon, How to read (2011).
28 Cod. 11006, fol. 3r.
29 Ibid., fol. 1v.
30 Cod. 11183, fol. 115v.
31 Cod. 11200, fol. 162r.

gold gulden.³² Handsch also heard that a buyer paid sixty gulden for the recipe for an electuary against all kinds of poison; it was said that it had proven effective against the plague.³³ And one Paduan physician purportedly even earned several thousand gulden with pills that supposedly protected against the plague for an entire month.³⁴

Not all "secret remedies" were kept secret. On the contrary, they were often passed on to students and colleagues without remuneration.³⁵ Speaking to his students, Willenbroch praised pills made with hound's tongue (cynoglossum) as a "secretum" that alleviated pain at night and encouraged evacuation in the morning.³⁶ Mattioli told Handsch "pro secreto" that the seeds and leaves of stinging nettle worked like magic to stop bleeding, as he had often seen himself with head wounds.³⁷ Numerous *secreta* were even published in print. Then, of course, they no longer gave their inventors and an initiated few an edge over the competition. By sharing proven *secreta*, however, the inventor was able to present himself as selfless, and he could also expect that his colleagues would reciprocate by passing on their own proven secret recipes. Ideally, the name of the remedy would remain tied to his own name and bolster his reputation. In the recipe books of laypeople, we find numerous formulas for remedies that were passed on under the name of the physician who (supposedly) invented them.

Paracelsianism and Chymical Medicines

Handsch's working life as a physician happened to unfold during a time when the teachings of Paracelsus (1493–1541) were finding increasing reception.³⁸ Of Paracelsus's major works, only his treatise on the French disease and his *Grosse Wundartzney* (Great Surgery) were in print during his lifetime, along with a series

---

32 Cod. 11251, fol 18r.
33 Cod. 11200, fol. 187r.
34 Cod. 11205, fol. 20v.
35 Cod. 11006, fol. 183v, on a proven secret remedy Alvise Bellicato in Padua gave away in his lecture ("in lectione pro experto secreto traditum").
36 Cod. 11183, fol. 486v.
37 Cod. 11207, fol. 146v.
38 The literature on Paracelsus and Paracelsianism is vast. The studies of Karl Sudhoff (esp. Sudhoff, Versuch (1898/99)) remain indispensable. Among the important more recent works are Pagel, Weltbild (1962), Grell, Paracelsus (1998); Williams/Gunnoe, Paracelsian moments (2002); Webster, Paracelsus (2008).

of astrological *prognostica*.[39] In the 1560s and 1570s, however, Alexander von Suchten, Adam von Bodenstein, Michael Toxites, Gerhard Dorn, and other proponents of a "new medicine" began to collect and publish the unpublished works, and to actively spread the word about his teachings. A notable number of medical professionals, but also princes[40] and other laypeople, began to take an interest in the Paracelsian teachings and especially in Paracelsian remedies.[41] As early as 1563, the physician and mathematician Georg Joachim Rheticus, who was himself very interested in alchemy, told the Nuremberg physician Joachim Camerarius from Cracow that he saw a burgeoning new school in Germany whose originator was Paracelsus.[42]

The Paracelsians presented their medicine as something fundamentally new, as a radical departure from traditional medicine as taught at the universities. They accused the proponents of such medicine of slavishly adhering to the words of Hippocrates, Galen, and Avicenna. For their part, the proponents of the Galenic-Hippocratic tradition countered such accusations with fierce criticism. In the early 1570s, Thomas Erastus made a move to settle the score, publishing his extensive and widely-read *Disputationes de medicina nova Philippi Paracelsi*.[43] Much of the scholarship and historiography of Paracelsus has foregrounded these tensions and in some cases adopted the self-presentation of the Paracelsians as the sole proponents of a new, empirically-based medicine who – finally! – were opposing the dusty book-knowledge of the Galenics, paving the way to a brighter future.[44] Thus Paracelsians and anti-Paracelsians have been presented as two warring camps and the attempt has been made to classify physicians who were active at the time as belonging to one or the other. In particular, efforts have been made to identify adherents of Paracelsus in order to map out his growing influence. Often no more than a certain knowledge of Paracelsian ideas or a simple interest in alchemy and distillation has been taken as proof of Paracelsian tendencies or even discipleship.

---

39 Paracelsus, Von der frantzösischen Kranckheit (1530); Paracelsus, Grosse Wundartzney (1536).
40 Trevor-Roper, Court physician (1990).
41 For a very useful introduction especially into early Paracelsianism, with an extensive bibliography see the editors' introduction to Kühlmann/Telle, Frühparacelsismus (2001), pp. 1–39.
42 Letter from Rheticus, 1 February 1563, ed. in Kühlmann/Telle, Frühparacelsismus (2001), pp. 77–78: "In Germania novam sectam pullulare video, auctore Theophrasteo Paracelso." At the time, the term "sect" ("secta") which is used primarily in religious contexts today, was taken, in particular, to refer to different philosophical schools like the Stoa and the Aristotelians.
43 Erastus, De medicina nova (1572/73); Karcher, Erastus (1957); Gunnoe, Erastus (1994).
44 On the meaning of "experience" in Paracelsus' works see Bianchi, Il tema (2002).

Looking at the writings of the self-proclaimed Paracelsians and the rebuttals of some of their opponents can indeed create the impression of two hostile and irreconcilable parties standing opposite each other across a deep divide. Taking this perspective comes with a danger of obscuring the many intermediate positions, however, especially when looking at the early days of Paracelsianism. Physicians with a Galenic orientation exhibited at times a selective openness to Paracelsian innovations, especially to the "chymical" remedies that were endorsed by the Paracelsians and which even then looked back on a centuries-old alchemical tradition. In recent times, authors such as Wilhelm Kühlmann, Joachim Telle, and Tilmann Walter have found significantly more nuance and complexity than is conveyed by the traditional dichotomous image.[45]

Yet, historical research continues to rely in large part on Paracelsian texts and on public polemics, and therefore on sources that tend to bring antagonisms into focus. So far, there has been a dearth of substantial studies on the reception and application of Paracelsian concepts and remedies in the practice of physicians who stood in the Galenic tradition. Handsch's notes only give insight into the world of a limited number of physicians working in the milieu of the Habsburg courts in Prague and Innsbruck. Nevertheless, they are illuminating. Even within this relatively small world, there were different positions and on the whole a remarkable openness for certain aspects of Paracelsian teaching and practice.

Georg Handsch himself has played a modest role in the historiography of Paracelsianism. Kühlmann and Telle, following Karl Sudhoff, have seen in him evidence of an "alchemo-Paracelsianism" in the court of Archduke Ferdinand.[46] Their

---

45 Kühlmann/Telle, Frühparacelsismus (2001); Walter, New light (2012).
46 Kühlmann/Telle, Frühparacelsismus (2001), pp. 457–459; the two found further evidenc for the Archduke's alchemo-Paracelsianism in his employment as court physicians of Mattioli, who, they claim, shared the aims of an "alchemia medica" (ibid., p. 457), and of Johann Willenbroch. They also point to a request of the Tyrolean government, in 1563, that the Carinthian estates procure various Paracelsian manuscripts; it is not clear, however, whether Ferdinand himself or one of his officials was behind this request. Handsch's notebooks do offer two other remarkable pieces of evidence, which Kühlmann and Telle did not know. They mention a "senex alcumista" (Cod. 11183, fol. 354r), who was called to the bed of the dying daughter of Frau von Loxan at the court in Ambras (he only prescribed some herbal remedies against putrefaction, however), and in another entry Handsch quoted under the heading "alcumistica" a certain "old Mathias" ("senex Mathias"), possibly referring to the same man (Cod. 11205, fol. 222v).

sources are two manuscripts by Handsch that include "Paracelsian material" in the Nationalbibliothek in Vienna,[47] as well as a manuscript with Handsch's "Medicinalia" in the Wellcome Library in London.[48]

Upon closer inspection, the London manuscript presented by Kühlmann and Telle proves to be unsuitable as evidence. It only contains, in a foreign hand and amidst numerous other "chemical" recipes, a brief instruction for the production of medical antimony which is signed (again in a foreign hand) with "Gregorius Handschius medicus Pragensis A° 1556". Handsch never used the first name Gregor (rather than Georg).[49] It therefore appears that he was merely quoted here for a little less than two pages.[50] By contrast, the Vienna manuscripts presented by Kühlmann and Telle – as well as other notebooks by Handsch – do contain several references to "chymic" medicines, indeed even lecture notes[51] as well as excerpts from the writings of Paracelsus about the French disease and from his work about the miners' sickness.[52] They clearly document Handsch's interest.

In printed works, taking a distinct position and setting oneself off from divergent conceptions and practices of other authors, necessarily played a salient role and was not infrequently the very reason for a publication. As opposed to this, Handsch's notes show in their openness above all, in their forgoing of a blanket devaluation or repudiation, just how blurred the boundaries were between the proponents and opponents of Paracelsian teachings. The fiery, often polemical debates found in printed works hardly find expression in Handsch's notes. In everyday medical practice, it turns out, the opposition was far less pointed than the polemical writings of Adam von Bodenstein or Thomas Erastus would have us believe, as would the historiography on Paracelsianism that followed. Clearly we must not consider physicians of the period to have been Paracelsian just on the basis of some Paracelsian or alchemical passages they penned.

---

47 Cod. 11200 and Cod. 11206.
48 Wellcome Library, London, Western Manuscripts 330.
49 Ibid., foll. 18v-19r.
50 In his commentary on Dioscorides, Mattioli mentioned a recipe for antimony that he had from Handsch and reported about Handsch's positive experiences with taking antimony in times of plague (Mattioli, Commentarii (1565), p. 1348). Presumably thanks to Mattioli, Handsch was still quoted (as "Giorgio Hendschio") around 1650 in testimony of the beneficial effects of antimony against the plague (Serpetro, Mercato (1653), p. 162).
51 Cod. 11205, fol. 130r, "in Paracelso", on a solution of antimony; ibid., fol. 151v, "dicit Theophrastus", on the blood cleansing effects of antimony.
52 Cod. 11206, foll. 134r-143r, excerpts from "Von der französischen Kranckheit", Nürnberg 1552; some further notes follow under the heading "Ex libello de ligno Guaiaco" (ibid., foll. 143r-144r).

As can be concluded from Handsch's notes, Handsch and the physicians he worked with – they included mainly the personal physicians to the Archduke – were only minimally interested in Paracelsus's new medical theories and were most certainly not interested in his theology. One would search in vain in Handsch's notes for more detailed accounts of Paracelsian concepts such as the *archeus*, the inner and the outer body, and the three Paracelsian principles sulfur, salt and mercury which were to take the place of the traditional four natural humors in the body. Only with reference to Johann Willenbroch (whose therapeutic approaches Handsch criticized vehemently on many occasions) do Handsch's notebooks suggest a more extensive adoption of Paracelsian concepts. Willenbroch traced diseases to "tartar",[53] and explained to Handsch that it was not always true that contrary heals contrary.[54] At one point, Handsch commented that Willenbroch seemed to follow Theophrastian medicine when Willenbroch advocated for a different therapeutic approach in a patient: Willenbroch held that fluids had collected in the sick person's stomach as well as a certain spiritus that liquified the food and turned it into winds or flatulence.[55]

Most physicians with a Galenic training who were interested in Paracelsianism quite clearly were not attracted by the new concepts. Rather, they hoped to learn about new, improved, and more effective medicines. Handsch, Mattioli, and other physicians in their professional environment expressed openness toward "Paracelsian" medicines, and toward "chymically" produced medicines on the whole so long as they promised to cure diseases more effectively.[56]

The image of slavish trust purportedly invested by learned physicians in the works of Avicenna, Galen, and Hippocrates, in opposition to which Paracelsus, in his *Labyrinthus* of 1553, positioned the light of nature as the true source of knowledge, was, as will have become sufficiently clear, a grotesque caricature. Not only Paracelsus but also the Galenic physicians were increasingly voicing skepticism about Avicenna's *Canon*.[57] In both their teaching and practice, they too had long come to the conclusion that personal, empirical observation of patients was to be a central methodological guidepost in diagnostics and

---

[53] Cod. 11206, fol. 15v: "Sequitur in hoc Theoprastum de Tartaro."
[54] Cod. 11183, fol. 372r; "quod contraria contrariis curentur"; Ferdinand II had burnt his finger with sealing wax and Willenbroch advised him to hold the finger close to a fire.
[55] Ibid., fol. 160v, "qui videtur sectari Theophrasticam medicinam".
[56] Nancy Siraisi (Siraisi, Medicine (2012), p. 499) has arrived at the same conclusion: "Many more practitioners seem to have made some use of Paracelsian remedies than espoused Paracelsus's belief system as a whole."
[57] Kühlmann and Telle have rightly underlined this shared critique of Avicenna and "Arabic" medicine (Kühlmann/Telle, Frühparacelsismus (2001), pp. 470–472).

therapeutics. And their esteem for the Hippocratic and Galenic teachings and remedies was founded not least of all on the conviction that this medicine had proven its validity empirically over the course of centuries. Given this appreciation for empiricism, even the most convinced Galenists had good reason to explore the effects and uses of chymically-produced and Paracelsian medications, whose outstanding effects had been touted in numerous reports.

This was true all the more when Paracelsians promised effective remedies against ailments for which traditional treatment was known to fail almost inevitably – diseases such as the plague, gout, epilepsy, dropsy, and leprosy.[58] In this context, the physicians' interest in Paracelsian and chymic medicines was no different than their interest in old and new medicinal plants and in numerous *experimenta* and *secreta,* which were said to have a powerful effect against certain diseases, without there being any explanation for these effects.[59] As we will see, this empirical outlook led some physicians even to accept that amulets and healing charms could be effective: After all, there were numerous reports by physicians and other credible witnesses attesting to their successful application.[60]

In a dedicatory letter to Handsch's employer Archduke Ferdinand, Adam von Bodenstein praised the refined and purified medications of the Paracelsians as more beneficial than the coarse substances of Galenic medicine, which had yet to cure any patients suffering from leprosy, gout, or the French disease, or who were crippled.[61] And indeed Paracelsians were eagerly advancing the production and medical application of "quintessences" and of other "chymically" produced medicines. According to neoplatonic doctrine, the *quinta essentia* stood above the elements, was indeed of a "celestial nature".[62] Willenbroch compared it with the human soul.[63] In practice, however, the term "quintessence" referred to medicines whose faculties or essence – which transcended the four elementary primary qualities and remained concealed – one could attempt to distill and thus concentrate and free of admixtures.

---

58 In his dedicatory epistle to Paracelsus, Bergsucht (1567), the editor declared the successful cure of podagra, epilepsy, leprosy and dropsy – diseases that were widely deemed incurable – the touchstone for the efficacy of Paracelsian medicines; Handsch excerpted the passage (Cod. 11206, fol. 161v).
59 Kühlmann and Telle have found a similar approach, for example, in the case of Rheticus and reject the claims of some scholars that he was an enthusiastic follower of Paracelsus (Kühlmann/Telle, Frühparacelsismus (2001), pp. 102f.).
60 Cf. the chapter on witchcraft and magic below.
61 Dedicatory epistle, 24 December 1571, in Bodenstein, Metamorphosis (1572).
62 Cod. 11207, fol. 89v.
63 Cod. 11205, fol. 2v.

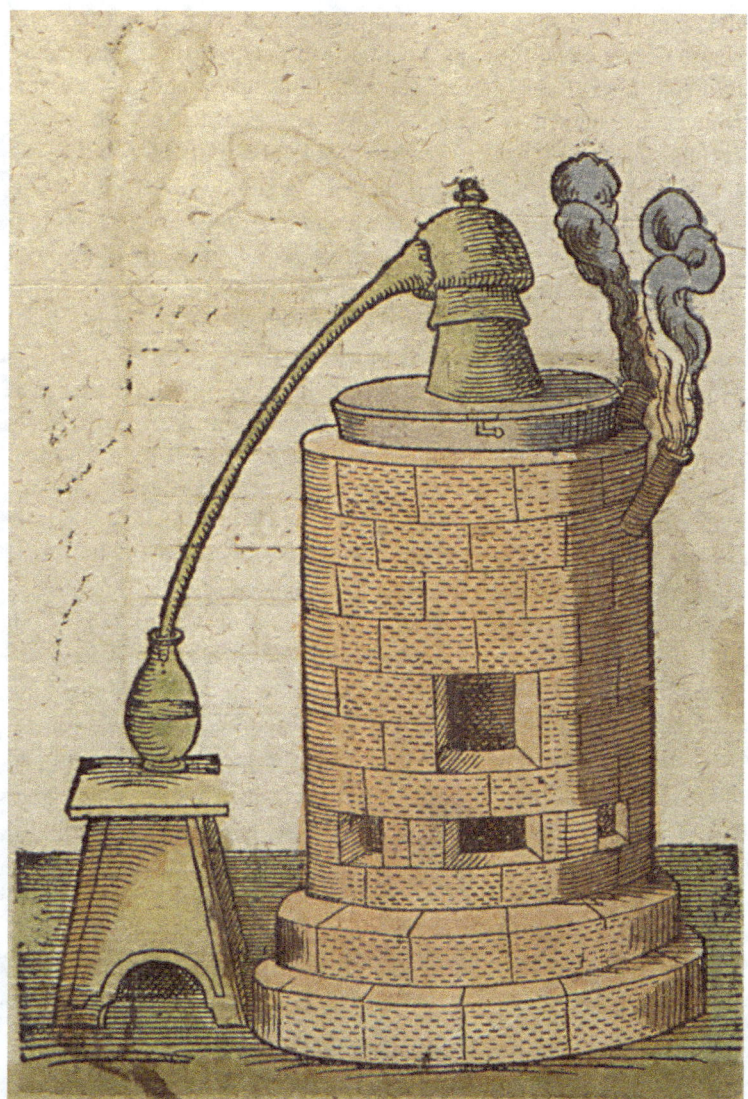

Fig. 10: Distilling oven (balneum Mariae) in: Pietro Andrea Mattioli, Kreutterbuch, 1611, Universitätsbibliothek Erfurt, Sign. 13 – MA 2° 23t.

The production of such quintessences was not a unique feature of Paracelsian medicine. The processes and apparatuses involved had been known for a long time, not least of all from the art of distilling spirits. At the theoretical level, Jean Fernel in his influential works had increasingly drawn attention to "occult" qualities and powers and to the ancient Galenic concept of diseases and medications whose effects could only be explained with respect to the "total substance", the *tota substantia*.[64] Diseases of the total substance could not be attributed to humors or to elementary qualities. They were specific, had their own essence. When Handsch, having read Paracelsus's work about the French disease, uncharacteristically wrote about Paracelsian theory, his comment very much followed in this vein: "He attributes the causes of the diseases to the specific substantial qualities."[65] Medicines and poisons that took effect through their total substance similarly had at their command specific – and ideally particularly powerful – faculties which could not be attributed to the primary, elementary qualities and which could only be identified and verified empirically.[66]

The physicians in Handsch's professional environment made widespread use of quintessences, which they understood as remedies whose specific effects were simply concentrated through distillation. Gallo's rhubarb quintessence, for example, was by no means an ethereal substance, but rather was quite pungent, sweet, brownish, and of medium consistency. As Gallo explained, he only called it "quinta essentia" because others did the same.[67] Mattioli very often used his personal quintessence with patients, even with an abbot suffering from the hiccups, which then immediately stopped.[68] When Ferdinand II was suffering from stones, his physicians gave him scorpion oil with a few drops of quintessence.[69] From the "chymist" Jacobus Gallus, Handsch learned how to make a whole array of essential oils "per alcumisticam [sic] artem". They each had their own indications for different diseases, and Gallus discussed with him such things as using oil of vitriol to treat hot fevers.[70] Philippine Welser, too, had her own quintessence.[71]

It is telling that Handsch called Mattioli's "quintessence" simply "aqua vitae", which was the contemporary term for brandy.[72] Michael Schrick's treatise *Von den*

---

64 Bianchi, Occulto (1982), pp. 188–212; Richardson, Generation (1985).
65 Cod. 11206, fol. 134r.
66 Cf. Argenterio, De morbis (1556), p. 217, on the *humores*: "Sunt qui in occultis, malignisque qualitatibus naturam obtinent, vitiataque sunt forma, quales sunt, qui in aere pestilenti gignuntur, aut a venenis tota substantia laedentibus inficiuntur."
67 Cod. 11207, fol. 89v.
68 Cod. 11207, fol. 27r and fol. 85a v.
69 Cod. 11204, fol. 54r.
70 Cod. 11205, foll. 128v-134v, cit. fol. 128v: "Quae a Iacobo Gallo chymista habuerim et didicerim". It is unclear whether the man's name was "Gallus" or whether "Gallus" has to be translated as "Frenchman", as the first name "Jacques" and the fact that Handsch mentioned previous activities in France suggest.
71 Cod. 11183, fol. 481v.
72 Ibid., fol. 135v.

ausgebrannten Wassern (On Distilled Waters), written in the fifteenth century, was reprinted many times in the sixteenth century and reached a wide audience. In it, Schrick presented distilled (and for the most part non-alcoholic) waters from dozens of different plants and described their applications.[73] The appendix to Handsch's German translation of Mattioli's commentary on Dioscorides showed the reader various types of distillation ovens and described the method by which the "subtlest and best part of the herbs [was] separated from the coarsest".[74] Made of tin or glazed clay, the "Rosenhütte", for example, allowed the distiller to place vessels with fresh, minced herbs in water or wine on hat- or bell-shaped structures that were arranged in several levels in a circle. If a fire was kindled in the oven, the heat would cause steam to rise into the little hats. It would then become liquid in the cooler parts of the hat and the distillate would run off into the vessel via an outlet or spout and could be collected.[75] Distilling with less intense heat was possible using a *balneum Mariae*, or *bain-marie*, whereby the contents of the distillation flask were heated from below in a copper bowl filled with water, which was heated with fire (cf. Fig. 10).[76]

The central innovation advanced by the Paracelsians was the widespread use of mineral and metallic preparations. With Paracelsianism, they attained a standing in medical treatment that was unprecedented. But even the most avid advocates of Paracelsian medicine[77] conceded that these substances already had held a place in older medicine. Handsch wrote that even Galen had used arsenic or similar substances to treat disease in individual cases.[78] In Padua, Falloppia strongly recommended *oleum vitrioli* to his students as a remedy for worms,[79] and this substance was also prescribed in Handsch's environment in Prague for a number of different diseases.[80] According to Sigismund Melanchthon, learned physicians were generally aware of

---

73 Schrick, Von den ausgebrannten Wassern (1481); Brunschwig, Destillierbuch (1512); Brunschwig, Buch (1519).
74 "Ein kurtzer leichter Begriff und Unterricht, künstliche Destillier oder Brennöfen mit zugehörender Bereythschafft zu machen", in: Mattioli, Kreutterbuch (1563), foll. 570v-574r.
75 Ibid., foll. 570v-571r.
76 Ibid., fol. 572r.
77 Dedicatory epistle of the architect Samuel in Paracelsus, Bergsucht (1567).
78 Cod. 11238, fol. 141r, on Galen's recommendation of clysters with arsenic against intestinal ulcers; according to Handsch's Padua notebooks, a certain Ludovicus – perhaps Tremenus – prescribed such a clyster but with limited success.
79 Cod. 11251, fol. 40v.
80 According to a letter from Conrad Gessner to Johannes Muralt, Muralt used oil of vitriol against diseases of the uterus; Gessner was critical, however, because of the corrosive effects (www.aerztebriefe.de/id/00000251, S. Weidmann).

its use around 1570.⁸¹ In one place, Handsch even expressed skepticism about Falloppia's use of a herbal remedy, writing that mineral remedies would have been a better choice.⁸²

When physicians with a Galenic background voiced their criticism of the metallic or mineral medications used by Paracelsians, they were not attacking the metallic, mineral or otherwise chemically-prepared substances as such, but were speaking up about the dangers associated with them and the hyperbole concerning their effectiveness. Caspar Hofmann, for example, stated in 1575 that while some liked to sing the praises of oil of vitriol, the ingestion of such a caustic, acrid substance came with great dangers. He had seen patients die in agony from it.⁸³ Even the aged imperial court physician Johannes Crato explained that although he certainly used chymic remedies with success, he opposed the claim that they worked miraculously, and he would not be moved to assent to the doctrine as a whole.⁸⁴

The fiercest disputes revolved around extremely toxic antimony, known in German as "Spießglanz". Particularly in France, it was a major point of contention between the Paracelsians and the proponents of orthodox medicine.⁸⁵ In Prague and many other cities, on the other hand, physicians were significantly more at ease when dealing with the new substances, including even antimony. While antimony was controversial, it was by no means only accepted by the self-proclaimed followers of Paracelsus. Mattioli, for example, used antimony to treat patients and discussed its production with Handsch.⁸⁶ Handsch himself gave some patients in Leipa antimony, especially women with disordered menstruation. With some, he found, it produced good effects.⁸⁷ He wrote that if someone expressed misgivings about antimony, one could reply that science ("scientia") knows no enemy except the ignorant.⁸⁸ A "chymicus" showed him

---

81 Letter from Sigismund Melanchthon to Joachim Camerarius, Nürnberg, 13 January 1570, (www.aerztebriefe.de/id/00000054, S. Wenning).
82 Cod. 11251, fol. 67v.
83 Letter from Caspar Hofmann to Johannes Hermann, Frankfurt [an der Oder], 1 June 1575, published in Scholz, Consiliorum (1594), pp. 380–82.
84 Copy of a letter from Johannes Crato von Krafftheim to Joachim Camerarius, Breslau, 28 January 1585 (www.aerztebriefe.de/id/00008399, S. Wenning).
85 Debus, French Paracelsians (1991), pp. 21–30, and on the ongoing conflicts in the seventeenth century, ibid., pp. 95–99; Nance, Turquet de Mayerne (2001), pp. 25–30.
86 Cod. 11205, foll. 131v-132r.
87 Ibid., fol. 122v.
88 Ibid., fol. 132v

how it was produced. It was not a simple process. The raw antimony had to be heated on a hot coal fire for several hours to separate the arsenic and sulfuric parts.[89] The work was also dangerous, as the apothecary Jeremias impressed upon Handsch and Mattioli when he showed them the production process ("calcinatio").[90] To protect oneself from the rising vapors, it was necessary to plug one's nose. He told them about a physician who had a special hood made that exposed only the eyes. The toxic vapors were likely also the reason why the apothecary availed himself of a portable stove that could be used outdoors.[91]

Handsch tried, by himself and with Mattioli, to produce medicinal antimony, but he failed various times.[92] Conrad Gessner, too, attempted to produce it during these years but ultimately had to ask for help from the Nuremberg physician Dr. Herold.[93] Joachim Camerarius, the founder of the Nuremberg *Collegium medicum*, requested detailed instructions for the production of antimony,[94] and even the well-known astronomer Tycho Brahe wanted to learn about the process.[95]

In one entry, Handsch even wrote down verses from the *Carmen elegiacum* by Michael Toxites, a well-known advocate of Paracelsianism. The work was a poetic riposte to the criticism of the Augsburg physician Lucas Stenglin about the use of antimony.[96] Here Handsch learned that when the antimony was "purged" in the fire, it was no longer toxic. The fire rendered it innocuous. At the same time, Toxites held that the illnesses physicians were dealing with were more severe than in earlier times due to widespread gluttony – the excessive enjoyment of meat, fish, and the like. Moreover, there were new "contagia" which were not mentioned in the old books. For these reasons, metallic medicines such as antimony were necessary as they were equipped with more powers than herbal remedies. And some traditional medicinal plants such as hellebore were incidentally

---

89 Cod. 11183, foll. 147r-152v.
90 Ibid.
91 Cod. 11205, fol. 132v.
92 Ibid., fol. 131v and fol. 132a v; in a marginal note, Handsch mentioned his failed attempt at making medicinal antimony "apud comitem", possibly referring to his time as a student in Padua with Comes de Monte.
93 Letter from Conrad Gessner to Hieronymus Herold, 27 January 1565 (www.aerztebriefe.de/id/00000249, S. Weidmann).
94 Letter from Gabriele Beati to Joachim Camerarius (1580) (www.aerztebriefe.de/id/00000385, U. Schlegelmilch).
95 At any rate, Heinrich Wolff promised Brahe that he would do everything so that Brahe could learn how to make antimony (copy of a letter, 11 November 1571, www.aerztebriefe.de/id/00004487, U. Schlegelmilch).
96 Cod. 11183, foll. 291r-293r; cf. Toxites, Spongia (1567); on the frontispiece, Toxites called himself explicitly a "Paracelsi discipulus".

also poisonous and potentially harmful. To complement the verses, Handsch also excerpted relevant passages from a letter Michael Toxites had written to Mattioli.[97] Here too, Toxites praised the effects of antimony, which could help heal almost any disease. Caution was only advised with patients whose brains were weak and with those for whom the vomiting caused by antimony was dangerous due to a tightness in the chest and veins. What was important, of course, was correctly preparing it. Paracelsus himself had described different antimony preparations, of which the white and red antimony flowers ("flores antimonii albi et rubentes") were the most excellent. A tincture made from the reddish antimony flowers cleansed the blood in such a way that an illness could not easily occur. This was the antimony liquid ("liquor stibii") that some earlier philosophers had mentioned but about which they had not gained complete knowledge.

In Handsch's notebooks, antimony figures simply as a promising medicinal product to be used with caution, which – like many other "tried and tested" remedies – produced good effects when used with certain diseases.[98] Handsch's own brother was first purged with antimony before he received external treatment for his scabies.[99] Handsch himself took antimony during a plague epidemic and experienced a laxative effect.[100] He observed the same effect in a patient to whom he administered antimony when the man was experiencing signs of paralysis in his leg. He had learned about the beneficial effects of antimony in another case with a patient who was experiencing similar symptoms.[101]

The opposition, at least in these early times, between traditional Galenic medicine and the "new" Paracelsian medicine also proves to be less pronounced than is suggested by the polemical disputes if we look at the evidence documenting the actual practice of physicians who explicitly espoused Paracelsian doctrine. In one of his notebooks, Handsch gave a detailed description of a *consilium* by Paracelsus for Bernhard Reichlinger in Augsburg.[102] Reichlinger was suffering from intense pain during urination and was only able to empty his bladder – if at all – with the help of a catheter. Paracelsus explained to the patient that the cause of his complaints was yellow bile. As treatment he recommended *trochisci*

---

97 Cod. 11183, foll. 293r-294r: "In literis ad Matthiolum". Toxites is not explicitly named as the author but the entry follows immediately after an entry on Toxites' *Carmen* and seems to have been written with the same ink and quill.
98 Ibid., fol. 292r; Cod. 11204, fol. 46r, on the successful use on a dropsical patient.
99 Cod. 11207, fol. 64r; the entry carries no date but goes back to Handsch's time with Gallo, around 1555.
100 Cod. 11183, fol. 124v.
101 Ibid.
102 Cod. 11200, foll. 240v-241v, "Consilium D. Theophrasti Paracelsi", with additional notes by Handsch.

(large cookie-like pills) made from physalis alkekengi (bladder cherry) and olibanum (frankincense). To improve urination, Reichlinger was also to use a secret remedy for fourteen days, a "heimlich Stück" or "secret piece" as Paracelsus called it: this was finely crushed pure crystal, to be mixed into white wine and drunk. This would drive all the yellow bile that was making him sick out of his body. His stones would be gone. If, against all expectations, he still had trouble urinating in spite of the remedies, he could tie a small satchel of saffron on his "pipe" (penis) and then the urine would flow.[103] It seems the yellow saffron was to pull the yellow urine out of the body. Paracelsus's explanation of the medical condition might just as well have been the explanation of an "archconservative" Galenist, just as his treatment with plant-derived substances could have come from one. The only procedure that was somewhat special was the use of crystal as a *secretum* and the external application of saffron with the help of a little satchel, which, as we will see, was documented for other physicians of the time as well.

To give another example, the way in which, according to Handsch's notes, an unnamed "physician of the Theophrastian discipline" explained the intense abdominal pain of a member of the Tucher family to him could have easily come from an opponent of Paracelsus. Having performed a thorough examination of the urine, the man explained that the patient's bile was corrupted in such a way that it was no longer of service to the liver, and that it was spoiling both liver and blood.[104]

Even someone like Bartholomäus Carrichter, who made explicit use of Paracelsian concepts like the three principles of mercury, salt, and sulfur[105] and the "tartaric fluids",[106] does not seem immediately subsumable as Paracelsian when we look at the way he treated his patients. In historical research, Carrichter is widely considered a Paracelsian and was coopted as such by Michael Toxites.[107]

---

103 Alternatively, Paracelsus recommended using the blood of a hare and a fox, in equal quantities, which had been dried in a baking oven.
104 Cod. 11183, fol. 158r; almost identical: Cod. 11206, fol. 15v.
105 E.g. Biblioteka Uniwersytecka Wrocław, Collection of the church library of Maria Magdalena, M 1024, fol. 1v, on an Augsburg citizen with an obstruction of the *nervus opticus* "ex resolutione crassi mercurii a resplendenti sulphure terrestri", and ibid., fol. 6r, on various symptoms of an "exustio mercurii et sulphuris".
106 Biblioteka Uniwersytecka Wrocław, Collection of the church library of Maria Magdalena, M 1024, fol. 4v
107 On Carrichter and his (alleged) Paracelsianism see Telle, Carrichter (1997).

Yet, his extensive practice journal from around 1560[108] contains countless diagnoses and explanations that could have easily come from the case histories of orthodox Galenic physicians. Sometimes Carrichter made direct reference to the four natural humors. He identified a quartan fever caused by an obstruction of the spleen in a patient with a sanguine temperament,[109] an excess of mucus in the body[110] or black bile,[111] cases of melancholy[112] and of melancholic hypochondria, itching caused by burnt black bile,[113] headaches or joint pain caused by black bile[114] and so forth. In addition came other classical humoral-pathological diagnoses such as "dripping catarrh" (*catarrhus destillans*),[115] a putrefaction of the lungs,[116] and an obstruction of the mesenteric veins. In the vast majority of cases, therapy involved plant-derived remedies rather than chemical medicines. Carrichter was known to have a profound knowledge of plants and was said to have shown Mattioli more than a hundred plants, which Mattioli then published in his commentary on *Dioscorides*.[117] Carrichter himself became well-known for his own herbal book, in which he made a point of specifically considering the astral influences during the collection of herbs.[118]

As the extensive *consilia* of Leonhard Thurneisser, court physician to Elector Johann Georg of Brandenburg, show, this self-professed proponent of Paracelsianism also relied on Galenic concepts to a great extent when interpreting and explaining illness. Thurneisser traced his patients' illnesses to "böse Flüsse" ("bad fluxes"), vicious mucus, rising vapors, obstructed veins and organs, and so forth. Like that of his Galenic colleagues, his treatment aimed primarily at "cleansing" the body, the blood, or individual organs such as the uterus, at "opening" the body with purgatives and at "strengthening" certain organs. The most important difference vis-à-vis orthodox Galenic practice was the additional use of valuable

---

108 National Library of Medicine, Bethesda, Ms. E63; Biblioteka Uniwersytecka Wrocław, Collection of the church library of Maria Magdalena, M 1024 (the two manuscripts are in large parts but not entirely identical).
109 Biblioteka Uniwersytecka Wrocław, Collection of the church library of Maria Magdalena, M 1024, fol. 3v.
110 Ibid., fol. 17v and fol. 20r.
111 Ibid., fol. 5r, fol. 14r and fol. 17r.
112 Ibid., fol. 16r.
113 Ibid., fol. 19v and fol. 22v.
114 Ibid., fol. 19r and fol. 21r.
115 Ibid., fol. 23v.
116 Ibid., fol. 21v.
117 Letter from Conrad Gessner to Johannes Crato, 1 August 1563, according to Helmich, Briefe (1938), pp. 34–35.
118 Carrichter, Kräutterbuch (1609).

and expensive medicines such as corals and gems, to which Thurneisser ascribed special healing powers.[119]

Since they needed to accommodate the medical notions and the expectations of their patients, it is not surprising that Paracelsian physicians were ready to avail themselves of Galenic explanatory models and purgative remedies, when dealing with patients and their relatives. For laypeople, the hope that the new or rare substances advanced by the Paracelsians, such as "chemical" medicines, would have miraculous effects certainly had its place. But complex new theories of disease, such as the doctrine of the three Paracelsian elements were much more difficult to communicate.

To summarize, a certain openness among learned physicians toward Paracelsian medicines must by no means be taken to prove that they were followers of Paracelsianism. The notion of a radical alterity of Paracelsian medicine – its irreconcilable opposition to the medicine of "Galenic" physicians – is untenable, certainly with respect to the 1560s and 1570s when Paracelsian literature and ideas were increasingly finding an audience. Those primarily responsible for drawing the distinction were the self-proclaimed proponents of Paracelsianism. Like Handsch and his colleagues, the Paracelsian proponents hoped for a new and more effective art of medicine. But they also wanted to position themselves in the health market as the advocates of a new medicine that was especially promising because it relied on new concepts and remedies. They wanted to secure for themselves the support of princes and other wealthy patrons, and some Paracelsians were very successful in their efforts.

Experimental Drug Trials

In their search for new and improved medicines, physicians were very aware of the great methodological difficulties involved in truly establishing efficacy. They agreed with Galen that when a disease took a favorable course after a certain medication had been administered, this could only serve as proof of its efficacy to a very limited extent. It was necessary to repeat the trial and to observe the patient, and even then, there was no guarantee of certainty. Reading Galen's commentary on the Hippocratic aphorisms, Handsch wrote, "Even testing a medicine six or seven times does not permit a general conclusion".[120] Much like the

---

119 Staatsbibliothek Berlin, Ms. germ. fol. 99, 420a, 420b, 421a, 422b, 423a, 423b, 424, 425 and 426.
120 Cod. 11200, fol. 126r: "Medicina etiam sexies vel septies probata non facit universalem propositionem."

way that the emergence of homeopathy in the early nineteenth century gave rise to the first known double-blind trial in medical history,[121] the spread of Paracelsianism and the reports of the miraculous – and for many physicians suspect – curative powers of Paracelsian remedies, such as theriac and various "secret remedies",[122] sharpened the focus on the issue of reliable drug testing in medicine.

Handsch made note of several reasons why one had to take care not to make hasty generalizations and draw conclusions prematurely:

1) It was common knowledge in medicine that the efficacy of a remedy was always dependent of the specific circumstances of the case – the patient's physical constitution, his or her living conditions, way of life and diet, the time of year, the point of time within the course of the disease, and other external factors.
2) The trust the patient had in the medication and/or the physician could have a great influence on the healing process. Today we would speak of the placebo effect. "It is the firm belief which sometimes heals", Handsch wrote.[123]
3) As a rule, most remedies at the time were composed of a mixture of medicinal plants or other substances. This made it difficult if not impossible to arrive at irrefutable conclusions about the efficacy of particular ingredients. Back in his university days, Handsch when discussing with his fellow students referred to a methodological principle of drug testing, which was later underscored by Samuel Hahnemann, the founder of homeopathy, and which has essentially retained its validity today: "When we want to gain experience about the faculties of a particular plant, we have to use it on its own".[124]
4) The observed favorable effect of a medicine could be merely an indirect "accidental" consequence. For example, Handsch wrote, if many stools were passed after a medicine was administered, this did not necessarily mean that the medicine had a laxative effect and could be used with future patients with this indication. A medicine that was known to strengthen the stomach could ultimately produce the same visible outcome. In itself, it did not have a laxative effect, but the stomach now had a greater expulsive power thanks to the medicine.[125]

---

[121] Stolberg, Homöopathie (1996). The randomized, controlled double-blind clinical trial (in which neither the physician nor the patient knows whether the drug in question is a placebo or the active substance) is widely considered the gold standard for assessing the efficacy of a remedy today.
[122] Bayle, Thériaque (2011).
[123] Cod. 9671, foll. 122v -123r, "fixa fides est quae sanat interdum"; see also Cod. 11207, fol. 154v, on the efficacy of amulets, in particular.
[124] Cod. 11240, fol. 99r.
[125] Ibid.

In other words, only studies with specific medicinal substances that involved patients with similar complaints and, better yet, studies that made comparisons with patients who were receiving no treatment, promised a degree of certainty. In particular, they could control for the influence of the natural favorable course of a disease, the most important reason for an error of judgment by far.

The idea of testing for efficacy, especially that of poisons and antidotes in comparative trials on humans and animals, goes back to antiquity.[126] In sixteenth-century medicine, the value of comparative trials was common knowledge. For example, Lehner told Handsch that he had tested a poison on two pigeons giving the poison to both but the antidote only to one of them – which survived.[127] And a man named Bräutigam told Handsch how one could tell the difference between expensive, real powdered unicorn horn, which was considered to be a powerful antidote, from the imitation powder made from dried horse bones: One had to give two pigeons mercury sublimate and then one of them the powdered unicorn horn as an antidote. It could be expected that only the latter would survive.[128]

Records of comparative trials on people are extant from as early as the fifteenth century. The Portuguese king João II was severely ill and his physicians diagnosed dropsy in 1494. They considered a treatment at a healing spring to be advisable, but found themselves in a fierce dispute about whether the healing spring in Óbidos was more appropriate than the one in Monchique. To settle the question, the story goes, "many" dropsical patients, each accompanied by a physician, were sent to the two natural springs to test and compare their efficacy against dropsy. When one of these patients quickly improved in Monchique, however, the king did not wait for the results of the trial.[129] In 1485, a similar trial had been done already under Queen Leonor to determine which of the three healing springs near Óbidos should serve as a location for a thermal hospital. Three patients suffering from the same disease were each sent to one of the three springs.[130]

By and large, the conditions for systematic comparative studies on humans remained unfavorable until well into the eighteenth and early nineteenth century. Before that time, there were hardly any hospitals with a larger number of victims of the same disease on whom the physicians could have performed comparative

---

126 Touwaide, Galien (1994); a very useful introduction into the historical development of clinical trials from antiquity until today, with numerous sources, is offered by the James Lind Library (https://www.jameslindlibrary.org/).
127 Cod. 11207, fol. 3v.
128 Cod. 11183, fol. 243v; today the horn of the "unicorn" is commonly believed to have been the tusk of a narwhal.
129 Resende, Crónica (1798), p. 272; cf. Mauser, Geschichte (2013), pp. 88f.
130 Mauser, Geschichte (2013), p. 41.

trials, withholding established medicines or therapies in order to exclude the influence of the natural course of the disease on the outcome. Moreover, early modern physicians prided themselves of basing their treatment not only on the diagnosis and the presumed pathological processes within the body, but of taking also into account the patient's individual constitution, temperament, way of life, and so forth, and modify the therapy accordingly.

Within a limited scope, however, comparative drug trials on humans were carried out systematically as early as the sixteenth century as part of the search for effective antidotes. The aim here was not only to have effective medication to treat the accidental consumption of toxic plants or mushrooms, or the bite of a poisonous animal. The deadly effects of devastating epidemics – the plague above all – were also often traced to a more or less specific morbid poison that entered the body. And for rulers, moreover, there was always the looming threat of being poisoned.

Physicians knew from experience that poisons, be they of plant, animal, or mineral origin, often could not be successfully combatted with the traditional evacuative remedies. Strong poisons, they concluded, had specific powers that transcended the elements and issued from their "total substance".[131] They could thus only be overcome, in turn, with a remedy whose powers were stronger than those of primary and secondary qualities. Such "occult", supraelementary powers could only be established or refuted by empirical observation.

In the case of poisonous plants and fungi that might be used for poison attacks, testing for the efficacy of antidotes proved to be particularly difficult. Poisonings from accidental ingestion of poisonous substances were rare, and it was even rarer that an antidote was on hand. A different way was found to conduct the research, however: giving first the poison and then an antidote to criminals who had been sentenced to death.[132]

Gabrielle Falloppia witnessed such a test in the 1540s in Ferrara. A cardinal from Ravenna had obtained the recipe for the celebrated *oleum Clementis*, an oil which Pope Clement VII was said to have composed in 1527 and which was praised for its miraculous effects against an epidemic pestilence that ravaged Rome at the time. The cardinal asked the Duke – presumably Ercole d'Este – for his permission that the oil be tried on a man who had been condemned to death. Antonio Musa Brasavola, who himself did not believe that the antidote would work, gave the prisoner a strong poison which contained sublimate of mercury. The man complained

---

131 Cf. Bianchi, Occulto (1982).
132 On the following see Stolberg, Tödliche Menschenversuche (2014); Rankin, On anecdote (2017). Rankin recently published a monograph on the topic (Rankin, Poison trials (2021). Unfortunately, it came out when this English edition of my book was already being prepated for print; not surprisingly, we have dealt with some of the same trials.

that it felt as if a fire were burning inside him and after several hours he collapsed and seemed half-dead. At this point, the oil was applied, and within half an hour he recovered. He lived for another five days, plagued by constant hiccoughs. According to Falloppia, even Brasavola was now almost ready to admit that the man would have survived for good if he had, in addition, been given an emetic and something to soften the caustic effects of the poison.[133]

Georg Handsch was personally involved in one the most widely publicized trials of this kind. In the winter of 1561–62, Pietro Andrea Mattioli tested the effectiveness of a powder in the possession of Archduke Ferdinand II. This archducal powder had allegedly been effective on many people. It had been tested, for example, on a man who was sentenced to death, and was believed to have proven successful. The man was first given arsenic and then, as he began to shake and his face began to swell and he seemed close to having a seizure, he was given the antidote. He vomited, survived, and was pardoned. In 1561, when Emperor Ferdinand I was spending time in Prague, it was decided that the efficacy of the archducal powder would be tested against aconite or monkshood, the most powerful plant poison at the time. In his notes, Handsch gave a detailed eye-witness account of the procedure and the results, and he described this first trial in his German translation of Mattioli's commentary on Dioscorides.[134]

The subject of the trial was a young man who had "forfeited his life with theft", as Handsch put in his published account, and who was to die the next day at the gallows. According to Handsch the man participated in the trial "very willingly indeed [. . .] because he preferred to die (since it was going to come to this) in a quiet place with few and honest people around rather than being hanged for all the world to see". He was promised that if he survived, he would not be executed.[135] In the presence of the imperial and archducal physicians, the man ingested a powder made from the root of the monkshood plant, which grew in the Bohemian mountains. When the man did not feel any effects from the poison, the physicians concluded that Bohemian monkshood was not as powerful as monkshood from faraway places, and that the poison in the roots had moved into the blossoms, leaves, and seeds. He was taken back to the dungeon. Several hours later, Mattioli gave him aconite blossoms and leaves in addition, and now the man began to experience serious symptoms. He felt pressure near his heart, and he fell to the ground like an epileptic and soiled himself. When he came to and

---

133 Falloppia, De tumoribus (1606), fol. 68v.
134 Mattioli, New Kreutterbuch (1563), foll. 472v-473r.
135 Ibid., fol. 473r, "dann er wolte lieber sterben (so es ja dahin gerhaten würde) an einem stillen Ort, unter ehrlichen und wenig Leuten, dann das er solt offentlich vor allem Volck erhenckt werden".

stood up, he had no memory of the fall. At this point, Mattioli gave him the antidote in wine, the "archducal powder" – a mixture of different plants[136] – and called on Handsch. Neither of them could feel the man's pulse. His face was running with cold sweat and he complained of cold. The physicians left him behind on a bed of straw, intending to return in an hour and a half. But just half an hour later, they were given the message that he had vomited and died.[137]

As we learn from Handsch's notebooks, another, slightly older young man had better luck, a few weeks later. He was given aconite root and, when the first signs of poisoning appeared, some bezoar. Bezoars, solidified clumps of hair and other substances that form in the stomachs of animals (and humans), were widely considered to have special powers to counteract poison. The man developed severe symptoms. His pulse raced and was weak and irregular. He vomited six or seven times. He complained of visual impairment and a coldness in his head, showed temporary signs of paralysis in his arms, but could speak the entire time. In the evening his complaints were gone. The following day, the Emperor sent him six talers and, it seems, pardoned him.[138]

Handsch was also present in 1564 when physicians gave monkshood and (arsenic-containing) nux-vomica to another young man who was sentenced to death. "My head feels strange, as if I were drunk" the man complained. His pulse became irregular. Then he too was given the "archducal powder". He vomited violently after sticking his finger in his throat, and had a bitter taste in his mouth. He threw his head back and his eyes bulged dramatically. He vomited again and again and was weak and fatigued. He had the feeling that his arm was liquifying. After five hours, Handsch left him. When he visited him the next day, the man was sitting at the table reading the Gospel. He was a free man.[139]

We also have records of a similar trial which was carried out in Florence in 1567. On the orders of Cosimo de' Medici, two men who had been sentenced to death for murder were used as subjects to test an antidote which several physicians had recommended to the prince. The two men received poison – the sap of monkshood, it was presumed – and then an antidote. They developed severe symptoms of poisoning, but survived. They were spared execution, but were sentenced to a lifetime of work on a galley.[140]

---

136 In Cod. 11183, fol. 190r, Handsch listed the ingredients.
137 Ibid., fol. 126r-v.
138 Ibid., foll. 127v-128v.
139 Ibid., fol. 128* r-v, inserted slip of paper.
140 Andreozzi, Leggi penali (1878), pp. 49f.; Andreozzi based his conclusion on the documents of the *Compagnia del Tempio*; in the *Archivio criminale* he found the names of the murderers and evidence for their having been pardoned.

In Paris too, a poison trial of this kind was carried out during these years, with explicit reference to Mattioli's trials in Prague. According to the account by the famous surgeon Ambroise Paré, the French king had been shown a bezoar from Spain that allegedly counteracted poisons of all kinds. Paré was incredulous. Poisons acted in different ways, he held, and therefore required different antidotes. At his behest, a cook who had been found guilty of stealing two silver bowls from his employer and sentenced to death would be used to test the effect of the bezoar. Having been promised that he would be pardoned if he survived the trial, the cook consented to taking first the poison and then some of the bezoar to test its efficacy. An apothecary administered the poison and the antidote. The poison – according to Paré it was likely mercury sublimate – produced immediate effects. The cook vomited and his condition worsened dramatically. His bowels were burning like fire, he wailed. In the end, as Paré wrote, the man broke out in a cold sweat and crawled on the floor on all fours with his tongue hanging out. Paré then gave him oil to drink to weaken the effects of the poison, but it was too late. After seven hours of torturous pain and screaming, he died.[141]

Alongside these non-comparative trials, records of comparative studies have survived from as early as the beginning of the sixteenth century. They followed the model of the above-mentioned trials with pigeons. In his commentary on Dioscorides, Mattioli recounted how he, as a young physician in 1524, was present in Rome when none other than Pope Clement VII had a topical oil tested which was said to act as an excellent antidote to poisons quite possibly the same oil Brasavola tested in Ferrara. Two men condemned to death were given aconite, but only one was rubbed with the oil in the days that followed; he survived. The other man, however, who was not treated with the oil so as to "test the power of the aconite poison", died in agony.[142] During his time in Padua, Handsch mentioned a similar story without naming the source or the people involved. Two men who had been sentenced to death served as subjects. One received a higher dose of aconite along with an antidote and survived, while the other received only a lower dose of the poison, without an antidote, and died.[143]

Further records have survived of a particularly sophisticated study that was carried out in the late 1570s in Germany.[144] Here, the human trials were preceded by a comparative trial on animals. A certain Andreas Berthold, probably a mine owner, had a large-scale operation selling *terra sigillata* from Silesia.

---

141 Paré, Œuvres (1575), p. 939.
142 Mattioli, Commentarii (1565), pp. 1095f.
143 Cod. 11240, fol. 142r, "Hystoria de duo damnatis"; perhaps this was the abovementioned trial under Pope Clement but the two accounts differ considerably.
144 Stolberg, Tödliche Menschenversuche (2014); Rankin, On anecdote (2017).

Also known as *bolus armenus, terra sigillata* had been considered an effective remedy for poison and the plague since antiquity. Gallo praised its effects "against putrefaction" ("contra putredinem").[145] But it was expensive because it came from distant Armenia. In petitions and advertisements, Berthold explained that his native *terra sigillata* was even more effective than the imported product. It was a true arcanum against many poisons and diseases – and he wanted to prove it. He first suggested to the Basel *Collegium medicum* that they test the efficacy in an animal trial, but it appears his application was unsuccessful.[146] He fared better in northern Germany. In Jülich and at the Kassel palace, he was able to initiate trials with five pairs of dogs who would serve as trial subjects. One dog in each of the pairs was given only poison, while the other was also administered Berthold's Silesian *terra sigillata*. The results seemed to prove Berthold right. All of the five dogs that had received the bole survived the poison, while without it, four of the five other dogs died.

Encouraged by the favorable results from the animal trials, Count Wolfgang von Hohenlohe in Langenburg initiated tests on humans. He had the procedure and the findings documented in a *Testimonium*, which Berthold put into print in 1583, giving us quite precise information about what happened. A thief who had been sentenced to death, a certain Wendel Thumblardt, ingested in the presence of Count Wolfgang and his nephew Georg Friedrich as well as the entire court half a drachm of mercury sublimate followed by a drachm of *terra sigillata*. This allegedly took place at the express wish of the man, who had been promised pardon by the count should he survive. The count's court physician Georg Pistorius and the apothecary Johannes Lutzen stayed with Thumblardt and monitored his condition. According to their account, Thumblardt developed severe symptoms after ingesting the poison, yet he survived.[147]

From today's perspective, these trials, even if some of the subjects came away with their lives, darkly recall the inhuman experiments in Nazi concentration camps. By all appearances, however, the physicians – and this is true of Handsch as well – did not believe they were doing anything wrong. Even Michael Boudewijns, who was strongly influenced by Catholic theology, did not categorically reject such trials in his *Ventilabrum medico-theologicum*,[148] and, if Mattioli's account is accurate, the pope himself was behind one of the trials. As

---

145 Cod. 11205, fol. 530r.
146 Letter from Andreas Berthold to the *collegium medicum* in Basel, 26 December 1579 (www.aerztebriefe.de/id/00001987, A. Döll/T. Walter).
147 Berthold, Terrae sigillatae (1583); Berthold, Compendium (1589); Berthold, Nützlicher unnd nothwendiger Bericht (1597).
148 Boudewijns, Ventilabrum medico-theologicum (1666).

is so often the case in the history of ethical norms in medicine, the standards accepted and used to assess and judge moral behavior have changed profoundly. For one thing, voluntary participation was emphasized, something that agrees with modern ideas to a certain extent. In Handsch's words "The poor person took the poison very willingly indeed".[149] By participating in the trial, the subject stood to receive a milder punishment, perhaps even a pardon – if things went well. And if he died of the poison, he and his relatives would at least be spared the degrading death at the gallows. Moreover, it was usually emphasized that a trial had been ordained by a ruler or at least explicitly endorsed by one. In other words, from the perspective of the period, these people had already forfeited their lives. No one at the time seriously contested the ruler's right to punish criminals with death for their crimes. Their lives were totally in his hands. And finally, not least of all, the trials served the common good – as was pointed out again and again.[150] For this reason, Johann Heinrich Meibom understood them to be in harmony with the Hippocratic Oath, which did not, he explained, forbid the physician from giving poison to a person condemned to death to test its effects, or those of an antidote, if this served the goal of being able to help others in the future.[151]

The search for new and more effective remedies was a high priority. For similar reasons, someone like Gabrielle Falloppia, too, had no misgivings about killing a total of nine men with opium, and about acknowledging this publicly, in front of his students. After all, knowledge was gained in these instances about the effects of opium; in fact, the men did not show the symptoms that were to be expected according to Dioscorides. And above all, their perfectly intact corpses were ideal for subsequent dissections which would allow the anatomist to make new discoveries and promote medical knowledge.[152]

On the whole, the number of "test subjects" in the trials named above was very small. And such experiments had no place in the practice of ordinary physicians. But they impressively show how an appreciation had grown in the sixteenth century for controlled empirical observation as a source of reliable knowledge.

---

149 Cod. 11183, foll. 125r-128*v: "Der arm Mensch nam das Gifft willig und gern"; similarly Paré, Response ([1575], p. 12, "tel poison fut pris par le brigand de bonne volonté".
150 Letter from Graf Wolf von Hohenlohe, 25 January 1581, published in a Latin translation in Berthold, Terrae sigillatae (1583), no pagination: "utilitatem totius humani generis"; and in an English translation in Berthold, Wonderfull and strange effect (1587), pp. 32–35: "for the commoditie and benefite of all Christendome".
151 Meibom, Hippocratis magni Orkos (1643), pp. 128–130.
152 Cod. 11240, fol. 78r.

Case Histories: Observation at the Bedside

The growing significance of empiricism and of personal observation in the medical practice of the sixteenth century also found vivid expression in another field, namely in the rise of medical casuistry. Increasingly, the individual case history entered the stage as a major source of knowledge alongside theoretical discussions and commentary on traditional authoritative texts. The individual case no longer served primarily as an *exemplum* to illustrate a general theory. Making precise observations about countless cases and noting them down – the symptoms, the external circumstances, possible triggering factors, the genesis and development of the disease, and the course it took under medical treatment – would, it was hoped, result in new knowledge. It would place diagnosis, prognosis and treatment on an ever more solid foundation.

Handsch's extensive notes powerfully illustrate this turn toward casuistic observation at the bedside. In thousands of entries, he documented experiences and insights – his own, and those of others – about the effects of remedies, the significance of certain diagnostic and prognostic signs, and other aspects of medical practice. In addition, he also wrote down entire case histories, summarizing them after the fact, or returning to a case in a number of entries or documenting the various visits in chronological order, as in a practice journal, with almost daily notes. Not infrequently, he complemented his notes as time went on with observations and insights coming from comparable cases, noting them down in the margins or providing cross-references to entries on other patients. In this, he was seeking to arrive in an inductive manner, as we would say today, at general conclusions, for example about the value of a diagnostic or prognostic sign or the use of a medication for a particular disease.[153]

In their sheer magnitude, Handsch's notebooks are unique. But many other physicians seem to have also made it a habit to note down their observations and experiences in medical practice, to document the medical cases they treated. They did this in practice journals and notebooks, as well as in collections of case histories from their own practices, which they extracted from their notes. European archives and libraries today hold a substantial number of such handwritten records,[154] and this despite the unlikelihood of the survival of this kind of material. Even lecture notes, which would have been taken down by the thousands by students at the time and were of obvious value to other students and physicians, are extant only in

---

[153] Historical overview in Milton, Induction (1987).
[154] Stolberg, Medizinische Loci communes (2013) gives references to a range of manuscript sources.

very limited numbers. There is little doubt then that taking notes on individual patients and cases was common practice among learned physicians.

The turn toward medical casuistry, toward the individual case history, was also reflected in the world of publishing and epistolary exchange. After the first beginnings around 1550,[155] collections of printed medical *observationes, casus, enarrationes,* and *historiae* became an important genre that was widely read and quoted. We do need to make a distinction here. Some of these collections and observations of individual cases belonged first and foremost in the domain of natural history. They concentrated on *observationes rarae*, that is they dealt with unusual clinical pictures and rare pathological phenomena such as bizarre congenital deformities which readers in all probability would never encounter in their own practice. They reflect the contemporary interest in observing miraculous phenomena and (apparent) deviations from the laws of nature.[156]

Some of the most successful and oft-quoted collections, however, contained cases that might easily be encountered by other physicians in their practices. Prominent here were above all German and Dutch physicians in wealthy mercantile and imperial cities – salaried municipal physicians such as Pieter van Foreest in Alkmaar and Felix Platter in Basel,[157] as well as, in the seventeenth century, self-employed physicians who had extensive urban practices, such as Tulpius in Amsterdam, Heer in Liège, Hechstetter in Augsburg, and Thoner in Ulm.[158] These urban physicians saw large numbers of patients over the years, often including many less well-off and poor patients, especially if the physicians were also responsible for providing medical care in hospital. It was therefore possible for them to draw on their personal experience in treating hundreds if not thousands of patients who covered the entire spectrum of known diseases.

Medical case reports have long been of interest to historians.[159] Starting with the numerous individual case histories that are documented in the Hippocratic *Epidemics*, they have a millennia-old history. Examining early modern *observationes, casus* and *curationes*, more recent historical research has highlighted and

---

[155] Amatus Lusitanus, Curationum (1552); in 1562, Girolamo Cardano, in an unabashed self-aggrandizing manner, published a series of reports about difficult cases he had (allegedly) successfully cured (Cardano, Opera (1562), pp. 118–137) under the heading "De curationibus et praedictionibus admirandis".
[156] Daston/Park, Wonders (1998).
[157] Valleriola, Observationum (1573); Foreest, Observationum (1603–1606); Platter, Observationum (1614).
[158] Tulpius, Observationum (1652); Hechstetter, Rararum observationum (1624); Heer, Observationes (1645); Thoner, Observationum (1649).
[159] Temkin, Studien (1929); Laín Entralgo, Historia (1961).

delineated the different types of published case histories as well as their different functions.¹⁶⁰ But the focus on printed sources easily obscures the fact that published collections of *observationes, casus,* and *curationes* were not the cause but already the consequence of a previous turn toward the individual case and toward empirical observation at the bedside in ordinary medical practice. Decades before the first collections of *observationes* and *curationes* went into print, case histories assumed a new importance in physicians' notetaking practices and in university teaching.

Along with the increasing orientation toward empirical knowledge in the study of nature as a whole, several factors were advancing this development more specifically in the field of medicine. With the rise of humanism, in which learned physicians played a very active part, there was a valorization of *historia*, of the observation and description of individual things and phenomena, over and above the Aristotelian ideal of *scientia* based in the knowledge of causes.¹⁶¹ Some extant medical case histories are even explicitly categorized under the heading "Historia", and Handsch, too, used the term "historia" or rather "hystoria" for both general historical depictions and for specific reports and stories about medical cases, such as a "Hystoria" of a sick matron who was "cured by superstitition".¹⁶² The parallels between medical case histories and other forms of historical accounts are indeed close at hand. Like other historical events – in the case of wars, the comparison is particularly apt – the origin and development of the individual case of illness could be told as a chronological sequence of events, determined by a multitude of individual circumstances. And just as historical accounts of past events aimed to arrive at possible lessons for future action in similar situations, medical histories offered the hope that through them knowledge could be gained that could be useful when treating similar cases. In fact, they owed their popularity largely to this fact.

A key catalyst and driving force of the medical turn toward the individual case and the practice of writing case reports was by all appearance the clinical, bedside training that emerged in northern Italian universities in the 1530s at the

---

160 Nutton, Case histories (1991) – I am grateful to Vivian Nutton for letting me read the manuscript of this lecture, which unfortunately was never published; Pomata, Praxis historialis (2005); Stolberg, Formen (2007); Pomata, Sharing cases (2010); Pomata, Observation rising (2011); Pomata, Word (2011); these papers also offer extensive bibliographies of printed editions of *curationes* and *observationes*.
161 Pomata, Praxis historialis (2005).
162 Cod. 11240, fol. 104r: "Hystoria de matrona aegrota, quae per superstitionem curata [fuit]"; further examples are ibid., fol. 74r; Cod. 11205, fol. 204v and fol. 223r; Cod. 11207, fol. 23r, fol. 72r and fol. 199r; Cod. 11210, fol. 199v.

latest, influencing generations of future physicians, including many who came from north of the Alps. Men such as Giovanni Battista da Monte in Padua and Antonio Musa Brasavola in Ferrara – where Amatus Lusitanus was active, whose *curationes* were among the earliest printed collections of case histories – were known as first class humanists and experts on the scholarly literature that had survived from antiquity. Their teaching, however, like that of Fracanzano in Padua and Elideo Padovani in Bologna, for example, focused on the individual case. In the *collegia*, the public discussions of cases in front of the student body, as held in Padua, and at the bedside, budding physicians learned how to draw conclusions from their observations of sick people, and how to apply their general, theoretical knowledge to individual cases of illness in a manner that was methodologically stringent, making the search for the internal and external causes of the disease their starting point.[163] Significantly, the first handwritten records of medical case reports from this period that have survived were penned by students, by prospective physicians, that is, rather than by experienced practitioners. The collection of case histories from the practice of Musa Brasavola and other medical professors in Ferrara, which I have cited several times, can be dated to around 1545 at the latest.[164] And the earliest known example of a collection of case histories that are explicitly characterized as *observationes* – which in printed collections later on was to become the most common term – is yet something else that originates with Georg Handsch. Under the heading "Observationes ex praxi doctorum Patavinorum", he filled approximately forty pages in 1551–52 with notes about cases he had seen with Trincavella and other professors.[165] In the same notebook, he included detailed descriptions of seven cases of illness he encountered in Vicenza with Comes de Monte late in the summer of 1552. Among the headings used here we find, for example, "Tercia observatio de hydrope ex retentis menstruis", about a dropsical peasant woman, and "Quinta observatio de febre interpollata remedioque post purgationem febrem fugante", about the successful treatment of a febrile woman.[166]

---

163 Bylebyl, The manifest and the hidden (2004).
164 Biblioteca Ariostea, Ferrara, Collezione Antonelli, Ms. 531; on the date see Part I, note 251.
165 Cod. 11238, foll. 95r-114v; it is not certain that the heading refers to the entries until fol. 114v; these pages are all devoted to such individual case histories, however. A similar heading, "Observationes in praxi medica apud Bellicatum, Helidaeum, Montanum et alios", is found on the first page of one of Johannes Brünsterer's student notebooks. He studied in Padua in the late 1540s already but the heading was probably added later only by Johannes Hesse, who married Brünsterer's widow, in 1555 (on Brünsterer see Stolberg, Teaching anatomy (2018), p. 76, note 10).
166 Cod. 11238, foll. 115r-118v and foll. 70r-74v; the heading of another, shorter passage in this notebook (ibid., foll. 124v-125v) uses the corresponding verb "observare": "Ex praxi D. Comitis de Monte observata".

Self-Observation: The Physician's Body as a Source of Knowledge

Not only in Handsch's student notes but also in his notes from his working life as a physician, much attention is devoted to individual cases of illness and observations of specific patients. But it is also striking how often he included notes about his own personal, physical condition and illnesses. He described himself as not particularly robust. He had a tendency to faint, though he had never actually collapsed.[167] And again and again, he depicted his own experiences with illness. He suffered from fevers a number of times and in his later years he was plagued by stones.

Handsch did not limit himself to simply depicting or describing his complaints. He used his observations of his own body to arrive at general conclusions. Feeling his own pulse, for example, showed him that the pulse before a febrile attack was "hidden" ("occultatus").[168] This insight helped him predict the onset of febrile attacks in patients and to impress these patients and their relatives with an exact prognosis and diagnosis. Once, when Handsch believed he was suffering from an obstruction of the spleen, he found a sandy, reddish, soft sediment in his urine, which turned to paste when rubbed between the fingers. He interpreted this as an excreted humor that had been overheated in the liver and could not flow into the spleen due to the obstruction. The examination of his own urine thus provided him with evidence that sandy urine did not always indicate stone disease.[169] Even Handsch's occasional notes about masturbation take their meaning from this epistemic practice. They are among the earliest known ego-documents on the subject and are thus of interest to historians of sexuality as well. The note-taking here did not serve as an outlet for confession or a means of self-scrutiny, as we sometimes find in later ego-documents. The entries were short, factual, and free of value judgments. They dealt primarily with the consistency of the semen and with the consequences of semen loss to his health and body.[170]

Handsch was not alone in this habit of careful self-observation. Other physicians, too, documented their own illnesses in detail and in a style consistent with the *observationes* physicians penned about their patients. Much like Handsch, Andrea Gallo used his observations of his own body and urine to counter Mattioli

---

167 Cod. 11207, fol. 29v.
168 Cod. 11205, fol. 69v, "ut in me cognovi".
169 Cod. 11210, fol. 92v.
170 Cod. 11183, fol. 434v and fol. 459v; Cod. 11205, fol. 74v, fol. 81r, fol. 193r, fol. 218r and fol. 513r

when the latter concluded from a patient's red urine that he was suffering from a fever. Strongly colored, red urine was considered to be a sign of excessive heat in the body, but Gallo knew from his own experience that this sign was deceptive. He explained that his own urine was sometimes red when he was not suffering from a fever.[171] And not in a journal, but as part of his collection of other medical cases, Bartholmäus Carrichter gave an account under the heading "pro mea persona", describing the hemoptysis, intense bowel complaints, tertian fever, dizziness, and trembling he developed after attending a banquet at an abbot's in 1558. The abbot had first served him light, but then very strong wine. Carrichter's description of the therapy and the course of his illness is detailed.[172] Girolamo Cardano told of how he first freed himself, and then many other patients, from an excessive flow of urine, while the patients in the hands of other physicians died.[173] Martin Ruland described the intense bleeding from hemorrhoids that plagued him for many days, even months, at a time. He felt very weakened from the great loss of blood, inasmuch as the blood that was flowing was not black and thick as was common in such cases, but was red, that is, natural blood. He treated his complaints with a small satchel of red cloth containing crushed acorns or oak leaves which had been cooked in strong vinegar.[174]

For his part, Caspar Weckerlin in the early seventeenth century added to his own handwritten "Observationes" a detailed depiction of his own "hypochondriacal" complaints, that is symptoms that were located in the upper abdomen. He had been suffering from asthma or shortness of breath for almost four years. It was worse when he lay on his left side, and he was experiencing pain. He was plagued by intense coughing, especially when reclining, and was forced to stand up. His face was pale, his appetite poor, and he had noticeably lost weight. In the evening, he felt a glowing heat. He salivated profusely and often needed to vomit, especially after drinking wine. Not only this, but for a year he had also been experiencing a sad mood, had been sleeping poorly and had a strong rumbling in his stomach. Added to this was a heavy head and catarrh. He suspected *apepsia*, an insufficient digestion of food in the stomach, and the development of burnt, black-bilious blood in the liver, which was obstructing it.[175]

Medical notes of this kind about a physician's own body and its diseases are not fundamentally different from those about a physician's patients. In many respects, the physician's own body fulfilled the same function as a source of

---

171 Cod. 11207, fol. 151v.
172 National Library of Medicine, Bethesda, Ms. E63, fol. 180v.
173 Cardano, Opera (1562), p. 129.
174 Ruland, Curationum (1578), p. 16.
175 Det Kongelige Bibliotek, Copenhagen, Ms. Gl. kongl. S. 4° 1694, fol. 63r, 29 July 1616.

empirical medical knowledge. It became an object which the physician met with the same distancing, knowledge-seeking attitude as he did when he encountered the bodies of patients. But there is an important difference. When working with patients, physicians had to rely on what patients told them, and could only hope that they described their physical sensations correctly. But physicians believed themselves to be far better trained in recognizing even subtle signs and physical changes which the layperson might miss or consider irrelevant. Thus, to physicians' minds, their own bodies were a source of knowledge that was much more dependable, and could help them better understand their patients' bodies. What Christopher Lawrence found for the natural philosophers in the seventeenth century, was equally true for many Renaissance physicians already: they "regarded themselves as highly reliable reporters of their own sensations and, for this reason, acutely perceptive of goings-on in other bodies".[176]

The prominent place of the physician's own body in Handsch's notes and in those written by other sixteenth-century physicians thus substantiates for medicine the findings of Werner Kutschmann's study on the role of the perception of the naturalist's own body in premodern science. According to Kutschmann, the human body during the Renaissance was "still a measuring stick and a model for 'natural' knowledge". It was only in later times, "in the course of the development of methodologically-constituted experimental science (which was proficient in the use of instruments and technology)" that the body was "displaced from its leitmotif function and faded out".[177]

Post-mortems

A further field in which the growing significance of empirical approaches in learned medicine made itself distinctly felt and was expressed with particular clarity was the growing practice of post-mortems, that is the dissection of the bodies of deceased patients (Fig. 11). Until very recently, historical research greatly underestimated the prevalence and relevance of post-mortem findings in Renaissance medicine. Works on the history of pathological anatomy have placed great emphasis on the autopsy reports that appeared here and there in Antonio Benivieni's *De abditis non nullis ac mirandis morborum et sanationum causis* of 1507.[178]

---

176 Lawrence, Medical minds (1998), p. 166.
177 Kutschmann, Naturwissenschaftler (1986), cit. p. 15; summary of his major arguments in Kutschmann, Naturwissenschaftler (1991); see also Shapin/Lawrence, Science incarnate (1998), esp. the editors' introduction (pp. 1–19).
178 Benivieni, De abditis (1994).

Benivieni's work and Théophile Bonnet's *Sepulchretum sive anatomia practica, ex cadaveribus morbo denatis* of 1679 are today considered classics of medical literature.[179] In their analysis of these works historians have largely focused on the findings that hold up in the eyes of modern medicine, however. This narrow focus has eclipsed the extent to which post-mortems were practiced on an everyday basis, within and outside the academic context, and the relevance that learned physicians attached to autopsy findings as early as the sixteenth century.[180]

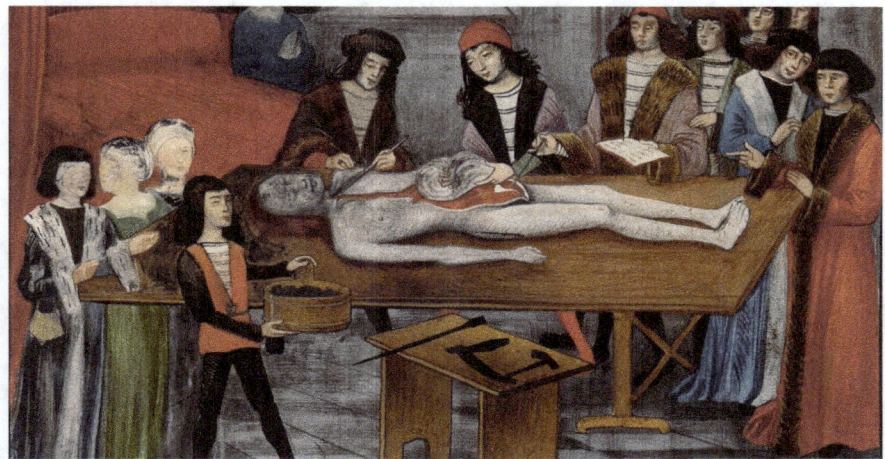

Fig. 11: Unknown artist, Guy de Chauliac performing a dissection, gouache after a 15th-century illuminated manuscript, Wellcome Collection, London.

Already a look at the printed medical sources shows quite well that post-mortem findings came to be widely appreciated, not only in Italy but also north of the Alps.[181] In the case histories of Jean Fernel (1497–1558), for example, of Pieter van Foreest (1521–1597), or Volcher Coiter (1534–1576) there are multiple accounts

---

179 Bonnet, Sepulchretum (1679).
180 The major exception is an important, seminal study of post-mortem reports from the sixteenth and seventeenth centuries by Nancy Siraisi (Siraisi, Segni (2001)). Siraisi doubts the value of these autopsies, however, and seems to underestimate their epistemic potential and the importance they had in the eyes of contemporary physicians as a source of new knowledge about the body and its diseases. For a study of the interpretation of post-mortem findings in sixteenth- and early seventeenth-century medicine and their relevance for medical practice see Stolberg, Post-mortems (2017).
181 In England, autopsies on deceased patients seem to have been performed less commonly, however (Wear, Knowledge (2000), p. 148).

of the changes that were found when the bodies of those who had perished of their disease were opened post mortem.[182] Other authors at least wove the findings of individual autopsies into their published observations[183] or they collected them in a chapter specially devoted to the subject.[184] Around 1600, even an ordinary municipal physician like Jean Chifflet in Besançon was able to supplement his sixty medical *observationes* with the findings of approximately two dozen autopsies.[185] Insights were also gained when the bodies of princes were opened for the purpose of embalming or to rule out a possible poisoning.[186]

Without a doubt, reservations about dissection were widespread in the population. But some relatives wanted to learn the true cause of death. Chifflet even mentioned the post-mortem of a patient who had explicitly requested it before he died.[187] And the published post-mortem findings almost certainly represent only the tip of an iceberg. Undoubtedly, numerous autopsies either produced no clear pathological changes worth publishing or these findings were unsuitable to showcase the exceptional diagnostic skill of the author of a printed case history. In their letters, physicians occasionally mentioned autopsies without saying anything more about the results. Even during epidemics, some physicians attempted to come closer to understanding the nature of the pestilence and its causes by opening up bodies, and did so without publishing their findings.[188]

Handsch's personal notes give us a very similar picture. But in addition they give us a good impression of the multitude of sources on which physicians could draw to learn of dissection findings, and they show the significance of

---

182 Fernel, Universa medicina (1644), collection of *consilia*, in the Elector the appendix of the separately paginated part *De abditis rerum causis*, pp. 247–397; Foreest, Observationum (1634); Coiter, Externarum (1573).
183 E.g. Dodoens, Medicinalium observationum (1581), pp. 13f., p. 43, p. 48, pp. 61f., pp. 67–69, pp. 105f., and p. 123; Sassonia, Pantheum (1603), p. 161; Brasavola, In octo libros aphorismorum (1541); Houllier, De morborum (1567), p. 60, Trincavella, De ratione (1575), p. 352; Boscius, De lapidibus (1580), fol. A3r–v, citing Falloppia and Johannes Pfeil, a personal physician of Moritz of Saxony Donati, De medica historia (1588), foll. 264r-267v.
184 Solenander, Consiliorum medicinalium (1609), p. 493.
185 Chifflet, Singulares observationes (1612); as far as the dates are indicated, Chifflet assembled most of these *observationes* in the 1590s.
186 See, e.g., the letter from Nikolaus Kistner to Johannes Posthius, 24 June 1574, in which he reported about the dissection of the deceased King Charles IX of France, in which massive changes in one of the pulmonary lobes were found but no evidence of poisoning (Kistner, Opuscula (1611), pp. 991–993, www.aerztebriefe.de/id/00013774, C. Hauck).
187 Chifflet, Singulares Observationes (1612), fol. 32v, "viventis iussu".
188 Thus Johannes Dryander (1500–1560), in 1547 wrote to Graf Wolrad von Waldeck even about several dissections he had performed on victims of the current "pestilential fever" (Wolff, Kartographen (1990), pp. 8f; www.aerztebriefe.de/id/00025350, U. Schlegelmilch).

autopsies as an essential foundation and an important corrective in medical practice. Numerous entries go back to Handsch's university days. The professors in Padua repeatedly told students about the observations they had made when dissecting the bodies of deceased patients. Bellocati, for example, told his students about a dropsical patient in whose liver blisters or cysts had formed.[189] And Handsch heard from Falloppia that when he cut open the corpse of a patient who had died of pleurisy, he saw that an apostema, that is a local accumulation of morbid matter or pus, had formed, and that the pleura, usually so delicate and thin, had grown two finger-widths thick. Falloppia added that similar changes could sometimes be observed with the meninges. Falloppia was not prepared to believe that the pus from such an encapsulated apostema could make its way into the lungs and be coughed up, as other physicians claimed. But later he had opened up two patients whose entire chest cavities were filled with pus while the pleurae were completely intact. He concluded that the morbid matter could evidently penetrate the pleura in a miraculous, hidden manner and find its way to the lungs.[190] Falloppia also told his students about his postmortem findings in patients who had suffered from stone disease: the stone was always in the renal pelvis and never in the substance of the kidney.[191]

In his years as a practitioner, Handsch repeatedly noted down autopsy findings. Some of them were relayed to him by others. Extraordinary findings were widely circulated, it appears. For example, Handsch wrote down the pathological changes that had come to light during the autopsy of the body of Emperor Ferdinand, who after an illness lasting ten months – the diagnosis was catarrh and hectic fever – was so emaciated that he was almost a skeleton and could no longer stand. The physicians not only found a large quantity of sand in the kidneys, but also an indurated, dried-out pulmonary lobe that had become attached to the spine.[192] From a history of Poland, written by an unnamed physician, Handsch learned about how King George had suffered from extremely swollen feet, a typical symptom of dropsy, which at the time was generally traced to a damaged liver. When his abdominal cavity was "disemboweled" ("exenteratus est"), the liver proved to be spoiled ("corruptum") and in the gall bladder there was a stone the size of a pigeon egg.[193]

---

189 Cod. 11183, fol. 22r.
190 Cod. 11210, fol. 14r.
191 Ibid., fol. 4v.
192 Cod. 11183, fol. 196v; in the light of such extensive pulmonary changes, modern physicians would suspect above all pulmonary tuberculosis or perhaps a carcinoma. The Emperor's corpse was embalmed afterwards.
193 Cod. 11205, fol. 323v.

In the above-mentioned cases, the autopsy findings matched the clinical picture and confirmed the physicians' suspicions. But not uncommonly, unexpected findings reminded physicians that they had to be careful with their diagnoses and prognoses, and were thus particularly valuable for future practice. As a cautionary example that might help him avoid public humiliation, Handsch noted down the *historia* of an Augsburg cardinal who died in Rome while in the intensive care of several physicians. The physicians had diagnosed a stomach disease and had given him numerous medicines which caused him to vomit many times and with such violence that a vein burst. The autopsy, however, revealed that there were no pathological changes in the stomach whatsoever. Instead the cardinal had a large kidney stone. The treatment had been completely wrong. Handsch concluded his entry with a reference to the son of Lorenzo de' Medici who, after the death of his father, ordered that his father's physician be thrown into a well.[194]

Handsch sometimes also received post-mortem reports from his mentors and colleagues in Prague. Gallo told him about a dissection which confirmed that the woman in question had an apostema of the liver, as the physicians had suspected.[195] From Mattioli he heard that cancer was sometimes discovered in the body on autopsy.[196] This was an important insight because, as we have seen, in the vast majority of cases, cancer could only be diagnosed in living patients because – as with breast cancer – it could be felt through the skin or if the skin itself was affected, or because – as with uterine cancer – cancerous matter was discharged to the outside of the body.

It appears that Handsch himself never performed a dissection, yet in his immediate environment, especially during his time at the Ambras court, he witnessed the dissection of deceased patients multiple times. A female patient in the *gynaeceum,* for example, suffered from dropsy when she was alive. She had felt pain when pressure was applied to the area above her liver. And indeed, the autopsy showed that her liver was enlarged and indurated. It had a rough surface and two pea-sized stones were found in the gall bladder.[197]

Surprises were in store during the autopsy of a man who succumbed to his injuries in Innsbruck. It seems that a horse had kicked him in the abdomen. The man's scrotum was extremely swollen and gangrenous. When the archducal

---

194 Cod. 11183, fol. 445r.
195 Cod. 11207, fol. 6v.
196 Cod. 11183, fol. 286v.
197 Ibid., fol. 289r; the estimated date results from an entry a few pages earlier (ibid., fol. 286r): "Oeniponti A. 67". The term "gynaeceum" may have referred to the *Damenstift* in Hall, a kind of school for young ladies from the aristocracy; it was founded in 1567 but opened its doors in 1569 only.

surgeon Hildebrand dissected the body, a wound about three finger-widths wide was found in the stomach wall, however. Vomiting and other typical signs of a stomach wound – as described by authorities such as Celsus – were missing. It was assumed that matter had flowed from the wounded stomach down to the scrotum. "Much happens in sick people that is not written about", Handsch concluded, adding a "nota bene" in the margin.[198]

In May 1571, Hildebrand also performed a post-mortem in Innsbruck on the body of a young man from Trento who had suffered from a dry cough, shortness of breath, and a heaviness in the chest. In the stomach area, a palpable induration had been found on the left. Based on the palpatory findings, the physicians had suspected an apostema of the stomach, yet the autopsy revealed that the stomach was fully intact. The liver, on the other hand, was very hard and of a leaden color. It did not have its natural shape and pustules had formed on its surface. The gallbladder was swollen. In the chest cavity, there were large quantities of blood and water. The substance of the lungs ("substantia pulmonis") had largely dissolved in the area near the heart; all that remained were a few filaments.[199]

Presumably in the same year, the court surgeon Hildebrand performed another dissection, this time on a heavy drinker who had developed a painful tumor in the area of the lower ribs. From the outside, it felt like a drum. The growth had been opened and within a month close to forty pounds of blood and pus were drained with a cannula, along with small particles of more solid substance that resembled spoiled brain matter. The autopsy revealed a greatly enlarged liver that could hardly be held with two hands, including a fist-sized apostema full of stinking pus. The liver was so large that it almost reached the stomach region. Hildebrand explained here that pain or other complaints that seemed to come from the stomach could also have their origins in the liver.[200]

Handsch also gave an account of the autopsy on the body of a ten-year-old boy at the Innsbruck hospital around that time. Two stones that were almost as large as chicken eggs were found in the bladder.[201] In the case of a tailor, who had suffered from shortness of breath without a cough as well as massive convulsions, and who ultimately succumbed to a colic attack, the intestines proved to be largely intact – the bowels were considered to be an important site or cause of colics. The liver exhibited only blackish particles, but no apostema. It

---

198 Ibid., fol. 409v; Handsch's notes are in a rough chronological order, suggesting that this post-mortem was performed in 1569.
199 Ibid., fol. 412r.
200 Ibid., fol. 412r.
201 Ibid., fol. 445r.

had, however, become joined with the diaphragm. And above all, parts of the lungs were "corrupted".[202]

Handsch's account of the autopsy of Hans Reiter in February 1574 is particularly detailed. The man had not been able to walk for quite some time. A treatment with guaiacum had been of as little benefit as a visit to the healing spring in Partenkirchen. In the end, he suffered from severe respiratory distress, could hardly speak, and ultimately died of asphyxia. Willenbroch, who was the last to treat him, had suspected muscular paralysis in the chest and legs. When Hildebrand opened the body at noon the following day, however, it was the lungs that showed massive changes. Especially the right lung was "corrupted", purulent, and spongy. According to Hildebrand, these pulmonary changes were the cause of the illness. In the renal pelvis, there were also small, hard stones, but not the ulcers which, according to Willenbroch, were the cause of kidney stones. The "nerves" ("nervi"), which ran downward next to the kidneys, were of a "flaccid" ("flaccida") consistency and seemed as if "cooked" ("quasi cocti") – a finding that, even if Handsch did not explicitly say so, would have, in the perspective of the time, confirmed Willenbroch's suspicion of a paralysis of the leg nerves.[203]

With this case, Handsch also wrote down a few technical details regarding how the court surgeon performed the dissection. It is possible that he wanted to acquire the necessary manual skills himself. The face of the dead man was covered, as we see in later depictions of anatomical demonstrations in the Netherlands (cf. Fig. 3). Hildebrand opened the abdomen with two incisions, forming a cross in the umbilical region. Before cutting through a vein, he tied it off to prevent blood from spilling out over the site.[204]

Within about a decade in Innsbruck, in other words, Handsch documented a series of autopsies. Because no comparable sources from this time are available for other towns and courts, it remains unclear whether the tally of dissections in Innsbruck and Ambras was particularly high, perhaps due to the presence of the experienced Hildebrand. On the whole, however, there can be little doubt that autopsies on deceased patients were a far more common occurrence in the sixteenth century than has commonly been assumed.

The main reason why historians have, with few exceptions, paid little attention to the numerous autopsy reports that are extant from as early as the sixteenth century, even in print, and to the appreciation afforded to them by contemporary physicians, is once again a simplistic, indeed flawed understanding of early

---

202 Ibid., fol. 288v.
203 Ibid., fol. 468r-v.
204 Ibid.

modern humoral pathology and its complexity and flexibility. If most diseases at the time had truly been attributed to a disrupted balance of the body's four humors, then autopsies would indeed have promised very little insight into the nature of a deceased patient's disease. Obviously, autopsies help uncover pathological changes primarily when a disease causes typical, visible local changes to individual organs or body parts. As we have seen over and again in this book, both physicians and laypeople mainly attributed diseases to pathologically altered humors or other fluid morbid matter, however, which frequently accumulated in certain parts or organs. Accumulations of morbid matter were visible to the naked eye in an autopsy, and as Handsch's descriptions of autopsies go to show, the vast majority of the specific pathological findings described by physicians who performed autopsies on deceased patients could be interpreted in terms of such local deposits.

Sometimes the morbid matter accumulated in a cavity, for example in the lungs or abdominal cavity. And just as it could be found on the outer skin, morbid matter could also collect in small blisters that formed on the surface of an organ. Even more frequently, it could harden in a particular place, build up in it and ultimately obstruct the organ in question. Indurations and enlargements of the liver, the stomach, or the spleen, which the physicians had palpated from the outside when the patient was alive, were now, in an autopsy, plain to see as indurated and enlarged organs. Sometimes the physicians found, as with Hans Reiter, that the organ's substance itself was altered. A lung or the liver might disintegrate and decay. The boundaries between decaying, corrupting organs and local accumulations of corrupting morbid matter were blurred. After all, according to Galenic doctrine, the *parenchyma*, the very substance of organs, derived from blood and other fluids that permeated the walls of the vessels and solidified.

The most conspicuous and often unmistakable finding – something that takes a prominent position in sixteenth-century autopsy reports and in Handsch's notes as well – was stones. In the living patient, stones or concretions sometimes occurred under the skin, particularly as gouty tophi, or they were excreted as kidney or bladder stones with the urine. Post-mortems showed that such concretions could form in the gallbladder as well, or even in the liver or the lungs.[205] Their genesis could be explained in two ways. Under the influence of heat, for example in a hot liver, local accumulations of humors could dry out and solidify to such an extent that they turned into sand or stones. Alternatively, just as lime deposits were known to form in the drains of some thermal baths, stones could also come

---

[205] E.g. Leonhard Dold in a letter to Sigismund Schnitzer, [Nürnberg] 1602 (printed in Hornung, Cista medica, p. 441) reported about the dissection of a corpse with stones in the liver and in the left kidney.

from the tiny particles that had dissolved in the blood or humors, coming together over time as ever larger concretions. As Handsch knew from his discussions with Willenbroch, this explanation nicely corresponded to the Paracelsian doctrine of "tartar". These tiny particles could get caught in the urinary tract, a place where stones tended to form, but they could also form small stones in the liver, which then showed up in the gall bladder.[206]

Even when no pathological finding was present during a dissection, important insights could be gained on occasion, and in some cases the opinion of a traditional authority could be corrected. For example, Handsch gathered from his reading of Galen that with cases of dropsy, the liver was always weak. Willenbroch, however, pointed him to a famous Roman anatomist who, when performing an autopsy on a deceased dropsical patient, discovered a completely clearn and healthy ("purissimum") liver.[207]

Observations made with dead animals could also provide valuable clues about similar pathological changes in humans. Handsch, for example, saw a pig's liver at his father's house whose surface was covered in blisters. The pig had seemed healthy when it was alive, he added. The implication was that blisters of this kind – in animals as in man – could also be harmless in nature.[208] Handsch also found it worthwhile to note down what he had heard from a butcher about the changes in the liver and lungs of sheep and cows. The butcher explained that these two organs could not only have blisters, which gave off water when they were cut with a knife, but sometimes the organs themselves were rotten or there were accumulations of morbid humors ("apostemata") from which pus ("sanies") issued when opened up. Handsch added here that one could presume that the same thing sometimes happened in humans.[209] When a peasant woman presented with a greatly distended abdomen, Handsch contradicted the previous diagnosis of a lay healer who suspected an infiltration of the liver with tiny stones (and therefore likely ascites). The *empirici* simply liked to talk this way, he wrote. He did admit, however, that the liver was sometimes interspersed with stones: he had seen it in the livers of sheep.[210]

---

[206] Cod. 11183, fol. 163v.
[207] Ibid., fol. 43r; he changed "corruptione" into "imbecillitate", i.e. "weakness".
[208] Ibid., fol. 22r.
[209] Ibid., fol. 188r: "Sic aliquando in homine credendum."
[210] Cod. 11205, fol. 408v.

Facticity

As we saw in Part I, medical students and physicians were very well-versed in the humanist notation technique of *loci communes*. Many of them compiled such *loci communes* since their youth, collecting quotations from ancient poets and authors, but also documenting their medical collectanea and practical experiences. For the latter, sequential *loci communes* were particularly suitable. Here, the author did not organize his notes alphabetically or order them as he would structure them in a book. He simply wrote his entries one after another, filling the pages as he went. The result resembled what was called *adversaria* at the time, a notebook in which entries on the most varied subjects were gathered without any sort of order.[211] However, the authors still adopted the central, constitutive element of the *loci communes* method: they assigned keywords or subject headings and used these again for future entries on the same subject. Generally, these keywords or subject headings (*capita*) were highlighted by writing them larger or in capital letters or by using ink of a different color, or a special marking on the page or in the margin. In this way, entries on a particular subject were easily recognizable as such (cf. Fig. 2) and were quickly identified when the author look for notes on a certain topic. In addition, an index or register could significantly facilitate future searches for different entries that shared the same keyword.

Handsch had good reason to use the sequential *loci communes* method when he practiced as a physician, as did other physicians and natural historians.[212] Sequential *loci communes* offered a very flexible, open tool. They put no restrictions on the choice of new keywords. In medicine and natural history especially, this had great advantages. With the shift towards empirical observation in medicine, the knowledge of specific substances, body parts, pathological phenomena, medicines, objects, and processes gained greater and greater significance. Using the sequential *loci communes* method, new subject headings could be added ad libitum, for example about a hitherto unknown medicinal plant or a hitherto overlooked anatomical structure.

Notebooks that applied the *loci communes* principle served as more than memory aids. They also held considerable epistemic potential. Elsewhere I have analyzed these epistemic effects in more detail, as "pluralization", "categorization", and "decontextualization".[213]

---

[211] In his guide to excerpting, Albert Kijper used the term "tumultuarie" (Kijper, Medicinam (1643), p. 265).
[212] In the seventeenth century, the Silesian physician Martin Kerger explicitly recommended this approach (Kerger, Methodus (1695))
[213] Stolberg, Medizinische Loci communes (2013).

Pluralization: Using a given keyword to collect passages on a particular subject from the works of different authors, or indeed even of one and the same author, rendered the plurality of observations and opinions immediately visible. Assembling passages on the same issue from different texts in this manner showed virtually at one glance where the cherished ancient authorities contradicted each other or even became entangled in contradictions in their own writings. Awareness of such pluralism and contradictions encouraged the use of ones own senses in order to decide which opinions and observations could be trusted, rather than just relying on the works of authorities.

Categorization: The *loci communes* method contributed to the reorganization of existing categories and to the creation of new ones. The mere act of choosing a certain *locus* or keyword and assigning entries from various sources to it could create new knowledge.[214] This was especially true for medicine and natural philosophy. After all, there was nothing about individual observations and insights that intrinsically implicated the choice of a given *locus* or heading. Choosing a more or less general heading or category was based on abstraction, and this abstraction could follow very different interests and criteria. In botany and zoology, for instance, different varieties of plants and animals could be construed as separate entities or grouped together as one. This was more than just an intellectual question. For example, the decision could have very specific implications for their therapeutic application: as experience taught, different plants, even if they looked almost identical, often had different specific medicinal properties. A fortiori, the act of assigning individual empirical observations on patients with similar symptoms to disease categories such as "scurvy", "cancer", "tertian fever", "hysteria", and "dropsy" had significant and far-reaching implications for the understanding and treatments of diseases as such. It reinforced the significance of ontological conceptions of disease, according to which disease entities could be distinguished from each other just like plants or animals.

Decontextualization: with good reason, none other than Francis Bacon (1561–1626), who has been considered by many to be the intellectual father of the often-invoked "scientific revolution" of the seventeenth century, emphatically recommended "the disposition and collocation of that knowledge which we preserve in writing" in the form of a "good digest of common places".[215] Medical

---

[214] Sharpe (Politics of reading (2000), p. 191)) gives a concise summary of the creative role of the notetaker: "as he selects, paraphrases, arranges, glosses, cross-references and indexes, he performs a very individual reading and interpretation".
[215] Bacon, Twoo bookes (1605), p. 106.

and natural-historical notebooks that follow the *loci communes* method have an important place in the history of an increasing appreciation of "scientific facts." As Lorraine Daston and others have underlined, the appreciation of "facts" is not a timeless phenomenon. It was only in the course of the early modern period, with the rise of a empirical approaches in science, that "facts" took on a key position. A central characteristic of facts, or more precisely, of their communication in language, with words, is their brevity, and it has sweeping epistemological implications: ideally such brevity reflects the pure, neutral, unconditioned, theory-free status of "facts". Facts do not follow a prescribed order. Like cards in a deck, they can always be shuffled at random and then rearranged in a different order. Thus, they can serve in new and very different ways as building blocks and as empirical evidence for an unlimited array of arguments, theories, explanatory models, or classifications.[216]

The parallels between these epistemic processes and the nature and function of notebooks following the *loci communes* method are plain to see.[217] The characteristic features of the entries were brevity and decontextualization. Passages from larger works and empirical observations were torn from their original context and assigned to individual keywords as the author saw fit. By adapting the use of *loci communes,* one of the central humanist cultural practices, to suit their own needs, physicians and natural historians helped create and maintain a mental habitus in which factual statements and snippets of knowledge played a key role. Just as school boys and students of philosphy and the liberal arts learned to organize and record short quotes and crucial passages from the works of ancient poets and philosophers according to *loci,* physicians and natural philosophers began to record short, concise statements and insights from the book of nature, without immediately fitting them into a given classification system that was predetermined by a particular theory.

---

[216] Daston, Perché (2001).
[217] In the words of Daston, Taking notes (2004), p. 445, "the Renaissance humanist practice of excerpting short, pithy quotations from long texts for florilegia and commonplace books bears a close resemblance to the excerpting of short, pithy facts from the continuum of experience"; in her analysis of Jean Bodin's (printed) *Universae naturae theatrum* Ann Blair, Humanist methods (1992), p. 545, had already argued along similar lines.

Medicine and the "Scientific Revolution" of the Seventeenth Century

We have seen, then, how learned Renaissance physicians turned to empiricism, not only in anatomy and botany but also and especially so with respect to questions of medical practice. This striking shift in medical epistemology and methodology found expression in the dedicated search for pathological changes by means of autopsies. It made itself felt in a burgeoning esteem for medical casuistry and for the knowledge gained through induction that came out of this, as opposed to knowledge deduced from general theorems. It was reflected in the development of the *loci communes* method into an instrument of recording empirical observations. And, in close connection with botany, it became manifest in the effort to verify the effects of medicinal plants and mixtures of drugs, which went so far as to include deadly experiments with persons sentenced to death.

The turn toward empiricism on the part of learned physicians is all the more remarkable as it threatened a central foundation of their professional authority and status. The more the scales tipped from *ratio* to *experientia*, the more problematic it became for the physicians to distinguish themselves from the *empirici*. The shift towards empirical approaches brought them dangerously close to the many healers against whom they unremittingly inveighed, claiming that they only treated patients based on experience, with the implication that they often treated only the symptoms while leaving untouched the true causes of disease, which only the learned "rational" physicians knew how to identify.

The growing esteem for empirical knowledge in medicine over and above book knowledge, as Hal Cook has pointed out, ultimately had far-reaching consequences for the development of the natural sciences as a whole. A striking number of Royal Society members and of the protagonists in the so-called scientific revolution of the seventeenth century on the whole were physicians.[218] From medicine they brought with them both a pronounced interest in the concrete, specific qualities and faculties of things found in nature, as could only be discerned by precise observation, and with methodological tools that allowed for a systematic verification of these properties. Essential epistemic practices of the *scientia nova,* as advocated in the early seventeenth century by Francis Bacon (1561–1626),[219] who has been celebrated as the pioneer of empiricism

---

218 Cook, Victories (2010); similarly also Ragland, "Making trials" (2017).
219 Bacon, Twoo bookes (1605).

and father of the scientific revolution, had long been introduced and successfully applied in medical practice. And the idea of utilizing nature and asserting man's dominion over nature was a central feature of medicine as an eminently practical discipline. Tellingly, a medical practitioner, the physician and humanist Girolamo Cardano (1501–1576) put this idea in a nutshell half a century before Bacon: "The study of philosophy as such is a beautiful thing [. . .] but its fruit is the science of natural things which gives rise to the arts, [the science] of propulsion through fire and water, and of the unloading and pulling machines, as well as the knowledge of the qualities of things and causes."

Part III: **Physicians, Patients, and Lay Medical Culture**

The rise of the learned medical profession

In the late fifteenth century, in the Holy Roman Empire as elsewhere on the European continent, learned medicine began to acquire a distinctly more prominent place in people's everyday lives. The number of educated physicians rose markedly and physicians began to establish themselves also in smaller towns, where no physician had practiced until then. In doing so, they made learned medicine accessible to wider segments of the population and in their everyday practice, they increasingly found themselves face to face with people from all social classes. A major driving force of this development was the growing demographic, economic, and cultural importance of the urban bourgeoisie and their appreciation for learning and education. Many burghers were ready and willing to consult a learned physician when they were ill and to remunerate him accordingly. Moreover, with their votes in the municipal council, they improved the prospect of a sufficient income for physicians also outside the large and prosperous trading cities. This was because, following the Italian model,[1] more and more cities and towns were beginning to hire municipal physicians. Especially in smaller towns, where physicians could not expect to find many affluent patients, a salaried position as a municipal physician now offered them a certain degree of financial security. It encouraged learned physicians to settle in these towns insofar as they could hope to supplement the usually modest salary paid by the town physician with earnings from their private practice, and thereby make a sufficient living overall. In the process, the urban middle classes came to recognize education and a secular profession as a means by which their own sons might climb the social ranks. Medicine became an attractive career option. The growing number of graduates of medical programs at universities in turn improved the accessibility and impact of learned medicine in the contemporary society.

---

1 Palmer, Physicians (1981).

ⓐ Open Access. © 2022 Michael Stolberg, published by De Gruyter. [CC BY-NC-ND] This work is licensed under the Creative Commons Attribution-NonCommercial-NoDerivatives 4.0 International License.
https://doi.org/10.1515/9783110733549-014

Private Practice

After three years of study in Padua and the completion of his doctorate in Ferrara, Handsch returned home via Trento.² It was time to establish his career. For a young physician, however, this was anything but simple. As a rule, patients preferred experienced physicians with a good reputation who were known for their successful treatment of numerous patients. Accordingly, fresh out of university in 1577, the *doctor medicinae* Johann Schwartz complained that he was hardly able to gain experience in Tübingen, where he had settled to practice medicine. The few patients who sought the advice of a learned physician were almost all seen by the local, experienced practitioners, meaning that as a young and little known physician he had hardly any work.³ Handsch knew that he had to expect similar problems. Early on, in his collection of sayings, he noted down this proverb: "People prefer to go to the tailor than to the tailor's apprentice".⁴

Indirectly, this widespread preference for experienced physicians can also be inferred from the letters physicians wrote to municipal authorities when they were applying for the position of municipal physician. Applicants frequently emphasized not only their university education, preferably at a famous university, but also their practical experience.⁵ The Wasserburg physician Georg Haindlacher, for example, underlined in 1549 that in his fourteen years of medical practice, he was consulted by so many patients and had become so practiced and experienced that he was a match for other physicians, by which he meant those in Augsburg in particular.⁶ Likewise extolling his experience in 1606, Jacob Berckhmüller wrote that he had not only studied at different universities, "but also practiced in the medical field at the renowned and praiseworthy Hospital Santa Maria Nuova in Florence and in other places to such an extent that now, with divine assistance, I have cause to apply my *talentum*."⁷ Urban Schlegel, for his part, pointed

---

2 Cod. 9650, foll. 25v-26v, copy of a letter to Matthaeus Collinus from Trento in the summer of 1553, announcing that he hoped to be back in Prague in the fall.
3 HStA Stuttgart, A 282, Bü. 1301, undated letter from Johann Schwartz to Duke Ludwig of Württemberg, received 4 April 1577. Schwartz therefore wanted to go to Esslingen, where only one physician was active.
4 Cod. 9671, fol. 74r.
5 Schlegelmilch, Promoting (2019).
6 Letter from Haindlacher, Augsburg, 1549: "mit solchem Vleiß gebraucht gebraucht unnd in ein solche Practic unnd Erfarnhait kommen" (www.aerztebriefe.de/id/00001294, S. Herde).
7 Letter from Berckhmüller, Augsburg, 7 March 1606 (www.aerztebriefe.de/id/00001973, S. Herde).

to the practical experience he had gained in hospitals in Munich.⁸ In their letters of recommendation, physicians' previous employers likewise praised them with words like "an experienced and lauded medicus".⁹

Competition was particularly stiff in larger cities like Nuremberg, Augsburg, Prague, Basel, and Zurich, which dangled the prospect of a lucrative practice due to their large populations of wealthy citizens. The population of Prague, for example, was about 20,000 at the time, and included numerous members of the nobility and wealthy citizens.¹⁰ However, newcomers had to hold their own against a host of established, experienced physicians, not to mention the countless barbers, barber-surgeons, and lay healers who also offered their services. As Handsch summarized the situation concisely: "In large ponds one catches large fish, [but one] may also drown in them".¹¹ There were young physicians such as Felix Platter, who by his own account was able to assert himself over a good dozen other *doctores medicinae* in his home city of Basel within a short period of time, soon counting among his patients sick people from the leading families of the city and the surrounding area. Platter had studied at a renowned foreign university, however, and his family as well as his future father-in-law, the surgeon and councilor Franz Jeckelmann, were well-known and influential in Basel. Thus, he could draw on a well-developed network of social connections. Moreover he knew well, it seems, how to effectively showcase his anatomical and uroscopic abilities.¹²

For a young, inexperienced physician, the competition encountered in smaller cities and market towns was less threatening. In these places, he could hope for smoother sailing. At the same time, however, they were home to fewer well-to-do families who would be able to secure him the income he hoped for with their generous remuneration. Even in Innsbruck, with the nearby archducal residence in Ambras, Handsch found: "If you want to survive in Innsbruck, you will have to mend much and eat little."¹³ Moreover, while the competition from other learned physicians in smaller cities and market towns might be less substantial, the young physician still had to assert himself over the local barbers, barber-surgeons, and

---

8 Letter from Schlegel, Augsburg, 15 November 1618 (www.aerztebriefe.de/id/00001983, S. Herde/T. Walter).
9 Stadtarchiv Augsburg, Collegium Medicum, Karton 4, testimonial of Pfalzgraf Wolfgang Wilhelm zu Neuburg, 1615.
10 Albrecht, Prag (2012), p. 1658; Ledvinka/Pešek, Public and private lives (1997); Pešek, Prague (1997).
11 Cod. 9671, fol. 60v.
12 Platter, Tagebuch (1978), pp. 338–356.
13 Cod. 9671, fol. 58r.

lay healers who, often in the absence of any university-trained physicians, had provided healthcare in many places for a long time and satisfied their clientele.

Despite such difficult beginnings, the large majority of medical graduates eventually worked in their own practice. Some, like Platter, stayed in their hometowns. Many moved to other places. Some were active in a single location for a long time or until their death. For others, the first move only marked the beginning in a series of way stations as these physicians climbed – in the ideal case – to ever more attractive and profitable positions over time. Physicians here were paradigmatic for a new and historically highly significant social phenomenon, and perhaps even acted as trailblazers: they were the members of a mobile profession whose success – both professional and economic – and standing in the urban society were primarily owed to their education and their academic degree rather than their family background and inherited fortune. Supported by the cultural capital[14] of their academic training, many of them could establish a professional life for themselves as strangers working far from home without the support of family and friends, and some accumulated considerable wealth.

Handsch was among the less successful physicians. It is possible – though there is no solid evidence – that he first attempted to gain a foothold in his hometown of Leipa when he returned from Padua. In his hometown, of course, he was known and his family was well-established. At any rate, soon after his return from Italy we find him back in Prague. It appears he was once more working in Collinus's school in the Angel's Garden, waiting, as he wrote in an epistolary poem, for the Archduke Ferdinand to return to Prague with his personal physician Andrea Gallo, who, for all we know, had paid for Handsch's studies in Padua. At that point, he hoped to live in Gallo's house and work with him.[15] From May 1555 to July 1556, Handsch lived with Gallo,[16] accompanied him on his visits to numerous patients and he also sometimes treated them on Gallo's behalf. He also had contact with Gallo's colleagues, especially Pietro Andrea Mattioli, who would play a crucial role in Handsch's later career. Handsch also assisted Gallo in other ways. He contributed to a detailed *consilium* that Gallo was writing regarding the "fluttering of the heart" ("tremor cordis") from

---

14 Bourdieu, Les trois états (1979).
15 Cod. 9821, fol. 247r-v, *epistola poetica* to Hoddeiovinus, 16 January 1554, written in Prague where "tantisper residebo, Ferdinandus/ Dum princeps rursus Pragensem migret in urbem/ Illius tunc cum medico Doctore, manebo/ Andreae Gallo fautore meo atque patrono/ Excellente, suas quoniam me sumet in aedes/ Inque suam praxim, sic innotescere possum/ Egregieque artem medicam deducere in usum."
16 Cod. 11207, fol. 1r; the whole notebook documents his time with Gallo.

which the king, the future Emperor Maximilian II, suffered.¹⁷ In 1556, he prepared Gallo's extensive plague treatise for printing.¹⁸

Working as an assistant or *famulus* to an older physician allowed Handsch, like other *doctores medicinae* fresh out of university, to watch how an experienced physician proceeded at the bedside. Handsch's comprehensive notes from his time in Prague impressively document this learning experience. He recorded numerous cases, noted down prescriptions given by Gallo and other physicians, and monitored the course and success of their treatments.¹⁹

Despite his acquaintance with Lehner, Gallo, Mattioli, and Collinus, Handsch was unable over the course of several years to establish a lucrative practice of his own in Prague, however. He was under no illusions about his failure. Eight years after receiving his doctorate, he loathed the thought of continuing to work in Prague as a physician for remuneration that was poor and shameful ("indigna et exigua praemia") and faced with the detestable crudeness ("detestabilem barbariem") and ingratitude of the people. He hardly had enough money for modest clothing and food, he wrote.²⁰ His poverty, in turn, as he saw it, was a major reason of the poor esteem in which he was held, and for the rather limited authority his patients granted him. A physician of only moderate erudition, he complained, who made an illustrious appearance became more popular than one who was truly learned but lived in modest circumstances. The present time was so corrupt, that what was inside a person was measured by what was on the outside.²¹ A physician who could not afford a certain style of living may indeed have raised eyebrows and for good reasons, too: It could be expected that if a physician cured many patients, he should achieve a degree of affluence that was evident to the eyes. Staying poor suggested the opposite.

---

17 Cod. 11158; Tobias Heusinger, Würzburg, is currently concluding his work on a dissertation on Maximilian's *tremor cordis* (Heusinger, Das zitternde Herz [2021]).
18 Cod. 9821, foll. 270v-221r, *epistola poetica* to Hoddeiovinus, Juli 1556; presumably Handsch was referring to the *Fascis de peste* (1567) which was published only after Gallus' death.
19 Cod. 11207.
20 Cod. 9650, foll. 76v-78r, copy of a letter from Handsch to Pietro Andrea Mattioli, 26 April 1561.
21 Cod. 9650, foll. 63v-67v, copy of an undated letter from Handsch to a parish priest ("parochus") in Leipa; he must have written it around 1560/61, since he mentioned only three volumes of *Farragines poematum*, which were in press but not the forth volume, which appeared in 1562.

Municipal Physicians

Most physicians depended primarily on the remuneration they received from patients to make a living. Many, however, additionally entered contracts of employment. Some agreed to provide medical care for the patients of a hospital or the residents of a monastery or convent in return for an annual remuneration. In most cases, however, especially in smaller towns, it was the position of a "Stadtarzt", a town physician that gave physicians status and a degree of economic security.

There already existed a certain number of *Stadtärzte* in the Germany of the late Middle Ages. Well-known examples are Amplonius von der Buchen (1403–1438) in Nördlingen, Hermann Schedel (1410–1485) in Augsburg and Hartmann Schedel (1440–1514) in Nördlingen and Amberg.[22] In those times, a *Stadtarzt* was not necessarily a learned physician. In the fourteenth and fifteenth centuries, barber-surgeons who learned had their trade as a craft could also be appointed as *Stadtärzte*.[23] By the sixteenth century, however, many towns decidedly preferred to employ medical practitioners with a university education.[24] Some town councils so strongly believed in the *doctores medicinae* and the superiority of learned, academic medicine that they appointed physicians who had only just graduated and had little or no practical experience. Smaller towns sometimes went to great lengths to woo learned physicians away from other places or from the services of a prince. Inquiries were made to other municipalities or physicians and other learned men in other places were asked to help convince a potential candidate. Finding town physicians became easier in the course of the sixteenth century, as more and more physicians graduated with doctoral degrees. Less attractive towns, far away from the major centers, however, still might have to go to some lengths in their pursuit of a suitable physician. For example, as late as 1593, the town council of Reval (today's Tallinn in Estonia) sent an apothecary to the German town of Lübeck, on the other side of the Baltic Sea, in search of a suitable physician.[25]

In spite of the obvious significance – also above and beyond the history of medical care in a narrower sense – the history of municipal physicians in the

---

22 Pfeil/Walter, Reichsstadt (2017); Kintzinger, Status (2000), p. 63; Laschinger, Dr. Hartmann Schedel (1993); Fischer, Hartmann Schedel (1996).
23 Kintzinger, Status (2000), pp. 68–69.
24 See e.g. Uhlig, Suche (1938), on town physicians in Zwickau.
25 Letter from Petrus Burdanus to the municipal authorities in Reval, Lübeck, 15 July 1593 (www.aerztebriefe.de/id/00035087, S. Schlegelmilch); see also Uhlig, Suche (1938).

German-speaking areas has not been adequately studied so far.[26] Occasional references can be found scattered across countless local-historical and biographical works. Georg Handsch's notes are not of much help here either, as he never held the position of town physician. Insights can be gained above all from the many employment contracts for town physicians that have survived, sometimes along with the extant correspondence between town physicians and municipal authorities. In their letters to colleagues, acting town physicians sometimes also described their situation and the challenges they faced. A systematic analysis of such documents has yet to be carried out. In what follows, I will draw primarily on about 200 contracts which the Würzburg project on "Early modern physicians' letters" has assembled in its online database.[27]

The obligations and the remuneration of municipal physicians were quite similar from one place to another. It seems that the position of town physician was already so well established in the sixteenth century that municipal authorities for the most part had quite clear ideas about what could be expected from a town physician and what he should be offered for his services. In one and the same town, the new contract for the future office holder frequently was almost identical with that of the previous one, or only minor details were changed, especially with regard to the physician's salary, not concerning his duties. In Frankfurt am Main, for example, the certificate of appointment for Nikolaus Bälz as municipal physician from 1465 differed only minimally from that for Peter Uffenbach and Johann Hartmann Beyer from the end of the sixteenth century.[28]

The most important obligation of a municipal physician is easy to overlook in hindsight because it may seem obvious: as with the Italian *medici condotti* and the Spanish municipal physicians,[29] learned town physicians in the German lands were to provide medical care for the population, by day and by night, for rich and for poor, as the contracts usually said. As a rule, this went hand in hand with the obligation to reside in the town and more or less strict rules regarding times of absence. In many places, the physician was not allowed to leave the city even for a night unless he had the express permission of the mayor or another

---

26 For an overview of extant work on town physicians in the seventeenth and eighteenth centuries and for case studies on individual town physicians from that time see Schilling/Schlegelmilch/Splinter, Stadtarzt (2011), pp. 99–133; Schlegelmilch, Magnificent work (2015), pp. 151–168; Schlegelmilch, Ärztliche Praxis (2018); on the fifteenth and sixteenth centuries, see Kintzinger, Status (2000), esp. pp. 70–73.
27 See www.aerztebriefe.de.
28 See www.aerztebriefe.de/id/00004035, T. Walter, www.aerztebriefe.de/id/00004230, T. Walter and www.aerztebriefe.de/id/00004232, A. Döll/T. Walter.
29 Nutton, Continuity (1981); López Piñero, Medical profession (1981), p. 95.

town official. The concern was that the town physician might otherwise spend a lot of time at the country estates of his wealthy noble patients instead of attending to patients in town.

Many municipalities also tried to ensure contractually that the services of the town physician were affordable to more than just a well-off minority. Employment contracts routinely demanded that the physician not overcharge his patients, indeed, that he practice due restraint when it came to his financial demands. In some municipalities, the mayor or town councilor reserved the right to determine the fee in cases of dispute and the town physician obligated himself by contract to comply with this decision.[30] Sometimes this was taken further and an upper limit for fees was established. Matthias Gabler, municipal physician for Esslingen, for example, was only permitted to ask at most eight pfennigs for uroscopy and medical advice or a prescription, and just as much for visiting patients in their homes.[31] Jörg Hayndlocher's contract for his position as town physician of Dinkelsbühl laid out almost identical sums in 1556.[32] In Frankfurt, Nikolaus Bälz in 1465 and Johann Steinwert in 1500 were permitted to charge a maximum of twelve hellers for uroscopy, and the same was true for Ludwig Graf and Adam Lonitzer fifty years later.[33] The municipal physicians of Lindau were not allowed to take more than three batzen for a house call in 1584.[34] These were all modest sums that almost every family could afford if they had to.

In addition to this, some municipal physician contracts forbade physicians from making deals with individual apothecaries. This helped protect the other apothecaries who were not privy to the deal, but at the same time it served the interest of patients. It prevented the apothecary from directing them to a physician with whom he was in cahoots and who would allow him to charge exorbitant prices or even collect a commission on each prescription. The 1502 appointment contract for Johann Steinwert as well as that for Gerhard Zwihl, dated 1622, explicitly forbade the latter.[35] As Handsch learned, the concern was not unfounded. Some

---

30 Contract of Karl Baumann in Burghausen, 13 July 1576, www.aerztebriefe.de/id/00023275, T. Walter.
31 Contract, 11 March 1529 (Stroh, Aerztliche Bewerbungen (1920), pp. 34–36).
32 Greiner, Dinkelsbühler Arzt-Instruktionen (1935).
33 See www.aerztebriefe.de/id/00004035, T. Walter; www.aerztebriefe.de/id/00004158, T. Walter (Steinwert); www.aerztebriefe.de/id/00004170, T. Walter (Graf/Grave, 12.4.1548); www.aerztebriefe.de/id/00004173, T. Walter (Lonitzer, 4 October 1554).
34 Contracts of Abraham Mürgel and Peter Eckholt, 11 November 1584 (www.aerztebriefe.de/id/00002339, T. Walter).
35 Contracts of Steinwert www.aerztebriefe.de/id/00004158, T. Walter) and Gerhard Zwihl Frankfurt 1622 (www.aerztebriefe.de/id/00004233, A. Döll/T. Walter).

physicians had agreements with apothecaries, he wrote. They wrote secret codes on their prescriptions like "D" or "T" – presumably for "duplex" and "triplex" – which indicated whether they expected to collect double or triple their fee from the apothecary. Doctor Raisthner in Lemberg went about things in this way, Handsch learnt.[36]

In places where there was no pharmacy, on the other hand, town physicians might explicitly be told to set up an apothecary's shop themselves in order to ensure that the necessary medicines would be available. The town of Flensburg in 1603, for example, appointed Dr. Johannes Leuß municipal physician while obligating him to establish an apothecary's shop with all necessary provisions within six months. His prices were to follow those laid down by regulations in Hamburg. In return, the town guaranteed him a monopoly on the sale of medicines, spices, sugar, and the like in Flensburg.[37] In the following fifty years, the *Ratsapotheke*, an apothecary's shop presided over by the Flensburg town council, was always run by the town physician, who embodied these two roles.[38] In other places, too, – Göttingen is a well-documented example – the town council entrusted the town physician with the running of an apothecary's shop.[39]

The obligation to provide of medical care in times of plague was a tender subject.[40] Some towns explicitly forbade the municipal physician from fleeing.[41] More rarely, a town physician was exempted from his duty to care for those suffering from the plague, or he had to compensate the town if he left this work to others. According to his 1548 certificate of appointment in Augsburg, Adolph Occo was allowed to leave the city in times of plague, but in return he had to put forty gulden annually – almost half of his salary of one hundred gulden – in the alms box.[42]

Often the municipal physician would also commit to treating poor patients for free and some were to provide cost-free medical care to town officials as well.[43] In some places, he was additionally obligated to provide medical care

---

36 Cod. 11207, fol. 327v.
37 Kraack, Anfänge (2006), pp. 287–9.
38 Kraack, Anfänge (2006), Ibid., p. 287 and p. 294.
39 Meinhardt, Magister Adamus Seidel (1966).
40 On the situation in England and the Netherlands, see Grell, Conflicting duties (1993).
41 Contract of Georg Pistorius (draft), Esslingen, 1561 (www.aerztebriefe.de/id/00030634, T. Walter).
42 Contract, 1 November 1548 (www.aerztebriefe.de/id/00002490, S. Herde).
43 Contract of Ludwig Graf, Frankfurt am Main, 12 April 1548 (www.aerztebriefe.de/id/00004170, T. Walter).

for sufferers of the French disease. His duties furthermore could include caring for the residents of local hospitals. However, larger cities like Augsburg tended to specially appointed physicians to who worked in institutions for the care of patients with certain ailments such as the French disease.[44]

A second important role of municipal physicians, as routinely stipulated in their contracts, was helping to maintain public health. They were often, for example, assigned to examine lepers, or at least participate in such examinations.[45] Leprosy at the time – unlike today – was considered extremely contagious, and thus it seemed urgently necessary to remove lepers from the town community. Some municipal archives still contain medical records of leprosy examinations, which demonstrate the town physicians' routine participation in this task.[46] A few municipalities also obligated their town physicians to examine the local midwives. An early example is Freiberg in 1524.[47]

As a rule, municipal physicians were also charged with supervising the local apothecaries. In some places, this meant biannual or annual apothecary visitations,[48] which usually involved the physician as well as delegates from the town council.[49] In other places, it was explicitly stated that this duty was to encompass not only such biannual or annual "general visitations" but to include "private visitations" as well.[50] If we look, for example, at Sommerfeld's 1523 appointment to Zwickau and at Graf's 1548 appointment to Frankfurt, we see how municipal physicians were specifically asked to supervise the production of complicated medicines and/or medicines that were intended to keep for

---

44 Stein, Negotiating (2009).
45 E.g. contract of Matthias Gabler, Esslingen, 11 March 1529 (Stroh, Bewerbungen (1920), pp. 34–36); contract of Adolph Occo III, Augsburg, 24 May 1564 (www.aerztebriefe.de/id/00002838, S. Herde); contract of Abraham Mürgel and Peter Eckholt, Lindau, 11 November 1584 (www.aerztebriefe.de/id/00002339, T. Walter).
46 The Stadtarchiv Augsburg, e.g., has a collection of such documents.
47 Contract of Franz Pormann, Freiberg, 16 September 1524 (www.aerztebriefe.de/id/00025297, T. Walter); in Augsburg and Lindau, this was the case, at the latest, since 1564 and 1584 respectively (contract of Jeremias Martius, Augsburg, 11 November 1564; www.aerztebriefe.de/id/00002839, S. Herde; contract of Abraham Mürgel and Peter Eckholt, 11 November 1584, www.aerztebriefe.de/id/00002339, T. Walter).
48 Contracts of Franz Pormann, Freiberg, 16 September 1524 (www.aerztebriefe.de/id/00025297, T. Walter) and Peter Eckholt, Lindau, 18 December 1576 (www.aerztebriefe.de/id/00002565, T. Walter).
49 Thus explicitly in the contract of Georg Frederaun, Goslar, 13 November 1569 (www.aerztebriefe.de/id/00002399, T. Walter).
50 Contracts of Abraham Mürgel and Peter Eckholt, Lindau, 11 November 1584 (www.aerztebriefe.de/id/00002339, T Walter); Eckolt used the terms "general" and "private" in an earlier letter, Isny, 2 August 1579 (www.aerztebriefe.de/id/00002571).

a long time, such as "dissolving medicine" and syrups, making sure that a date of manufacture was provided.[51] The granting of such authority to municipal physicians gradually led to a shift in the balance of power between physicians and apothecaries. It is revealing that it was not an apothecary but Valerius Cordus, a young physician in Nuremberg, who created the *Dispensatorium,* the first official pharmacopoeia, that is a list of official medicines which the city's apothecaries had to make and keep in stock.[52]

In some respects, the office of the municipal physician thus has an important place in the history of public health. Yet, we must not overstate the significance of municipal physicians within health policy, their influence on public health. They were not yet responsible for administering state health policy, the way the salaried public health officers in the late eighteenth and nineteenth centuries were. It was mayors and town councilors who held and used the power to make decisions and shape policy in matters of public health and even in times of pestilence. The municipal physicians were respected for their learned knowledge. If necessary, their advice was sought, their expertise put to use. Ultimately, however, they were civil servants, like other municipal employees. In municipal archives, we are thus likely to encounter them not as decision- and policy-makers, but as supplicants asking for a modest pay raise, a better apartment, or official protection against non-certified healers.[53]

As a rule, municipal physicians were appointed for a limited period of time. This practice helped ensure that the physician would discharge his duties adequately. The municipal physician, for his part, had a chance to demand a higher salary when the time came to renew his contract. Here, he could implicitly or explicitly threaten to look for a more lucrative position elsewhere if his demands were not met. The usual period of employment was three[54] or four years. Sometimes it was only one year,[55] and then again a more generous limit could

---

51 Contracts of Johann Sommerfeld, Zwickau, 28 November 1523 (Herzog, Physikat-Bestallungen (1848), pp. 194–195) and Martin Holzapfel, Augsburg, 12 June 1590 (www.aerztebriefe.de/id/00003145, S. Herde).
52 Cordus, Pharmacorum (1546); for a detailed analysis of the developments see Murphy, New order (2019).
53 Nutton, Continuity (1981), p. 31; Palmer, Physicians (1981); on the later development see Cipolla, Public health (1976).
54 E.g. contracts of Nikolaus Bälz, Frankfurt am Main, 28 November 1465 (www.aerztebriefe.de/id/00004035, T. Walter) and of Cosmas Diechtel, Frankfurt, 14 November 1520 (www.aerztebriefe.de/id/00004165, T. Walter).
55 E.g. contracts of Jung, Augsburg, 18 December 1510 (www.aerztebriefe.de/id/00002488, S. Herde), of Jacobus Conradi, Frankfurt, 27 March 1500 (www.aerztebriefe.de/id/00004157,

be agreed upon – five, eight[56] or, in the case of the famous Janus Cornarius, as much as ten years.[57] At times, a trial period was agreed upon for both sides. If both parties desired, the contract could generally be renewed. This is, in fact, what happened in many cases, and quite often for the remainder of the physician's career.[58] Only exceptionally was a municipal physician appointed for life, however, like Johannes Castner in Amberg in 1546.[59]

In many biographies of sixteenth-century German physicians, the position of municipal physician – the *physicus ordinarius* – was an important stepping stone in their career, and many physicians were employed by municipalities over the course of their entire professional lives. By all appearances, in other words, the office of a town physician was an attractive career option. This is reflected in the numerous letters in which physicians requested such a position, for example because they had heard that the current municipal physician was severely ill or had just died.[60] The salary paid to municipal physicians was only part of the reason why it was a sought-after position. Some municipal physicians received one hundred gulden annually, and even more if they stayed in their position long enough.[61] But many towns paid an annual salary of around fifty gulden only in the sixteenth century, and in some places it was as low as twenty,[62] thirty[63] or forty gulden.[64] Even someone like Otto Brunfels in Bern had to make do with an annual salary of sixty gulden.[65] In the case of Janus Cornarius, the

---

T. Walter), and of Georg Frederaun, Goslar, 13 November 1569 (www.aerztebriefe.de/id/00002399, T. Walter).
56 Adolf Occo II, Augsburg 1548, for five years (www.aerztebriefe.de/id/00002490, S. Herde); Leopold Drinckel, Augsburg 1553, for eight years (www.aerztebriefe.de/id/00002779, S. Herde).
57 Herzog, Physikat-Bestallungen (1848), pp. 195–198.
58 E.g. contracts of Siegmund Grimm, Augsburg (1511) and Johann Tieffenbach, Augsburg (1531) (www.aerztebriefe.de/id/00002539 and www.aerztebriefe.de/id/00002489, S. Herde).
59 Contract of Johannes Castner, Amberg, 24 May 1546 (www.aerztebriefe.de/id/00020270).
60 A supplication by Raymund Minderer to the Augsburg town council (20 August 1616) was successful (www.aerztebriefe.de/id/00001525, S. Herde).
61 According to Wolfangel, Ayrer (1957), p. 15, Heinrich Wolff at first received 100 gulden and later 200.
62 Contract of Johann Boel, Frankfurt am Main, 5 December 1469 (www.aerztebriefe.de/id/00004038, T. Walter).
63 Contract of Bechtold Bach, with 60 gulden and 15 Batzen per year, Frankfurt am Main, 28 February 1589 (www.aerztebriefe.de/id/00004231, T. Walter).
64 Wolfangel, Ayrer (1957), p. 15, on Melchior Ayrer's first contract (1549); later his salary was raised by 12 fl and he received, in addition, 20 fl and later 40 fl for visiting patients in the hospital.
65 Request to the Strasbourg magistrate to be exempted from his school services, October 1533 (www.aerztebriefe.de/id=00000779, U. Schlegelmilch).

authorities in Zwickau in 1546 explicitly pointed to the physician's fame to justify paying him a salary that was higher than average for the area: one hundred gulden instead of forty. And in this case, the salary was not only for his medical work. He was also tasked with the supervision of the local school, presumably the famous Zwickau Latin school.[66] In addition to their salaries, municipal physicians could expect fringe benefits such as tax reductions or the provision of wood, grain, or wine,[67] or the were given rent-free accommodation.[68] But even with all of this, the income as a town physician was nothing to write home about. In comparison to the income that could be reaped with a successful private practice, the salary of a town physician offered only a basic income. The Zwickau town physician Hiob Finzel, for example, who kept a detailed record of his medical earnings, owed at most twenty percent of his total annual income to his salary as a municipal physician (sixty gulden and some firewood) in the late sixteenth century; between 1573 and 1588, this total income averaged 435 gulden annually.[69] Obviously, this also means that equating a physician's municipal salary with his total annual income when comparing the earnings of different professional groups would lead to serious misjudgment.

We have seen, then, how the financial benefits taken by themselves hardly explain the attractiveness of the position, especially since the obligation to remain within town limits prevented municipal physicians from treating wealthy patients outside the town over the course of days and weeks, in return for a more or less lavish payment. Clearly, the position of town physician came with other benefits. Many municipal physicians worked in smaller towns, where the position secured them not only a basic income but also gave them a certain monopoly. In some cases, the town physician's contract even guaranteed such a monopoly. In Freiberg, for example, a 1524 certificate of appointment stipulated that only the municipal physician was allowed to practice "Leibarznei", meaning that as opposed to the barbers and barber-surgeons, only he would be allowed to practice internal treatment, using medicines the patients had to ingest.[70] Even in those places where other learned physicians had set up practice – in the same

---

66 Contract of Janus Cornarius, Zwickau, 18 September 1546 (www.aerztebriefe.de/id/00014028, A. Döll/T. Walter).
67 Letter from Tobias Baltz to the town of Esslingen, Juli 1579; Baltz received among others four buckets of wine per year (www.aerztebriefe.de/id/00030644, T. Walter).
68 Letter from Tobias Baltz to the town of Esslingen, 16 December 1573, asking for a more suitable accommodation (www.aerztebriefe.de/id/00030642, T. Walter).
69 Cf. Stolberg, Accounting (2021).
70 Contract of Franz Pormann, Freiberg, 16 September 1524 (www.aerztebriefe.de/id/00025297, T. Walter).

town or nearby – the municipal physician could always hope that the authority of his position would give him an edge over the competition and attract wealthier patients from the bourgeoisie and nobility.

Of course, some municipal physicians were not spared the painful experience of their private practice not bringing in what they had hoped – or had been promised. Especially in times of rising prices, some of them were hardly able to get by on their salary combined with the fees they received from their patients. But the fixed contractual periods, the limited average life expectancy, and the considerable number of positions for municipal physicians that were created in the sixteenth century all meant that there was usually a chance to find a better and more lucrative position somewhere else if need be. When negotiating the renewal of a contract, some municipal physicians were very frank about the more attractive offers they had received from other towns or cities, and sometimes they even asked to break their contract because better circumstances awaited them elsewhere. In 1533, Johann Neefe, for example, requested to be released from his duties after six years of service as a municipal physician in Annaberg because he wanted to make a change for the better. Not four weeks later, he was appointed municipal physician in Joachimstal.[71]

---

71 Letter of release from the contract, 2 October 1533 (www.aerztebriefe.de/id/00023841, T. Walter).

Court Physicians

A second position that was aspired to by doctors of medicine was that of the court physician, or in German *Leibarzt*. The term has been the source of many misunderstandings in historical writing. In traditional usage, a *Leibarzt* was simply the opposite of a *Wundarzt* or surgeon. To this day, "Leib" refers to the lived body as a whole. The domain of the *Leibarzt* was the diagnosis and treatment of internal diseases using medicines that patients needed to ingest.[72] A *Wundarzt* on the other hand was responsible for the local treatment of wounds and injuries, for small surgical interventions and generally for those "external" diseases that primarily found expression on the surface of the skin or were treated externally, for example ulcers and other skin changes. Accordingly, municipal physicians who had graduated from a university were sometimes referred to as *leibärzte* on their certificate of appointment. The term *Leibarzt* or *Leibmedicus,* had since the late Middle Ages been increasingly reserved for "personal" physicians, however, who were entrusted with providing medical care for emperors, kings, popes, princes, or other members of the nobility (and usually for their families and servants as well). Sometimes the *Leibarzt* was distinguished from the *Leibchirurg* or "personal" surgeon. But at times even a barber surgeon without an academic degree could be referred to as a *Leibarzt*, meaning a medical practitioner who took care of a ruler or some other high-ranking person. In the following, the term *Leibarzt* will be translated as personal or court physician in the sense that was becoming established at the time, that is to say a university-educated, learned physician in the service of a ruler, nobleman, or high-ranking clergyman.

Court physicians have long been of interest to historians. Older research was mostly limited to more or less short biographical outlines of famous court physicians or the physicians at a particular court.[73] Over the past decades, more and more work has been done on the figure of the court physician from the perspective of social history, with studies of the medical practice of court physicians and of their interaction with the respective rulers and those around them.[74] We can now draw on valuable studies about England, France, and Italy in particular.[75]

---

[72] See also Bünz, Leibärzte (2005), pp. 156f.
[73] Beierlein, Sigismund Kohlreuter (1954); Kostenzer, Leibärzte (1970).
[74] Nutton, Medicine (1990); Andretta/Nicoud, Être médecin (2013); for an overview of the scholarship on this topic see also Lammel, Hofmedizin (2018).
[75] Nance, Turquet de Mayerne (2001); Lane Furdell, Royal doctors (2001); Lunel, Maison (2008); Andretta, Roma (2011), pp. 285–347.

With respect to the German-speaking areas, the focus has continued to remain on biographical approaches, however.[76]

Part of the reason for this lies with the sparse source material. Sources that could shed light on the role, the tasks, and the position of court physicians are – apart from a handful of well-known and therefore well-documented figures – relatively few and far between. Certificates of appointment with detailed descriptions of physicians' duties are not extant for court physicians to the same extent that they are for municipal physicians. In the domestic archives of noble families, we primarily find documents that refer to payment and other financial matters. Alongside the certificates of appointment and Handsch's relatively detailed notes on his time as a court physician in Prague and Innsbruck, letters exchanged between court physicians and their employers are particularly revealing, allowing for insights into the work of the court physician and into the relation between court physicians and their noble patients.

When it came to the conditions and tasks which fell to the lot of a princely court physician, there were great differences depending on the employer. In many places, a distinction was roughly drawn in contemporary terminology between personal physicians "at the court" and those "from home". The personal physician "at the court" (in German "zu Hofe" or "am Hofe") was a "courtly" physician in the true sense of the word. He took part in life at the court, belonged to the princely household and generally had to be available at all times so that he could give assistance should his ruler or another patient at the court require it. In some cases, he was expected to accompany the ruler on travels and military campaigns as well. A personal physician "from home" ("von Haus aus") on the other hand generally only had to come to the court a few times a year, or when he was called to attend to a specific case of illness. He could otherwise carry on with his practice as usual, and his daily life as a physician did not differ significantly from that of other physicians. A letter regarding the appointment of the Rothenburg physician Bernard Stieber from the early seventeenth century describes and exemplifies such contractual conditions: he was to attend to his prince, the Count Georg Friedrich von Hohenlohe Weikersheim four times annually, each time staying at the court for three days. For the rest of the time, he was only obliged to come to the court when the count sent for him because he himself or a family member was sick. For these visits, Stieber would be paid separately, just as he would be when he saw the count's servants. He

---

[76] Graf-Stuhlhofer, Humanismus (1996); Zitter, Leibärzte (2000); Aumüller, Professor (2011); Kotthorst, Gelehrte Mediziner (2018). See, however, the recent collective volume ed. by Hilber/Taddei, In fürstlicher Nähe (2021).

was required, however, to consult by letter at all times, even when he was travelling.[77] Finzel's practice journal shows that families of the landed gentry around Zwickau, too, would sometimes secure the services of a learned physician by awarding him a modest annual salary. Thus, Wolf von Weisbach paid Finzel seven talers for a "half year's salary", Heinrich von Enda paid him ten talers for a "half year's salary", and Jörg Albrecht von Witzleben even gave him an "annual salary" of thirty gulden.[78]

Depending on how frequently the physician was actually sent for and how high his salary was, a position as personal physician "from home" could be highly attractive. His salary might be more modest than that of personal physician "at the court". Stieber, for example, received only wine, carp, and pike as a basic remuneration for his service and for his four annual visits to the court.[79] In 1512, Guttenberger, a personal physician "from home" in Frankfurt an der Oder, received forty gulden plus provisions when he attended to the Brandenburg elector Joachim or his wife at the court or on travels.[80] But being appointed court physician – at least where an eminent, powerful prince or even a king or emperor was concerned – meant distinction and honor for the physician in question. It opened many doors for him. If a great prince trusted a physician with his health, this had to mean that the man knew his craft. It was with good reason that court physicians made explicit reference to their positions on the title pages of their publications. Court physicians who were especially well-respected and well-known could further count on a substantial salary, even if they worked "from home". Their salary was sometimes significantly higher than that of the average town physician. For example, when Paul Luther was appointed Saxon elector Christian's court physician "from home", his annual salary was 200 gulden, which merely obligated him to see the elector when he fell ill and to consult with the other physicians employed by the elector.[81] Reiner Solenander's annual salary when he was working as a court physician for Wilhelm, Duke of Jülich-Kleve, was of a similar order of magnitude. He received 200 talers plus fifty malters of grain for his

---

77 Contract of Bernard Stieber, Schloss Schillingsfürst, 23 April 1623 (www.aerztebriefe.de/id/00010240, T. Walter).
78 Ratschulbibliothek Zwickau, Ms. QQQQ1, p. 39 and Ms. QQQQ1a, p. 42 and p. 385.
79 Contract of Bernard Stieber, castle of Schillingsfürst, 23 April 1623 (www.aerztebriefe.de/id/00010240, T. Walter).
80 According to Löwenstein, Biographien (1848), pp. 290f.
81 Richter, Genealogia Lutherorum (1733), pp. 761–63.

cattle, firewood, and feed for his two horses. He was required, however, to spend three months of the year at the court with his colleague Johann Weyer.[82]

It appears that physicians at the archducal court in Prague and Innsbruck were appointed as court physicians "at the court". Andrea Gallo and Pietro Andrea Mattioli both had their own household in Prague, and Handsch too would later live not at the Ambras Castle, but in nearby Innsbruck. Various entries in Handsch's notebooks describe, however, how his court physician colleagues would go "in aulam" without a particular reason after finishing up other work, and how high-ranking patients would later seem well again "in aula". These entries suggest that the Archduke's personal physicians routinely found themselves at the court and were involved in courtly life.[83] Even on All Saints' Day, Mattioli went to do his "duty" at the court in Prague ("in aulam ad servitium"), Handsch noted,[84] and, as Mattioli complained to Ulisse Aldrovandi, he had to accompany the Archduke when he travelled or went to war.[85] When their help was needed, they had to be at the ready. In Ambras, the Archduke sometimes called for his court physicians in the early morning hours or even in the middle of the night if his stone disease troubled him or he felt his heartbeat become irregular.[86] Sometimes they even had to keep watch over him for several nights, as in the autumn of 1568, when Ferdinand had massive, bloody diarrhea.[87]

Famous physicians "at the court" could expect more generous remuneration, particularly if they had already acquired fame and respect. Caspar Neefe, for example, who was court physician to the Saxon elector Augustus, received 400 gulden annually for eight years, plus ten ells of fine English cloth, courtly attire for his servants and, twice a year, a plump pig. And because he was unable to make any earnings outside this service, the elector additionally allowed him and his heirs to borrow as much as 3,500 gulden, on which he had to pay an annual interest rate of 5%, which seems to have been considered low.[88] As the most senior court physician of Archduke Ferdinand II, Pietro Andrea Mattioli received 400 talers annually,[89] more than the 300 gulden, for example, which

---

82 Contract of Reiner Solenander, 3 August 1559, ed. in Wackerbauer, Dr. Reiner Solenander (1932/33), p. 105.
83 E.g. Cod. 11183, fol. 129r (on Mattioli); ibid., fol. 111r-v, on the Lord of Donin, who suffered from quartan fever and with whom Handsch later talked "at the court" ("in aula").
84 Ibid., fol 159v.
85 Letter from Mattioli to Aldrovandi, Regensburg, 19 January 1557 (in Italian), ed. in Raimondi, Lettere (1906), pp. 148–152.
86 Cod. 11204, fol. 55r and Cod. 11240, fol. 61v.
87 Cod. 11204, fol. 34v.
88 Ed. in Lesser, Die albertinischen Leibärzte (2015), pp. 71–73.
89 Kühnel, Andrea Matthioli (1962), p. 67.

the renowned scholar Caspar Ursinus Velius earned per year as the appointed historian at the Vienna court.[90] Younger and lower-ranking physicians, it should be added, sometimes had to make do with a significantly lower salary. In 1520, Johann Franck was appointed court physician of the Hessian landgrave Philipp and paid one hundred gulden annually; in addition, he and his servants were provided with room and board at the court as well as courtly attire.[91] Younger court physicians could at least expect pay raises and bonuses if they proved their worth. When he was hired at the Innsbruck court in 1542 at the young age of around thirty, Giovanni Pietro Merenda (d. 1567) was likewise paid a salary of only one hundred gulden annually. Ten years later, he was earning six times that.[92] As long as they did not have to accompany the ruler on travels, even a position "at the court" also appears to have offered the opportunity to treat patients outside the court and thus gain a further source of income. This was particularly attractive because their position tended to bring them into frequent contact with potential patients from the nobility, and it worked out particularly well when the physicians retained their own household in the city while remaining available to call on their noble patients at any time.

In smaller cities with a much smaller potential clientele among the upper classes, physicians could not as easily round out a moderate salary as a court physician with income from their practice outside the court. Not every court physician necessarily became wealthy. After his many years of service, the Württemberg *hofmedikus* Christoph Schwartz left his widow – as she lamented after his death – merely a small house with an orchard.[93]

For Handsch, being appointed court physician to Archduke Ferdinand II (Fig. 12) was both the high point and the end point of his career. There are no records of the exact date,[94] but he would have been hired in the late

---

90 Letter from Georg Tannstetter to Joachim Vadian, ca 1527, ed. in Arbenz /Wartmann, Vadianische Briefsammlung, part 7 (1913), pp. 20f. (www.aerztebriefe.de/id/00017428, M. Kohler/T. Walter).
91 Hauptstaatsarchiv Stuttgart, A 20 Bü 47, copy of Franck's contract, Kassel, 3 October 1520.
92 On Merenda see Bachmann, Merenda (1953), pp. 7–8; Oberrauch, Medizin (2012), pp. 375–377.
93 Hauptstaatsarchiv Stuttgart, A 282, 1302, supplication, submitted on 4 April 1621; Schwartz, his widow added, had had considerable expenses for the treatment of his diseases.
94 The earliest trace of Handsch which I have so far been able to find among the documents of the archducal court in the Tiroler Landesarchiv in Innsbruck dates from 1572 (collection of copies of outgoing letters, "Geschäft von Hof", 1572, fol. 345v, "Doctor Jörg Hanndtschius"); further entries on Handsch are ibid. 1575, fol. 130r and ibid. 1576, foll. 501r-502r and fol. 802r-v.

1560s. Presumably[95] he came to the position through his work with Pietro Andrea Mattioli, who enjoyed great esteem as an archducal court physician. After Handsch's patron Andrea Gallo died in 1560, Handsch had offered to translate Mattioli's commentary on Dioscorides into German for him.[96] They came to an agreement and in 1563 Handsch's German translation of Mattioli's famous work was published.[97]

The most important task of a court physician was to care for the health of the ruler and his family. This was a great responsibility. The illness and death of a ruler, a successor to the throne, or the wife of a ruler – especially if she had not yet borne an heir to the throne – could have far-reaching consequences for subjects and for the royal court but also for the state and the population at large. An indication of the paramount significance of safeguarding the ruler's health is found in the considerable religious tolerance that even the Habsburgs showed with respect to hiring court physicians. Here, getting the best physicians outweighed denomination. Johannes Crato (1519–1585) and the Saxon court physician Johann Neefe (1499–1574), for example, enjoyed the Emperor's trust as court physicians, although neither made a secret of their Protestant orientation. Presumably, Georg Handsch as well benefited from this tolerance. He had, after all,

---

The archducal archives from that period are quite voluminous, however, with a number of volumes for each year. I have not yet been able to go carefully through all of them.

95 Handsch himself claimed, shortly before his death in 1578, that he had served the Archduke for 25 years. At first glance, this would seem to be corroborated by the copy of a *consilium* of Renato Brasavola from Ferrara in the Österreichische Nationalbibliothek in Vienna (Cod. 11155, foll. 1v-24v), dated 14 February 1554, in which Brasavola praised Willenbroch and Handsch as the Archduke's highly learned physicians. The date on the copy is undoubtedly wrong, however. Willenbroch was still a student in Padua in 1556 (Favaro, Atti, vol. 1 (1911), p. 13). Brasavola also mentioned that he acted on the order of his lord, Duke Alfonso d'Este but Alfonso was neither Duke nor his lord in 1554. It was only in 1559, after the death of his father, that he took over. Probably the 25 years of services to the Archduke which Handsch claimed referred to his work with and for Andrea Gallo after his return from Padua. At any rate, according to his own notes, Handsch started working in Innsbruck in 1567. In early 1567, one of the Archduke's personal physicians, Giovanni Pietro Merenda (Bachmann, Merenda (1953), p. 9) died and in the same year Mattioli requested that he be allowed to take his leave (but offered to continue his services until the following year). Quite possibly, there was thus a vacancy. Handsch's notes in a special notebook he devoted almost exclusively to the health of the archducal family (Cod. 11204) begin on 6 September 1568 (ibid., fol. 34r).

96 Cod. 9650, foll. 142r-143r and foll. 76v-78r, copies of letters from Handsch to Mattioli, 12 February and 26 April 1561; in the second letter, he detailed his offer: for free board and lodging and 100 fl. per year, he would translate Mattioli's herbal into German and also assist Mattioli in other scholarly activities. On the same day, he asked Johann Willenbroch to put a good word in for him (ibid., fol. 76r-v).

97 Mattioli, New Kreutterbuch (1563).

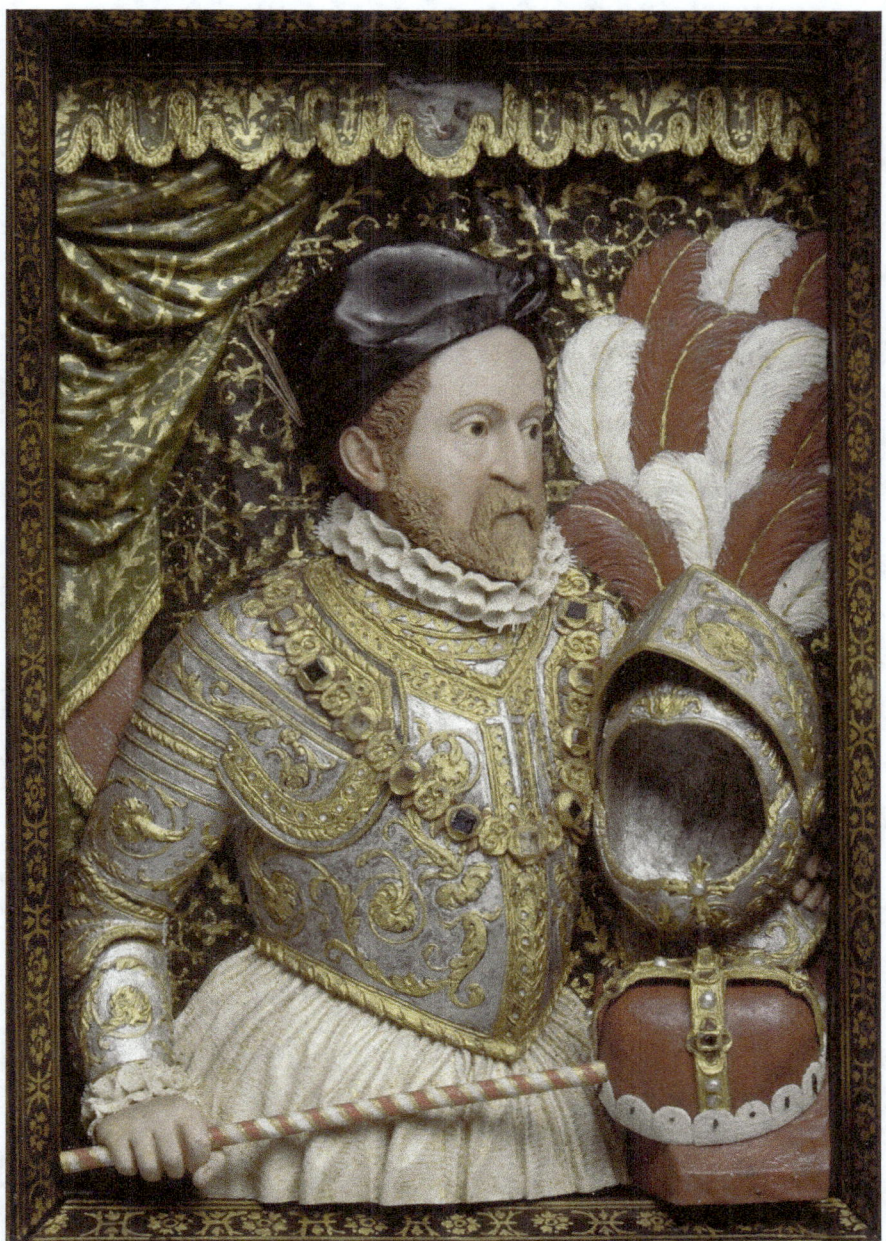

Fig. 12: Francesco Segala, relief portrait of Archduke Ferdinand II, around 1580, Kunsthistorisches Museum, Vienna, KK 3085.

attended the school in Goldberg, which decidedly embraced Protestant educational ideals.[98] He quoted from Melanchthon's works multiple times,[99] and his notes and poems on religious issues – which, admittedly, are rather few and far between – evince clear sympathies for the doctrine of the Reformers,[100] which he in one place bluntly characterized as the "true religion" as opposed to the papacy.[101]

Protecting the health of a ruler and his family was a demanding job. To begin with, preventive care – warding off illness through suitable nutrition and a salubrious way of life – was afforded much more attention in the medical practice at courts than it was in private practice. In the letter of appointment written by the Palatine elector Philipp for his court physician Adolf Occo, it was impressed upon Occo that he was to alert the ruling family if ever they were given food to eat that could be harmful to them, and in this way prevent illness.[102] The papal court physicians even regarded it as their duty to agree upon a *regimen* that was adapted each day to suit the pope's current physical condition.[103]

In their typically very detailed handwritten consultation letters for noble patients, court physicians accordingly gave meticulous dietetic instructions on a regular basis, and also recommended an array of preventive medications. Leonhard Thurneisser, for example, wrote a six-page letter advising his mistress, the Brandenburg electress, to have bloodletting and cupping done three days before or after each full moon. He warned her emphatically not to stand at the window before getting dressed in the morning, which would allow the air to enter her body via the pores; she was only to breathe the air in. She was to refrain, at least now in April with its hazy and "sharp" air, from drinking milk. Along with the letter, he sent eight different medications or secret remedies aimed at prevention: a water against the greying and falling out of hair and against mites; another to strengthen the brain, memory, reason, and vision, which was also to help against the "bad fluxes" which could settle in the temples, teeth, cheeks, and arms; a remedy she was to apply to her "body" to help with eructation, to cleanse and "renew" the uterus, and that would keep her heart from fluttering and prevent sadness, fear,

---

98 Absmeier, Schulwesen (2011), pp. 110–128.
99 Cod. 9671, fol. 18r. "Crede mihi sapere est, non nimium sapere"; see also Cod. 11183, fol. 71v, and, already in his Padua years, Cod. 11210, fol. 2r, fol. 11r, fol. 16v, fol. 37v and further entries with references to various passages in Melanchthon's *De anima*.
100 E.g. Handsch, Widmungsgedicht (1554); Cod. 9821, foll. 260v-261r.
101 Cod. 9821, foll. 11v-15v.
102 Letter of confirmation with a copy of the conditions of the contract, ed. in Mone, Krankenpflege (1851), pp. 273–75.
103 Andretta, Roma medica (2011), pp. 285–88.

and melancholy; another remedy for the bath and as a mouth rinse, which would prevent scurvy, cleanse the blood and cause it to flow at the right time, and would simultaneously strengthen the nerves, the seed, and the nature of the body as a whole, as well as consume and drive out "bad moistures"; an oil to be rubbed into the skin that would open the veins, strengthen the heart, dissolve obstructions of the liver, assuage melancholy, expel mucus from the stomach and cleanse the intestines and the gall-bladder; corals for inflammation and obstruction of the liver, lungs, heart, and vessels, for bad mucus and to "open" the body; pearls for viscous fluxes of the brain, to strengthen the memory, vision, hearing, and reason; and finally a "Schlagwasser" ("apoplectic water") made with amethyst that would open all obstructions, reinvigorate the suffocated vital spirits that had "almost died away", and that was a surefire secret remedy against apoplexy, paralysis, and all diseases of the head and heart.[104]

If their noble employers did fall ill despite these efforts, court physicians basically adopted the same diagnostic and therapeutic practices they used with other patients. The body of a king, after all, obeyed the same laws as that of the common mortal. There were, however, slight differences in emphasis. In addition to medicines, physicians relied more heavily on dietetic measures when treating rulers and other high-ranking patients, not only for prevention, but to treat illness as well. One reason for this must have been the knowledge that rich and powerful patients found it easier than less affluent contemporaries to purchase the food and drink recommended by physicians and to change their lifestyle according the physicians' instructions. But such detailed instructions were doubtlessly also designed to demonstrate that the physician was capable of controlling every detail of the disease and thus curbing its development. The message was that the physician was not powerless in the face of the illness, but rather were able to exert a very precise influence over it.

When noble patients received medical treatment in a narrower sense, it tended to be particularly thorough and painstaking. Here too, there was a confluence of the physicians' knowledge of the ruler's financial means – no medicine was too expensive – with their desire to make it clear that they would leave no stone unturned to heal his or her illness. From the perspective of the period, rulers could therefore consider themselves privileged with regard to matters of health. They could seek the advice of the most famous medical authorities of their time or even have them come to their court, and did not have to spare any costs. If we consider this medical treatment anachronistically from the perspective

---

[104] Staatsbibliothek Berlin, Ms. Bor. 682, foll. 10r-12v, "report" ("Bericht") by Thurneisser to the Electress, around 1575.

of modern medicine, for a moment, we arrive at a significantly more shaded view, however. On the one hand, the knowledge that they had access to the advice and medical care of the best physicians doubtlessly helped rulers deal with the threat of illness. But on the other hand, physicians frequently disagreed about medical matters, and they tried to distinguish themselves in the presence of the ruler by prescribing many, special medicines. In hindsight therefore, when we imagine a ruler surrounded by a crowd of court physicians, we may quite rightly feel some pity for him or her. From today's perspective, it would have been better for their health in many cases if the rulers had not subjected themselves to such thoroughgoing treatment measures, which were often accompanied by severe side effects. These measures could hardly – again, according to modern standards – have a curative effect, but instead threatened to weaken the patient, for example through ample bloodletting or by bringing on massive diarrhea, which may, at times, even have accelerated the death of the patient.

If, despite all medical efforts, a ruler's health worsened, his personal physician, surrounded as he often was by envious and jealous contemporaries, had to fear that he might fall into disfavor. "Omnia sunt longa in aula, praeter praecipitum" – "Everything lasts long at the court, except the [fall into] the abyss", Georg Handsch learned from the imperial court physician Andrea Camuzio (1512–1587).[105] On the other hand, in her study of court physicians at the Sforza court, Marilyn Nicoud found only few references to serious tensions or signs of mistrust on the part of the dukes or those in their entourage.[106] My findings on court physicians in the German-speaking areas point in the same direction. It appears that in their daily interactions rulers essentially trusted their physicians. Without a doubt, the lavish gratifications granted to Mattioli and other court physicians when they retired from service at the court may be understood as genuine expressions of gratitude.

A relation of trust was also established insofar as the ruler and his entourage generally made sure to let little about the ruler's illnesses come to the surface. This was certainly true when his or her life was in jeopardy. If the news did get out, there was a looming threat of unrest at the court and among subjects. But not only this: internal and external enemies might take advantage of the momentary weakness and engage in aggressive behavior, or in the worst case launch a military attack. Some appointment contracts explicitly stated that the physician must maintain confidentiality, both with respect to illnesses of the ruler and his family, and with respect to everything that the physician might hear and see

---

105 Cod. 9671, fol. 21r.
106 Nicoud, Medici (2013).

at the court.¹⁰⁷ Accordingly, Elector Johann Georg explained to his court physician Leonhard Thurneisser that it would be very inconvenient to him and did not seem advisable "to surround ourselves, now that we are growing old, with strange physicians, and thus reveal our complexion and our nature to everyone."¹⁰⁸ The situation was particularly serious, from the point of view of the court, when there was the danger of physicians leaking the information that a ruling prince's mental health was in peril. The letter of a ducal official to Reiner Solenander is to be read accordingly, it seems. Solenander was treating the mentally ill Johann Wilhelm, Duke of Jülich-Cleve-Berg. Repeatedly and with great emphasis, the official impressed upon Solenander that he was to maintain confidentiality, and very bluntly warned Solenander that if he did not obey this command, he would be putting his life on the line.¹⁰⁹

We have seen, then, that in the ideal case the position of princely court physician entailed a special relationship of trust and opened a privileged line of access to the ruler. It was an attractive career option and a unique chance to rise on the social ladder. Royal and imperial court physicians usually did not come from noble families. They owed their position to nothing but their education and the accounts their contemporaries gave of their specialized knowledge and medical skill. And yet in some respects, they came closer to the ruler than anyone else, often interacting with him on a daily basis, even conversing with him over a shared meal.¹¹⁰

There was, however, a significant downside to being a court physician. Ultimately, the physician was a servant of the court and could count on being treated as such. The letters written to the court physician Thurneisser by the Brandenburg elector vividly attest to this. They are noticeably brief and the tone is often brusque, commanding. In one of them, it was stated that a huntsman was sick and that Thurneisser was to go see him in Spandau.¹¹¹ Always written using the "du" the informal German form of address, the letters became more urgent when the elector himself or his wife fell ill. In July 1579, the elector informed Thurneisser that he "almost felt nauseous and had flying heat" the

---

107 Löwenstein, Biographien (1848), pp. 290f., summary of the contract of Eberhard Guttenberger as a personal physician to the Elector Joachim I, 29 April 1512; contract of Otto Bötticher as a personal physician to the Elector Georg Wilhelm, 1 May 1622 (www.aerztebriefe.de/id/00004058, U. Schlegelmilch).
108 Staatsbibliothek Berlin Ms. bor. fol. 680, fol. 17r, letter from the Elector, 8 February 1578.
109 Letter from Hofmarschall Wilhelm von Waldenfels to Reiner Solenander, 10 January 1595, in: von Lahr, Original-Denkwürdigkeiten (1834), p. 142.
110 Nutton, Introduction (1990), p. 2.
111 Staatsbibliothek Berlin Ms. bor. fol. 680, fol. 3r, 14 July 1574; similarly ibid., fol. 5r, 17 May 1576.

previous night und his back was bad as well. Thurneisser was to distill the urine that was sent with the letter and to make his diagnostic judgment, and then come to him in the afternoon or at the latest in the evening.[112] And when the electress was suffering from, among other things, "intense pains" in her head and the elector complained of a jerking pain in his abdomen, Thurneisser was instructed to come immediately.[113] It even happened that Thurneisser was summoned to the court on short notice without any explanation whatsoever.[114]

On top of that, rulers were rarely satisfied with appointing just one court physician. As a result, those physicians who ranked low in the hierarchy of the court physicians were faced with a second tier of subordination. Handsch gave a vivid description of what this could entail. In 1574, the wife of the archducal chancery scribe was suffering from colics. According to Handsch, she was first treated by a Dr. "Achilles" in Steinach – presumably this was Achill Jelmus – and was then also seen by Willenbroch and Handsch in Innsbruck. Soon there was a disagreement. Willenbroch allowed the patient to drink wine, but Achilles considered this dangerous. Handsch recommended a decoction he had been given by his mentor Gallo, but he was unable to assert himself. To the chagrin of his colleagues, Willenbroch, who clearly ranked highest, prescribed a series of bloodlettings. Handsch complained sorely that "Willenbroch did not proceed methodically and according to the rules of the art [. . .] but in his own manner, and we were forced to relent."[115]

Not only this, but life at the court with its complicated hierarchies followed its own rules to which court physicians, like everyone else, had to submit. One of the sayings and expressions in Handsch's collection reads, "Much waiting happens at the court."[116] In the same place, he noted "Ferre moras, frenare iramque, docemur in aula", meaning roughly, "Tolerating delays and harnessing our anger is what we are taught at the court."[117] In 1586, Willenbroch bitterly complained to Theodor Zwinger about the "merciless servitude" ("serivitutem inclementen") he faced as archducal court physician in Innsbruck. He wrote that he could barely feed himself and his family and must not write about this in more detail because even just complaining was dangerous.[118]

---

112 Ibid., fol. 19r, 14 July 1579.
113 Ibid., fol. 27r-v, 2 August 1582.
114 Ibid., fol. 23r, 23 May 1580.
115 Cod. 11183, fol. 479v: "Villebrochius non processit methodice et secundum canones, more suo et nos coacti fuimus connivere."
116 Cod. 9671, fol. 20v.
117 Ibid.
118 Letter from Willenbroch, 15 November 1586, Universitätsbibliothek Basel, Frey-Gryn Mscr. 11, fol. 85r-v; http://doi.org/10.7891/e-manuscripta-7721; listed in the catalogue as addressed to an unidentified recipient ("Brief an N.N.") but clearly written to Theodor Zwinger, whom

In some places, it fell to the court physician to carry out further medical duties. In the sixteenth century, the prince-bishops of Würzburg, for example, assigned their court physicians with caring, like a municipal physician, also for the population at large, rich and poor alike, in return for suitable payment.[119] Employed as the court physician to the bishop of Olmütz, Lorenz Span was expected not only to provide medical care for his employer and his servants, and to accompany him on travels; he also had to be available to attend to the residents of the entire town.[120] The findings are similar for secular rulers. The court physician of the Count von Hohenlohe was responsible for providing medical care to the count's subjects and for supervising the apothecary's shop in the town of Öhringen.[121] Just as was evidently the case for many municipal physicians in smaller towns, being appointed as a court physician could give physicians a monopoly on the medical care for the local population. Eucharius Seefried, who held the office of Hohenlohe Court Physician in the 1580s, successfully lodged a complaint about the curtailment of his income when a municipal physician was hired in Öhringen in the wake of an epidemic. The counts granted him an additional 106 gulden annually, as well as a large amount of grain, hay, and straw.[122]

Some rulers were also looking for something more than medical expertise when they hired a court physician. They appreciated the value of their court physicians' knowledge of natural philosophy and history, especially if this knowledge promised certain economic advantages. Julius, Duke of Braunschweig-Wolfenbüttel, for example, hired a physician specifically because he was considered as knowledgeable "in minerals and other things", charging him with not only caring for the ducal family but also for miners, smelters, alum makers, and other workers in the mines and mineral works. Not only this, but he was to set up an apothecary's shop with the help of a laboratory assistant.[123] Johannes Crato and Joachim Meyer, too, were hired as both court physicians and "mine physicians" in 1579–81.[124] Leonhard Thurneisser even owed his career as a court

---

Willenbroch addressed as the author of the famous *Theatrum* (cf. Zwinger, Theatrum vitae (1586)).
119 Contracts of Johann Stoll, 1527 (www.aerztebriefe.de/id/00019750, U. Schlegelmilch), Kaspar Dierbach, 27 December 1533 (www.aerztebriefe.de/id/00019760, U. Schlegelmilch) and Johann Vischer, 23 April 1534 (www.aerztebriefe.de/id/00019761, U. Schlegelmilch).
120 Wondrak, Span (1983), p. 240.
121 Contract of Gregor Fabri, Öhringen, 17 December 1554 (www.aerztebriefe.de/id/00010217, T. Walter).
122 Letter from Seefried, Nördlingen, 5 June 1579 (www.aerztebriefe.de/id/00034170, H. Langrieger).
123 Wellner, Bergmedicus (1984), pp. 36–38.
124 Ibid.

physician and printer in Berlin in large part to his book *Pison*, in which he described the natural resources of the Brandenburg territory. It caught the attention of the Brandenburg elector, and when the electress was ill and recovered under Thurneisser's treatment, Thurneisser, who had never studied medicine, was appointed court physician.[125] The elector later accepted Thurneisser's offer to instruct the *provisor* (presumably the court apothecary) in the production of his secret remedies, on the condition that "you do not teach this art and these tinctures to anyone but our apothecary".[126] When Martinus Rhenanus was appointed *medicus extraordinarius* to the landgrave Moritz von Hessen-Kassel, he was explicitly expected to make his alchemical knowledge available while maintaining secrecy about these arts to the outside world.[127]

Georg Handsch, too, put his natural philosophical knowledge to good use. At the request of Archduke Ferdinand II, he authored a five-volume *Historia animalium*.[128] In it, he described at length the habitat of animals, their nutrition and reproductive habits as well as the species-typical behaviors. While Conrad Gessner in his famous *Historia animalium* included a lengthy discussion of the fauna of the new world,[129] Handsch focused almost exclusively on animals that were native to Bohemia or could at least be seen there on occasion. In a broad sense, then, his work focused on the natural resources of his ruler's territory.[130] Later, his depiction of contemporary practices of pisciculture in Bohemia, Moravia, and Silesia would be extolled.[131] As his poems for Hoddeiovinus show, Handsch was able to draw on his personal observations of fish pond designs he had seen at the country estates of noble families.[132] Ottokar Schubert, however,

---

125 Thurneisser, Pison (1572); on Thurneisser's biography see Moehsen, Leben (1783).
126 Staatsbibliothek Berlin, Ms. bor. fol. 682, fol. 3r-v, letter from the Electress Katharina of Brandenburg, Küstrin, 17 April 1571. On the widespread interest in alchemy among contemporary rulers, see Moran, Alchemical world (1991).
127 Contract, 1 January 1594 (www.aerztebriefe.de/id/00021254, U. Schlegelmilch).
128 Cod. 11130, Cod. 11141, Cod. 11142, Cod 11143 and Cod. 11153; one of Handsch's poems carries the title "In historiam animalium, institutam ab Archiduce Ferdinando" (Cod. 9821, fol. 310r); for a detailed assessment of this work, which never made it into print, see Simons, Theatrum (2009), pp. 141–154.
129 Gessner, Historia (1551–1558); the fifth and last, incomplete volume appeared posthumously, in 1587.
130 This included some exotic animals such as the camel, the lama, the baboon and the crocodile which Handsch seems to have seen with his own eyes on various occasions. He saw a crocodile, for example, in 1548 in a church in Budina and remarked with amazement on its ability to move the teeth in its lower jaw (Cod. 9666, fol. 16v).
131 Handsch, Elbefischerei (1933).
132 Cod. 9821, foll. 256r-257r; Collinus et alii, Quarta farrago (1562), foll. 400v-401r.

would later identify those passages from Handsch's *Historia animalium* as having been copied from Johannes Dubravius's *De piscinis* from 1547.[133] As far as we know today, only the descriptions of the various native species of fish were penned by Handsch himself.

With their comprehensive humanist education and their linguistic and analytic skills, court physicians were also hired by some rulers to write about the history of their court. The contemporary rulers were aware of the significance of a positive representation of the history of their dynasty, their reign, and their territory for the legitimization of their rule. They encouraged history writing of this kind and some even appointed an official court historian, who was sometimes a physician. Johannes Cuspinian, Wolfgang Lazius, and Johannes Sambucus, for example, each combined the office of imperial court physician (and professor at the university in Vienna) with the tasks of a court historiographer.[134] Handsch, too, described himself in his will as "medicus et historicus".[135] Allegedly he promised the Archduke a historical account of the House of Austria.[136] Whether he actually wrote it, however, is unknown.

---

133 Handsch, Elbefischerei (1933), p. 2; cf. Dubravius, De piscinis (1547).
134 Siraisi, History (2007).
135 Tiroler Landesarchiv, Innsbruck, Ferdinandea 164, Handsch's will, 17 February 1578.
136 Hirn, Erzherzog Ferdinand II. (1885), p. 363.

Everyday Practice

The Physicians' Clientele

For a long time, historians believed that until the eighteenth century, learned physicians treated almost exclusively noble, rich, and educated patients.[137] More recently, various authors have argued, however, that more patients also from the less affluent parts of society sought the advice of a learned physician than commonly assumed.[138] In fact, even the collections of published case histories, whose authors liked to emphasize their own rank by describing how they treated elite patients, show that also ordinary people such as craftsmen, farmers, merchants, and servants most definitely sought the advice of learned physicians as early as the sixteenth century.[139]

Robust quantitative statements about the predominant clinical pictures and diagnoses, the makeup of medical clientele, the intensity of treatment and similar questions are only possible on the basis of practice journals or comparable sources in which a physician noted down every medical case in his practice over a given period of time. We may assume that many physicians at the time kept a practice journal, if only for the purpose of bookkeeping. But for the time before 1600, there are unfortunately only very few surviving journals of this kind. And the few that are known – for example the *Receptarium* of Hartmann Schedel in Nördlingen and Amberg from the late fifteenth century, and the practice journals of Georg Palm and Johannes Magenbuch in Nuremberg from the early sixteenth century – are furthermore essentially limited to listing the names of the patients and the prescribed medicines.[140] Because these names are often

---

[137] See the seminal and highly influential study by Jewson, Medical knowledge (1974).
[138] E.g. Jütte, Ärzte (1991), p. 100; recently, Klaas/Steinke/Unterkircher, Daily business (2016), pp. 91f. have offered concrete evidence for this.
[139] For bibliographies of early modern printed collections of case histories see, e.g., Stolberg, Formen (2007) and Pomata, Sharing cases (2010).
[140] Fischer, Hartmann Schedel (1996), with an edition of the manuscript (Bayerische Staatsbibliothek, Clm 290); Stadtbibliothek Nürnberg, Ms. Cent. V, 10b and Germanisches Nationalmuseum, Nürnberg, Hs 100.822 (Georg Palm); Universitätsbibliothek Heidelberg, Cpl 1895–1 (Johannes Magenbuch); Assion/Telle, Magenbuch (1972); König, Palma (1961). The journal of the Augsburg physician Philipp Hoechstetter (1579–1635) is a rich source for contemporary life in general but yields hardly any information about his medical practice (Herz, Tagebuch (1976)). Sources for other countries are similarly scarce. In her survey of surviving practice journals in England, Lauren Kassell has found only fragmentary notes from the fifteenth and sixteenth centuries (Kassell, Casebooks (2015)). The situation is markedly better for the seventeenth century. On Petrus Kirsten's early seventeenth-century practice in Breslau see Ofenhitzer, Praxisalltag

known from other contemporary sources, these practice journals at least provide the evidence that these physicians predominantly treated patients who were members of the local elites. But as Fischer has established for Hartmann Schedel, patients from all social classes occasionally sought the advice of this learned physician.[141]

Although Handsch mentioned numerous patients in his notebooks, they do not serve as a reliable reflection of his practice. We cannot, for one thing, assume that he made a note of all or even most of the patients he saw. Secondly, many of his entries concern patients treated by Gallo, Mattioli, and other physicians, and it is often unclear who was the primary physician in each case. Nevertheless, his notebooks do give us an impression of the makeup of the medical clientele served by this circle of physicians. As court physicians, Gallo and Mattioli in Prague mainly treated members of the Habsburg Court and the Bohemian nobility. But according to Handsch's notes, there were also many "common" folks among their patients, and the same was true later when Handsch practiced in Innsbruck. Seeking and receiving medical advice from learned physicians were, according to his notes, also pupils and students, goldsmiths, brewers, and peasants ("rustici") and even the occasional "poor lad in the hospital". There were, furthermore, cooks, kitchen boys, stable hands, and others with "lower" occupations who in many cases apparently worked at the court in Prague or – as Handsch sometimes stated explicitly – in the service of another noble master. With a noticeably large number of patients, Handsch did not add a "D." to their names in his notes, which stood for "Dominus" or "Domina", an epithet reserved for high-ranking members of society.

The practice journal of Handsch's first medical teacher, Ulrich Lehner, seems to have survived in completion for the years 1546 to 1549. Under the title "Practica D. Ulrici" Handsch copied this journal including the names of the patients, their

---

(2015); Sabine Schlegelmilch has analyzed the practice journals of Johannes Magirus and Johann Heinrich Bossen (Schlegelmilch, Ärztliche Praxis (2018)); for England, the rich notes of the Paracelsian physician Turquet de Mayerne (1573–1655) have survived for the years from 1603 until 1653 (Nance, Turquet de Mayerne (2001)). In quantitative terms, none of these sources matches the practice journals of Simon Forman (1552–1611) and John Napier (1550–1617) in the late sixteenth century (MacDonald, Mystical Bedlam (1981); Traister, Notorious astrological physician (2001); Kassell, Medicine (2005); https://casebooks.lib.cam.ac.uk/). It is a rich and fascinating source but neither Forman nor Napier had studied medicine. They were no *doctores medicinae*. Moreover their largely astrological practice was very untypical of the practice of the overwhelming majority of contemporary physicians. Practice journals from the seventeenth to the nineteenth centuries, are the principal source for the the contributions in Dinges/ Jankrift/ Schlegelmilch/ Stolberg, Medical practice (2016).
141 Fischer, Hartmann Schedel (1996), p. 90.

clinical pictures or diagnoses, as well as Lehner's prescriptions, which were presumably of central interest to Handsch.[142] Lehner was "only" a *magister*, not a *doctor medicinae*. He ran a very successful practice in Prague, however, and moved in the same circles as Gallo and later Mattioli. What is remarkable in Handsch's copy of his journal is the classification, which was presumably originally Lehner's, of patients according to social class, namely as *barones, nobiles,* and *plebeios*. This betrays a clear consciousness of the significance of such class differences. Unfortunately, the classification, at least in Handsch's copy, was not carried out consistently. The occupation and position of the patients are named often but not always, making a statistical analysis difficult. But the journal clearly shows that Lehner, too, treated patients from all social classes. Noble Bohemian families and eminent clergy such as the abbot of the Strachov monastery, as well as the families of court employees of all ranks made up the majority of his patients. However, we also find a fisherman, a butcher, a goldsmith, an organist, various merchants, *magistri*, and patients who are recorded as only "mulier", "iuvenis" or even as simply "someone" ("quidam"). Several "Jews" as well sought his advice; it is possible but not confirmed that Lehner was Jewish himself.

The by far most comprehensive extant sixteenth-century practice journal of a *doctor medicinae,* from which I have already quoted various times here, is Hiob Finzel's *Ratiocinium* from 1565 to 1589. Because he also used it to calculate his income, we may assume that the records are complete and that only the odd unpaid consultation is missing.[143] Finzel was first a municipal physician in Weimar, where he fell into disfavor for political reasons, and then he served as court physician in Eisenach from 1569 to 1571. In 1571, he became the municipal physician of Zwickau, where he was able to establish a successful practice. He stayed there until his death in 1589. An analysis of his practice journals from the seventeen years in Zwickau – from January 1572 to December 1588 –yields a total of 8,746 consultations.

As a rule, the patients' ages are not identified. Child patients can at least in part be recognized through identifiers such as "filiolus" "(little son"), "filiola"

---

[142] Cod. 11006 and Cod. 11247; Handsch added some notes of his own, e.g. on some patients of Gallo's, and excerpts from his reading. I intend to undertake a more detailed analysis of Lehner's practice journal elsewhere.

[143] Ratschulbibliothek Zwickau, Ms. QQQQ 1, Ms. QQQQ 1a and Ms. QQQQ 1b; for a detailed description and analysis of this source see Stolberg, A sixteenth-century physician (2019), and on its use as a tool for accounting Stolberg, Accounting (2020). I want to express my thanks Hannes Langrieger who supported me decisively in the statistical analysis of this journal.

or "Töchterlein" ("little daughter"), "Kindelein" ("little child"), or "Megdlein" ("little girl"). These were terms Finzel used for his own children until they reached the age of approximately ten years. These terms appear in at least 271 consultations. A further 83 entries concern "boys" ("pueri"), and significantly more, 272, "girls" ("puellae"). In addition to these, there are further entries on patients whom Finzel characterized solely as daughters or sons, which would have included at least some children and adolescents. By all appearances, then, infants and children were underrepresented, but they were most definitely seen at times by physicians and not just left to their fate as older generations of historians have claimed. In her study of Peter Kirsten's Breslau *Rezeptdiarium* from between 1612 and 1616, Franziska Ofenhitzer arrived at a similar conclusion. A good 18.5 % of the patients whom Kirsten gave prescriptions were children.[144]

To the extent that sex can be determined on the basis of the first name or other details, male patients were in the majority, accounting for 4,863 consultations (56.6 %) as opposed to 3,701 consultations (43.4 %) for female patients. This proportion, too, was not untypical of the time. Of the patients, whose treatment by Benedetto Vittore an unidentified student recorded in the early 1540s, fifty-five (57 %) were men and forty-one (43 %) were women.[145] In Palm's Nuremberg practice, 63.4 % were male as opposed to 36.6 % female, and with Kirsten's Breslau *Rezeptdiarium*, the respective relation was particularly unbalanced, with 70.7 % to 29.3 %.[146]

Finzel's practice journal offers some clues about the social standing of his patients. About 8 % of the patients (who accounted for a disproportionately large percentage of the consultations) came from noble families. This is doubtlessly a lower proportion than in the practices of Lehner, Gallo, Mattioli, Willenbroch, and Handsch, which were all very closely connected to the court. Among the approximately 3,000 patients whose occupation or status was indicated in one way or another by Finzel, there are numerous members of the town's bourgeoisie: town councilors, officials, teachers, clergy; 170 patients came from the households of pastors alone. But there were also dozens of craftspeople such as millers, coachmen, blacksmiths and nail smiths, cloth dyers, cobblers, potters,

---

144 Ofenhitzer, Praxisalltag (2015), p. 91.
145 Biblioteca comunale Aurelio Saffi, Forlì, Fondo antico, Ms. 94; the notes mostly document cases in the spring of 1540, the spring of 1541 and the fall and winter of 1541/42 and thus do not offer a complete record. There is no indication, however, that the notetaker selected certain cases on the grounds of the diagnosis or the patient's sex. Presumably, the notes simply reflect the time periods in which he accompanied Vittore.
146 Stolberg, Sixteenth-century physician (2019).

tailors, bookbinders, chandlers, and furriers, as well as a number of tavern owners and musicians. 733 patients worked in agriculture or Finzel simply referred to them as "country folks" or "peasants" ("rusticus", "rustica").[147]

It becomes very clear from Finzel's bookkeeping that broad sections of the population were able to afford the help of a physician. Wealthy patients sometimes paid him several gulden, while from most others he received only one, two, or at most three groschen for a consultation.[148] For comparison's sake, a hare cost six to eight groschen if we go by indications given by Finzel, a large cheese, nine. According to northern German sources, a chicken or ten eggs cost about one groschen at about that time, while a pound of butter cost one and half groschen, and a journeyman carpenter earned four groschen daily.[149] Naturally, the cost of the medicine came added, but in general most families were certainly able to ask a physician for his advice if they believed it was worth it.

Routines and Practices

We do not know much about the daily work routines of medical practitioners during this period. We have to rely predominantly on the anecdotal references provided by physicians and patients and on the information that can be indirectly inferred from practice journals and other documents reflecting medical practice.

Just trying to establish where the physicians saw their patients presents significant difficulties. As opposed to today – this much is clear – the practice of house calls prevailed. A messenger was sent to the physician, who called him to the sick person's bedside. The physician betook himself to the patient and this – considering that it might involve longer distances, poor weather conditions (especially in winter) and difficult terrain – could be attended by certain strains and dangers, and it also cost him time. It is incorrect, however, to claim or to presume, as historians of early modern medicine have widely done, that learned physicians only made house calls. House calls were undoubtedly

---

147 Bernhard Unger († 1594) also mentioned the "rusticos" he treated when he practiced in Biberach and, more specifically, a remedy he sometimes ("saepius") successfully used when they could not speak, after a stroke (Universitätsbibliothek Freiburg, HS 99, fol. 94r, marginal annotation).
148 In Montpellier, the fee for a house visit was between 20 sous and a livre, in 1523 (Lingo, Rise (1980), p. 55).
149 Voigtlaender, Löhne und Preise (1994).

standard in the case of affluent patients. While practices with regular consultation hours may have only been introduced on a wide scale in the nineteenth century,[150] a closer examination of early modern sources offers ample evidence that already at this time physicians also practiced in their own house.[151]

One clear indication of this are the numerous reports (and complaints) of physicians about the widespread expectation on the part of patients that any medical practitioner worth his salt would be able to make his diagnosis simply by looking at the patient's urine that was sent to him. Surviving accounts of patients and their relatives furnish further proof that they often did nothing more than send urine to the physician's house. Uroscopy, after all, held the great advantage that the physician did not have to make his way to patients, or they to him. He could examine the urine in his own office, write his orders, and give them to the waiting messenger.

Uroscopy was unique insofar as it did not require a personal encounter between physician and patient. The physician needed only to inspect the urine, and then he could convey his diagnosis to the messenger orally and, if necessary, give him a prescription for the apothecary. Contemporary correspondence and physicians' notes show, however, that also personal encounters between physicians and sick people took place not only in the houses of the patients. At closer analysis, this is not surprising. As we have seen with the example of Finzel, hundreds of patients from the surrounding villages sought his assistance. It is almost certain that many of them went to see the physician in his house rather than calling for him and potentially facing a much higher fee for his visit.

But even townsfolk went to see the physician in his dwelling if their health allowed. In the late 1550s, Felix Platter reported that, as a young physician in Basel, when he was still living in his father's house, he "questioned" patients in his chamber or, in the cold winter months, in the "downstairs hall", which we can assume was heated.[152] And when Baltz, the municipal physician of Esslingen, requested more suitable accommodation from the town in 1573, his express reason was that those who currently sought his medical advice had to climb the stairs to his little room and then go down them again afterwards. Baltz even suggested that physicians sometimes hospitalized patients in their own houses. For such purposes, he complained, his current accommodation was too small.[153] In the early seventeenth century, Turquet de Mayerne likewise saw patients in his

---

150 Vieler, Arztpraxis (1958); Heischkel, Welt (1967).
151 Klaas/Steinke/Unterkircher, Daily business (2016), pp. 73–75.
152 Platter, Tagebuch (1976), p. 330.
153 Letter from Tobias Baltz to the magistrate of Esslingen, 16 December 1573 (www.aerztebriefe.de/id/00030643, T. Walter).

home office. He received them sitting at his desk, surrounded by books, pictures, and a wax model of human anatomy.[154] We do not know to what degree physicians' wives supported their husband in these circumstances but it seems likely that they did.

The significance of the apothecary's shop as a further site of medical practice can only be vaguely reconstructed from the sources we have. Here and there, we find hints that physicians spent so much time in apothecary shops that people went there to call them to a patient or to deliver urine to them. At this point, however, we cannot tell how common this was in the sixteenth century. As we have seen, municipal physicians – a position held by many physicians – were often explicitly held not to give preference to one apothecary over another. A physician who spent much of his time in one specific pharmacy clearly would have appeared to favor it.

It remains unclear how much of a physician's time was taken by his medical practice. In their letters, physicians sometimes complained that because of their patients, they had no time left for anything else – in particular, for replying to letters. Except in times of epidemics, this of course may have served as a pretext or excuse, however. The few practice journals that have survived from the time before 1600 give us a very different picture. Hartmann Schedel's *Rezeptdiarium* documents 1,135 individual prescriptions in a time frame of about four years. Even if we assume that he only prescribed medicines to every second patient, which is unlikely, this would mean he had less than two consultations per day.[155] Looking at Hiob Finzel's practice journal of a hundred years later, we hardly find more: just an average of not even three consultations daily. And examining medical practice journals from the seventeenth and eighteenth centuries, the numbers continue to be similar. It was only in the nineteenth century that the number of patients seen per day rose significantly.[156]

Epistolary Medical Practice

A peculiar form of medical consultation emerged at the time, thanks also to improved postal services, gaining some currency among the upper classes, particularly when an illness was prolonged: this was consultation by letter, based on

---

154 Nance, Turquet de Mayerne (2001), p. 24.
155 Fischer, Hartmann Schedel (1996), p. 87.
156 Klaas/Steinke/Unterkircher, Daily business (2016), table on p. 78.

a written account of the patient's complaints.¹⁵⁷ Sometimes this correspondence followed on the heels of an in-person exchange, for example when a patient had seen a physician at his place of residence but had then gone home again, or if a physician had visited a wealthy patient at his country estate but then had to return to his practice and could henceforth only occasionally call on the patient again. More frequently, the communication was exclusively by letter. For patients who lived in places where they had no access to a learned physician they felt they could trust this was a welcome alternative to the care of a local barber-surgeon or a popular healer. Others wrote to a renowned physician because they were not satisfied with the diagnosis and treatment of their local physician or to hear a "second opinion".

A typical consultation letter consisted of two main parts. After a short outline of the clinical presentation, the physician would explain the medical condition, describe the pathophysiological processes he had determined were at work in the body, and only then would he, as the circumstances required, present his diagnosis and prognosis. The second, generally more extensive part of the consultation letter consisted of therapeutic and dietetic instructions. As a rule, this included lengthy advice about proper nutrition and lifestyle, as well as recommendations for medicines and other measures such as bloodletting and baths.

Some patients also sent their urine, trusting that an experienced physician would be able to arrive at a precise diagnosis just on the basis of uroscopy. The Berlin Paracelsian Leonhard Thurneisser turned this into a very lucrative business model. Numerous wealthy patients sent him their urine, along with a gold coin and a brief description of their complaints. They asked him to examine the urine using his special urine distillation process, to identify their illness on this basis, and to send them suitable medicines. An ordinary physician like Handsch, too, might be sent urine and asked for a uroscopic diagnosis by letter. In one of his letters, he regretted that he was unable to provide a judgment about the color of the urine because the flask had been damaged.¹⁵⁸

When famous, remote physicians were consulted, the patients often left it to their local physician to write the history of their disease and describe their

---

157 On the widespread practice of consulting by letter and the countless patient letters that have come down to us from the early modern period see Stolberg, "Mein äskulapisches Orakel!" (1996) and idem, Experiencing illness (2011). For the time from the late seventeenth century onwards see also Weston, Medical consulting (2013). Patient letters from the sixteenth century have not yet been examined systematically.
158 Cod. 9821, foll. 51r-52r, 12 April 1559.

current complaints.[159] For the local physician in charge this may sometimes have been a humiliating experience, a sign of distrust. Especially in protracted, difficult cases, however, it could also be in the local physician's own interest to seek such advice. If the treatment did not deliver the desired outcome, he did not carry the full burden of responsibility. As a rule, the physician who was seeking advice, even when he was writing on a patient's behalf, could furthermore expect to be addressed in a respectful tone by his colleague. Certainly, he had to be prepared for the possibility that the distant physician would somewhat modify his diagnosis or treatment – if only to justify the fee for the requested epistolary consultation. However, an unwritten rule ensured that the advising physician would not be hard on the local attending physician, fundamentally criticizing his diagnosis or therapeutic approach or even questioning his competence. This was in his own best interest if he wanted his medical colleagues to request his epistolary advice in future cases.

Handsch, too, sometimes offered consultations by letter, and he even collected these letters, apparently hoping to publish them. To a certain Viderinus, for example, he gave precise instructions about how he was to treat his chronic illness and even specified the days he was to take his medicines depending on the planetary constellations.[160] In the practice of successful, respected physicians, writing medical consultation letters could demand considerable attention and generate significant income. Composing a detailed consultation letter was a challenging and time-consuming task. Consultations for noble patients could be as long as a dozen pages or more. A handwritten copy of Renato Brasavola's epistolary consultation for Archduke Ferdinand II is almost fifty pages long.[161] An consultation on the prevention and treatment of stones, which was probably also written for Ferdinand, goes on for more than a hundred pages.[162] And Andrea Gallo's consultation on the "trembling of the heart" of the later Emperor Maximilian II comprises as many as 180 pages.[163]

---

159 Copy of a *consilium* by Trincavella, with a summary of the *historia morbi*, in Cod. 11238, foll. 168–177v.
160 Cod. 9650, foll. 31v-33r, 18 July 1556.
161 Cod. 11155, foll. 1r-24v.
162 Cod. 11083; cf. Oberrauch, Medizin (2012), pp. 368f. The author was an unidentified doctor.
163 Cod. 11158.

The Physician-Patient Relationship

Historical scholarship on the physician-patient relationship in the sixteenth and seventeenth centuries, has so far largely relied on normative, deontological texts, which outlined how physicians and patients should behave.[164] Deontological works such as Gabriele Zerbi's *De cautelis medicorum*,[165] Leonardo Botalli's *De officio medici*,[166] as well as the literature on the *medicus politicus*[167] that blossomed after 1600 provide valuable insights into physicians' self-understanding and into the way physicians wanted to be seen by others.[168]

Whether such normative texts can be seen as a reflection of lived practice, however – of the interactions between physicians and patients that took place on a daily basis – is a different question. At times, the very recommendations for the "right" behavior already reveal certain tensions, for example when it is recommended to physician readers that they stay away from the terminally ill and not treat children, pregnant women or those with eye diseases because treating such cases was difficult and could lead to a tarnishing of one's reputation.[169]

If we want to arrive at a realistic picture of the physician-patient relationship we need to resort to sources that describe the actual interactions, as they took place on an everyday basis. Unfortunately, such sources are rare and the historical scholarship on this issue is so far very unsatisfactory for the Renaissance period.[170] We have only fragmentary knowledge – even with respect to the educated upper classes – of how physicians and patients actually interacted and dealt with one another, what they said and did in everyday medical practice in the sixteenth century. We know very little, for example, about differences in the bedside manners of physicians when they were dealing with male as opposed to female patients.[171] And the nature of the interactions between learned physicians

---

[164] Historical overviews in Laín Entralgo, Relacion (1964); Elkeles, Arzt und Patient (1992); Sawyer, Friends or foes? (1995); Belmas/Nonnis Vigilante, Les relations (2013); Pancino, Doctor and patient (2015).
[165] Zerbi (Opus perutile) ([after 1494]).
[166] Botalli, Commentarioli duo (1565).
[167] Castro, Medicus-politicus (1614); Hoffmann, Medicus politicus (1708); on the genre, in general, see Eckart, Anmerkungen (1992).
[168] On ideas about the doctor-patient in medieval deontological writing (based, in particular, on the early manuscript tradition) see MacKinney, Medical ethics (1952).
[169] Zerbi, Opus perutile ([after 1494]).
[170] This includes recent surveys such as Pancino, Doctor and patient (2015).
[171] Olivia Weisser has arrived at a similarly negative conclusion for seventeenth-century England (Weisser, Ill composed (2015), p. 18).

Open Access. © 2022 Michael Stolberg, published by De Gruyter. This work is licensed under the Creative Commons Attribution-NonCommercial-NoDerivatives 4.0 International License.
https://doi.org/10.1515/9783110733549-019

and patients from the lower classes – perhaps even with peasants or farmhands, or with simple tradespeople and journeymen – is almost entirely obscured.

Although Handsch's notes are oriented on everyday practice and experience and are richly detailed in many respects, close descriptions of face-to-face encounters between learned physicians and patients are the exception; I will be presenting two detailed descriptions further along. However, in hundreds of entries he wrote down explanations and phrases that he could use in his dealings with patients and their relatives or that he or his colleagues had actually used in particular cases. With great care, Handsch furthermore noted down the mistakes that he himself or physicians in his professional environment had made when interacting with patients and their relatives. Repeatedly he even described the words and actions of patients and their relatives, their responses to physicians' recommendations and actions, and the way in which they approached the physician. Although they are written from the perspective of a physician, and although the boundaries between his descriptions of lived reality and wholesale statements or even gross overgeneralizations are not always clear, his notes are of unique value to research on the physician-patient relationship in the sixteenth century. Supplemented by sources such as the above-mentioned practice journal of Hiob Finzel as well as pertinent references in ego-documents, Handsch's notebooks shine welcome new light on essential aspects of this relationship.[172]

Interactions

The modern reader of Handsch's entries concerning bedside manner will immediately notice a distinct degree of reserve. One would search in vain for emotional statements let alone demonstrations of pity for suffering patients, as have been documented for some physicians of the eighteenth century with its "culture of sensibility".[173] Rather, the patient emerges in large part as a foreign, stubborn, and sometimes downright hostile interlocutor who approaches the physician with skepticism, who often questions his advice or even flatly rejects it, who might cast him off in the end, and who fails to express the necessary gratitude. The physician, by contrast, seeks to be seen as a saviour or angel (Figs 13, 14) and turns to a variety of strategies to safeguard his authority and his economic interests vis-à-vis his patients and their relatives.

---

172 On what follows, see also Stolberg, Doctor-patient relationship (2021), which largely draws on the same sources.
173 Stolberg, Experiencing illness (2011), p. 95; Barker-Benfield, Culture of sensibility (1992).

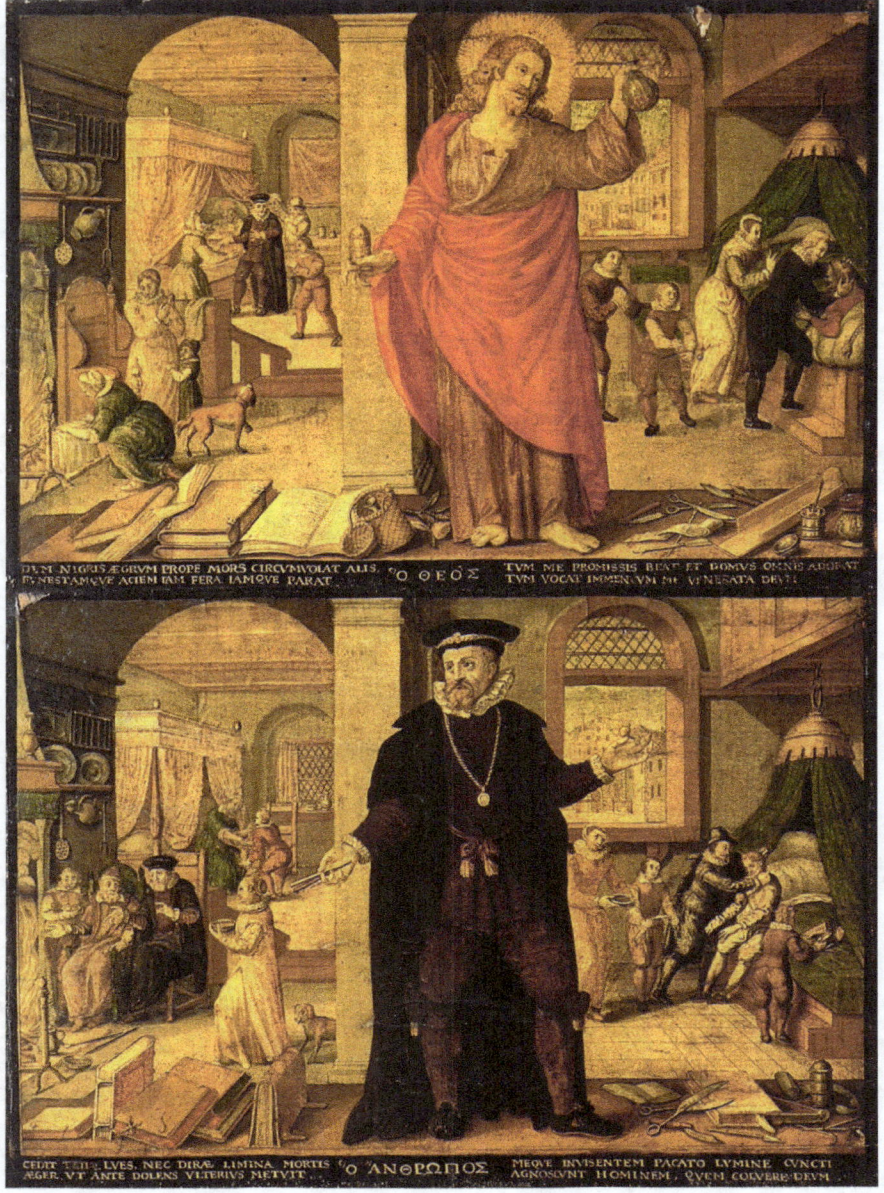

Fig. 13 and 14: Egbert van Panderen (1581–1637?), The medical practitioner as Christ, angel, man and devil, Wellcome Collection, London.

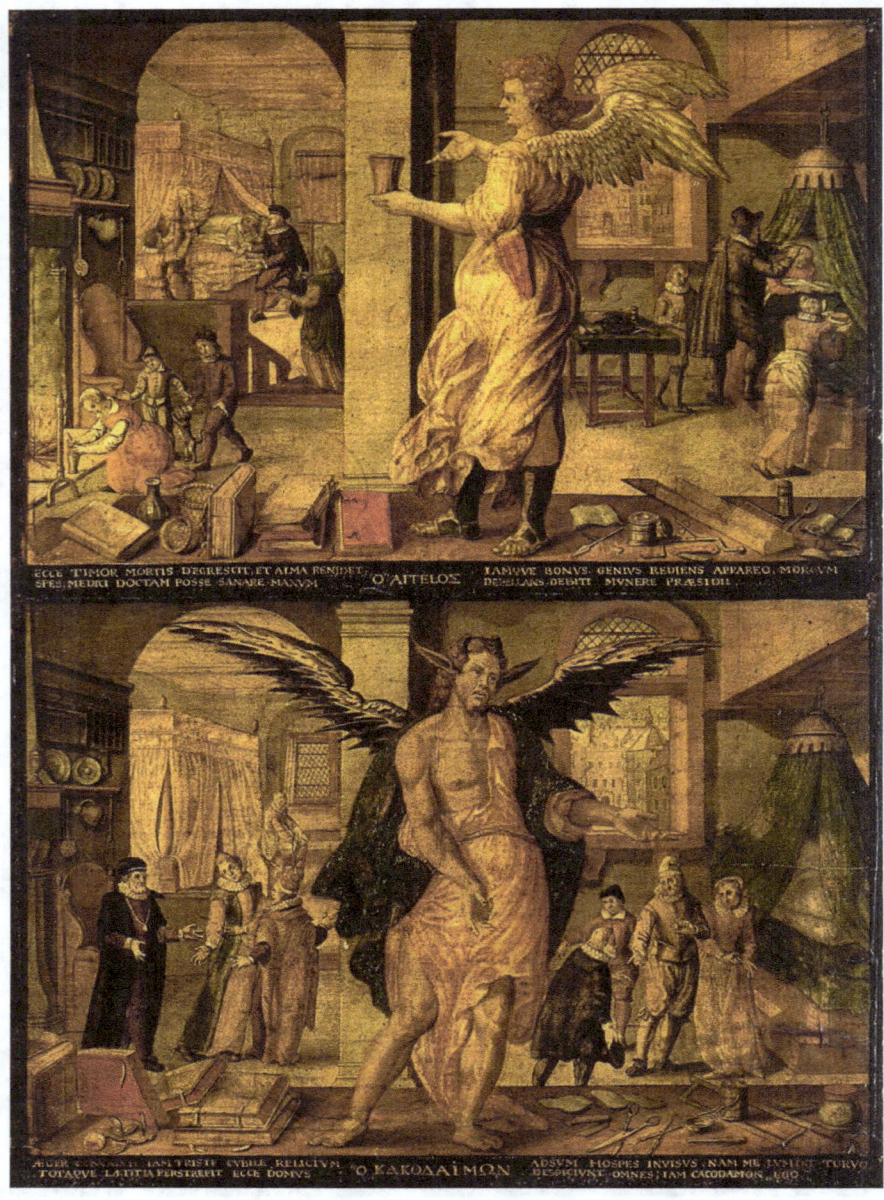

Fig. 13 and 14 (continued)

A qualifying statement must be added right away: there were different groups of patients. On the one side of the spectrum, the distinctions between clientele and friends could be very blurred. Quite frequently patients who asked a learned physician for his medical advice were at the same time his friends, acquaintances, or relatives. "I was called because he was my friend" a young physician in Bologna reported; at the time he usually accompanied with his teacher Benedetto Vittore to see Vittore's patients.[174] When patients were also friends and close acquaintances, the physician-patient relationship was doubtlessly more personal and characterized by mutual trust. At the other end of the spectrum, there were the urban lower classes and the numerous country people who by all indications consulted a physician only rarely. Hiob Finzel's practice journal as well as numerous entries in Handsch's notebooks do show that even simple peasants sought the advice of a learned physician far more often than previously assumed by historians. However, the evidence provided by both physicians indicates that there was little room for establishing something like a personal relationship. The physician saw many of these patients only once. If the medicines he prescribed worked, there was no need to come back. And if it failed, it made sense, for patients with limited financial means that they try their luck with another healer or turned to home remedies. The sporadic nature and impersonal character of these encounters with patients from the country finds vivid expression in the way in which Finzel in particular made note of these people in his journal. They remain, as a rule, nameless. Usually he went no further than to note their places of residence, and sometimes not even that. Handsch, too, who otherwise so carefully noted down the name, rank, and sometimes family relations, made do with a simple "farmer" or "peasant" ("rusticus") for dozens of rural patients, supplemented at best with a note about where or with whom he had seen the patient. Several of his entries even point to a serious dissociation from, and denigration of, country people on the part of the learned physician. The "peasant" ("rusticus") was "like cattle", he once noted; all that was missing were the horns. Further: peasants know how to shed tears, but not how to spread cheer. These sayings counted among many such adages and expressions Handsch collected and therefore may not necessarily have expressed his personal views.[175] However, Handsch also wrote of his intention, to test the uncertain effects of opium on "some peasant", thus indicating a striking distinction regarding the respect and consideration he owed to patients of different social classes.[176]

---

174 Biblioteca comunale Aurelio Saffi, Forlì, Fondo antico, Ms. 94, fol. 54r, 28 August 1540, "fui vocatus, quia erat meus amicus". He treated patient's fever himself, without Vittore's support.
175 Cod. 9671, fol. 21r.
176 Cod. 11205, fol. 223r: "His ergo positis, omnino experiar in aliquo rustico".

What was crucial for a physician's professional and economic success above all were patients from the middle and upper classes (Fig. 15). Handsch documented the interactions with them in greater detail in his notebooks. The conditions forestablishing a trusting and personal relationship were significantly better with these groups. With an average of only two or three consultations per day, there was ample time for extensive conversations, and the house calls that were typical for these classes strengthened the private, intimate character of the relationship. As a rule, the physician saw the patient in the *hypocaustum*, a room that could be heated, if necessary.[177] Unlike Finzel, Handsch visited some patients every day over an extended period of time. Rich, noble patients even had physicians stay at their country estates for several days or even weeks. Multiple times, Handsch spent quite a few days with the Baroness of Hungerkasten when she was ill, for example. Most families from the upper nobility in Bohemia had such country estates.[178]

It goes without saying that physicians had to do their best to maintain the trust and goodwill of patients and their relatives. They were well aware that, first of all, their demeanor was important. One of Handsch's maxims was: "Do not make yourself unworthy. Retain your authority".[179] It was essential to maintain modesty, soberness, circumspection, and a pleasant human warmth, combined with prudence, steadfastness, truthfulness, and patience, and furthermore – and here Handsch repeatedly had to face reproach – one had to avoid drunkenness.[180] Naturally, the physician was not to rush, thus showing that he took his patients seriously. "Nota bene", Handsch wrote, "if a physician shows himself to be obliging, hardworking, and friendly, he will earn a name for himself and people will say that he has been reliable and diligent."[181] It was not enough to carefully inspect the urine. The physician also had to ask the patient many questions, and listen to what the patient had to say "patiently and attentively"

---

177 Cod. 11183, fol. 242v; in Roman times, the term "hypocaustum" referred to the heating of rooms from sources of heat in rooms underneath. Handsch and his contemporaries used "hypocaustum" as a general term for a warm, heatable room, however, as added adjectives such as "calidum" ("warm") or references to an oven that could be lit in that room indicate. Junghans, Zeitpunkt (2017), pp. 29–31 has arrived at the same conclusion for Luther's writing about "hypocaustum meum".
178 Pánek, Nobility (1997), pp. 274–276.
179 Cod. 11240, fol. 2r.
180 Cod. 11205, fol. 560v: "Modestia morum, sobrietas, diligentia, blanda humanitas cum gravitate coniuncta, constantia et veritas, frugalitas. [. . .] Et in summa cave ebrietatem, ut etiam Hofrichterus, M. Ulricus et D. Gallus obiecit."
181 Ibid., fol. 690v.

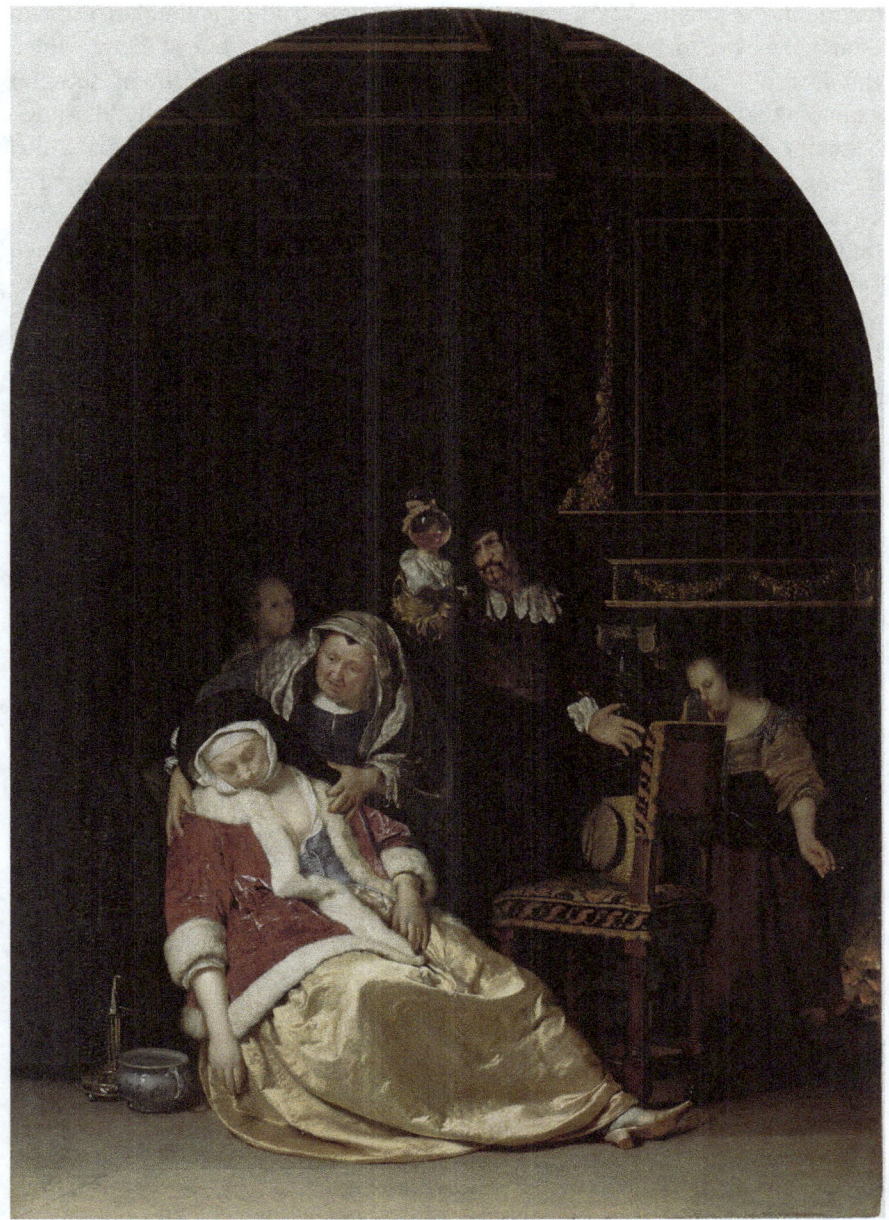

Fig. 15: Frans van Mieris, The doctor's visit, 1667, Paul Getty Museum, Los Angeles.

("patienter et attente").[182] To demonstrate his care ("ad ostendendam diligentiam"), he was to feel the pulse not only at one wrist but at both, which Handsch did.[183] Handsch even considered small gestures worthy of note, for example that one shook the patient's hand upon leaving.[184] Ideally, dignified behavior that commanded respect and asserted authority was accompanied by a manner that was engaging and considerate. In Handsch's words: "The physician is graced not only with experience, but also with humanity and affability" – he added the German word "Holdselickeit" ("sweetness") – which "allows him to encourage and console a patient."[185] He had heard that the reason why his colleague Jacobus Camenicenus had many patients was because he was "blandiloquus", that is, he knew well how to use words.[186] Another physician, by contrast, was called an ox by his clientele. He pressed so hard on a patient's wrist when taking the pulse that he left a bruise.[187] It appears that Handsch himself was not always adept at dealing with patients. He received serious criticism from his father, according to whom he was unfriendly to people, careless in his treatment, and did not bring the treatment to a conclusion, thus endangering his livelihood.[188]

Once a physician had gained the initial trust of a patient and his or her relatives, the conditions for a long-term relationship were essentially in place. Physicians benefitted from a conviction that was widespread among educated laypeople, namely the idea that if a physician was familiar with a person's physical constitution and medical history, there was a better chance that his treatment would be successful. Finzel treated some patients over the course of many years, and there are records of close to 200 visits for certain families in his practice journal. Contemporary ego-documents by patients, for example

---

[182] Cod. 11200, fol. 56v.
[183] Cod. 11206, fol. 149v; cf. the chapter on pulse diagnosis.
[184] Cod. 11205, fol. 513r.
[185] Cod. 11206, fol. 178v: "Medicum non tantum decet experientia, sed humanitas & affabilitas."
[186] Cod. 11205, fol. 129v.
[187] Cod. 11203, fol. 237r; Handsch only used the first name, Ludovicus, presumably referring to Ludovicus Tremenus. The wife of the semi-comatose ("lethargicus") Wilhelm called Ludovicus "an oxen" ("eyn Ochsen") (ibid., fol. 272r). Handsch thought that Ludovicus had acted with good intentions and wanted to stimulate the patient's numbed senses in this way. It remains unclear, however, why he pressed the wrists so hard for this purpose that they looked bruised rather than pinching the skin, for example.
[188] Cod. 11205, fol. 425v, "patris monitio"; Handsch had decided not to continue his treatment of a podagric woman as too laborious because the next pharmacy was four miles away.

the notes of the Cologne councilman Weinsberg, likewise indicate that families tended to keep calling the same physicians when a family member was ill.[189]

In many cases, however, the relationship between physicians and patients outside the closer circle of friends and acquaintances had little in common with our familiar image of the paternal family physician who cared for patients, even whole families, from the cradle to the grave. This is shown by Handsch's notes and Finzel's practice journal alike. Not only country people, but well-off craftspeople, merchants, clergy, teachers, and other patients from the educated middle classes in town sought the advice of the physician only sporadically according to Finzel's journal. They were content with one, two, or at most three consultations, and it was the exception rather than the rule that they returned to the physician when they fell ill again at some later point. In his notebooks, Handsch did record various cases where he or other physicians treated patients over the course of days or weeks, attending them once or twice a day. For more than twelve days, he treated an unmarried woman who was suffering from daily febrile attacks.[190] But in Handsch's notes, too, it is striking how only very few patients have entries dedicated to them that span longer periods of time – and those who do tend to be from the nobility.

Authority in Jeopardy

Finzel and Handsch do not explain why the interactions between physicians and patients were often limited to a short period of time or indeed to a single visit. Of course, patients with acute diseases may quite simply have gotten better and felt no need to come back. But patients often suffered from long-standing, chronic diseases. When they did not get better with the medicines a physician had prescribed many of them did not come back, it seems. Instead they sought the help of another physician, a barber surgeon or some unlicensed medical practitioners. "They hop from one to the other", Handsch described this widespread behavior.[191]

There were good reasons for this. For many people, the trust the educated classes invested in learned medicine as such went hand in hand with a good dose of skepticism about the ability of the individual physician. Moreover, standardized treatment of different diseases according to the "rules of the art" existed

---

189 Jütte, Ärzte (1991).
190 Cod. 11207, fol. 209r.
191 Cod. 11205, fol. 290r.

to a very limited degree only. Experience taught that when consulted about the same case of illness, different physicians would frequently arrive at different diagnoses and treatment recommendations, and sometimes even express overt criticism of a colleague's judgment. In the contemporary perspective, it therefore only made sense to try one's luck with several different physicians provided that these physicians, on the whole, enjoyed a good reputation.

When patients did not recover or their condition even worsened – as often happened with more severe or prolonged illnesses – the cause for doubt and distrust was all the greater. Sick Malwitz, for example, told Handsch about being treated with guaiacum, first by Gallo, then by Mattioli. Although he did not have any noticeable skin changes, the physicians were convinced – probably due to his genital discharge – that he was suffering from the French disease. After the treatment, however, he was much worse: "I felt much healthier before than now that I have lain in the wood." And he believed he knew the reason. The guaiacum, which had a heating and desiccating effect, was – as a court physician to the Duke of Cleve had told him – harmful in his case because his liver was already hot and dry.[192]

When it seemed that they were unable to cure the patient, physicians could urge patience. Handsch wrote down phrases to use on such occasions: one could not cut down a big tree in one stroke;[193] it was a "dogged disease";[194] prolonged illnesses "like to take plenty of time".[195] They could also give an excuse, pointing to divine providence. Willenbroch, for instance, told the ill Blasius that he must bear the cross that God had laid upon him. God punished those He loved, he said.[196] Without God's blessing, the peasant, too, slaved away for nothing, Handsch explained to Count Sigismund von Berka.[197] Another formulation he presumably noted down with a view to future use was: "I will do what is human and possible, and will ask for the help of God the Lord."[198] And further: "Health is not a rabbit I can pull out of a hat; I do as our art allows, but one has to grant the Lord his power."[199]

---

192 Cod. 11207, fol. 222r.
193 Cod. 11206, fol. 179v, "nicht mit einem Streich abschlagen".
194 Ibid., fol. 184r, "beharrliche Kranckheit".
195 Ibid., "ire bequeme Zeit haben".
196 Ibid., fol. 180r.
197 Ibid., fol. 127r.
198 Ibid.: "Ich wil thun, was menschlich und möglich ist, und wil Gott den Herrn in Hülff nemen."
199 Ibid., fol. 180v: "Ich kann die Gesundheit nicht aus dem Ermel schütteln, ich thue was unser Kunst vermag, aber man mus unserm Herrgott auch sein Gewalt lassen."

But how were patients and their relatives to decide if ongoing ill health was due to the nature of the disease, divine providence, or medical incompetence? Sooner or later it only made sense from their point of view to try their luck with a different physician or healer who was perhaps better equipped to identify the true nature of the illness and to cure it. Without meaning to, learned physicians encouraged this attitude. They tended to emphasize their ability to tailor their treatment to the patient's physical constitution and specific life circumstances. Yet, these efforts necessarily heightened the differences between the recommendations given by different physicians for the same medical case. Many physicians furthermore boasted about the particular effects of their *experimenta* and *secreta*, about the medicines and mixtures of drugs which in their own experience had proven effective. If the promised effects of one physician's medicine failed to materialize, patients could therefore always hope that perhaps another healer had a more suitable and effective remedy in his arsenal.

Diagnostic and Prognostic Uncertainty

On the whole, physicians and patients alike believed that medicine had at its disposal the necessary means to cure diseases. The key to a successful practice, to attracting patients – especially those patients from wealthy and aristocratic circles – in the circumstances that have been outlined was word of a physician's good results in treating illness. This is also shown by comments made by laypeople in letters and other ego-documents when they sought to assess the qualities of different physicians. From their perspective, being treated by a good, experienced physician could make all the difference. When word got around that a physician had cured numerous patients, even of severe diseases that had perhaps been declared incurable by others, he could count on more patients finding their way to him. Nothing was better able to bolster a physician's reputation and authority in the eyes of future patients than stories of sick people he had cured, ideally against all expectations. As a student, Handsch already noted that his teacher Comes de Monte had been accorded "great glory and honor" for his treatment of a woman with dropsy from obstructed menstruation.[200]

A physician could lose the trust of patients and their relatives as easily as he had gained it, however. Making the initial diagnosis was already fraught with challenges. Many patients and relatives expected an immediate, clear judgment, well before it was actually possible for the physician to arrive at one in his own

---

[200] Cod. 11238, fol. 71r.

estimation. As we have seen, many people even believed that a truly skillful physician was able to name the complaints in question simply by examining the urine. This could easily go awry. Handsch once diagnosed a girl suffering from febrile heat and vomiting with a *febris continua,* and wondered if she also had worms. Two days later, the girl developed the rash that was typical of measles, and Handsch was reproached by the father who told him that he should have known about the measles by looking at the girl's urine.[201]

Physicians could resort to certain practical tricks to avoid potential humiliation following obvious misdiagnosis. Handsch entrusted his notebook with a number of these. If in doubt, the physician was well advised to diagnose widespread – and thus more probable – complaints and illnesses. With women, he could hardly err if he said to them, "It sometimes goes to your feet". This was because with the widespread uterine complaints, but also with diseases of the liver and the spleen, the legs would typically swell.[202] It was also a safe bet to say, "It sometimes goes up to your chest and you have difficulty breathing, especially when climbing stairs."[203] In the springtime, when prolonged fevers were common – this Handsch learned from Lehner – he could quite confidently conclude just by looking at the patient's urine that there was a fever and say that it was a "hidden, inner, heating fever", in case the patient had no corresponding symptoms.[204] Older people often concocted their food insufficiently and had much liquid in their bodies and heads. With them, he could speak of a "weak, poorly digesting stomach" and fluxes,[205] and "of a weak and liquid head" which carried the risk of a stroke or that fluid was dripping down into their legs, making them heavy.[206]

In many cases, especially as the disease developed, one could avoid misjudgment that would later be patently obvious by diagnosing occult pathological processes within the body, for example an obstruction of the liver or spleen. Patients and their relatives were rarely able to judge such a diagnosis, but it was acceptable to them if it seemed sufficiently plausible and accorded with the changes the patient perceived. If a physician diagnosed a "hidden" fever, or "inner measles" in times when the measles were going around, he could hardly

---

[201] Cod. 11207, fol. 42r.
[202] Cod. 11205, fol. 435v ("Es kompt euch bisweilenn ynn die Fuß") and foll. 433v-434r.
[203] Ibid., fol. 435v: "Es kompt euch auch bisweilen kegen der Brust, habt ein schweren Athem sonderlich wenn yr die Stigen auffsteiget." Similarly ibid., fol. 534v.
[204] Cod. 11206, fol. 25v, "heimlich, innerlich, hitzende Feber".
[205] Cod. 11205, fol. 542r, "schwachen, ubeldeuenden Magen".
[206] Ibid., fol. 433v: "Von eynem schwachen und flussigen Haeupt und ist zubesorgen, der Schlag wirt sich einmal ruren."

go wrong. If the symptoms of a fever became manifest, or the rash typical of measles broke out, he had said the right thing ("bene dixisti"). And if not, he could not be blamed: the fever or measles had remained hidden inside the body.[207]

Another trick Handsch noted down was that the physician should, if possible, try to find out more about the illness and its potential causes before he even set foot in the sickroom. This, he added, would make it seem is if he already possessed a quasi-supernatural, divine knowledge about the person's illness when he approached the patient, helping him to gain the patient's trust.[208] Treating a sick man by the name of Skala, Handsch experienced firsthand just how useful the information of third parties could be. Based on the complaints described by the patient, Handsch was about to speak of a liver obstruction or a constricted lung – both were diagnoses that were difficult to refute – in the hope that he might later hear something that would allow him to recognize the cause of the illness and to arrive at a "truer" ("verius") judgment. But before he spoke to the patient, a maid happened to tell him something about the man's stomach. Consequently, he explained to the patient that his stomach was not digesting food sufficiently and was also incompletely closed at the top, allowing many vapors to rise up from there when he was sleeping. Because these vapors could not exit through the thick roof of the skull, they condensed and became water and flowed down as catarrh into the lungs.[209]

Putting the physician's authority and credibility most at risk was prognostic assessment. Many medical diagnoses were not verifiable for patients, and if a patient did not recover, there could be various reasons why; therefore, a misdiagnosis was not necessarily at the root of it. But whether or not a physician had correctly predicted the course of the disease was something that even uneducated laypeople could recognize, and the chances of disgracing oneself were accordingly high. It was ultimately difficult to determine with certainty how the disease would unfold on the basis of the current clinical picture, or even just to predict the effect of specific therapeutic measures accurately. Handsch learned from Musa Brasavola that Hippocrates had already alerted physicians to the uncertainty of prognosis. Even the best physicians had to experience with embarrassment ("cum pudore") how their predictions proved to be wrong. To remain on the safe side, then, it was best for the physician to dispense with making prognoses entirely. Handsch had heard that it was almost impossible to wrest a prediction

---

207 Ibid., fol. 213v.
208 Cod. 11200, fol. 56r.
209 Cod. 11205, foll. 274v-275r.

from some famous physicians, for example Leoniceno and Manardi in Ferrara.[210] This was a privilege, however, that only great medical luminaries could afford, because the majority of patients and their relatives expected and demanded a clear prognosis from their physicians – if only because it helped them determine whether the medical treatment with its attendant costs and strains was worthwhile. It was difficult for the physician to turn down this request entirely.

The question of prognostic assessment had a preeminent position in Handsch's rules for a successful practice, which he time and again drew attention to with an "ad cautelas" in the margin. By his own admission, Handsch had repeatedly made grave errors in this regard. The basic rule was easy to grasp: the physician was not to audaciously promise the success of his treatment and the recovery of the patient. If the patient were not cured – and here Handsch was cautioning himself – the physician would lose "esteem and faith".[211] Certainly, even from a strictly medical point of view, it was acceptable, indeed advisable, not to take away the patient's last hope. After all, negative affects such as sorrow and anger were considered to have strong physical effects that could exacerbate the illness. In his conversations with relatives, however, the physician was well-advised not to shield them from the seriousness of the situation.

What was more: in his own interest, it was better for the physician to exaggerate the seriousness and make it seem as if the illness were difficult to cure. Handsch wrote that if the physician did this and the patient recovered, money and honor would be bestowed upon him. And if he died, there would be less criticism.[212] This was Mattioli's modus operandi. He "always portrays the illness to the sick and their relatives as greater than it is, because this, as he has said, is good for physicians."[213] Along these lines, another motto Handsch wrote down in Latin was: "Always make the illness great to those giving support (but to the sick [make it] small), because if he becomes healthy again, you will be accorded greater praise [and] if he dies, you will likely be excused because you had warned of the danger."[214] To those giving assistance to the patient, one could say such things as, "Truly, he is in a bad state of repair; a cause for concern; dangerous; he is hanging

---

210 Cod. 11183, fol. 332v, "quod nemo potuit ab eis extorquere prognosticum"; similarly Cod. 11205, fol. 494r.
211 Cod. 11205, fol. 410v, "aestimationem et fidem".
212 Ibid., fol. 212r: "Simula difficilem esse morbum".
213 Cod. 11206, fol. 128v: "D. Matthiolus apud astantes semper pluris facit morbum quam est, quia dicit bonum esse pro medicis."
214 Cod. 11207, fol. 229r, "magnificias semper morbum apud astantes (apud aegrum vero parvifacias), nam si sanatur maior laus tibi erit, si moritur excusatior eris quia monuisti de periculo."

in the balance".[215] But when it came to the patient, one was to "console him entirely, not make him frightened, not desert him."[216] When a fourteen-year-old girl with a fever was increasingly deteriorating, he consequently gave the parents hope. Yet, he told their maid that the sick girl would die. When the girl indeed did succumb to her illness, the maid told the parents that Handsch had predicted the girl's death and, as he noted explicitly, "they appreciated this."[217]

Even when he was convinced that a patient's medical condition was irremediable, indeed terminal, the physician did well to refrain from clear, unambiguous statements. He could, after all, be mistaken and the illness could, against all expectations, take a favorable turn. Following Mattioli's example, he could say in such cases, that the patient was "not without danger".[218] In a different place, Handsch noted a further phrase he could use to get himself out of such corners: "Death is at the doorstep, but I don't know whether or not he'll come in."[219] If a patient was seriously ill, it was furthermore advisable to send a boy ahead of oneself, so that when he made his call, the physician would not encounter a deceased patient, making it obvious to everyone that he had not expected the imminent death. Or he could first walk by the patient's house and check if the windows were open. Opening windows was common practice when someone died.[220]

In practice, however, Handsch found it difficult to comply with this rule. He suggested that he sometimes wanted to spare the patient the painful truth, and be pleasant to them instead ("gratia blandiendi"). But other times – here he was honest with himself – it was sheer vanity ("vanitas")[221] when he believed that he could make a precise diagnosis by looking at the symptoms, or indeed that he could predict the time of death. With words like "be more careful in the future",[222] he repeatedly and sometimes with capital letters brought himself back to his senses, admonished himself to practice reserve, and set the intention

---

215 Cod. 11206, fol. 100v: "Es stehet warlich baufellig mit ym, sorglich, gefehrlich, auf der Wag."
216 Ibid., "allwegen trösten, nicht feyge machen, yn nicht verlassen".
217 Cod. 11183, fol. 140r.
218 Cod. 11207, fol. 217r.
219 Cod. 11205, fol. 212v: "Der Todt stehet vor der Thur, ich weis aber nicht, ob er hereyn wirt komen".
220 Cod. 11206, fol. 116r; on the practice in Innsbruck see Cod. 11183, fol. 410r. The custom of opening a window when someone is dying survived far into the twentieth century. Presumably, it served to facilitate the soul's journey from the body to the heavens. For the same reason, tiles were lifted from the roof in some areas, when someone was dying; cf. Stolberg, Heilkunde (1986), pp. 282f.
221 Cod. 11183, fol. 331v.
222 Ibid., fol. 332r.

of no longer "making audacious promises and prognoses".[223] Yet, again and again, he made the same mistake of promising too much or omitting to communicate the seriousness of the situation, giving the patient hope – as was his duty – but then failing to at least tell the patient's family the fatal prognosis.[224]

He left a bad impression, for example, when he said of a seriously ill boy in Collinus's private school that if he survived the night, he would live for a long time to come. For several days Handsch, knowing of the boy's dire condition, had found out from a scout whether the boy was still alive before he made his visit, thus ensuring that it would not look as if he had not foreseen the boy's death. This time he did not consult the scout. The boy survived the night, but when Handsch returned in the afternoon, he found him lying dead in his room.[225]

Things also turned out badly for him in the case of a sick fishing warden named Hosska. He had to admit that he and his hapless methods had been anathematized because Hosska had died in his care. The patient he excused himself, had ingested none or only a little of Handsch's medicines. Handsch's mistake, indeed his failure or "offence" ("meum delictum") had been to misjudge the seriousness of the situation despite the old man's weakness and deathly pale face, and to have not warned the man's wife about the looming death, not even when she made a point of asking if the disease was terminal, so that she could know if it made sense to continue giving him medicines. He had actually wanted to give the man antimony but did not get the chance because the man suffocated from his *catarrhus* just an hour after Handsch's last visit. In the future, he decided once more, he wanted to tell bystanders that the patient's life was in danger.[226]

He also found himself repeatedly making the opposite mistake of giving an all too self-assured prognosis of imminent death. He marked the case of a fever patient named Kretzel with "error", commenting, "I told him he would die". The sick man lay in bed utterly weakened, delirious, with a brown-coated tongue and suffering from diarrhea – but he recovered.[227] When a peasant fell and seriously injured himself, he said to the man's wife that he was "not going to beat about the bush, because you desire to hear the truth; so I will say that he will die", whereupon the woman began to cry. A year later the man was still alive. Admonishing himself once more to practice reserve, Handsch wrote, "Therefore do not be too rash and daring when making your prognosis". In this case at least, he

---

223 Cod. 11205, fol. 276r.
224 Cod. 11183, fol. 50v.
225 Ibid., fol. 332v.
226 Cod. 11205, fol. 255v.
227 Ibid., foll. 127v-128r.

had added the consoling remark that he only judged by human reason. God was powerful. He was able to wake the dead, and to heal the sick all the more.[228]

Money

The question of remuneration posed great challenges for the physician-patient relationship and the physicians' public self-fashioning. Expecting money and asking to be paid to treat patients tended to muddy the image they wanted to present to the public, and could potentially cause considerable conflict in their dealings with patients and their relatives. While physicians, like lawyers, were commonly alleged to be greedy, physicians did their fair share of complaining about the ungratefulness of patients. As Handsch hinted, some did not pay at all. "No recompense" he elaborated in one entry; there was "no gratitude".[229] In Finzel's practice journal, we find a considerable number of entries in which he did not note down payment. Only some of them concerned patients whom he saw several times or indeed for an extended period and who would presumably not have paid for each consultation separately. As Finzel used the journal to calculate his annual income, we may assume that he documented all of his earnings. We thus must conclude that in fact hundreds of patients simply did not pay him or were offered pro bono treatment to begin with.[230]

It is important to keep in mind that those who acquired wealth at the expense of others were committing a far greater offence in sixteenth-century societies compared to today. This was true not only of money lending for interest. Recent work on the history of accounting has shown that merchants, even those doing business in prospering trading cities, believed that they had to justify themselves before God for the profits they made by reselling goods at a higher price than what they had paid. This was one of the reasons why contemporary manuals on how to keep account books recommended using religious elements such as an appeal to God on the first page and to include religious symbols such as the cross.[231] Hiob Finzel followed these recommendations in his practice journals, putting small crosses along the upper edge of the page, appealing to God, and writing pious poems at the beginning or the end of each year.[232]

---

[228] Ibid., foll. 420v-421r.
[229] Cod. 11206, fol. 183r.
[230] Ratschulbibliothek Zwickau, Ms QQQQ1, Ms QQQQ1a and Ms QQQQ1b.
[231] Aho, Confession (2005).
[232] A more detailed treatment of this issue can be found in Stolberg, Accounting (2020).

In some respects, the income a physician earned from treating the sick, was particularly offensive. After all, he profited from the suffering of his fellow human beings. And, even worse, he earned more if his treatment did not lead to a timely cure but dragged on – possibly due to his own errors. Today, the payment physicians receive is referred to in German as an "Honorar", literally an honorarium, that is something conferred as an honor. Encapsulated in the term is the understanding that a physician's help cannot be remunerated in the same way that other goods or services are. However, this term and the message it sends was not established in the sixteenth century. The common Latin expression used to describe a physician's fee, which Handsch used as well, was, tellingly, "merces", derived from "merx", or merchandise, and closely related to "mercator", the merchant.[233]

While Handsch's notes do not include specific figures for the payments he or his colleagues received from patients, Finzel's practice journal allows us to study the income of a common municipal physician in private practice quite closely. As mentioned above, what is immediately striking is the large number of patients who only paid him a very modest fee. A large majority gave him not more than two or at most three groschen for a consultation. One has to be careful with general statements, yet this seems to indicate that physicians – or at least town physicians like Finzel – made their services accessible to the populace at large and were willing to adapt to their patients' financial circumstances. More affluent patients, by contrast, paid Finzel considerably more. One, two, or even five talers or gulden, the equivalent of about twenty to one hundred groschen were not uncommon, and some noble patients even paid considerably more.[234] In one case, the treatment of even a simple servant warranted a gold coin, paid to Finzel by the man's employer.[235]

We hardly know anything about the ways in which physicians "billed" their patients and about the extent to which patients knew how much they would have to pay. As we have seen, some towns set a – usually very modest – maximum fee which the municipal physician could demand from poor patients. Physicians who were not in the service of a town were, by all appearances, free

---

233 The relevant section in Zerbi, Opus perutile ([after 1494]) was titled "De mercede medici accipienda". Sometimes, Handsch also used the term "praemium" (Cod. 11205, fol. 312v and fol. 573v; Cod. 11206, fol. 183r).
234 Ratschulbibliothek Zwickau, Ms QQQQ1a, p. 299 and p. 310 and Ms QQQQ1b, p. 77 (on the wife of the Margrave of Brandenburg, who gave Finzel 20 gulden); four gulden was also the amount young Sebald Welser gave to the Nürnberg physician Melchior Ayrer for his repeated advice (Wolfangel, Ayrer (1957), p. 22).
235 Ratschulbibliothek Zwickau, MS QQQQ1a, p. 47.

to charge whatever they considered adequate and the only limit would have been, in the long run, that a physician who was known to charge exorbitant fees would no longer be consulted. In Münster, the town magistrate found, in fact, that some patients hesitated to consult a physician because they were uncertain about the cost. It decreed that physicians were, in principle, entitled to four batzen per visit or a taler per week but added the advice to ask the physician beforehand whether he would be content with this fee.[236]

More affluent patients seem to have considered it a matter of course, even a question of honor, to remunerate the physician according to their station and their financial abilities. This situation is confirmed by the fact that Finzel, in many cases, noted down payment in kind, for example with cheese, butter, fish, meat, or more rarely, beer and wine. One might think that payment in kind was widespread among common people, especially peasants, who practiced subsistence farming, but this would be mistaken, as Finzel's journal tells us: almost exclusively it was the nobility and members of the upper classes who reciprocated in this way. While Finzel converted the value of the natural produce in groschen and gulden to calculate his annual income, his noble patients likely did not consider the produce they gave him payment at all, thinking of it instead as gifts which they graciously granted him and which also served to highlight their social status. When they sent Handsch a hare, a haunch of venison, different kinds of birds, or wild boar meat, they were expressing something about their privileged position. It was they who usually held the exclusive hunting rights, at least to bigger game. Even the cheese loaves, valued up to sixteen groschen, which Finzel received from them, presumably emphasized their rank insofar as they pointed to the command they held over subservient farmers.

In the course of a professionalization process that lasted hundreds of years, one of the decisive successes achieved by learned physicians was a detaching of the assessment of, and payment for, medical efforts from the success of the cure. Physicians practicing in the Renaissance were already working to establish this point of view among patients and their relatives. But recipients of medical care largely continued to regard them like other craftsmen who were paid for their goods or services. When a treatment did not bring the desired result, patients and their relatives held that the physician had not rendered the service they had expected, he therefore had forfeited his entitlement to a generous reward. According to Handsch's account, some clients were not even willing to

---

236 Stadtarchiv Münster, A-RatsA_A II Nr. 20, minutes of the town magistrate, vol. 42 (1610), fol. 230v.

settle their debt with the apothecary when the medicines prescribed by the physician did not have the desired effect.[237]

The physicians here were encountering a behavioral pattern that the sick and their families also exhibited towards other medical practitioners. And contrary to the learned physicians, some barbers, barber-surgeons, and lay healers were willing to make concessions. According to Handsch, some were prepared to sign a *pactum,* a healing contract, with their clients which made their payment conditional, to a degree, on the success of their treatment. For example, one barber who was treating a patient for a painful abscess was to receive three talers in total: one up front, one if the abscess got better, and another one if it healed completely.[238] Another agreement stipulated the payment of fifteen talers to a barber for the three-week treatment of a young man suffering from the French disease.[239] This practice has been documented for other places as well, especially in cases where healers took legal action against a patient or his or her heirs to recover outstanding fees.[240] A lay healer called Jakob Schäffer, a former cowherd from the Stuttgart area, recounted in 1592 how he was called to a sick man with a chronic abscess that other healers had attempted to cure in vain, and that he "offered to try and help", without, however, promising a sure "cure or healing". He sent to the apothecary for "several things" to give the sick man, asking that the patient, for the time being, pay only for these medicines. Ultimately, he was unable to help the man who therefore did not have to pay him for his services.[241] One agreement, signed in 1528, stipulated that a Zurich surgeon was to receive twenty gulden if he succeeded in making a sick woman healthy enough that she could go to church again without pain or cane, otherwise he would get nothing.[242] And, as agreed upon in a *pactum,* the Bamberg prince-bishop even paid the sum of 175 gulden to an Englishman who cured a nun. She had been suffering from a cancerous ulcer for three years, and the treatment took three months.[243] As late as the late seventeenth century, a draft tax bill on Württemberg barbers

---

237 Cod. 11205, fol. 676v.
238 Ibid., fol. 245v. See also ibid., fol. 267v, on the "pactum" between a Jewish healer and a paralyzed nobleman; Handsch did not indicate the amount.
239 Cod. 11183, fol. 77v; the man had initially sought Handsch's counsel.
240 Cf. Gianna Pomata's detailed analysis of the relevant documents of the *protomedicato* in Bologna, in Pomata, Promessa (1994), esp. pp. 61–128.
241 Hauptstaatsarchiv Stuttgart, A 209, Bü 725, letter of supplication from Schäffer; he ran an extensive medical practice and had been accused of witchcraft.
242 Wehrli, Bader (1927), p. 68.
243 Letter from Sigismund Schnitzer to Andreas Libavius, Bamberg, 2 February 1603, printed in Horst, Observationum (1628), pp. 463–465; Liphimeus, Warnung (1626) pp. 52–54, also mentioned this practice, here in connection with an itinerant theriac peddlar who (allegedly)

stipulated that they would receive only half of the agreed-upon fee if they amputated legs or feet and the patient died.[244]

In the absence of an explicit agreement, some clients still believed they were entitled to withhold payment from a healer if they did not recover as promised or, worse yet, their condition deteriorated further under the treatment. In a case documented for the year 1525 in Nuremberg, for example, a mother was unwilling to pay the eight gulden charged by a surgeon for treating her little daughter for an evil disease over the course of twenty-seven weeks. She complained that he had crippled the child with his medicine, so it could not stand.[245] In Zurich, the case of a widower went on record who denied a physician payment for treating his deceased wife, "because he killed his wife and now wants to cheat him out of his chattels as well".[246]

Physicians, too, had to be prepared for the possibility that patients would ask them to sign this kind of agreement. To do so went against their professional self-image, however. From their point of view, these agreements were degrading, demoting them to the level of an ordinary salesman or service provider. Handsch wrote down what his reply might be "if they want to sign a contract".[247] He would caution them not to bargain with the physician the way they would with a mercenary or landsknecht;[248] he was "no merchant" and did not desire to "sell his art".[249] Considering that other healers accepted such requests, it remains questionable whether his patients took these objections to heart. Nor might they have been content with his assurances that "I will do what I can but I would not promise you anything and I never have in all my life".[250] Georg Pictorius even believed that the Hippocratic Oath prohibited such contracts. He claimed that it

---

promised a nobleman to cure him against a certain fee and died when, on the patient's request, he took the purgative himself first which he had prescribed.
244 Hauptstaatsarchiv Stuttgart, A 228, Bü 68.
245 Stadtarchiv Nürnberg, B 14 II, 20, fol. 100r; the municipal court sided with the surgeon but reduced the amount the mother owed him from eight to six gulden.
246 Cit. in Wehrli, Bader (1927), p. 68, "derwyl er ime syn Husfrowen umbracht und welte ime jetz ouch um sin Gutt bringen."
247 Cod. 11205, fol. 215v: "Si volunt pactum facere"; ibid. fol. 291r, "si volunt facere pactum ante curationem".
248 Ibid., fol. 215v.
249 Cod. 11206, fol. 117v.
250 Ibid., fol. 127v: "Ich wil thuen was mir möglich ist, aber das ich euch solte was versprechen, das habe ich mein Lebtag nicht gethan."

said "that no one is to make a contract with a sick person for the sake of the matter, as someone who is sick would promise to give his fortune, and thus people would be gravely overcharged."[251] And as late as 1636, Ludwig von Hörnigk in his publication *Politia medica* cautioned the learned physician: "He must not negotiate or barter with the patient about the cure for an affliction or demand a specific fee before the cure is completed (in cases where this is possible)." Lawyers, after all, were paid no matter how the legal proceedings ended.[252] In Italy, Orazio Augenio, too, stressed that a physician who was unable to heal a patient but fought the disease with all available means was carrying out his task very well indeed.[253]

Even in cases when there was no specific agreement, letters sent by patients to physicians indicate that even upper-class patients believed that the "physician's fee" should in part be decided on the basis of the success of his efforts. If Thurneisser "helped" him, he would "reward him faithfully and well", Valten von Schaplo promised the Elector of Brandenburg's court physician.[254] Another said that he would show "his full gratitude" if Thurneisser's treatment, "with divine grace" would help him.[255] A third patient promised that "If God the Almighty will bestow his grace and blessing, good fortune and salvation, and I will recover," Thurneisser's efforts and labor would be amply remunerated.[256] And there were still others who promised rich rewards if they "experience help and recovery".[257] In its own way, the notion that more money was owed to the physician when his treatment was successful is also reflected in Handsch's observation that "many" patients who "recovered" pretended "to still be sick for the purpose of giving nothing or giving less to the physician".[258]

---

251 Pictorius, Von Zernichten Artzten (1557), fol. XVIv, "das keiner mit dem Krancken umb der Ursach willen vorhien soll pacisciren, dieweil einer, so kranck, alles verhies zuo geben das sein Vermögen were, unnd die Leut dardurch hart würden ubernommen."
252 Hörnigk, Politia medica (1636), p. 7: "Doch soll er die Schwacheit zu Curiren nicht uberhaupt mit dem Patienten dingen oder handlen, oder ein gewisen Lohn vor geendigter Cur (wann die möglich ist) fordern."
253 Augenio, Epistolarum (1602), fol. 88v.
254 Staatsbibliothek Berlin, Ms. germ. fol. 420a, fol. 163r, letter from Valten von Schaplo to Leonhard Thurneisser, 1571.
255 Ibid., foll. 175r-176r, undated letter from Nicles von der Linde.
256 Ibid., fol. 216r, letter from Britt von Schlieben [?], 8 August 1571; he already sent 20 taler with his letter, however.
257 Staatsbibliothek Berlin, Ms. germ. fol 420b, foll. 470r-471r, letter from Hans Kottwitz [?], 18 February [1575]; further examples ibid., fol. 245r-v.
258 Cod. 11205, fol. 676v.

Self-Confident Patients

The perception of physicians as "service providers" and the ever-present threat – which was often unspoken but could also be explicitly stated – of dispensing with the attending physician and seeking counsel from other healers if the diagnosis or the cure did not meet expectations also had a profound impact on the position of the patient in the physician-patient relationship. From the physicians' perspective, the ideal patient "submitted"[259] to their medical opinion and "obeyed".[260] When the Archduke declined to proceed with a suggested treatment, Mattioli held that, when it came to his health, the patient had to entrust himself to the physician as if he was the helmsman on a ship.[261] But this was wishful thinking. In practice, Jakob Oetheus in Eichstätt found, many physicians complained "that most patients are quite unwilling to obey and to submit to the physician's orders", which was "not only harmful to the sick but also very much interferes with physicians' decisions regarding treatment and its accomplishment".[262] Handsch noted down phrases that the physician could say to make a patient follow his instructions, including, "Your life is in your hands. If you follow [my instructions], you will get well, if not, you will be going on the scrap heap"[263] or "If you don't follow, you will be followed to the churchyard."[264] It seems doubtful, however, that he ever dared make such drastic statements to his patients. After all, as we see in Handsch's notes all too clearly, everyday medical practice was marked by a precarious and complex balance of power. Patients and their relatives pinned their hopes on the physician but at the same time, they met him with great self-confidence. The physician for his part was always aware that he might be replaced by another healer and therefore had little choice: he had to do his best to meet the expectations and wishes of his clients and, if necessary, he had to compromise against his better judgment.

If a physician wanted to convince a patient of his diagnosis and the therapy he was recommending – and thereby indirectly convince him of his competence – he first of all had to describe the disease process clearly and provide good reasons for the way he intended to treat it. As becomes very clear from the physician's notes as well as from epistolary consultations, many clients expected to hear these kinds of explanations, and they listened and paid attention

---

259 Cod. 11207, fol. 170v: "Submisit se patiens iudicio medico".
260 Cod. 11205, fol. 691r.
261 Cod. 11206, fol. 133r.
262 Oetheus, Gründtlicher Bericht (1574), dedicatory epistle.
263 Cod. 11206, fol. 691r.
264 Cod. 11205, fol. 282v.

to them. The Latin jargon that might be used by physicians to underscore their erudition could not be palmed off on them. They mistrusted physicians whom they did not understand.[265]

Handsch's notebooks drive this point home very clearly. Handsch, who otherwise wrote almost exclusively in Latin, put down the exact wording of hundreds of phrases in German, which he and his colleagues had used to communicate medical conditions or that he considered useful at least for this purpose. The large number of these entries speaks for itself. They give expression to the conviction that an plausible and comprehensible explanation of the medical condition and rationale of the physician's treatment was of utmost importance for winning the trust of the patients and their families. Sometimes, Handsch also wrote down how the patients responded to his explanations. When patients or their relatives returned to him, bringing the money for the medication he had recommended, this confirmed for him that he had found the right words.[266] Here and there he even marked his entries on these vernacular explanations with a simple "placuit" or "non displicuit": Handsch's statements had been appreciated and he could hope that similar phrases would prove successful with other patients as well.[267]

Frequently, the immediate, perceptible effect of the prescribed treatment helped the physician to establish the plausibility of his diagnosis and treatment plan in the mind of the patient and bystanders. For example, when a physician prescribed emetics or laxatives, the appearance and the smell of the matter that was brought up or passed with the stool illustrated vividly how highly impure, spoiled, harmful substances and possibly also worms had indeed accumulated in the stomach, in the lower abdomen, or in the body as a whole and had needed to be evacuated. Handsch recounted about the merchant Fabian that, after taking a purging agent several times, the sick man had personally lifted stringy mucus from his stool using a piece of brushwood "and he liked it".[268] When patients were bled, the physician could afterwards show them the bloodletting bowl and point out the phlegmy or blackish burnt nature of their blood as proof that it had been right, indeed even urgent, to prescribe bloodletting.

Handsch's notes also show that the physician always had to be prepared to meet with objections. Some patients had their own ideas about their illness. For example, when Handsch located the cause of a female patient's breathlessness

---

265 Cf. French, Medicine (2003), esp. pp. 118–122.
266 Cod. 11206, fol. 17r, fol. 35v and fol. 39v.
267 E.g. Ibid., fol. 39v and fol. 40r; see also Stolberg, Kommunikative Praktiken (2015).
268 Cod. 11183, fol. 180r.

in her head – according to current doctrine, catarrhs developed there, then emptied into the respiratory passages – she did not agree. She was convinced that the actual seat of the disease was in the lower regions of her body, which, incidentally, physicians, too, did commonly suspect was the true, ultimate origin of catarrhal matter.[269] Some laypeople, as mentioned, also found it difficult to understand why a physician would prescribe a laxative for a patient who was already eating hardly anything and accordingly had little to excrete.[270] Here, the physician could try to convince them that his remedies targeted the morbid matter specifically, helping to excrete it alone.[271] When it came to "female troubles" ("Frauensachen"), the physician's advice was sometimes at odds with what women knew about their own bodies. When, after she had been bled, Handsch advised the sick wife of a lapidary to interrupt breastfeeding for a couple of days and give her infant almond milk instead, she refused. She said this would make her breasts hurt from the incoming milk. She also refused when Handsch then suggested that she let off some of the milk and collect it in jars, and continued to breastfeed her child.[272]

Some ideas had taken root so deeply in lay culture that physicians felt as if they were going up against a brick wall. For example, female patients very commonly and categorically objected to taking medication directly before or during menstruation and paused treatment that was already in progress.[273] "Women will not accept medication during menstruation", Handsch noted down when he was a young physician.[274] This refusal, too, could be understood in the context of humoral pathology. Physicians themselves agreed, in principle, because many medicines had an expelling, purgative effect. Taking them during menstruation, women risked disturbing the natural, health-preserving downward flow of impure, corrupt matter into the uterus and then out of the body.

The prudent physician, as Handsch had to learn personally, also avoided giving certain diagnoses and using certain disease names. The mere mention of "acute fever" could set off warning bells for laypeople because it meant to them the possibility of pestilential fever.[275] As we saw earlier, physicians furthermore had to be very careful when diagnosing the French disease as this almost inevitably led to the question of the route of infection, which we presume would

---

269 Cod. 11205, fol. 242v.
270 Ibid., fol. 287v.
271 Cod. 11206, fol. 180v.
272 Cod. 11183, fol. 46v.
273 Cod. 11207, fol. 221v.
274 Ibid., fol. 189v: "Fluentibus menstruis mulieres non accipiunt medicamenta."
275 Cod. 11205, fol. 276r.

have been found morally reprehensible. This in turn might well have endangered the patient's prospects for marriage.[276]

Learned physicians faced particularly challenging difficulties with respect to the substantial trust laypeople placed in uroscopy. In the scholarly literature of the Middle Ages, the diagnosis of illness from an inspection of urine was still lauded as a major source of authority for physicians.[277] As we have seen, however, doubts about this began to emerge in the medical literature. What was questioned first and foremost was the patients' expectation that physicians should be able to identify diseases and pregnancies and even the patient's age and sex from urine alone, without any additional patient information. Critics cautioned of the danger of an embarrassing false diagnosis or prognosis. It could so easily happen that a physician diagnosed a terminal illness and then, following treatment from a barber or blacksmith, the patient got better again and walked the earth for years to come! And how embarrassing it was when a physician identified and treated a case of obstructed menstruation and several months later the woman gave birth! Medical writers cautioned that people might even put their physician to the test, for example by giving him false information about the sex and age of the patient or by slipping him the urine of a cow, or indeed Malvasia wine.

The problem for the physicians was that other healers commonly diagnosed diseases and pregnancies simply from the urine people sent them, and patients were often satisfied with their judgment. Fruitlessly, learned physicians railed against the "piss prophets" or "urine prophets" who used all kinds of "fraudulent" tricks to arrive at their diagnoses, shrewdly questioning the messenger, for example, or listening from behind a curtain while their wives sounded out the messenger.[278] In this situation it was inevitable that physicians, whether they wanted to or not, sometimes had to diagnose diseases from urine alone if they did not want to lose their patient's trust. Handsch learned it the hard way. When a blade smith sent his urine and did not give Handsch anything else to go by, Handsch was unwilling to commit. He let the man know that, by itself, urine was deceptive – and that concluded their interaction. The blade smith looked for help elsewhere. Months later, he came back to Handsch, this time in person, consulting him about complaints in the stomach area. He praised an old woman ("vetula") and her excellent uroscopic assessment of his previous condition. She had explained to him, "You drank too much, drank too often when you were not thirsty, and this extra drinking gave it to you". She also told

---

276 Cf. the chapter on the French disease.
277 On the following see also my detailed analysis in Stolberg, Decline (2007) and Stolberg, Uroscopy (2015).
278 See e.g. Hornung, De uroscopia fraudulenta (1611); Hart, Arraignment (1623).

him that he was sad because his wife had died and that he sometimes had complaints of the loins. The man said that this was indeed the case when he was sitting down. Handsch had to acknowledge that the man liked ("placuit") the old uroscopist's assessment.[279]

In other cases, Handsch did not even try to convince the messenger, and with him the patient, that uroscopy by itself was unreliable. He gave in. In his notes, he frankly admits that he sometimes only pretended to be looking at the urine a messenger gave him.[280] Instead, he relied on plausible and most probable diagnoses. For example, if he learned from the messenger that the patient was a tailor, he could – likely considering the tailor's many hours of sitting – diagnose an obstruction of the spleen or liver. He added that one could generally use the term "obstruction" ("oppilatio") quite often.[281] If he was able to find out that the patient was older, he could be confident in stating that he had "fluxes in the head and that the fluxes fell down into the chest, stomach, loins, and limbs",[282] or that he had stomach complaints and produced a lot of sputum, especially in the morning.[283]

With women, determining a uterine complaint was a safe bet.[284] When urine was once taken to Handsch from four miles away, and he was only told that it came from a woman, he, according to his own notes, only pretended that he had inspected it and then, in his "usual way",[285] announced a general diagnosis that would be useful to many female patients: the woman had phlegm in her uterus and therefore her menstruation was obstructed. She also sometimes had complaints in the area of the loins and in the legs and found breathing difficult. The person who delivered the urine confirmed everything and wanted to know whether the lungs or liver were affected. This was not surprising to Handsch, because after all, they – and here he was likely referring to the traditional uroscopists – were in the habit of saying that the lungs, the spleen, or the liver were rotting, were "obstructed, swollen, filled with mucus, ulcerous, withered, and shrunken".[286] Sometimes Handsch deliberately abstained from giving an obvious diagnosis, such as

---

279 Cod. 11205, fol. 222r.
280 Ibid., fol. 435r, "finxi me aspexisse".
281 Ibid., fol. 208.
282 Ibid., fol. 424v; similarly but even more elaborately ibid., fol. 433r, on the urine of the old Jew Markus.
283 Ibid., fol. 208.
284 Ibid..
285 Ibid., fol. 435r, "dixi solito meo more".
286 Ibid., fol. 435r; "verstopfft, verschwollen, verschleimet, geschwurig, absemert, geschwindt"; "absemert" probably derived from the old German word "semmern" for "emaciate" and "geschwindt" clearly refers to the "schwinden" ("consumption") of the affected part.

mucus in the uterus, to avoid giving the impression that he always arrived at the same result ("ut variarem").[287]

It was further possible to reduce the risk of giving an obvious misdiagnosis if one claimed that the complaints – supposedly identified from the urine – were either already present or would soon become manifest.[288] One could also avoid saying, "The water further shows . . . ", and instead ask: "Does she not sometimes complain about . . . ?" or, "Has she never complained?"[289]

In one entry Handsch even described a *Ceremonia pro simulanda diligentia,* a little diagnostic ritual designed to create the impression that he was working with great care, while in reality he was not basing his diagnosis on uroscopy at all. This was occasioned by a urine sample that was supposed to be that of a woman in a village who had not borne children for several years and was suffering from various ailments: "Hold the flask and inspect it carefully and say the following: 'Her time is not arriving naturally the way it should be'. Hold one finger under the flask and look at your fingernail and say, 'She has complaints in the area of the loins and sometimes it goes to the legs'. [. . .] Move the matula in a circular motion and say, 'If the slime is stirred up, it rises as vapor to the stomach and the heart, which sometimes causes her complaints and she breathes with difficulty, especially when she goes up the stairs.' Put your finger on the other side. 'When the vapors from the slime in the mother rise up higher, they reach the head and make the brain sick.'" And because he knew that the woman had not had a child in several years, he added, "With the slime, she cannot have children, because nothing can take hold in a place that is slimy and slippery; you cannot get wax to stick to a wet table."[290] He noted down that the separate steps of the *ceremonia* should be accompanied with utterances such as, "The water also shows . . . ".[291]

---

287 Ibid., fol. 436r.
288 Ibid., fol. 428v.
289 Ibid., fol. 429r.
290 Ibid., fol. 428r-v: "Halte das Harnglas und inspiziere es sorgfältig und äußere dich so: 'Yre Zeit hat sie nicht naturlich wie es recht sein solte'. Tu einen Finger unter das Harnglas und schaue auf den Fingernagel und sage 'Umb die Lennden ist yr schwer, und auch bisweilen kompt es yr ynn die Beyne'. [. . .] Bewege das Harnglas und lasse es kreisen und sage 'Wenn sich der Schleym erreget, so dempfft er auff kegen dem Magen und Herz, das beschweret sie auch bisweilen und sonderlich ist yr der Athem schwer, so sie eyn Stigen auffsteiget.' Halte den Finger auf die gegenüberliegende Seite. 'Auch so die Dempff aus der Mutter Schleym hocher auffsteigen, so kommen sie auch yns Haupt, und krencken das Gehirn'. [. . .] Si kan mit dem Schleym kein Kinder haben, denn wo es schleimig und schlipfrig ist, kann nichts hafften, Wachs kann man nicht ankleben an eynen nassen Tisch."
291 Ibid., fol. 429r, "das Wasser zeigt auch an".

Bitter Pills

Physicians often felt even more compelled to accommodate their patients' expectations and wishes when it came to devising a therapy. First, there was the taste of medicines, a subject that was of major importance in everyday medical practice. In those days, it could not be taken for granted that patients would receive medication whose taste was more or less bearable and whose smell and consistency did not constitute an absolute affront to the senses. Standardized, packaged medicinal drugs hardly existed at the time. The pharmacists usually held a range of common medicinal mixtures in stock. Many medicines were prepared *ad hoc*, however, according to the physician's instructions. As we learn from Handsch's notes, physicians also quite frequently prescribed medicine such as herbal decoctions which could be prepared in the patient's home, in the kitchen. Taste and consistency could therefore vary considerably, depending on the ingredients and the quantities prescribed by the physician, and depending on how they were prepared and administered. Composing suitable mixtures was far from banal, also because the ingredients in a mixture of drugs chosen for the individual patient did not always work well together. And some medicinal ingredients by themselves had a strong unpleasant taste that inevitably came through in a mixture.

Handsch dedicated many entries to the taste of different medicines, which underlines the importance of this aspect in everyday practice. One of his rules for a successful practice was that, if possible, a physician was to give gentle, reasonably palatable medicines so the patients would not refuse the treatment.[292] "When medicines are mild and gentle, they praise the physician", he noted.[293] Sometimes Handsch tested medicines on himself by putting some in his mouth so he could judge the taste.[294]

Some patients found the widespread medical syrups cloying. This was the reason why one young patient refused a syrup Handsch had prescribed.[295] An herbal decoction with syrup that Handsch recommended to a mason's wife who suffered from gout had a "highly unpleasant" taste ("sapor ingratissimus"), as he found himself.[296] Another female patient, to whom Handsch tried to give a herbal decoction that involved some very bitter plants, including chicory and

---

[292] Cod. 11207, fol. 1r: "Sis studiosus in exhibendis suavibus medicamentis, scis enim quantum alienati sint patientes ob ingrata pharmaca."
[293] Cod. 11183, fol. 116v.
[294] Cod. 11207, fol. 65r, fol. 95v and fol. 163v.
[295] Cod. 11183, fol. 116r.
[296] Cod. 11205, fol. 410v.

absinth, rejected the syrup in which it was administered as "very unpleasant". Not only this, but a wretched foam had formed on the surface.[297] And there were other medicines, such as *manus Christi*, a sugary mix, that some patients found unbearably sweet.[298]

Other remedies were very bitter. Again and again physicians had problems with cassia, a very commonly used, tried and tested laxative plant, and with the bitter *hiera picra*, which was produced from several different plants and was praised as an excellent medicine that cleansed and strengthened the stomach.[299] One patient let him know that the prescribed cassia had tasted awful but had later warmed his stomach nicely.[300] Handsch had the court apothecary Balthasar show him how to prepare cassia in such a way that it had a pleasant taste when taken by itself. But the apothecary cautioned him not to mix it with *hiera picra*: "It would be a pity to spoil such a lovely thing with hiera. I would rather eat pig dung than hiera; it is so repulsive".[301] Because he was to take *hiera*, the Archduke had once even sent for another physician instead, and, as Handsch added, the same had happened to Andrea Gallo, when he was treating a castellan.[302] Handsch himself thought the remedy was "abhorrent" ("abominabile") and was only willing to administer it with liquid, if he administered it at all.[303] One of his own patients, he found, detested him for prescribing it.[304] Gallo's *mixtura cordialis* as well was "nauseating", and some patients were reluctant to take it.[305]

Handsch also had an in-depth discussion with Mattioli about how to make opiates taste better, for example by mixing them with plum butter or fruit paste to neutralize the bad taste, or by giving them with Malvasia wine, as Handsch suggested. Another possibility considered by Mattioli was to mix them with athanasia. Later Handsch added that it was best to administer opiates as pills or mixed with cinnamon in wine.[306]

Choosing a better way to administer the medicine could sometimes make the taste more bearable. When one of Gallo's female patients refused to take *hiera picra* as a so-called *bolus* because of the bitter taste, he gave her the

---

297 Cod. 11207, fol. 209v.
298 Cod. 11205, fol. 147r.
299 Cod. 11207, fol. 158r.
300 Ibid., fol. 150v.
301 Ibid.: "Es ist schade, das man solch liblich Ding mit Hiera verterben sol. Ich wolt lieber ein Seudrek essen, dann Hieram, es ist gar widerwertig."
302 Ibid.
303 Ibid., fol. 55v.
304 Ibid., fol. 150v.
305 Cod. 11205, fol. 155r, "nauseabunda".
306 Ibid., fol. 94r-v.

medication in the form of a *pillula,* which still today refers to remedies that have a coating.[307] Handsch wrote that when cassia was administered as a drink, it swelled up so much that one needed to drink it in large volumes, and that made patients "abhor this kind of drink". He advised a patient to take cassia in solid form, because it was "sweet by itself", and then drink some water of violet.[308]

Physicians sometimes accommodated their patients in other matters of taste, too. For example, Handsch asked a sick man whether he preferred sour or sweet medication,[309] and with other patients he left it up to them whether to take the remedy in solid or liquid form.[310] He learned from another physician that the "matrons" preferred to take their purgatives if they were handed to them in spiced wine.[311] Further, physicians advised their patients about what they could do to counteract the bad taste. According to Camenicenus, it helped to rinse the mouth with vinegar before and after taking medication.[312] After taking a repulsive syrup – the sick Collinus, too, found it horrible – Mattioli recommended putting a few pomegranate kernels into the mouth, to swallow their juice and spit out the seeds.[313]

Some patients found just the appearance of a medicine distasteful. The sheer sight of a cough remedy prescribed by Handsch not only made the sick man Knebel nauseous; Handsch had to admit that he was disgusted himself.[314]

Strong-Willed Patients

Patients and their relatives not only had a say in the taste of medicines, but quite often also played a very active part in deciding upon the treatment in general. Frequently they demanded certain therapeutic measures and rejected others. When one patient asked to be given something for her stomach – she was experiencing pain in her upper abdomen – in addition to remedies for her fever and cough, Gallo gave her an ointment that she could rub on the stomach area before

---

307 Cod. 11207, fol. 208v.
308 Ibid., fol. 168r, "grausen vor eynem solchen Tranck".
309 Ibid., fol. 95v.
310 Ibid., fol. 51v.
311 Cod. 11205, fol. 222v.
312 Ibid.
313 Cod. 11183, fol. 204v.
314 Cod. 11205, fol. 107v.

eating.³¹⁵ Handsch, too, yielded in cases like this. Adam Bohdanski, for example, complained of a cold stomach and asked why Handsch was not rubbing his stomach with something, whereupon Handsch seems to have personally ("unxi") applied "stomach oils".³¹⁶ The matron Walpurgis, who had a fever and pain in her loins and then developed convulsive seizures, asked for bloodletting – and Willenbroch bled her, even though the illness, by Handsch's judgment, was bilious and therefore would more likely respond to treatment with emetics or laxatives. It was no surprise then that the result she had hoped for did not materialize.³¹⁷

Some patients did not even readily allow the physician to make the decision about which vein was to be used for bloodletting. In the case of the sick wife of Heidenreich, for example, the physicians wanted to let blood from the *vena saphena*, first on one leg, then on the other. She however, wanted to be bled from the popliteal vein.³¹⁸ In the case of a sick accountant, Handsch rejected the idea – because it was winter – of doing the bleeding from the *vena mediana* in the elbow, as the patient requested, preferring instead the much smaller *vena salvatella* at the back of the hand. A barber, however, explained that this was sometimes done even in the winter, and the patient got what he wanted in the end.³¹⁹

Sometimes other people's negative experiences could make a patient dubious. The Countess of Thurn, for example, did not want to take a remedy to strengthen the teeth because it contained the bark of *thus* (frankincense tree). Her maid, she reported, had lost two teeth from it. Gallo was able to reassure her: the effect of the bark was different from that of the plant as such. But as Gallo told Handsch later, the plant itself did not cause teeth to fall out either.³²⁰

Other patients were forceful in their demands for specific medicines. When the menstruation of Collinus's sick wife did not arrive on the expected day, she urged Handsch to give her medication. As she refused liquid remedies on principle, and as Handsch had no solid, sweetened, and dried *confectum* at hand, he gave her a strong dose of antimony.³²¹ Another female patient wanted to get well again right away, and so he gave her an electuary to "dissolve" the morbid matter, without administering the preparatory remedies that were commonly given first to promote the concoction or "digestion" of the matter.³²²

---

315 Cod. 11207, fol. 59v.
316 Cod. 11183, fol. 96v.
317 Ibid., fol. 466v.
318 Ibid., fol. 379v.
319 Cod. 11207, fol. 92r.
320 Ibid., fol. 160r.
321 Cod. 11205, fol. 251v.
322 Cod. 11207, fol. 152r.

"Do everything with a good conscience", Handsch wrote, reminding himself to show some reserve with demanding patients. He wanted to respect the rules of the art ("canones curativos") and not carry out treatments without using the necessary medicines simply to do the patient a favor ("in blandimentum aegri").[323] Whenever decisive action was called for, he wanted to be brave, and when it was not, he wanted to say no: one should not allow patients to get their way just to be pleasant ("propter blanditias concedere").[324] In practice, however, he found it difficult at times to observe his own rules. He allowed one patient, for example, to drink cold water from a well, just because he wanted to please him, though he knew that this was not the right thing in this case.[325] To be pleasant, he gave a scribe who was suffering from a fever and severe breathlessness less of the medicine than was necessary. When, contrary to Handsch's prognosis, the illness ended in death, people rightly held him in contempt, he thought.[326] He also admitted that, with some other patients, he prescribed medication or actively intervened in other ways only because he did not want to look bad. To avoid giving the impression that he was not doing anything ("ne nihil agere videar"), he gave something to the wife of Collinus that he happened to have with him: an essence of rhubarb.[327] He even admitted to having treated a patient with severe stone complaints for eight days, more "for appearance's sake than according to the rules", using oil of chamomile and *hiera picra*.[328] Against one of the fundamental rules of medical therapy, which said that very cold and very hot days were ill-suited for treatment – a rule Handsch's teachers liked to stress – Handsch gave a medicine to the wife of Collinus when it was bitter cold. He wrote that he did this "for appearances" ("ad speciem aliquid agendum") and without an assured method, "to be amenable" rather than out of conviction.[329]

Patients frequently also had very clear ideas about what they did not want. Enemas, it seems, were especially unpopular.[330] Handsch had heard that young women in the Netherlands had no reservations. They liked to be given enemas before they went dancing, "to be light".[331] And in Italy, the courtesans used the

---

[323] Cod. 11205, fol. 541r.
[324] Cod. 11207, fol. 231v.
[325] Ibid.
[326] Cod. 11205, fol. 541r.
[327] Ibid., fol. 250r.
[328] Ibid., fol. 263r, "potius fuit ad videri quam ad regulam".
[329] Ibid., fol. 251r.
[330] Ibid., fol. 268v, "laici illi, qui clysteres abominantur".
[331] Ibid., fol. 200v.

same remedy to be more "agile" ("agiliores").[332] The sick, however, were apparently often very reluctant. When Handsch wanted to give an enema to fourteen-year-old Friedrich von Kunritz, who had dysentery, the patient was adamant in his refusal ("obstinate recusavit").[333] With another sick boy, Handsch did not even try because he "might detest" it ("forsan abhorrebit"), even though an enema seemed indicated. He gave him a remedy that the boy could take orally as a first line of action, having decided that he would only take recourse to the enema if the medication did not yield good results.[334] Gallo had a similar experience. Because a woman plagued by colics refused being administered medicines via an enema, he prescribed her pills instead.[335] Mattioli, in particular, was nevertheless fond of prescribing them,[336] but he could get away with it more easily because of his status.

It remains unclear why enemas apparently were often met with obstinate refusal. A young Englishman told Gallo of his worry that an enema might weaken him.[337] But possibly some patients experienced the whole procedure as unpleasant or even embarrassing and humiliating. Jakob Fugger's son was unwilling to accept even a suppository.[338] Handsch's notes further show us that enemas also came with certain risks if they were not administered by a capable hand. Stories about this may have circulated. The sick archivist Matthias experienced such massive and sustained bleeding following an enema that he, by his sister's account, almost fainted and seemed close to dying. Mattioli, who had prescribed the enema, suspected an injury due to "bad use of the instrument".[339] A captain related that his grandfather had cried out in pain and died when he was given an enema.[340]

Understandably, patients sometimes showed reluctance when it came to interventions that were necessarily painful. Even the pain of bloodletting – for which a blade was used to cut through the skin and the wall of the blood vessel – should not be underestimated. There were patients who were afraid of it. Handsch knew a man called Tuchel who said that, his feet trembled before he let blood.[341] And it

---

332 Cod. 11206, fol. 118v.
333 Cod. 11183, fol. 105v.
334 Cod. 11207, fol. 195v.
335 Cod. 11238, fol. 63r.
336 Cod. 11183, fol. 135r.
337 Cod. 11238, fol. 128r, "dixit se debilitatum a clystere".
338 Cod. 11207, fol. 25r.
339 Cod. 11183, fol. 118v; Handsch referred to the patient as a "chartarius", a term used for archivists but also for people who sold paper. The patient had severe pain the upper abdominal region and died soon after.
340 Cod. 11205, fol. 150v, under the heading: "Mortuus ex clystere".
341 Cod. 11183, fol. 88r.

was said about some patients that they experienced so much fear that the blood did not flow when they were cut; physicians and laypeople alike assumed that fear made the blood and the spirits withdraw to the heart. To counteract this effect, the arm with the opened elbow vein was put in warm water.[342]

Not surprisingly, patients wanted to be all the more actively involved when the promised effect of a treatment did not materialize or they experienced undesirable effects. The wife of a lapidary removed poultice Handsch had prescribed the very next morning because she thought that it drew too much fluid out.[343] Another patient did not want to put up with the poultice he had been prescribed because the stinging was too much to bear.[344] Some patients put their physician's patience to the test. After one or two applications, a sick young nobleman was unwilling to tolerate further compresses for his belly. He claimed they were not good for him: "My belly rumbled more and was hardened". The sick young man was then given hellebore as a syrup, but he was not content with that either. After he took it, he complained, that he was dizzy, had no stool and was anxious. A purging agent finally caused him to produce four to six stools per day. Now the patient said he was getting weaker and the treatment was not helping much, "because my stomach is still gurgling and my head hurts with dizziness."[345]

From the physicians' point of view, a patient's "disobedience" not only jeopardized his or her health but also the physician's standing and reputation. Ultimately the physician would be held responsible when a patient did not get better. In exceptional cases, Handsch gave up. He took his leave from the sick Baron von Meseritz because "he did not want to obey".[346] Handsch likewise finally stopped going back to Spaner, who suffered from colics and *epilepsia,* because he "did not listen and made a mess of everything."[347]

At times physicians could profit from their patients' lack of "obedience". Handsch found out, for example, that one of his female patients drank Malvasia wine, which she had not told him. He did not believe that this was harmful, but when in the following days she was faring very poorly, he pretended

---

342 Ibid., fol. 243v.
343 Ibid., fol. 47r.
344 Cod. 11207, fol. 221v.
345 Cod. 11183, fol. 434r; "denn es korret ym nach [sic!] ymmer ym Leibe, und das Heupt thet wehe mit eynem Schwindel"; the term "korren" (also: "kerren") usually referred to gurgling sounds in the abdomen. The patient died three years later, from excessive drinking, Handsch believed.
346 Ibid., fol. 114r, "dum obedire noluit".
347 Ibid., fol. 321v, "quia non obediebat et omnia confundebat."

("praetexui") that this came from drinking the wine. His treatment, at any rate, could not be faulted now.[348] In other cases, one could blame a patient who did not recover completely by saying, "You went outside too soon".[349] On one occasion, he was able to defend himself well by pointing out that the patient had rejected taking the prescribed soporific because of its unpleasant camphor smell.[350]

Physicians could even plan ahead and use a patient's predictable recalcitrance to serve their own purpose. When he gave opiates, one of Handsch's *cautelae* ran, he would tell patients not to eat or do certain things that he knew they would find difficult to resist. When the pain came back – the way it usually did because the measure in question was only a "cloaking" treatment ("cura palliativa") – he would blame the patient for not doing as he was told.[351] In another entry, he explained that a physician could resort to a mere "cura palleativa", when he felt unable to heal the patient, and when the patient relapsed, he could claim that the patient had not respected his dietetic instructions.[352]

Undesirable Effects

If a patient got significantly worse under treatment or the treatment produced major undesirable effects, a physician could count on the patient's resistance to continuing with the treatment and could expect to be fiercely reproached. This could happen to any physician. Handsch, too, encountered bitter complaints, for example, when he treated someone suffering from the French disease with mercury fumigations. The patient was faring worse than he ever had, and stated that he would rather die, and he never experienced the flow of saliva that was supposed to take the morbid matter out of his body. Afterwards, Handsch's own brother reprimanded him and told him that he should not pursue a treatment like this if he did not know what he was doing.[353]

Especially with the widely used herbal remedies, the action of a medicine could vary widely, even if it had been carefully dosed. Factors such as the plant's quality, age, place of origin, as well as the plant parts that were used, along with the patient's physical constitution could make a difference. Mistakes could easily

---

348 Cod. 11205, fol. 298v.
349 Cod. 11206, fol. 171r.
350 Cod. 11205, fol. 300v.
351 Ibid., fol. 306r.
352 Ibid., fol. 223r.
353 Cod. 11183, fol. 254r.

happen. Especially when it came to evacuating morbid matter, the right choice and the dosing of the remedy was very much a balancing act. Patients and their relatives expected and asked for a strong, noticeable effect, and from a medical perspective, too, a drastic evacuation in many cases was considered essential to curative success. However, the effect could also be all too powerful.

Patients were willing to accept some quite unpleasant attending symptoms. Time and again, without giving any indication that there was dissatisfaction or protest, Handsch noted down cases like that of the sick wife of a chancery scribe, who passed twelve large, mucous stools following the administration of a laxative, and felt weak.[354] An acquaintance told him that he had passed fifty stools after a barber had given him a purgative to prepare him for treatment with mercury. He had discharged blood and been so faint and tired that he had to rest for eight days. Yet, he continued the treatment.[355]

When, however, the negative attending symptoms predominated from the perspective of the patient, physicians had to be prepared to face resistance and criticism. A phrase Handsch wrote down in this context was, "The doctor has ruined him".[356] The wife of a man called Baptist cursed the remedy she had been given (or the physician who prescribed it), because she felt bad ("male sensit") after taking a mixture of rhubarb powder and "opening" roots for her white discharge; even so, she had praise to spare ("laudavit") for other remedies.[357] Handsch's colleague Willenbroch brought upon himself the "great indignation" ("magnam indignationem") of a noble female patient – which, Handsch thought, was perhaps not entirely unjustified – when he applied a poultice with Spanish flies to her feet. It seems he meant only to warm the feet, but blisters formed and the woman experienced severe pain.[358] In other cases, the response from patients and their relatives is not documented but is easy to imagine. Fröhlich, for example, was given cassia by Handsch when he was sick. The patient subsequently had close to fifty bowel movements and died several days later.[359] A young nobleman produced close to thirty stools after taking a powerful laxative. This left him very weak and he soon died.[360] An old woman even had close to a hundred stools after taking cassia. She

---

354 Ibid., fol. 458r.
355 Cod. 11205, fol. 244r.
356 Cod. 11206, fol. 185r: "Der Doctor hat in verterbt".
357 Cod. 11183, fol. 399r.
358 Ibid., fol. 6v.
359 Cod. 11207, fol. 202v.
360 Ibid., fol. 214v; the physician in charge was a certain Dr Kunstat, whom Handsch mentioned repeatedly.

ultimately died as well.[361] In retrospect, it cannot be said whether the medical therapy contributed to or even caused death in these cases, but the physicians could hardly blame the bereaved if they held them at least partly responsible.

In one of his more detailed entries, Handsch described his unfortunate encounter with the sick Baron von Meseritz. The old gentleman suffered from severe febrile attacks. He complained of a great heat and in his layman's ignorance ("imperitia laicorum"), as Handsch wrote, he wanted something to be done about it right away. But Handsch was unwilling to even let him be fanned by a boy. The next morning the patient said that he had sweated so much that he had to change his shirt twice. He developed a piercing pain in his knees, as if the morbid matter had moved there, as Handsch remarked. But then Handsch found a murky deposit in the urine, which he interpreted as indicative of a "critical" transformation and excretion of the morbid matter. He therefore believed the disease was subsiding and predicted a marked improvement for the following day. But he was wrong. The old man sent for him and complained vehemently. Handsch wrote, "I had assured him that he would be quite fresh that day but he was very faint, had not slept at all, and his head was like an empty pumpkin". He criticized Handsch for not giving him any medication, instead "feeding [him] hope about his strong nature". But now one could see just how strong he was, he said. He had not had a moment's peace in the night and he claimed he had "become run-down due to negligence". He demanded a tonic but Handsch did not have any with him, "so now he was breathing anger". Handsch sent a messenger to fetch a soporific from an apothecary in a nearby town, but the apothecary did not send anything good. The following day, the sick man was weak, and angrily discontinued treatment with Handsch. Handsch learned later that he went to Prague, had himself treated by Mattioli, and recovered but his wife succumbed to a terminal disease. In his final conversation with the patient, Handsch defended himself. If he had promised him that he would be better the following day, he had only done what all physicians do. It was only proper to give a sick person hope, "because this is how he can take heart, can endure the disease with more cheer and overcome it". He had not given him medication, for one thing because this was to be avoided during the dog days, and for another because he had wanted to first get a better idea of the disease, and when there were signs of a critical excretion, he did not want to get in the way of nature. Handsch admitted in his personal notes that he had made mistakes. He should not have prematurely assured the patient that he would get better and fully recover. If, against all expectations, this turned out not to be true, it diminished the authority of the physician ("diminuitur authoritas

---

[361] Ibid., fol. 152r.

medici"). So as not to avoid accusations of neglect, he decided that he would always give medicines in the right order and according to the rules of the art ("canones") and make sure to give medicine at the right time. In future, he also wanted to ensure that he always had tonics with him, since he had been trusted less because he did not have one with him.[362]

The Sense of Shame

People's modesty or sense of shame posed another challenge especially when the patients were women. As Handsch suggested repeatedly, even talking about menstruation was a source of embarrassment for women, which was also reflected in the widespread use of metaphors, euphemisms, and roundabout expressions. With their patients, the physicians used expressions like "time of the month" or simply "your time"[363] or they even took recourse to poetic turns of phrase like "roses" or "time of the roses".[364] Handsch's colleague Merla wanted to know from a patient "whether she had her justice".[365] Handsch noted down some suitable expressions for his own use, such as "your attribute", "she has come into her time" or "the roses are not going at the right time", and "she does not have her justice".[366] He could explain complaints by saying, for example, "The disease often occurs in women because they do not have their roses in the right way."[367]

Numerous entries in Handsch's notebooks as well as case histories in published medical *observationes* show at the same time that physicians certainly did ask women about their menstruation, regardless of the feelings of shame this could prompt, and that women on their own initiative sought physicians' advice when they thought their menstruation was not right. Menstruation was considered too important for women's health to be hushed, at least when it had

---

362 Cod. 11205, foll. 226r-229r: "Ich hett ym zugesagt, er solte den Tag gar frisch seyn, so er doch gar mattlos were, hette die gantze Nacht nicht geschlaffen, der Kopf were ym wie eyn lediger Kurbiß"; "vertröstet auff seyne starcke Natur"; "durch Nachlessikait verwarlost worden"; "da war er nach [sic!] erger gesinnet auff mich"
363 Ibid., fol. 627r, copy of a *consilium* bei Johann Neefe.
364 Ibid., fol. 503r and fol. 547v.
365 Cod. 11206, fol. 36r, "ob sie ire Gerechtikeit hett".
366 Ibid., fol. 39v, fol. 126v, fol. 176v and fol. 183v; Cod. 11207, fol. 189r: "Euer Eygenschafft"; "Die Rosen gehen nicht zu rechter Zeit"; "sie ist in ire Zeit kommen"; "Sie hat nicht yr Gerechtikait".
367 Cod. 11206, fol. 179v: "Die Kranckheit tregt sich offte zu bey Weibspersonen, darumb das sie ire Rosen nicht zu rechte haben."

become "disorderly". It is clear that husbands and wives talked about these things, so that men were able to tell the physician when their wife was expecting her next period,[368] or could pass on their wife's request to the physician that he do something to encourage her menses.[369] However, Handsch also mentioned a woman who at first did not tell him that her menstruation had stopped.[370] And he wrote that when a woman's husband was present, he could not ask her questions about menstruation.[371] In his experience, dealing with young women was especially delicate. He wrote about one case in which he had not dared, for reasons of shame ("propter verecundiam"), to ask about menstruation or bowel movements, or to palpate the upper abdomen. This was because young, unmarried women ("virgines") felt especially bashful in front of young physicians. In the end, he had to leave her uncured.[372]

Handsch's records further tell us that, even more so than with menstruation, genital discharge was associated with shame. He found that women kept the common experience of white or yellowish discharge to themselves. They concealed it "out of shame" or "admitted" it, if at all, only when the physician inquired.[373] Possibly there was a confluence here of notions of impurity – as were connected to menstruation – and ideas of incontinence, that is an insufficient control over one's excretions in general. Despite her severe illness and her repeated miscarriages, the wife of a private tutor also kept an ugly anal growth to herself at first.[374]

This woman, like many others, did seek medical advice in the end. In the final reckoning, the desire to be healthy often seems to have outweighed shame. What is more, Handsch's notebooks clearly disprove the commonly held belief that physicians left the visual examination and the touching of female genital organs to midwives and other female healers. He described at great length, for example, how he personally attempted to inject warm wine into the uterus of the sick Baroness of Hungerkasten, whom his famous colleague Neefe had diagnosed with a "bad cold moisture". Handsch used a catheter ("syphon") for the purpose, which he had received from Ulrich Lehner. He gave a close description of the long, round-tipped tube featuring a slit-shaped opening at its end, which,

---

368 Cod. 11183, fol. 82r.
369 Cod. 11205, fol. 490r.
370 Cod. 11206, fol. 35v.
371 Cod. 11183, fol. 10v, "propter praesentiam mariti"; similarly Cod. 11207, fol. 111r, "propter praesentiam viri".
372 Cod. 11207, fol. 210r.
373 Cod. 11183, fol. 460r; Cod. 11206, fol. 33r; ibid., fol. 107v.
374 Cod. 11183, fol. 368r.

remarkably, he compared to that found in the male glans. He added in his entry that he had read in a surgery book written in German that a "uterine clyster" should have two holes on the side, which is to say not at the tip. He further described how the woman had to lie on a table with her legs spread and afterwards lie in her bed for two hours. The attempt failed, however, and the wine flowed back out. The patient stated that, by feeling for it ("ex tactu") one could tell that the uterus was closed but it remains unclear whether Handsch was allowed to verify this.[375]

To the extent that learned physicians also did surgical work, we may even more safely assume that, if it was necessary and if the patient agreed, they did not refrain from treating the genital area of their female patients. When he died in 1643, Johann Georg Wirsung, who practiced medicine and surgery in Padua, left behind not only a "speculum anni [sic!]" for the examination of the anus but also a "speculum uterinum".[376]

When it comes to male patients, Handsch's notes give no indication that they showed signs of a pronounced sense of shame when they disrobed in front of the (likewise male) physician. With great matter-of-factness, he described, for example, how he palpated a man's groin and scrotum.[377] He treated a man presenting with small ulcers on his penis and a swollen lymph node in his groin by injecting white wine mixed with several drops of sulfuric acid under his foreskin.[378] And when mercury unctions were used to treat patients suffering from the French disease, a complete disrobing could hardly be avoided. Handsch gave an exhaustive description of a Jewish healer applying mercury unction to the different body parts of a naked patient, using his own hands to rub it into the gluteal fold, and on the genitals.[379] Only when a seriously ill man exposed his genitals for no discernible reason did Handsch explicitly note down that the man had not "blushed", which apparently could be expected under normal circumstances; the absence of blushing here seemed to indicate to him mental confusion due to the illness.[380]

Reading Handsch's notes, it becomes clear that a male sense of shame could primarily be witnessed in medical practice when the patient's virility or sexual morals were at issue. The merchant Fabian had waited six months before

---

375 Ibid., fol. 7r-v.
376 List of Wirsung's estate, edited in the appendix to Ongaro, Wirsung (2010), here foll. 14v-15r.
377 Cod. 11205, fol. 259v.
378 Cod. 11183, fol. 142v.
379 Ibid., fol. 117* r.
380 Ibid., fol. 106v.

he "confessed" to him ("confessus est mihi") that he also had an ulcer on his penis and a swollen lymph node in the groin, as Handsch added in the margin. He had sought treatment from a Jew and had recovered, but then he went back to the prostitutes.[381] Shame and honor had to be considered when treating a patient. A cure with guaiacum or mercury over the course of several weeks in a "French house" was hardly a possibility for men from higher classes. Thus, Mattioli treated a private tutor with a guaiacum decoction that he prepared at home. The position of a teacher of boys from the aristocracy, wrote Handsch, did not allow for his treatment to become public knowledge ("manifeste").

Shame and injured manliness also seem to have played a role with an older male patient who complained that he could no longer contain his winds. Especially when he was walking, they escaped him with a loud "purz, purz, purz" – presumably audible for everyone around; and sometimes his urine also flowed against his will.[382]

Even the sexually impotent sought the advice of physicians in spite of – or sometimes perhaps precisely because of – the fact that impotence was mortifying and shameful and could have serious consequences at the time, in the worst case the scandal of public legal proceedings for the annulment of marriage.[383] Handsch mentioned a number of impotent men who approached him and other physicians, along with some he had heard about in private conversations. Some newly-wed men – here he gave their names – had difficulties during the first weeks of their marriage.[384] A certain Hans Ferber, according to Handsch, did not dare get married a second time, even though he already had two daughters with his former wife.[385] Other men suffered from impotence for years and tried all kinds of things to overcome it, taking medicines or visiting healing springs. Inguinal or scrotal hernias were feared in this regard because they were linked to the danger of impotence and infertility.[386] Repairing hernias posed a great risk, because a testicle was often removed in the process. After he

---

381 Ibid., fol. 177r.
382 Ibid., fol. 222v.
383 Darmon, Tribunal (1985); Ründal, Mannschaft (2011).
384 Cod. 11183, fol. 87r.
385 Ibid., fol. 222v.
386 Cod. 11205, fol. 108r, among others on Hoddeiovinus who fathered children inspite of his hernia.

had undergone the procedure, one young husband mentioned with great relief that intercourse was diminished only a little or not at all.[387]

Some men expressed concerns not only about their male honor and their ability to have children but also acknowledged their obligation to satisfy their wives' desires. In a letter to Mattioli, an approximately forty-year-old nobleman wrote that he had begun early with "the work of the flesh" and had "practiced it much" as well. Starting twelve or fourteen years ago, however, his ability had declined more and more. His "male member had become unwilling to stand" and if it did, the semen had run out forthwith. He had tried many medicines and consulted various physicians in vain. Mattioli was to please help him "now that he had taken a young wife", so he may father children and "the wife's lust may be given its due". Mattioli prescribed him herbal baths, electuaries, powders, and other remedies. The outcome remains unknown.[388]

"Bystanders" and Caregivers

It is with good reason that, in the preceding chapters, I have often referred to patients as well as to their families or more generally to the "bystanders". When a physician made a sick call, he normally met not only the patient but family, friends, and acquaintances, all of whom took an interest. He might even find them standing around the sickbed when he arrived.

This "sickbed-society"[389] could help the attending physician by providing additional information. For example, he could learn from them that the patient was hardly eating anymore[390] or that his sweat reeked and stained the bedding yellow.[391] They could describe the quality of the sick person's stool for him[392] or corroborate Handsch's explanation that the cloudiness in the urine of a patient meant "much phlegm" by pointing out that the siblings were "all phlegmy", which suggested a certain predisposition.[393] If the patient was a child, the parents and the other bystanders were commonly the most important source of

---

387 Cod. 11183, fol. 451r.
388 Cod. 11183, fol. 158v and fol. 185r, with a partial transcription of the patient's letter; "das fleischliche Werck [. . .] viel geübet"; "ime das männliche Gliedt nicht mehr stehen wöllen"; "dem Weib ir Lust auch gebust werde".
389 Lachmund/Stolberg, Patientenwelten (1995), p. 124.
390 Cod. 11207, fol. 65r.
391 Ibid., fol. 92r.
392 Ibid., fol. 226r.
393 Cod. 11205, fol. 293v.

information. It was they who let the physician know, for example, about a three-year-old girl, that "she has a head cold and toward the evening she runs hot".[394] They might also describe an epileptic seizure for him which they had witnessed.[395] Or they might tell him that a little boy sometimes started to scream all of a sudden, and smelled "strange from the throat", adding, when Handsch's asked them, that he often rubbed his nose, which, for Handsch, was an important indication of a worm infestation.[396] Sometimes bystanders also lent a hand with the treatment. The wife of Adam Zyma, for example, held the clyster in her husband's anus, while an apothecary – apparently in Handsch's presence – poured in the liquid.[397]

The frequent presence of relatives and other bystanders undoubtedly had an impact on the quality of the physician's visit. Intimate, personal conversations between physician and patient were probably the exception rather than the rule. It also put more pressure on the physician to assert his authority. He had to win over not only the patient but also the whole "audience" with his demeanor, his explanations, and his recommendations. He had to stage himself and his abilities appropriately if he wanted to gain the trust of both the sick person and the bystanders.[398]

Frequently relatives, especially spouses, would even want to have a say in the choice treatment. In the case of a sick woman called Watzarka, for example, it was her husband who rejected Handsch's prescription of a purgative and a tonic along with the herbal footbath.[399] At another occasion, this husband also refused the use of an emollient, soothing remedy for his wife. He explained that he had no trust in Handsch, because Handsch had wrongly promised that an external treatment of the feet would draw the heat down.[400] In the case of the feverish Johann von Meseritz, it was the father who criticized Handsch because his son was doing worse and Handsch was not giving him any tonics.[401] When treating the widow of a certain Kneysel, who was suffering from suffocation of the womb, Handsch did not even dare to do cupping on the vulva to draw down the rising uterus "because of the women".[402] In another case, an old woman

---

[394] Cod. 11207, fol. 168r "Sie hat den Schnupffen und gegen dem Abend hizet si."
[395] Ibid., fol. 169r, "selzam aus dem Hals".
[396] Ibid., fol. 180r.
[397] Cod. 11183, fol. 44r.
[398] On the importance of theatrical elements at the patient's bedside see Lachmund/Stollberg, Doctor (1992), drawing on eighteenth- and nineteenth-century sources.
[399] Cod. 11205, fol. 287r.
[400] Cod. 11205, fol. 276r.
[401] Cod. 11183, fol. 114r.
[402] Ibid.

("vetula") prevented a young man with a swollen knee from taking the syrup a physician had prescribed.[403]

Among the "bystanders", those who were directly involved in the nursing care and who looked after the patient's wellbeing played a special role. Little is known to date about nursing care in the sixteenth century, which largely took place in private homes rather than in hospitals.[404] Handsch's notes tell us about sick-nursing and the relationship between physicians and nurses only occasionally, in no more than a few dozen entries, but they do help illuminate some aspects.

We know very little about the people who did the nursing or caregiving, the "adstantes" as Handsch sometimes called them. Sometimes, they were relatives, wives and mothers but also husbands.[405] In the case of more affluent patients, Handsch frequently also mentioned men and women of lower social status who were presumably in the employ of the patient's family or were hired specifically as sick nurses.[406] He sometimes referred to them only in general terms as servants ("servus", "puer"),[407] maids ("Magdt", "ancilla", "puella"),[408] but sometimes also spoke more specifically of "female helpers" or "by-standing women" ("mulier administra", "mulier adstans"),[409] and in some cases of a "nurse" ("mulier curatrix"), who was appointed to help a sick official or whose help a certain patient had to do without.[410]

The contemporary medical literature, for example Oetheus's deliberations on nursing care, emphasized the importance of good nurses who helped ensure that the physician's orders were carefully followed, prepared medicines and food according to his instructions, and informed him about changes in the patient's condition.[411] Oetheus and other authors contrasted this idea with the

---

403 Ibid., fol. 569r: "Non insumpsit sirupum obstante vetula."
404 Extant historical scholarship focuses almost exclusively on the more recent past; for a useful overview of treatises on nursing from the late seventeenth century onwards, see Panke-Kochinke, Geschichte (2003).
405 E.g. Cod. 11183, fol. 49r and Cod. 11205, fol. 268r (wife); Cod. 11205, fol. 234v (husband); Cod. 11183, fol. 417r and Cod. 11207, fol. 135r (mother).
406 Thus also Jütte, Weib (1989), p. 20.
407 Cod. 11207, fol. 116r, fol. 167v, "servus" and 226v, "puer".
408 Cod. 11183, fol. 28r, "Magdt"; Cod. 11205, fol. 298v, "ancilla"; Cod. 11183, fol. 223v, "puella".
409 Cod. 11183, foll. 406r, 423v and 424v, "mulier administra"; Cod. 11207, fol. 114v, "mulier adstans".
410 Cod. 11183, fol. 418v, "ut dicit mulier curatrix"; ibid., fol. 419v, "adhibita curatrice"; Cod. 11183, fol. 329r.
411 Oetheus, Bericht (1574), "die fremden Personen, welche der Krancken zu pflegen verordnet, solches mit grossem Verdruß und Unwillen thuon". The third part of this work is devoted

poor training, negligence and disobedience of those who were usually given that task. Not only "the strangers who were ordered to care for the sick person", they claimed, "do so with great annoyance and reluctance".[412] Even relatives occasionally longed for nothing more than for the sick person to die so they would be relieved of the trouble of attending and came into an inheritance. It was no wonder then that even by "their closest friends, they are moved closer to death than to health".[413] Oetheus complained that nurses in their ignorance quite often "turn and pull the patient away from obeying and doing the proper and necessary things as ordered by the physician".[414] He vehemently condemned their ignorance and their inability to "give the sick person even the least bit of useful advice". "Wantonly and impudently" they proclaimed that the patient should eat and drink what he liked and not take not what the physician ordered and toss it out.[415] Some even denigrated the physician so that the patient took "to disliking the physician, losing all trust in him, and becoming unwilling to obey and duly follow."[416]

According to Oetheus it also often happened that patients were "so delicate and soft or rebellious" that they would not tolerate anything, leave alone allow any pain to be inflicted on them. In such cases, those who nursed them were not to "pay court to the sick at all times" but if necessary "find some hard words". For if, for the reason that the patient was unwilling to have something or other done and complained of suffering, one were to forgo useful and necessary remedies, this would be doing the patient a great disservice.[417] In the seventeenth century, this criticism culminated in the accusation that sick nurses sometimes even sought to accelerate the death of seriously ill patients out of impatience or greed by pulling the pillows out from under their heads and backs or abruptly putting them in a horizontal position by other means.[418] Under the heading "removing the pillows" ("Die Kussen wegnemen"), Handsch already mentioned such practices in the mid-sixteenth century, without reproach, however, describing them simply as a means to literally help people with dying.

---

to nursing; in 1599, Johannes Oswald curated a revised, expanded edition (Frankfurt: apud Romanum Beatum).
412 Ibid., fol. 119r.
413 Ibid.
414 Ibid., fol. 122r, "den Krancken vom gebürlichem unnd notwendigem Gehorsam der jenigen Dinge, welche von dem Artzet geordnet, abzihen und abwenden".
415 Ibid., fol. 122v, "fräventlich unnd unverschampt".
416 Ibid., fol. 123r, "ein Widerwillen gegen dem Artzet fasset, und das Vertrawen zuo ihm gäntzlich fallen lasset, auch zuo dem Gehorsam unnd gebürlicher Volge unwillig wirdt."
417 Ibid., fol. 126r-v, "jederzeit dem Krancken hofieren"; "mit Worten hart sein".
418 Questel, De pulvinari (1678); cf. Stolberg, Active euthanasia (2007).

Someone – he forgot who – had said during a meal: "When they struggle with death and cannot die, one should take their pillows away to make them lie suddenly; then they will die." Handsch added without any undertones of indignation that this had been done similarly with an old and dying tutor; he was laid down on a straw mat on the floor.[419]

Handsch, too, occasionally criticized caregivers. For example, he upbraided a wife for her "negligence" when she did not get someone to give her paralyzed husband the prescribed enema. He acknowledged, however, that giving an immobilized and greatly overweight man an enema was difficult.[420] He also thought it was a poor decision when the mother of a severely ill, delirious young man suffering from a fever cooled her son's face with rose vinegar. In his view, it was essential not to drive the morbid matter back into the body with cooling remedies but instead it should be allowed to evaporate. Accordingly, he was surprised when the patient was back up on his feet again only three or four days later.[421] The case of Virginia von Loxan, a cousin of Philippine Welser, even led to a dramatic argument between the attending physicians and the "bystanders". Virginia had the measles, which were going around in Innsbruck at the time. As was common to promote sweating, the physicians advised keeping the woman as warm as possible in a heated chamber. Yet, Virginia complained about the great heat and wanted to cool down. She even asked the Archduke himself for a sip of beer and got it, "in the name of God" ("propter Deum"). Handsch learned that she also put her feet down on the cold floor and leaned with her bare back against a wall. The measles rash was visible only briefly and quickly faded – too quickly, thought the physicians. The young woman found it increasingly difficult to breathe and became delirious. She died one week after the onset of the disease. Now the physicians were faced with the harsh reproaches of the women who were present who blamed them for doing nothing to counter the great heat of the fever, for even increasing it and for giving the sick woman nothing as refreshment and nothing to fortify her. The physicians, on their part, claimed that the women's disdain for their advice was at fault. Presumably they thought that the external cold had made the skin and pores contract and had thus prevented the morbid matter from exiting; it had been driven back to the inside of the body and to the vital organs. This was the reason why the rash had gone away too quickly. They went on to say that all the other young women who came down with the measles around that time had recovered because they did not

---

419 Cod. 11207, fol. 182r: "Wenn sie mit dem Tod ringen, und nicht sterben konnen, so sol man yn die Kussen weg nemen, das sie gleich liegen, so sterben sie."
420 Cod. 11205, fol. 268r.
421 Cod. 11183, fol. 417r.

have so many and such "compassionate" caregivers ("adstantes"). The bystanders replied that these women had not been kept in such a hot chamber.[422]

In most of his notes on the subject, Handsch did not pass negative judgment. Rather, he expressed a certain esteem for the *adstantes* and the work they did: "Good care and a cheerful disposition", were central to a favorable healing process.[423] He even discontinued the treatment of a sick nobleman "because he had no one to attend to him."[424] In the case of a court chamber's messenger, he decided against a more intensive treatment and instead prescribed an oil because the man did not have a nurse ("curatrix").[425]

It was furthermore Handsch's experience that the information he could obtain from caregivers was helpful for his diagnosis, prognosis, and treatment. Caregivers could describe, for example, a patient's black colored urine,[426] or foul, sanious stool[427] when he was unable to see for himself. They could tell him the observations they had made while he was away, for example, a patient's vomiting and shortness of breath,[428] the approximately forty stools another patient produced in two days,[429] or the terrifying epileptic seizure a sick woman had had the moment the nurse sat her up. It had lasted the length of two Sunday prayers and she had flailed her arms enough to make the bed shake.[430]

Handsch went even further. He also appreciated the practical knowledge, the experience of the caregivers, noting down in many entries how they proceeded at the bedside. These notes evidently served the same purpose as his many entries on the effect of certain medicines or treatment methods, that is to say they could be useful in his own practice in the future. He wanted to be able to introduce with future patients those nursing procedures he considered helpful. He described, for example, how the *adstantes* put a wooden spoon between the teeth of severely ill and dying patients, presumably to facilitate airflow.[431] He even made an entry on the preparation of meat dishes for old patients who

---

422 Ibid., foll. 356v-357v.
423 Cod. 11206, fol. 124v: "Gutte Wartung, und ein frölich Gemüt".
424 Cod. 11205, fol. 258v: "Dieweil er keyn Aufwartung hett"; the reason why the man was hospitalized is not known.
425 Cod. 11183, fol. 329r.
426 Ibid., fol. 223v.
427 Ibid., fol. 424v, "mulier administra dicit fuisse quasi saniosas".
428 Ibid., fol. 28r.
429 Cod. 11205, fol. 298v.
430 Cod. 11183, fol. 423v.
431 Cod. 11205, fol. 236v; apparently this was not done as a means to prevent an injury to the tongue as it could easily happen in epileptic fits.

did not want to chew anymore.⁴³² He described with particular attention to detail how the caregivers worked to protect Christoph von Gendorf from "raw skin from lying", that is from bedsores. The sick man had become emaciated and was unable to move in bed due to his pain. They put a linen cloth under his hips, which helped collect his feces, but above all allowed them to turn him by holding on to the fabric on either side of his body. They also put soft deer leather down on the bed for him.⁴³³ Handsch learned at another occasion that the white ointment used by a barber for injuries was useful in treating skin that had opened up from lying.⁴³⁴

Based on their observation, caregivers sometimes offered a specific diagnosis or a prognostic judgment, which the physician could adopt for similar cases he might encounter in the future. Handsch found it noteworthy that with the sick Schrenck, for example, the nurse ("mulier curatrix") suspected an "epileptic disposition", because he had shaken his head and rolled his eyes.⁴³⁵ It was "as if the fit was approaching her", stated a caregiver ("mulier adstans") in another case.⁴³⁶ From the vomiting and the "sandy" urine of one of Handsch's adolescent patients, "the women" ("mulieres") concluded that he had stone disease.⁴³⁷

The Incurably Ill and the "Cura Palliativa"

A great challenge that physicians encountered regularly in their practice was the treatment of incurably ill patients. Over and over again, physicians had to experience how their medicine sometimes reached its limits.⁴³⁸ An oft-quoted couplet, which Handsch wrote at the beginning of one of his notebooks was "Contra vim mortis non crescit herba in hortis" or "No herb grows in the gardens against the power of death".⁴³⁹ In many of his notes, he wrote down words he could use to explain to patients, relatives, and bereaved family members why even the best medical help could do nothing at a certain point. "When the hour has come, no

---

432 Cod. 11183, fol. 34v.
433 Ibid., fol. 33v, "er möcht die Haut rohe liegen".
434 Ibid., fol. 40v, "ad excoriationem a iactura".
435 Ibid., fol. 418v.
436 Cod. 11207, fol. 114v, "gleich wie sie das Fressl wolt anstossen".
437 Cod. 11183, fol. 277v.
438 Cod. 9821, fol. 91r: "Non omnes medici possunt depellere morbos. Plus, quam fatorum vis, medicina nequit."
439 Cod. 11210, fol. 1r; as the words the physician could use when his patient died: Cod. 11205, fol 212v.

medicine will help",[440] was one of the phrases, or "If God is unwilling, I have no means",[441] or, in Latin, under the heading "When your patient is dying", "The physician is nature's servant, not Her master".[442]

Handsch learned early that certain diseases were usually incurable and that with them a radical cure that addressed the cause of the disease was essentially ineffective or even dangerous. Included here were most notably protracted stone and kidney complaints, consumption, cancer, dropsy, and long-standing gout, and with the elderly hectic fever, quartan fever,[443] asthma, and paralysis.[444]

In such cases, the physician was not condemned to doing nothing. Galen had already elaborated on a merely palliative treatment – aimed at pain and other subjective complaints and not at their causes – as an independent form of therapy.[445] Denoted as "mitigating" ("cura mitigativa"), "flattering" ("blanditiva")[446] and most widely as a "cura palliativa" – literally, a "cloaking treatment", understood here in a positive sense – this approach was firmly established in the medical literature of the Renaissance.[447] In fact, the notion of "palliative" treatment is much older than generally assumed. As early as the fourteenth century, the French physician Guy de Chauliac had recommended a "broadly conceived, preventive, and palliative treatment" for incurable diseases, or for when a causal therapy was too dangerous or was refused by the patient.[448] In 1543, the English edition of the well-known surgical work by Giovanni da Vigo explicitly juxtaposed the "palliatyue" with the "eradicatyue cure".[449] Handsch, too, in his notes used terms such as "cura palliativa", "cura pal[l]eativa" and "palliare" several times.[450] Sometimes a "merely palliative" treatment was mentioned in a negative, derogatory sense, when the treatment did nothing but literally cover up the symptoms. "If one only pretended to heal", is what Handsch called this.[451] But

---

440 Cod. 11206, fol. 116r: "Wenn das Stündle do ist, hilfft kein Artzney."
441 Ibid., fol. 126r: "So Gott nicht wil, kan ich nicht."
442 Ibid., fol. 115v.
443 "Hydrops et quartana medicis sunt scandala plana", Handsch noted (Cod. 11206, fol. 105r).
444 Cod. 11240, fol. 42r.
445 Galen, Opera (1822), vol. 18, pp. 59–61.
446 Cardano, De malo (1536), pp. 8–9.
447 For a detailed study see Stolberg, Cura palliativa (2007); Stolberg, Geschichte (2011), pp. 21–42.
448 Chauliac, Chirurgia (1559), foll. a2(v)-a3(v), "cura larga, praeservativa, et palliativa"; cf. Chauliac, Inventarium (1997).
449 Vigo, Workes (1543), fol. 43v, "we wyll speake of his cure aswel eradicatyue as palliatyue".
450 Cod. 9666, fol. 43v; Cod. 11205, fol. 223r; Cod. 11206, fol. 135v; Cod. 11207, fol. 32r.
451 Cod. 9666, fol. 43v: "Wenn man ym Scheyn heylet".

if a causal treatment that attacked the root of the disease was not possible, a "palliative" treatment became the means of choice, a duty even.

According to Vigo, there were some cases in which powerful remedies that targeted the disease cause would potentially kill the patient, while mitigating, flattering remedies – these were usually called "paregorica"[452] or "mitigantia"[453] – could prolong his or her life and take the pain away.[454] Especially for patients with a cancerous ulcer, forgoing a causal treatment – here usually a dangerous and rarely successful surgery – was recommended.[455] But also with consumption, with indurated tumors, with hidden cancer that had not yet penetrated the skin, and similar illnesses, the well-known Italian physician Girolamo Cardano cautioned that a causal treatment would do more harm than good and came with the great risk of ending patients' lives before their time. Vehemently, he denounced the "not so few" physicians who attempted a curative treatment here in spite of the danger. Some, he said, acted in this way because they did not want to believe that these diseases were incurable or at least hoped to bring about an improvement. But others, which was worse, were guided by their thirst for glory or by greed. He concluded that in such cases a mitigating treatment was indicated instead, one that did not weaken the patient, did not advance the disease and instead calmed the pain.[456]

The concept of the "palliative" treatment allowed physicians to continue attending to patients in good conscience and, though this might not be their primary goal, they could still count on being rewarded, even when the prospect of a successful outcome was remote. Yet, in practice physicians were often faced with a dilemma. With a palliative treatment that focused on the symptoms, they were able to reduce patients' suffering and ideally even prolong their lives. Yet, in a world in which the success and the reputation of a physician hinged on the outstanding cures attributed to him, treating incurable patients was fraught with risk. Even if the physician, speaking frankly at least to the relatives, conveyed the impossibility of curing the patient or even predicted imminent death, he always had to be prepared for the possibility that people would lay part of the blame on him and would believe that another healer might have been able

---

452 Cf. Houllier, De morborum (1572), fol. 136r.
453 Cf. Castelli, Lexicon (1598), p. 307.
454 Vigo, Workes (1543), fol. 43v.
455 Arcaeus, De recta (1574), pp. 99–101 and p. 102; Staatsbibliothek Bamberg, Ms. JH msc. med. 9, Nr. 8, undated account of a consultation by Venetian physicians and surgeons on a 83-year-old patient with a (presumably cancerous) tumor on his nose.
456 Cardano, De malo (1536), pp. 8f; in his notes, Handsch quoted from this work (Cod. 11205, fol. 405r).

to avert the unfavorable outcome. This danger was especially great for younger physicians who still had to establish a good reputation for themselves. They could almost count on having patients come to them who were more likely to do badly or indeed die in their care, after they had already tried their luck with other physicians in vain.

The radical solution to this dilemma was to refuse these patients as a matter of principle. "Do not accept incurable patients if you want to protect your reputation", Handsch wrote after reading the famous Giovanni Manardi.[457] Giovanni Battista da Monte likewise cautioned his students not to accept desperate cases in the early days of their medical practice.[458] Both were leading proponents of medical humanism, which held the classical authorities in great esteem, and in fact they were able to refer to them in this point. The position that physicians should not treat incurable patients had already been stated in the writings of Hippocrates and the Roman encyclopedist Celsus, who enjoyed great currency in the sixteenth century.[459]

However, when Hippocrates and Celsus voiced these concerns, it appears they mainly had the wellbeing of the patients and their relatives in mind who would be spared senseless interventions and expenditures. And early modern physicians could also find passages in the Hippocratic writings in which the treatment of incurable patients was not rejected but was rather explicitly deemed the task of the physician.[460] Not only this: the classical physicians were heathens. For a Christian physician, it would have been all the more unseemly to abandon the incurably ill to their fate. Leading physicians at the time, including Guido Guidi (1509–1569), Baptista Codronchi (1547–1628), and Orazio Augenio, declared it a high duty to assist patients even if their disease was incurable and death was on the doorstep.[461] As Laurent Joubert in Montpellier admonished his students, physicians lacked humanity if they believed that desperate cases should be left alone: love and piety, not striving for fame and money should guide their actions. Certainly, they were to forego powerful remedies like purgatives and bloodletting so as not to create the impression that they had hastened the death of the patient, which would discredit the medical remedies that helped so many. But Joubert

---

457 Cod. 11200, fol. 126r: "Ne suscipias morbos incurabiles, si famae tuae consultus esse cupis."
458 Da Monte, Consultationum (1565), col. 458.
459 Hippocrates, Peri technes, in: idem, Œuvres (1839–1861), vol. 6, pp. 2–26, here pp. 12–14 ; Celsus, De medicina (1657), pp. 282–283 (book 5, ch. 26.1).
460 Guidi, De curatione (1626), p. 121; cf. Wittern, Unterlassen (1979); von Staden, Incurability (1990); Prioreschi, Hippocratic physician (1992).
461 Guidi, De curatione (1626), p. 121; Codronchi, De christiana ratione (1591), p. 24; Augenio, Epistolarum (1602), fol. 87v; on Codronchi see also Bergdolt, Gewissen (2004), pp. 173f.

held that nothing could be said against mild remedies that alleviated the disease and supported nature, all the more so as often one could never be completely certain about an infaust prognosis.[462] Several decades later, Paolo Zacchia, personal physician to two popes, summarized this position when he wrote that humanity and Christian piety did not permit the physician to disregard people who asked for medical help by categorizing them as desperate cases. Rather, the physician had to take care of them and give them hope. If he could not cure the disease, he must at least fight its progression and alleviate the complaints that commonly made such diseases unbearable, through the use of medicines or at least by prescribing a suitable diet.[463]

We have little knowledge of how physicians in daily practice dealt with the dilemma sketched out above, how they dealt with incurably ill people. But the problem must have come up frequently. Illnesses like consumption and dropsy were widespread. Not surprisingly, Handsch brought up the subject repeatedly in his notebooks, and his notes about specific cases show which course of action he and his colleagues adopted with incurably ill patients. The resulting picture is complex and in some respects contradictory.

Whenever Handsch wrote explicitly about the treatment of incurable patients, his position was unambiguous: his concern about damaging his reputation and medical authority prevailed. As a student, Handsch had already noted down the cautionary words, "Do not take on incurable illnesses",[464] and he would remind himself of them often in subsequent years,[465] in part made wiser by painful experience.[466] His teacher Lehner, Handsch found, followed the same principle and never accepted someone as a patient when he knew that the person suffered from an incurable disease.[467] Lehner had treated the above-mentioned old man called Hosska, who suffered from *asthma;* but then he discontinued treatment, true to his guiding principle.[468] In the case of a man called Wisktanski, who suffered an acute stroke and was gasping for air, Lehner deliberately did not follow what would have been considered proper medical protocol ("secundum artem") for patients suffering from acute shortness of breath; he did not bleed

---

462 Joubert, Oratio (1580), p. 15.
463 Zacchia, Quaestiones (1651), p. 393.
464 Cod. 11240, fol. 42r: "Incurabiles morbos non suscipere."
465 Cod. 9666, fol. 27r: "Deplorata non sunt curandi"; Cod. 11205, fol. 268r: "Morbos incurabiles noli suscipere, ne merearis nomen mali medici"; similarly ibid., fol. 528v and fol. 690v.
466 Cod. 11205, fol. 690v.
467 Ibid.; see also ibid, fol. 236v and fol. 255v.
468 Ibid., fol. 255v.

him, because the relatives would have blamed him for the predictably unfavorable course. Struggling for air, the sick man suffocated within a day.[469]

As we begin to see here, a physician who needed to decide whether a disease was in fact incurable usually had to see the patient or follow the patient for a certain amount of time. It was therefore unavoidable that he would accept some patients whose disease ultimately proved to be incurable. But his guiding principle told him that when it became obvious that the disease was incurable, it was time to part company with the patient. It appears this happened regularly. Again and again we read of patients who were said to have been "abandoned" or "given up on" by their physicians or other healers. Sometimes such accounts refer to cases in which the author himself did not give up. By underlining the unfavorable prognosis given by his colleagues, he was all the more able to demonstrate his own therapeutic ability.[470] But there are also other examples, including in Handsch's private case notes, that show how physicians did in fact leave incurably sick patients to their fate at some point.

This was primarily the case for people suffering from the symptoms of consumption or, closely related, of an empyema, a collection of pus in the lungs. Considered by many to be consumptive, a young man from the accounting office at the Angel's Garden in Prague, for example, was abandoned by the physicians after months of unsuccessful treatment. However, when Handsch saw the pale and emaciated patient, he suspected nothing more than an obstruction of his entrails, especially the spleen. He gave him some medicinal herbs and the young man recovered.[471] When the consumptive wife of Korzaur, a mother of four, was being treated, all other physicians gave up hope when she began coughing up blood. Handsch continued to see her for several more weeks, but then he too "abandoned" her and she died soon after.[472] He likewise "abandoned" – as he put it himself – a chef who had been suffering from an empyema or consumption for three months. Handsch's experienced colleague D. Kunstat also did not expect that the man would recover.[473] Gallo, by Handsch's account, did not leave a severely emaciated dropsical man by the name of Gregor to his

---

469 Ibid., fol. 236v.
470 See also Cod. 11238, fol. 97v, on a poor patient in the hospital in Padua whom Trincavella treated by dietetic means only, after he had been "relinquished" by other physicians ("ab aliis medicis relictus") and Cod. 11251, fol. 37v, on the report of a physician by the name of Florianus who successfully cured a boy with *dysenteria* in the hospital in Bologna, whom all physicians had "relinquished".
471 Cod. 11183, fol. 136r.
472 Cod. 11183, fol. 81r, "postea reliqui ipsam".
473 Ibid., fol. 80v; after several months, the patient was still suffering but when Handsch encountered him again, three years later, he appeared to be cured.

fate, but he visited him infrequently and neglected to administer his medication properly. He, too, ultimately died.[474] In the case of an old peasant woman who developed a large, festering tumor, it was the barbers who refused to give her what would have been primarily a surgical treatment.[475]

At the same time, Handsch repeatedly documented the continued medical treatment of patients for whom there remained no realistic hope for a cure, revealing contradictions in the approach to incurable patients. The dropsical Moritz, for example, had a bloated belly, a sunken-in face, discolored yellow eyes, and a cough. Gallo stated that the cough was a bad sign as it indicated water in the lungs. Gallo, who had been seeing Moritz for four weeks with Handsch, gave him juice of iris despite the grim situation and on the following day merely expressed his regret that the remedy had only shown a mild evacuative effect. The patient died in the night.[476] Neither did Handsch relinquish his treatment of a dropsical man called Krafft until the patient died, even though he was coughing up blood and evacuating great amounts of blood with his stool and in the end needed to be sitting upright to breathe properly.[477] Handsch also helped the severely ill Balthasar Hirschberger until the man was prepared to reconcile with his brother and could receive his last rites.[478] And Willenbroch continued to treat the little son of Kaspar von Müllenstein with arum root when the patient was no more than skin and bones, his belly swollen, his face sunken in, and his breath stinking. The boy's death struggle went on for a day, and then he died in convulsions.[479]

One reason to continue treatment with patients who were by all appearances incurable, and even with the obviously moribund, was the possibility of misjudgment. "Nota bene: many emaciated [patients] healed", we can read in Handsch's notes.[480] He was telling himself that if he saw the signs of emaciation or dropsy, he was not to give up hope too soon. He then listed examples of patients who recovered against all expectations, like a dropsical postmaster whom Gallo had cured.[481]

---

474 Cod. 11207, fol. 214r.
475 Cod. 11183, fol. 22r.
476 Cod. 11207, fol. 70r-v.
477 Cod. 11183, foll. 394v-395r; Handsch stopped visiting him for eight days but the reason was apparently not that he had given up hope.
478 Cod. 11183, foll. 108v-110v.
479 Ibid., fol. 479v.
480 Cod. 11205, fol. 265v: "Merke: viele Abgezehrte geheilt".
481 Ibid., fol. 266r.

In other cases, the main reason why physicians continued their visits was a different one, and they sometimes stated it explicitly: they pursued a palliative treatment to relieve the patient's suffering. "With diseases that are difficult to treat, do a palliative treatment," we read in Handsch, who pointed to how Galen approached consumption.[482] When the "whore" ("meretrix") who lived next door vomited feces – this was called *miserere* and still today is known as the dramatic sign of an often fatal bowel obstruction – Ulrich Lehner stated that she would die but nevertheless gave her an enema.[483] Handsch himself praised a salve "for the palliation of leprosy".[484] And to the terminally ill young Friedrich von Kunritz suffering from heavy dysentery he gave common hound's-tongue (*cynoglossum*) for the pain, the insomnia, and the diarrhea.[485] For a sixteen-year-old severely dropsical boy in *Bruderhaus* in Innsbruck, Handsch prescribed antimony and a diuretic remedy. The boy's legs became less swollen and he felt "lighter in the chest". But then he no longer wanted to take the somewhat oily diuretic. His condition worsened and he died several weeks later.[486]

The most important palliative was opium, used as an analgesic and, depending on the case, as an antidiarrheal. Even if it amounted to no more than a "cura palleativa", wrote Handsch, the physician could sometimes give an opium preparation "for his own honor".[487] Using such a preparation, called *philonium*, Mattioli was able for a while to mitigate the pain of Hieronymus, who was suffering from severe colics. The pain returned, and the sick man wrote his last will and prepared himself for death but after a second dose of *philonium* the pain receded and he recovered.[488] Handsch gave a dropsical patient who already had water running out of his legs a remedy with opium for the pain; he died soon after.[489] Gallo had told Handsch that he had done a "curam palliativam" in dysentery cases ("dysenteria") and had received "much praise" ("multam laudem").[490]

From the study of Handsch's notes, the question of whether physicians at the time took on incurably ill or terminal patients or continued treatment when patients turned out to be incurably or indeed terminally ill can thus not be answered with a clear yes or no. Rather, what emerges is that even one and the same

---

482 Cod. 11240, fol. 36r.
483 Ibid., fol. 37r.
484 Cod. 11200, fol. 4v, "ad palleationem leprae unguentum".
485 Cod. 11183, fol. 106r.
486 Ibid., fol. 443r.
487 Cod. 11205, fol. 223r.
488 Cod. 11183, fol. 322r.
489 Ibid., fol. 46r.
490 Cod. 11207, fol. 32r.

physician attended to some of these patients, hoping to heal them or mitigate their agony, while with others he discontinued treatment and "abandoned" them.

At the Deathbed

As we see from some of the aforementioned cases of chronic, incurable illness, death had a strong presence in quotidian medical practice, a very strong presence even, not only in times of plague. In this respect, the collections of published medical *curationes* and *observationes* paint a picture that is substantially removed from reality. They report fatal outcomes only very exceptionally. This was a deliberate choice. Understandably, their authors or publishers selected cases for publication which allowed the reader to learn about the successful treatment of even serious diseases and which at the same time shone a light on the exceptional ability of the attending physician. Handsch's personal notes, by contrast, paint a different, much more differentiated picture. When treating patients with serious, acute illnesses, physicians frequently had to expect fatal outcomes.

To be sure, Handsch had decided that, as a matter of principle, he would not treat patients who were close to dying, so people would not attribute the cause of death to him.[491] They might otherwise say, "No sooner did he give him the medicine, he died".[492] Gallo had advised him early on that when the physician, realized that the illness was stronger than the body, than nature, he should hand the case over to the clergyman.[493]

However, this assumed that the physician could be certain that the patient would succumb to his disease, and in many cases, it was hardly possible to attain this certainty. Physicians could consult the vast medical literature written since antiquity, which named the characteristic signs of approaching death. In 1601, Prosper Alpinus (1553–1616) dedicated an entire volume to them.[494] There was the above-mentioned *miserere*,[495] and the famous *facies hippocratica*,[496] the sunken-inface of the dying. Pointed and cold was the nose of the dying Frau Lehner, Handsch learned from her son who was a physician himself. Her upper lip was pale, her lower lip reddened.[497] Medical laypeople, too, were familiar with some

---

[491] Cod. 11240, fol. 42r: "Item extreme affectu propinquum morti non medicatur, ne deinde mortis causam tibi ascribunt."
[492] Cod. 11205, fol. 202r: "So bald er ym die Ertznei geben, ist er gestorben."
[493] Ibid., fol. 271r.
[494] Alpinus, De praesagienda vita (1601).
[495] Cod. 11210, fol. 93r ; Cod. 11240, fol. 37r.
[496] Cod. 11205, fol. 301v.
[497] Cod. 11183, fol. 47v.

characteristic signs. Handsch found them noteworthy, writing for example, that bystanders at the sickbed interpreted the rattling breath of a severely ill person as a deadly sign,[498] as they did with sustained hiccoughing: "[when] a person is sick and gets a hiccough that lasts twenty-four hours or longer, it is a true sign of death".[499] When a young nobleman was dying, the wife of Handsch's mentor Collinus even believed that she was able to feel how his breath was cooler than usual when she put her hand in front of his mouth.[500] In several instances, Handsch wrote down the popular belief that someone who started to pluck non-existent crumbs from the bedspread was close to dying.[501] From Archduke Ferdinand II he heard, however, that "picking at the bedding" was not a sure sign.[502]

As aware as a physician might be of such signs in theory, it remained difficult or even impossible to predict death with certainty at the sickbed, let alone determine the likely time of death. Mattioli was still treating an archducal preacher with antimony two days before the man's death, and only when he saw him with Handsch on the evening before his death did both physicians predict the fatal outcome. The patient made his confession and died that same night.[503] Sometimes, the physician was called only when the patient was already in the throes of death. Handsch described repeatedly how he arrived at a patient's home and the patient was agonizing or already breathing his last breath. The old Baron von Meseritz had been lying in bed with his eyes closed for days when Handsch and a colleague – likely the Prague physician Thaddeus Hagecius of Hajek[504] – were called to see him. He was wheezing and his feet were twitching, and he died that same night.[505] Handsch also found Kekeritz, who was suffering from fever and *pleuresia,* with his eyes already half closed, "as if the light had gone out of them". Struggling for air, he lay in agony. Handsch stayed with the sick man who was not ready to accept that he had to die. Finally, he "took a deep breath" and they brought him the light – evidently the sacramental candle. He was dead a short while later.[506]

Accounts like these also illuminate how, in the care for the dying, spiritual and physical support were connected and the lines between the two were blurred.

---

498 Ibid., fol. 454r; the patient ultimately survived.
499 Cod. 11240, fol. 108v, "[wenn] eyner die Kranckheit hett, unnd kem yn ein Kluxen an unnd werete 24 Stunden aber [oder, M.S.] mehr, das ist ein gewarlich Zeichen des Todes."
500 Cod. 11205, fol. 270r.
501 In the case of sick Kretzel, for example, a certain Hensel said, "when he starts picking at his bed, it is over" (Cod. 11205, foll. 127v-128r, "wenn er wirt am Bette klauben, so ist es aus").
502 Cod. 11183, fol. 350v, "am Bette klauben".
503 Ibid., fol. 196r-v.
504 Handsch recorded only the first name, Thaddeus.
505 Cod. 11183, fol. 259v.
506 Ibid., fol. 27r and fol. 28r, "wie sie ym gebrochen weren"; "eynen grosen Athemzug".

In historical research it has often been assumed that the physician yielded the floor to the clergyman when things came to an end – as we saw with Gallo's advice. Handsch's notes and other contemporary sources tell a different story. They show that it was not uncommon for physicians to continue their treatment until the very end,[507] and that sometimes they even stayed at the deathbed when the clergyman came to administer the last rites. The reasons are plain to see. If one wanted to prevent a severely ill patient from dying without receiving his last rites and spiritual support, it was essential to call the clergyman, even if one was not sure that the patient would actually die soon. At the same time, given this prognostic uncertainty, especially with acute illness, it was certainly possible that the medical treatment would show a positive effect after all. Simply breaking it off would have been irresponsible. In striking contradiction to his plan to treat incurable patients, Handsch even declared that one should "not abandon a person as long as he is still breathing because spiro, spero, and thus we want to do our best and send to the apothecary".[508] He may have found such words useful, of course, to convince the bystanders of the necessity of continuing treatment, which in their eyes had become meaningless and therefore an unnecessary expense. Even in the case of the dying Hosska, whose death he did not predict, a case in which Handsch was cursed for his luckless efforts, he argued that he was not allowed to leave him, because as long as "he breathes, one is not to abandon a person".[509] To make sure that the patient "was not robbed of human help", Handsch, Andrea Gallo, and Adam Lehner treated an apoplectic man according to the rules of the medical art ("quae praescribit ars"), though they had little hope. The man died as expected.[510]

Handsch witnessed several times how a sick person ate what was believed to be his last supper, received his last rites, and then lived on. After a girl, in Ambras, who was expectorating blood had received her last rites, they had already opened the windows to make it easier for her soul to leave the house. Handsch, too, had given up hope. And yet, the girl recovered.[511]

With dangerously ill princes and other important figures, whose death would have far-reaching consequences for numerous people, even for an entire territorial dominion or a religious movement, it seems that physicians routinely left nothing

---

507 E.g. ibid., fol. 47v, on Mattioli's treatment of the dying wife of Ulrich Lehner.
508 Cod. 11205, fol. 420v, "einen Menschen nicht verlassen, weil [dieweil, solange, M.S.] er Athem hat, denn spiro, spero, darumb wollen wir thun das best, als wir können, wollen ynn die Apothekenn sennden"; similarly ibid., fol. 213r.
509 Ibid., fol. 255v, "er Athem hat sol man keynen verlassen".
510 Cod. 11183, foll. 245v-246r; Handsch recorded only his colleagues' first names, Adam and Andreas.
511 Ibid., fol. 448v.

untried to keep them alive as long as possible, even when they were clearly dying. The death of Philipp Melanchthon offers a vivid example. According to the account written by his personal physician, the sixty-three-year-old was close to dying. His pulse was becoming weaker, his extremities cold. He lost consciousness several times and the physicians tried, successfully at first, to bring him back using quickening, stimulating agents. When he regained consciousness, he said, as was later reported: "Ah, what are you doing? Why do you hinder my gentle peace? Just leave me my peace until the end, it won't be long now." He died soon after.[512]

Sometimes physicians and clergymen worked amicably together in attending to the spiritual and physical needs of the dying. A good example here is the deacon Johann Altenburger's detailed description of the death of Countess Anna von Sachsen, who was only forty-five years old. When the deacon was called to Coburg eight days before Anna's death to see the severely weakened woman who was plagued by coughing and vomiting, he came with the physician Michael Schön. Schön prescribed various medicines but then had to leave to attend a wedding. Anna took the medicines when they arrived from the apothecary's shop. But an hour later her face changed color and she became very fearful; she lost her speech and believed she was suffocating. When she recovered, she asked the deacon whether she should take the remaining medicine. He advised her to wait until the following day. This was when Schön came back and prescribed her different remedies, "which she praised highly, because they did her good". She had told the deacon several times that she would not "refuse proper remedies, so people could not say she was headstrong". And she stuck to this position. "If it helps, I will have God to thank, if not, I can hope for better things to come." When she was given a syrup to soothe her, she was unwilling to drink it. Now her condition deteriorated. She developed a strong sense of pressure in her chest, had several convulsive fits, and said things like, "I wish I were dead" or "Dear God, come and take me now". When the physician and the deacon spoke to each other in Latin in her presence, she asked them to speak openly: "I won't live long now". She died the following night. As is clear from this, the physician in no way gave up his place for the clergyman. He remained at the bedside until the sick woman finally rejected his medicines.[513]

---

[512] Müller, Philipp Melanchthons letzte Lebenstage (1910), with an edition of this account, ibid., pp. 47–87: "Ah, was macht ir, warumb hindert ir mich in meiner sanfften Ruhe? Lasst mir doch mein Ruhe bis an mein End, es wird nicht mehr lang weren."
[513] Thüringische Universitäts- und Landesbibliothek, Jena, Ms. Prov. fol. 26 (16), foll. 375v–392v.

Alternatives to Medical Treatment by Physicians

In today's Western industrial countries, academically educated physicians for the most part have a monopoly on healthcare. This is a relatively recent historical development. Despite their growing numbers, learned physicians until well into the nineteenth century represented only a small minority of healthcare providers. Throughout the entire early modern period, they existed alongside a great variety of other healers. Competing with them in the health market were barbers and barber-surgeons who were trained as craftsmen as well as lay healers of all stripes.[514] Not only this, but everyone in contemporary society had a certain basic medical knowledge at their disposal and could treat themselves with home remedies. In other words, when people fell ill, they had the choice between a range of alternative options – and quite frequently they would resort to more than one, in the course of time.

Self-Treatment and Domestic Medicine

In the sixteenth century, having a sound knowledge of the genesis and treatment of diseases was not the prerogative of professional healers. As is also shown by countless entries in Handsch's notebooks, basic medical knowledge was widespread in the population. For an educated minority, it was possible to turn to medical manuals and health guides written in the vernacular.[515] Some of the authors and editors of such works were severely rebuked for passing medical knowledge on to the uninitiated.[516] But the most crucial medium for the dissemination of medical knowledge among the lay population was – and this went for all social classes – the spoken word.[517] People discussed medical matters. They shared their positive experiences with certain medicines and treatment procedures. And they applied this knowledge when they themselves or their relatives or neighbors got sick.

---

[514] An important seminal study on the early modern healthcare market is Park, Doctors (1985); for a more recent overview, see Wallis, Medicine (2007) and for a case study on Cologne, see Jütte, Medical pluralism (2013), pp. 32–37.
[515] E.g. Gasser, Bericht (1544); Glaubitz, Zwo Haußtaffeln (1584); Starck, Krancken Spiegel (1598); Wittich, Praeservator sanitatis (1590).
[516] Telle, Arzneikunst (1982), pp. 43–48.
[517] Lindemann, Medicine and society (2010), pp. 121–122 has likewise concluded that "the most frequent sites of medical education (broadly understood) were families, households, and neighborhoods".

Open Access. © 2022 Michael Stolberg, published by De Gruyter. This work is licensed under the Creative Commons Attribution-NonCommercial-NoDerivatives 4.0 International License.
https://doi.org/10.1515/9783110733549-020

Time and again, Handsch noted down what laypeople had told him about their successful self-treatment. A goldsmith, for example, told him that a decoction of horse hair had alleviated the ulcer in his urethra after he had tried in vain to treat it with sulfuric acid.[518] Caspar Belwitz recovered from a paralyzed limb the same night that some women had given him lavender water to drink and had rubbed the affected limb with myrrh and mustard.[519] By his own account, a lapidary healed his mother's gangrene with alum, frankincense, and myrrh – and this while the surgeons were beginning to speak of amputation.[520]

Various domestic remedies were known in Handsch's own family and put to use when necessary. Handsch's stepmother explained to him that iris helped with infant stomachaches.[521] It was also his stepmother to whom he owed a remedy that could be given to children when they, like one of his nieces, rolled their eyes during seizures; it appears there was a concern that the child might become permanently cross-eyed. One had to chew caraway seeds and then breathe into the face of the child, who then would be able to see straight again.[522] One of the remedies Handsch's sister Apollonia praised was using linen dipped in salt water to cure headaches.[523] She also advised applying hare brain to the sore gums of teething children.[524] Handsch noted that his father ate roasted figs when he was developing a cough, and it helped.[525] During a fever epidemic, he drank sorrel water to fend off febrile attacks and tied creeping cinquefoil to the soles of his feet. Handsch's father explained that Georg's stepmother had done this as well when she had been ill with tertian fever, and he advised the local town clerk to do the same.[526]

Even those in the highest circles of society – people who could easily afford the help of a physician – were keen to acquire medical knowledge and sometimes engaged in healing practices of their own. As Alicia Rankin has demonstrated for Anna von Sachsen, Dorothea von Mansfeld, Elisabeth von Rochlitz, some noblewomen were particularly interested in delving into medical questions and producing medicines.[527] In Ambras Castle, Ferdinand's mother-in-law

---

518 Cod. 11183, fol. 188r.
519 Ibid., fol. 206r.
520 Ibid., fol. 2v.
521 Cod. 11205, fol. 122r.
522 Cod. 11183, fol. 207v.
523 Ibid., fol. 10v; Cod. 11251, fol. 39r.
524 Cod. 11183, fol. 240v.
525 Ibid.
526 Cod. 11207, fol. 210v; Cod. 11205, fol. 144r; usually Handsch simply referred to his "mother" ("mater") but his biological mother died in 1539 already.
527 Rankin, Panaceia's daughters (2013).

Anna Welser engaged in medical activities on a considerable scale. According to Handsch, she quite literally "prescribed" her domestic remedies to those who fell ill at the court and in the surrounding area.[528] One of her favorite medicines was a so-called "Stechwasser" made from unknown ingredients. She gave this, along with *rob sambucinum,* made from elderberries, to a sick lady at the court, as well as to a sick woman in nearby Weierburg.[529] In other cases she lent support by offering her medical advice and, at times, asserted herself over others. When a certain Eustachius was suffering from convulsions in his arms and legs, those caring for him wanted to hold him down and stop his movements. Anna Welser, however, would not allow it, saying that this could lead to paralysis.[530]

Anna Welser's daughter Philippine, the wife of the Archduke, also engaged in the healing arts. She often told Handsch about various remedies used routinely by the women in her hometown of Augsburg.[531] Still today, she is known for her book of medicines filled with recipes she collected from various sources.[532] She is said to have set up her own apothecary's shop at Ambras and to have produced various medicines with the apothecary.[533] For her ailing husband she had remedies made from valuable gemstones, pearls, corals, and unicorn horn.[534] She treated the wife of a chancellor with her "quintessence" and had a blistering plaster applied.[535] Like her mother, she did not limit herself to treating relatives at the court. Handsch noted down, for example, the various remedies she used to treat the cancerous ulcer of a barber. Initially, a horrid odor was released, but then the ulcer healed. Unfortunately, the man then developed dropsy and died.[536] Philippine also sent oil of absinth to a poor and sick man who was suffering from dropsy, leg ulcers, and worms.[537]

---

528 E.g. Cod. 11183, fol. 371r: "Vetula Welserin ordinavit ei Stechwasser".
529 Ibid., fol. 383v; Anna Welser asked for the same remedy in her own disease (ibid., fol. 362r).
530 Ibid., fol. 326r.
531 Ibid., fol. 398r.
532 Hirn, Ferdinand II. (1885), p. 484; Hirn, Ferdinand II. (1887), p. 327; Beer, Philippine Welser (1950); Größing, Kaufmannstochter (1992); Größing, Heilkunst (1998).
533 Hirn, Ferdinand II. (1887), p. 327.
534 Cod. 11183, fol. 444r.
535 Ibid., fol. 481v.
536 Ibid., fol. 461v; Handsch did not question the efficacy of the medicines. His only reservation was that the man should have been purged before. Presumably, he felt it was necessary to first free the body of the morbid matter in this way which could no longer be evacuated through the ulcer. In his eyes, this was the reason why the patient ultimately became dropsical and died.
537 Ibid., fol. 366v.

According to a cherished narrative, it was women first and foremost – the mothers of the household – who were formerly responsible for caring for the health of their families, using home remedies to treat their illnesses. This notion accords well with an image of female nature that continues to hold sway today: this is the perception of women as more attentive, caring, and empathetic than men, willing and able to devote themselves to the physical needs of their fellow human beings. Handsch's numerous entries on the medical knowledge of men – which they put to use not least of all in their treatment of relatives – call on us to exercise a certain degree of caution. There are not enough sources for the population at large that would allow for more precise conclusions to be drawn about the extent to which men and women respectively engaged in the healing arts within their families and neighborhoods. It is very obvious, however, that involvement in matters of health, including the treatment of relatives, was by no means essentially limited to women. Men, too, could play a very active role. This is shown, for one thing, by the collections of tried and tested household recipes used in self-treatment, which were compiled not only by women but also – and perhaps even primarily – by men.[538] Handsch's entries contain, for example, multiple references to the recipes and experiences a certain lapidary recorded in his recipe book.[539]

In cases where relatives asked for medical advice from a physician by letter, the active participation of men is especially evident. One father, for example, was worried about his son, who at the age of a year and a half was suffering from diarrhea in the middle of summer; Handsch copied excerpts from his letters. It had been going on for five days, wrote the father. This morning alone, the son had produced four very slimy, loose stools that had some blood mixed in as well. He went on to say that the boy had become very weak, his body hot. He was being breastfed by a wet nurse. Otherwise, he was not eating.[540] Two days later, he reported that the child was still hot and feverish, but was otherwise feeling better. His stool was becoming firmer and its color was beginning to look more natural. He therefore considered it time to do something about the diarrhea itself – evidently, he had so far considered it an expression of nature's efforts to rid the body of morbid matter. He enclosed the recipe for a plaster which he had received from his brother's wife. However, he wrote that until he heard from Handsch, he planned to use only

---

538 In her analysis of early modern English recipe-books, Elaine Leong has come to a similar conclusion. According to Leong, these compilations cannot be attributed primarily to the women in the household but were the product of a shared activity in which men and women participated; cf. Leong, Collecting Knowledge (2013); Leong, Recipes (2018).
539 Cod. 11183, fol. 45v and fol. 154v, "in libro gemmicidae scriptum erat"; ibid., fol. 155 "oleum Antimonii ex libro gemmicidae".
540 Ibid., fol. 271v-272r.

domestic remedies ("vulgaria remedia"). He had given the toddler a broth made with wheat beer and egg white, and the wet nurse, too, was given constipating food. And, following the advice of a certain Herr Schonfeld, who had used this remedy on his own son, he injected a warm infusion of mullein (*verbascum*) into the boy's anus. He added, however, that just as he was about to seal the letter, he saw that the feces were indeed still green, as Handsch could see from the enclosed linen cloths with greenish stool residue on them. This meant that it was unadvisable to limit defecation just yet. But he was asking for a recipe to counter the intense heat and the powerful urge to defecate.[541] Two days after this letter was written, Handsch went to the village, saw the little boy, and prescribed him, among other things, embrocations to be applied to the abdomen.[542] On the tenth day of illness, the child was feeling significantly better according to the father's account. He was playing again and no longer had such intense, foul diarrhea. But the father did ask for an invigorating remedy and compresses to strengthen the heart. He had seen how, in Germany, physicians often gave a so-called "Kraftwasser" – a drink that gave strength – in such cases. He furthermore asked for a remedy that would make the stool firmer and would take away the stomach pain and the heat. Of course, one had to take care not to treat the diarrhea too aggressively as the little boy was very susceptible to worms and one did not want to block their passage out of the body.[543] In response to these wishes, Handsch sent him Neefe's "strengthening water" and a cardiac fomentation (*epitema cordiale*). Three days later, the father reported that the boy's condition had, overall, improved even more. Yet when he wanted to sleep, he was constantly awoken by pain, and kept reaching for his anus while screaming. The father had had a look at the boy's anus and had seen that the skin truly was irritated, likely from the ongoing discharge of acrid matter. Clearly the boy also experienced pain during defecation, and his private parts were swollen. The father asked Handsch to get him an enema as quickly as possible to cleanse the bowels.[544] The following day, Handsch sent an apothecary to give the enema. But the apothecary was unsuccessful. All the liquid flowed back out immediately. Now, the father was furious with Handsch and the apothecary. He did not even try to apply the other remedies – an oil and a sage infusion – and instead sent for another physician. Two days later, Handsch learned that the child had died.[545]

---

541 Ibid., fol. 272r-272v, August 17.
542 Ibid., fol. 273r.
543 Ibid., August 20.
544 Ibid., fol. 274r, August 21.
545 Ibid., fol. 274r.

We find indications of a thoroughgoing interest in matters of health and home remedies on the part of men even in the highest social circles. For example, an extensive collection of medical recipes, extant in Gotha, is connected with the name of Johann of Saxony.[546] One of my own ancestors, Count Wolfgang Ernst zu Stolberg (1546–1606), also compiled such a book of recipes whose cover is magnificently adorned with his initials.[547] Handsch for his part noted down a large number of the insights and experiences conveyed to him by men from the court or from the nobility. Count von Helfenstein, for example, explained to him that the slimy matter on the surface of frog ponds worked well for *podagra*. He said it needed to be heated up and applied to the painful area with a piece of cloth.[548] And Handsch heard about the effects of a whole host of medicines and medical procedures from the captain of the castle of Brandeis, a position that was generally reserved for members of the nobility. In the case of fever, the patient was to walk over absinth plants, while with dysentery, a powder made with dried deer penis was beneficial.[549] When his burgrave ("count of the castle") became ill with fever, the captain gave him powdered unicorn horn, about which he said "it is as valuable as its weight in gold".[550] The captain even gave advice about obstetric matters. He had learned from his mother that the placenta would come out immediately if one held camphor to the woman's nose after she had delivered.[551]

Bearing in mind contemporary role patterns and gender norms, it is ultimately not surprising that men were interested and involved in medical matters and that they also treated their families. Men naturally had a concrete interest in treating their own illnesses if need be, but it went beyond this. As the heads of the family, they held the authority over the household. Furthermore, as opposed to women, men were significantly more likely to be able to read and write at the time – and hence to have access to health guidebooks and collections of recipes. It can be assumed, on the other hand, that it was predominantly women who prepared the medicines in their kitchens at home and that it was mainly they who nursed the sick.

---

546 Forschungsbibliothek Gotha, Memb. I, 111–113 (1515).
547 Privately owned.
548 Cod. 11251, fol. 157v; the entry probably refers to Georg von Helfenstein who worked as a teacher at court (*magister curiae*).
549 Cod. 11205, fol. 144r and fol. 148r.
550 Ibid., fol. 147r.
551 Ibid., fol. 150v.

Barbers and Barber-Surgeons

When patients did not want to rely on home remedies alone, and decided to seek the help of a professional healer, barbers and barber-surgeons were an important alternative to learned physicians in many places. In the Holy Roman Empire, barbers and barber-surgeons were usually organized in guilds and received a master craftsman's certificate following their training and apprenticeship, which allowed them to establish and conduct their own workshop. Their domain was not only grooming and body care, but they were also active, on a regular basis and often above all, as medical practitioners.[552]

The *Bader,* translated here as "bath-master", was the keeper of a bathhouse; the Latin designation was *balneator, balneatrix*. Since operating a bathhouse required a stove and a plentiful water supply the bath-masters were bound to their location. On certain days, the bathhouse would be heated, with a masonry stove or with large stones that had been laid in embers to heat. What was important in any case was that the stove could be stoked from the outside so as not to fill the bathhouse with smoke.[553] Hot stones could also be used to heat the water in the tubs.[554] In some places, a horn was blown or a metal basin was loudly beaten to signal that the stove, the room, and the water were hot.[555] In the better bathhouses, customers or patients entered a change room where they could lay their clothes. Women could cover their nakedness with a skirt or apron-like garment called a "Badehre" (lit. "bath honor"), while men were offered a decidedly short pair of trousers that barely concealed their private parts. Both sexes could also don a special bathing hat woven from straw.[556]

Customers could then take a warm bath in a wooden washtub. Often, herbs were added to the water, or a herbal decoction was used instead of pure water.[557] Bath servants and maids were sometimes on hand to pour water over the bathing clientele and to "rub" or "scratch" their skin. Bundles of oak or birch twigs, tied to

---

[552] On the history of barber-surgeons and bath-masters and their medical activities see Flamm, Bader (1996), Wehrli, Bader (1927) and the exhibition catalogue by Widmann/Mörgeli, Bader (1998), with numerous illustrations.
[553] Widmann/Mörgeli, Bader (1998), p. 61.
[554] Cod. 11183, fol. 253v.
[555] Wehrli, Bader (1927), p. 10; Widmann/Mörgeli, Bader (1998), p. 50.
[556] Wehrli, Bader (1927), p. 10; Flamm, Bader (1996), p. 17; Widmann/Mörgeli, Bader (1998), pp. 52f. and pp. 58f., with illustrations.
[557] Wehrli, Bader (1927), p. 20.

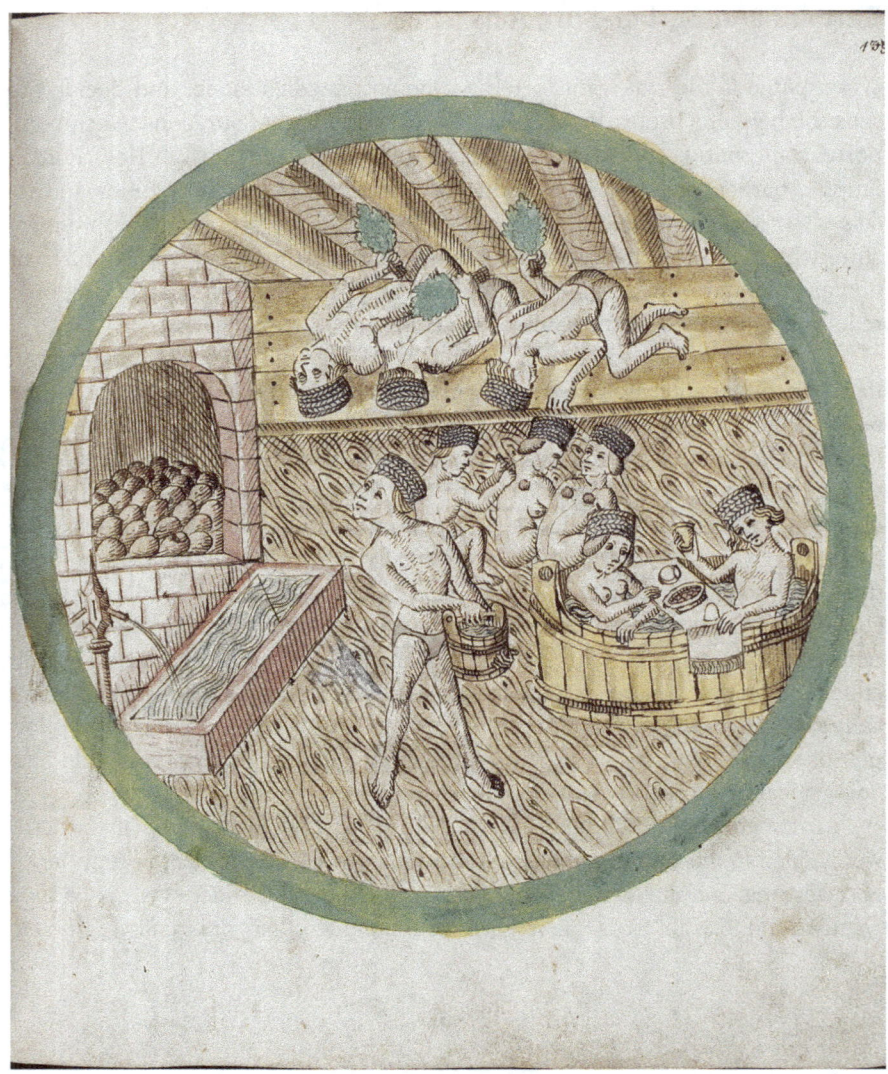

Fig. 16: Bath chamber with clients in a tub, on a sweating bench and undergoing cupping, Herzog August-Bibliothek, Wolfenbüttel, Cod. Guelf. 8.7. Aug. 8°, fol. 139r.

form fronds or brushes, served to "stroke" the skin and stimulate the flow of sweat.[558] Bathers could also have their hair washed, and in Padua, Handsch made use of the services of a barber-surgeon who removed his pubic hair and the hair in other places such as his thighs.[559] Depictions of naked women from this time suggest that the practice of hair removal, which today is often perceived as a new phenomenon, was widespread at the time,[560] perhaps encouraged by the aforementioned notion that hair came from excremental matter. Contemporary illustrations of people sitting in tubs with a board lying across, eating or holding one another while nearly naked show how bathhouses were also social places and sometimes more than that.[561]

More than taking baths in tubs, what was important for preventive healthcare were the so-called sweat benches. In the larger bathhouses, these wooden benches on which people would lie were arranged in several levels (see Fig. 16). It was hottest on the *Oberbank*, the upper bench,[562] below the ceiling, where the hot steam collected which was produced – just as it is today in steam baths or saunas – by pouring water on hot stones. Lying on the sweat benches, customers and patients could take hot steam baths that promised to cleanse the inside of the body of accumulated waste matter through a plentiful flow of sweat. Bathing in tubs, by contrast, was considered potentially dangerous when there was a buildup of impure matter in the body because bathing only mobilized the matter rather than evacuating it.[563]

The most important surgical "intervention" carried out by the bath-masters was prophylactic and therapeutic cupping. Even a high-ranking patient such as the Baroness of Hungerkasten sought out a bathhouse in which she could have cupping glasses applied to her shoulders to fight catarrh and headache by drawing the morbid matter down from the head.[564] The bath-master's portable lamp, whose small flame was used to heat the cupping glasses before they were applied to the skin, even served as a symbol of the profession. In contemporary depictions, bath-masters can be identified by the lamp and by their scanty clothing, which was owed to the heat in the bathhouse.[565]

---

558 Wehrli, Bader (1927), p. 9; Flamm, Bader (1996), p. 15; Widmann/Mörgeli, Bader (1998), pp. 68f.
559 Cod. 11006, fol. 187v.
560 Widmann/Mörgeli, Bader (1998), pp. 76f.
561 Ibid., p. 37.
562 Cod. 11210, fol. 62r.
563 Cod. 11183, fol. 399v: "Impura corpora et repleta non balneanda, quia funduntur humores mali"; similarly Cod. 11205, fol. 119r.
564 Cod. 11205, fol. 406v.
565 Widmann/Mörgeli, Bader (1998), p. 87, with an illustration.

In the Middle Ages, a barber quite often also worked in the bathhouse and was responsible for shaving and cutting hair. Some bath-masters hung up a barber's bowl of the kind that the customer had to hold under his chin during wet shaving, to advertise the work of the barber at their business.[566] By the sixteenth century, however, the barbers had become barber-surgeons and as such significant competitors for the bath-masters. Indeed they had largely – with the exception of cupping – displaced them from the curative arts in a narrow sense.[567] Tellingly, Handsch spoke much more frequently of barbers ("barbitonsores") than of bath-masters ("balneatores") in the context of patient treatment. Alongside hair cutting and beard trimming, the domain of the barbers was predominantly considered to comprise minor surgery, pulling teeth, and the treatment of wounds and injuries as well as external diseases such as ulcers and other pathological skin changes with ointments and compresses. Handsch gave numerous descriptions of such activities performed by barbers, for example stitching a head injury,[568] setting a dislocated arm,[569] and cutting open gums and extracting a tooth.[570] The most important surgical intervention for barber-surgeons was bloodletting, which for many seems to have constituted a central source of income. As a rule, it was to the barber-surgeons that learned physicians sent their patients when bloodletting was indicated.[571]

The barber-surgeons had a great advantage over the bath-masters insofar as they did not require a bathhouse. They could practice in the houses of their customers or patients, which suited affluent patients very well. Unlike the bath-masters, they furthermore did not suffer the consequences of the repeated severe shortages of wood.[572] And they were also not affected in the same way by the population's fear of contracting the new French disease. This fear has often been connected to the loose sexual mores in some bathhouses. But clearly, the crux of the matter was something else: given the disease concepts described above, there was a significant concern that the disease could be transmitted by the vapors that emanated from the skin, especially from profusely sweating people affected with the disease.[573]

---

566 Ibid., p. 79, with an illustration.
567 For surveys see Wehrli, Bader (1927), pp. 47–77; Flamm, Bader (1996), pp. 22–24.
568 Cod. 11183, fol. 164v.
569 Ibid., fol. 206r, "barbitonsor rectificavit brachium luxatum".
570 Cod. 11205, fol. 291v.
571 E.g. ibid., fol. 4v.
572 Wehrli, Bader (1927), pp. 32–34.
573 Widmann/Mörgeli, Bader (1998), pp. 158f.

Although the treatment of external conditions was considered their domain, in practice bath-masters and barber-surgeons often also administered medicines for internal use to their patients and ultimately practiced the full range of the healing arts. In many places, they were not forbidden from doing so. While the surgical activities of the barber-surgeons were protected by guild laws and other regulations, the internal treatment of illnesses – the domain of the physicians – often was not, in marked contrast to later times. It was only in a few places, like in Zurich in 1553, that barber-surgeons were outright forbidden from practicing internal medicine as early as the sixteenth century.[574] In rural areas, where the next learned physician could be quite some distance away, the bath-masters and barber-surgeons, along with lay healers, often provided the first line of treatment for any sort of ailment.

The practice of internal medicine on the part of the bath-masters and barber-surgeons was a thorn in physicians' sides. Some physicians picked their craftsmen competitors to pieces. In this regard, leading proponents of academic medicine were for once in agreement with Paracelsus, who polemicized against the bath-masters and feldshers who – he claimed – conducted themselves as surgeons, even "masters", despite lacking the necessary knowledge.[575] Johannes Lange found very similar words when lambasting the barber-surgeons of his time, writing that with no anatomical knowledge whatsoever and after having no more than seen a butcher slaughter a calf or a piglet, they were ready to abuse their patients with a knife and hot iron.[576]

In everyday practice, as Handsch's notes show, physicians and bath-masters and barber-surgeons often got along with one another and coexisted quite peacefully.[577] Many patients who were being treated by physicians for an internal disease such as the French disease also developed ulcers or abscesses or other skin changes which, because they were external complaints, fell in the domain of the bath-masters and barber-surgeons. And as we have seen, physicians for their part were sometimes asked for their advice about wounds and operable complaints such as bladder stones and hernias. Even in published case histories penned by physicians, there are numerous indications that learned physicians cooperated with barber-surgeons, indeed that they even treated patients together.[578] What is more, it was apparent to physicians – as Handsch's notes vividly show – that

---

574 Wehrli, Bader (1927), pp. 62f.
575 Paracelsus, Grosse Wundartzney (1536), conclusion ("Beschlußred", no pagination).
576 Lange, Medicinalium epistolarum (1554), p. 13.
577 Thus also Schlegelmilch, Blick (2019), pp. 75–76.
578 E.g. Cod. 11207, fol. 161r, on a severly injured man whom Mattioli treated "together with the barber-surgeons" ("cum barbitonsoribus").

they stood to learn something from barber-surgeons. Learned physicians actually had great respect for the knowledge and skills of established, experienced surgeons such as the court surgeon Hildebrand who practiced in Handsch's immediate environment. It was with good reason that Handsch made detailed notes of Hildebrand's methods for various surgical interventions.[579] Occasionally, Handsch even deferred to Hildebrand's opinion when it came to the treatment of internal diseases. When Handsch wanted to bleed a fever patient, for example, he ultimately did not do it because Hildebrand did not consider it necessary for a simple tertian fever.[580] Surgery, as a matter of fact, serves as a prime example of that close and mutually productive relationship between book-learning and craftsmanship in the early modern period, which Pamela Long and Pamela Smith underscored in their studies about other fields of knowledge and activity.[581]

Lay Healers

In their censure of the numerous lay healers, who treated patients in towns and in the countryside without formal education and without the permission of the authorities, medical authors were even more relentless. In printed works and in their petitions to the authorities, they condemned the "fraud" and the "murderous acts"[582] of these "bunglers". They warned of the great harm "people's best and most beloved treasure, namely life and health",[583] suffered through their doings. Sometimes they even named specific healers, demanding that an end be put to their "dirty tricks".[584]

It was with good reason that such polemics were chiefly written in the vernacular. The authors were seeking not only to warn sick people about the "fraudulent machinations" and the "dangerous ignorance" of the lay healers. A second and

---

579 See the chapter on surgery in Part II.
580 Cod. 11183, fol. 449v.
581 Long, Artisan/practitioners (2001); Smith, Body (2004).
582 As indicated already by the title in Horer, Artzney-Teuffel (1634).
583 Preface of the German translator of Foreest, Uromanteia (1620), p. 8; similarly, dedicatory epistle by Johannes Crato to Da Monte, Consultationum centuria secunda (1559); the critics frequently combined their attacks with a fundamental rejection of the diagnosis of diseases just from the the patient's urine, which many of these empirics (but also many physicians) practiced; examples are Clauser, Betrachtung ([1543]), Hornung, De uroscopia (1611) and, based on Foreest's diatribe, Hart, Arraignment (1623); on the context, see Barbara Elkeles, Medicus und Medikaster (1987); Stolberg, Harnschau (2009), pp. 187–195.
584 See e.g. the supplication by Jeremias Martius and other Augsburg physicians, 16 August 1573 (www.aerztebriefe.de/id/00002330, S. Herde).

decisive target audience was the authorities, who would have actually constituted the main readership considering the limited literacy of most of the population. It was the authorities who, through their "unobservant supervision" allowed "any fellow who comes along to go about his mischief and sinful murder".[585] To "put things right", the physicians demanded severe punishment for lay healers. Cordus, for example, lamented that forgers, who only conned people out of their money, were burnt at the stake, while those who robbed people of their lives were allowed to run free.[586] Sounding the same alarm bells, Ananius Horer wrote that anyone passing himself off as a baron would be punished, but not the person who pretended to be a physician.[587]

Already as students, budding physicians were initiated into the struggle against this opponent. An incident in Montpellier, reported by Felix Platter, is telling. An *empiricus* who was caught with medicinal ointments and powders was apprehended and led through the town by students. As punishment, he was forced to sit backwards on a donkey while those surrounding him scorched his face, hands, legs, and clothes with burning branches.[588] Under headings such as "Contra empiricos", quite a few entries in Handsch's notebooks show that he, too, had to some extent adopted the negative image that was being presented of lay healers in polemical treatises and petitions. We read, for example, "They want to be physicians, just as peasants want to be nobility",[589] or, "They practice medicine at random", or, as he added in Latin, "An incomplete physician is a complete murderer".[590]

For a long time, historians stood in the same camp as the learned physicians, bemoaning the "dreadfulness" of the "quacks" and "charlatans" who stood in the way of true – that is learned – medicine. However, if, for a moment, we consider this through the lens of modern medicine, it is by no means a given that the therapeutic outcomes of the *empirici* were inferior to those of learned physicians. Quite the contrary, from a modern perspective, administering a simple laxative or treating a disease with magical, sympathetic rituals would in most cases have been more salubrious than the extreme and likely damaging – again, from today's perspective – treatment that physicians sometimes gave their patients: drastic purgatives, numerous other medications, bloodletting, enemas, and further procedures. Renaissance physicians may have indeed been

---

585 Preface of the German translator of Foreest, Uromanteia (1620), p. 8.
586 Cordus, De urinis (1543), no pagination.
587 Horer, Artzney-Teuffel (1634), p. 29.
588 Germain, Les étudiants (1876), p. 38.
589 Cod. 11206, fol. 97r.
590 Ibid.

convinced of the dangers they were depicting so vividly and harrowingly. From a modern perspective, however, the struggle against the *empirici* was unmistakably also a central element of a more comprehensive professionalization and monopolization campaign that unfolded over the course of centuries.[591]

To do justice to the activities and the significance of lay healers, it is necessary to distinguish two groups. There were, first of all, those itinerant healers and vendors of medicine who advertised their services and remedies on market squares; Handsch saw them in Venice.[592] And then there were the sedentary lay healers. The distrust of the itinerant healers and vendors of medicine whom the physicians called *circumforanei* or *circulatori,* makes some sense, also in historical retrospect. By the time it was possible to determine whether their remedies were effective and their treatment successful or not and whether they were perhaps even cunning crooks, these itinerant healers were often long gone and could no longer be made accountable and punished. Vagrants usually sat on a horse so that they could flee, as Handsch put it laconically.[593] He also retold a story that offered evidence of their deceptive machinations: an acquaintance of his allegedly saw with his own eyes how one such itinerant healer drank from wine that had a living snake in it. Afterwards, the man's abdomen swelled up and he measured his girth with a rope. Then he drank the theriac which he was touting. His abdomen shrank back down, thus supposedly proving the effect of the theriac. Handsch, however, considered it impossible that the snake's poison would only cause the belly to swell without also severely affecting the heart and liver, and without causing the man to faint.[594] In some places, the municipal authorities had taken action against such itinerant healers and drug peddlers as early as the late Middle Ages insofar as they had demanded licenses or even required them to pass an examination conducted by the town physician. In larger municipalities, the medical faculties and the *collegia medica* gradually acquired the right to conduct examinations and to supervise medical activities.[595]

The itinerant healers and drug peddlers were colorful figures but they ultimately played a limited role in ordinary health care. By contrast, the sedentary healers – the *empirici, vetulae* ("old women"),[596] or the "Kuedocter" ("cow

---

591 See also Lingo, Empirics (1986).
592 Cod. 11240, fol. 36r and fol. 37v.
593 Cod. 11205, fol. 205r.
594 Ibid., fol. 134v; in another entry, Handsch bluntly referred to the "fraudes theriacantium empiricorum".
595 Sudhoff, Kurpfuscher (1915), with an edition of relevant sources; Wagner, Doctores (2008); Schütte, Medizin (2017), pp. 216–239.
596 Kinzelbach, Heilkundige Frauen (1999).

doctors"), as Handsch and other contemporary physicians called them[597] – played a central role in medical care, especially in rural areas where the large majority of the population continued to live. They were known and trusted. In fact, it is often difficult to draw a line between lay healers whose primary occupation consisted of their healing activities and the numerous medical laypeople who occasionally offered medical advice to neighbors and acquaintances. Because they were rooted in the community, these healers could hardly afford to deceive patients openly and deliberately.

When sick, people from all social classes would at least sometimes seek the advice and help of a lay healer. It is therefore not surprising that the physicians' polemics and petitions were rather unsuccessful in their principal aim, namely to move the authorities to enact drastic measures against the lay healers. Princes and others authorities had little reason to deprive their fellow citizens, their own families, and themselves of the possibility of consulting healers who were widely appreciated for their skill and success in treating patients. Handsch's notes are telling in this respect. Again and again, they make it clear that the clientele of lay healers was by no means limited to simple, uneducated people who lacked the financial means to consult a physician. Patients from the highest circles of society – the preferred clientele of the learned physicians – sought their advice. The archducal chamberlain Christoph von Gendorf, for example, did not have his sciatica treated by Andrea Gallo and Ulrich Lehner alone, but also consulted a lay healer, who completed the treatment using a poultice and could take credit for the cure.[598] When, in 1565, Sigismund von Berka took a fall while inebriated and injured his head and began experiencing symptoms of paralysis, he, too, sought the advice of a lay healer. The Berkas were one of two powerful noble families in Handsch's hometown of Leipa.[599] Johannes Schentigar told Handsch about a nobleman at the Habsburg court in Prague who first consulted a lay healer when he was suffering from tertian fever before turning to him, Schentigar.[600] Even famous medical experts like Johann Neefe had to contend with this type of competition. The Baroness of Hungerkasten for example, while she did have herself treated by him, also spent a month with an unnamed lay healer.[601]

---

597 Cod. 11205, fol. 408r and fol. 413r.
598 Cod. 11240, fol. 35v; also mentioned in Cod. 11210, fol. 61r; on Gendorf see Bůžek, Ferdinand (2009), pp. 55f.
599 Schober/Neder, Sechshundertjahrfeier (1929), pp. 2–10.
600 Cod. 11205, fol. 101v.
601 Ibid., fol. 613r.

Physicians thus had to expect that none of their patients – from simple farmers to even patients from the high nobility – would entrust themselves to their counsel alone, but would also turn to lay healers, sometimes even at the same time. Handsch's notes suggest that some noble patients, like the Berkas, even routinely sought the advice of lay healers, indeed that these lay healers more or less entered their service. There is mention of an "empiricus D[omi]ni Rosensis", of an "empiricus apud Berkam"[602] and of a "medicus empiricus" called Bacchus at the court of Emperor Maximilian II.[603] The latter was said to have diagnosed a "yellow, black, and white jaundice" in a noble female patient and to have treated it with a powder he made from a root which he gathered not far from the Prague castle.[604]

Handsch's father was a member of the town council and his son was a physician but in Handsch's own family, too, a lay healer was consulted regularly. Handsch called him "our empiricus" ("empiricus noster") or the "Leipa empiricus" ("empiricus Lippensis"). Apparently, this was one and the same person, likely a certain Lorenz.[605] Handsch mentioned him many times in his notes, and both his father and stepmother consulted him.[606]

The *empirici* were not only serious economic competitors; they also posed a threat to the status and authority of learned physicians and academic medicine. When these healers were able to cure patients, it called into question the superiority of the rational, scholarly medicine that the physicians were so vehemently and categorically defending. It was clear to the physicians that patients were looking for one thing above all else: being cured. And physicians could not deny that in the hands of the *empirici*, too, numerous patients became well again. Understandably, patients and those around them ascribed their recovery in such cases to the skills and remedies of the lay healer. In the worst case, physicians found themselves publicly exposed and shamed by such curative success. As a student in Padua, Handsch noted down, for example, the story of a man with an incessant nosebleed. The attending physicians were trying everything under the sun, but after twenty days, they declared the case hopeless. At this point, an old woman advised the patient to eat a fresh raw egg, including the shell. He did this, and five days later the nosebleed was gone.[607] In Prague,

---

602 Cod. 11251, fol. 116v.
603 Cod. 11183, fol. 154v and fol. 285r.
604 Ibid., fol. 285r.
605 E.g. Cod. 11205, fol. 116r, fol. 122v, and fol. 124r; Cod. 11183, fol. 142r.
606 It is not known whether there was a learned physician or an apprenticed barber-surgeon or bath-master in Leipa, at the time.
607 Cod. 11251, fol. 31v.

a man from the court told Handsch about his experience of having been diagnosed as consumptive by physicians, who considered him a desperate case. He was coughing and becoming emaciated. Then an old woman advised him to drink warm beer with a little butter every night when he went to bed. He followed these instructions for several months and recovered.[608]

Stories like these got around. In Trento, Handsch heard about a cardinal who hurt his foot when he fell from a horse in the Holy Land. For years he was treated to no avail by physicians until he finally followed the advice of a countrywoman ("rustica") and successfully cured his affliction with the remedies she recommended.[609] Another story was about a watchman who cured the Saxon Elector Friedrich of his *podagra* within a short period of time using a secret remedy. It was claimed the Elector said that if he had known of this remedy and its good effects he could have spared himself all the remedies from the apothecary's shop.[610] According to another of Handsch's entries, a *vetula* was said to have laughed at the medical doctors ("medicos doctores") because they were unable to gain the upper hand on a patient's bladder stone. She gave him a simple remedy made with the dried stems of beans and peas as well as bean flour in mutton broth and in this way cured the patient without any further medicine.[611] And in Italy, a *vetula* made a "scandal" out of the physicians ("ad scandalum posuit") by successfully treating the lame and gouty with a simple remedy of cloves, sage, saffron, and cream. Handsch clearly believed in the effects: he recorded the remedy in his *Liber experimentorum*, his collection of tried and tested medicines.[612] Handsch himself, too, suffered such humiliations. In the case of a female patient experiencing chronic colics, he ultimately had to admit that the treatment of a female lay healer was more successful than his own. Over the course of months, Handsch had tried numerous remedies, to no avail. Then an old woman cured the patient with a decoction of wild thyme (*serpyllum*). Handsch noted down that wild thyme was an "excellent remedy for colics".[613]

---

608 Ibid., fol. 116r.
609 Cod. 11251, fol. 7r.
610 Ibid., fol. 33v; presumably, Handsch was referring to Friedrich III (1463–1525).
611 Ibid., fol. 74r.
612 Ibid., fol. 85v.
613 Ibid., fol. 37v, "contra colicam experimentum optimum".

Learned Physicians and Lay Medical Culture

In an oft-quoted passage from the preface to his *Große Wundartzney*, Paracelsus presented his medicine in opposition to the book-learning and devotion to authority of the orthodox Galenic physicians. Everywhere he went he "asked diligently, researched" including "with bone-surgeons, bath-masters, the wives of learned physicians, necromancers [. . .], with the alchemists, in monasteries, with the noble and the humble, with the sane and the foolish".[614] Even though Paracelsus added that he was unable to learn some essential answers from these people, the passage has often been cited as evidence of his special position and his proximity to folk culture. Handsch's notes put the originality and significance of Paracelsus's statement in perspective. They show that some Galenic physicians also explored in great depth and took seriously the traditional and empirical knowledge of medical laypeople.[615] Unlike Paracelsus, however, who stylized himself as a man of the people, they were loath to admit it in public.

Learning from Laypeople

Handsch documented lay medical knowledge in numerous entries. Sometimes he described popular practices and convictions in general terms. In Tyrol, he reported, women allowed leeches in lake water to attach to their bare legs, and left them there until the water turned blood-red. This was an alternative to bloody cupping.[616] As a preventative against the plague, it was thought that one should eat theriac on toasted bread and then inhale the stench of a sewer with a wide-open mouth, keeping the air in one's mouth for a while; this offered protection for that day.[617] To treat the "Keichen" ("wheezing") of children who screamed, struggled to breathe and turned blue in the face, the children were sometimes placed in the hollowed-out body of a freshly slaughtered ox.[618] In

---

[614] Paracelsus, Grosse Wundartzney (1536), preface, "empsig nach gefragt, Erforschung gehapt"; "Beinscherern, Badern, gelerter Artzeten Weibern, Schwartzkünstlern [. . .], bey den Alchimisten, bey den Clöstern, bey Edlen und Unedlen, beyn Gescheiden und Einfaltigen".
[615] For a more detailed analysis see Stolberg, Learning (2014).
[616] Cod. 11183, fol. 495.
[617] Cod. 11251, fol. 111r; Handsch mentioned this popular Bohemian practice of inhaling foul odours from cesspools as a preservative against the plague also in other entries (Cod. 11205, fol. 80v; Cod. 11240, fol. 145r, "bohemi ad praeservationem olfaciunt cloacam").
[618] Cod. 11183, fol. 205r.

Open Access. © 2022 Michael Stolberg, published by De Gruyter. This work is licensed under the Creative Commons Attribution-NonCommercial-NoDerivatives 4.0 International License.
https://doi.org/10.1515/9783110733549-021

Leipa, people used pimpinella powder as a fortifier, adding it to their beer soup,[619] and used *manus Christi* as a cough remedy.[620] And it was a common belief ("vulgaris opinio") that if you were suffering from a "catarrh" you were not to get your head wet or take a bath.[621] Handsch also described in detail how women treated "Nabelverstürzung" – the term suggests a hidden or visible protrusion of the umbilicus, a clinical picture the physicians did not even know about. Their treatment involved running the hands from the navel toward the back and then pinching or pulling up the skin there, or pressing one's knee into the child's back in a seated position on the floor and pulling back the skin of the belly until "it" gave.[622] Fever patients were generally wrapped in a blanket so that the heat of the fever would leave the body; likely what was meant here was through perspiration.[623]

Much more abundant still were Handsch's entries about the medicines and home remedies that some lay healers used or recommended for the prevention or treatment of various illnesses. He collected some of them, along with the remedies he owed to his fellow physicians, in his *Liber experimentorum*, a collection of tried and tested medicines intended for use with his own patients.[624] Among them was, for example, a "surefire remedy" with which a monk treated *panaritia,* inflammations of the nail bed[625] and a "secret remedy" to encourage the flow of urine.[626] He documented the case of a boy whose pain from bladder stones was alleviated by a lay healer who gave him an ointment that smelled of balsam and juniper.[627] A fellow citizen of Leipa told Handsch that the smoke of burning absinth was a reliable remedy for headaches if it was blown into the person's mouth and ears.[628] Handsch owed the recipe for a "mild purgative that could also be used in pregnant women" to the widow of a royal judge; it was a decoction of senna, licorice, sage, hyssop, and other plants.[629] A female cook told him about the successful treatment of mouth sores with an electuary containing among other things honey and rust.[630] The wife of a certain Weitmüller

---

619 Cod. 11006, fol. 184v.
620 Cod. 11183, fol. 190r.
621 Ibid., fol. 397v.
622 Cod. 11205, foll. 117v-118r; further notes and cases in Cod. 11183, fol. 62r and fol. 138v.
623 Cod. 11183, fol. 474r.
624 Cod. 11251.
625 Cod. 11183, fol. 271.
626 Cod. 11251, fol. 31r.
627 Cod. 11205, fol. 105r-v.
628 Cod. 11183, fol. 240v.
629 Ibid., fol. 240v.
630 Ibid., fol. 135r.

cured cold fevers with St. Benedict's thistle.[631] She also told Handsch that chicory blossoms worked well for jaundice.[632]

In his Innsbruck years, Handsch expressed respect for the curative practice of his landlady. "My landlady knows many medicines", he wrote.[633] For example, a young woman with "sciatica" came to her house asking for advice. Handsch's landlady diagnosed a "cold flux" and prescribed warm juniper oil.[634] Within eight days, her treatment with St. Benedict's thistle was able to heal an ugly boil from which another patient had been suffering for years.[635] Handsch also learned from her that strawberry water was good if someone felt "tight around the chest".[636]

Handsch evidently took seriously the knowledge and the experiences of lay healers and even the treatment recommendations of common laypeople. In one case, he heard from a woman who had treated an ugly abscess on her leg with the leaves of a plant recommended by an old woman, and he went so far as to ask an apothecary to help him identify the plant.[637] This attitude stands in striking contradiction to the aforementioned attacks on the "murderous" misdoings of the "ignorant" *empirici* which physicians mounted in their published writings. Only seldom do we find instances in which a learned physician publicly credited lay healers, the *empirici* and *vetulae*, with successful treatment or at least took their recommendations seriously.

Considering the growing appreciation of empirical knowledge within academic medicine, there were good reasons not to outright reject the knowledge and experience of the lay healers. After all, their curative successes were confirmed by the testimony of numerous people. They could not simply be brushed aside. Handsch was thus in good company with his respect for what he could learn from lay healers. The famous Paduan professor Vettore Trincavella stated to his students that there were "sometimes old women who achieve much with their herbal decoctions".[638] From the no less famous Gabrielle Falloppia, Handsch

---

631 Ibid., fol. 243v.
632 Ibid.
633 Cod. 11251, fol. 112v.
634 Ibid.
635 Cod. 11251, fol. 114v.
636 Cod. 11251, fol. 112v, "eng umb die Brust".
637 Cod. 11183, fol. 45v.
638 Cod. 11238, fol. 88r.

heard that in a severe dysentery epidemic, the physicians had tried all kinds of remedies. The most effective one, however, came from an old woman who made it from cabbage and bacon fat; within three days, the sick were well again.[639] Falloppia also recommended the repeated local application of the menstrual blood of a virgin as an excellent means to reduce the size of excessively large breasts. An old woman had taught him this remedy, which, according to Falloppia, acted by its "total substance". He had experienced its effects numerous times.[640] Elsewhere, too, physicians occasionally approached lay medical knowledge with a remarkably open mind, without making public knowledge of it. The English physician John Symcotts made numerous notes in his private notebook about the knowledge he gained from female lay healers who had learned from their own experience; he repeatedly documented their treatment of patients. He even learnt from a woman beggar how to make a certain remedy.[641]

Physicians might even resort to lay healers in their own illnesses. Handsch was told by an old court physician who suffered from dropsy. It was not hurting him very much but when he reached under his ribs on the left, he noticed something like an egg. Breathing was difficult when he climbed stairs and his belly always swelled up after eating and was smaller again in the morning. He put his trust in the arts of an old woman healer who had supposedly healed many dropsical patients before him. The old woman gave him an oil to ingest and told him to soak linen in his own urine and apply it. Instead of his own urine, the man took that of a healthy boy. After eight days, he said, his spleen was healed, though he still felt weak.[642]

Writing about his encounters with lay healers, Handsch sometimes even explicitly used phrases such as "I learned that" and "he taught me". For example, in one entry he noted down what the *empiricus* of Leipa had "taught" him about the use of antimony. Handsch had given quite a number of patients antimony, but instead of it producing many bowel movements, as he expected and hoped, vomiting occurred. The *empiricus* told him he had to give mastic with it,

---

639 Cod. 11251, fol. 30r.
640 Falloppia, Tractatus (1566), fol. 51r (based on the notes of Falloppia's student Petrus Angelus Agathus); the old woman recommended more specifically the blood from the first menstruation of a virgin.
641 Poynter/Bishop, A seventeenth-century doctor (1951), pp. 54f. and pp. 80f.; in the eighteenth century, the Nürnberg physician Götz, for example, still made the empirical medical knowledge of ordinary women his own (Kinzelbach/Neuner/Nolte, Knowledge (2016), p. 109).
642 Cod. 11205, 220v-221r; Handsch called him Dr. Michael Cadanensis; presumably, "Cadanensis" was not his name, however, but indicated his place of origin, the town of Kaaden, today's Kadaň, not far from Annaberg.

and then he would achieve his aim.[643] The *empiricus* also "taught" him a recipe for a purgative that was often used "in cold fluxes".[644] From a miller near Innsbruck, Handsch "learned" that there was no better remedy for the "Breun" – presumably an inflammation of the throat – than the juice of three crabs.[645]

Some lay healers furthermore possessed specialized knowledge and skills that most learned physicians could hardly claim for themselves. The production of oily essences from juniper and other plants through distillation is an example.[646] Handsch praised the gentle procedure commonly used by the old women to distill rose water from petals, and he described it in detail.[647] He also gave an in-depth account of getting together with the *empiricus* in Leipa in 1558 to produce medicinal antimony.[648] Finally, as we have seen, the experience and specialized skills of lay healers were valuable not least of all when it came to a disease that had not been discussed by the ancient authorities, namely the French disease. In particular, Handsch mentioned a number of Jewish healers who treated sufferers of the French disease. He watched them work and noted down what they told him.[649]

A Shared World?

For a long time, medical historians painted a dichotomous picture of early modern medicine. There was, one the one side, the "true" medicine, practiced by physicians, which ultimately led to modern medicine. On the other, there was "folk medicine", which was largely passed on orally and shaped significantly by "superstitious" practices. This picture fit in with the overall notion of an elite culture and a "folk culture" existing parallel and in opposition to each other in premodern society. In more recent research in social and cultural history, these dichotomies have been fundamentally challenged.[650] In the course of this development, medical historians have criticized the term "folk medicine", and with it the idea

---

643 Ibid., foll. 122v-123r: "docuit me empiricus Lippensis."
644 Cod. 11205, fol. 519a v, "docuit me empiricus Laurentius".
645 Cod. 11251, fol. 112r; Handsch made that note in a section devoted to the proven remedies or "experimenta" "which I learnt in Innsbruck". The German term "Bräune" usually referred to diseases of the throat with symptoms that were similar to those associated with diphtheria today.
646 Cod. 11240, fol. 132r.
647 Cod. 11205, fol. 139v.
648 Ibid., fol. 131v and fol. 132a v.
649 See the chapter on the French disease.
650 Burke, Popular culture (1979).

that there was something like an independent medicine of the "common man" that could be seen as separate from academic medicine.[651] These recent studies instead paint the picture of a pre-modern medical world that was shared by learned physicians and common folk, in which no clear dividing line could be drawn between lay medical culture and learned medicine as practiced by physicians.[652]

The research presented here essentially confirms this thesis of a shared medical worldview. Certainly, there were some marked differences. While empirical knowledge was becoming increasingly valued, medicine as practiced by learned physicians continued to be based in great measure on book-learning. It drew on a complex theoretical edifice shaped by the classical Hippocratic and Galenic heritage as well as by Aristotelian philosophy, and it had at its disposal a sophisticated logical and methodological apparatus. Its disease categories were far more complex than those used by laypeople. Moreover, the learned medical literature – fever theories are a good example here – described, differentiated, and explained many disease phenomena and diagnoses for which lay medicine had no terminology and no equivalents. And not least of all, with the rise of anatomy, learned physicians were increasingly able to rely on detailed knowledge about the structure of the human body. Yet, in medical practice, in everyday encounters with patients and their relatives, the commonalities, as we have seen, continued to outweigh the differences. For the majority of cases, physicians relied on a very limited number of diagnoses such as "fever", "catarrh", or "flux", "obstruction", "dropsy", or "suffocation of the womb", all of which were familiar to laypeople. They also attributed most diseases to unclean, insufficiently concocted, rotting, or otherwise corrupted morbid matter that could be traced to a blockage or disruption of the flow of humors and the excretions; to a stomach that was either too weak, too cold, or overtaxed by food; and, more rarely, to an excessively heated liver or to a contagion that had entered the body from the outside. As physicians explained to their patients using metaphorical language that was readily graspable by laypeople, these pathogenic substances could spread throughout the blood or accumulate in certain places in the body. There, they could spoil further, harden to become tumors, or give off disease-causing vapors. Consequently, physicians as much as laypeople in most cases considered it of paramount importance for successful treatment that morbid matter be evacuated, obstructions be

---

651 Stolberg, Probleme (1998); Wolff, Volksmedizin (1998).
652 Nagy, Popular medicine (1988), p. 52; Gentilcore, Was there a "popular medicine" (2004) and, for France, Brockliss/Jones, Medical world (1997), esp. p. 16, have arrived at the same conclusion; looking at the situation in France around 1800, Ramsey, Professional and popular medicine (1998) still was not able to identify a clear demarcation line.

dissolved, and weakened organs – the stomach, the heart, and/or the brain – be strengthened.

The far-reaching agreement between the physicians' conceptions and practices and those of laypeople raises the question as to why these similarities existed. A comparison with the very different medicine of non-Western cultures, such as traditional Indian or Chinese medicine, suggests that one central factor was the shared cultural heritage of laypeople and learned physicians. Many of the fundamental ideas about the origin and treatment of diseases, as well as the understanding of the therapeutic use of many medicinal plants – which, taken together, formed the basis of the medical world of the Renaissance – had been handed down from antiquity. It is quite possible, likely even, that the physicians of antiquity, in turn, already seized on images, ideas, and experiences from the lay medical culture of their day and put them into writing. In subsequent times, laypeople doubtlessly adopted concepts from learned medicine countless times. This is difficult to prove for a lay medical culture that was largely passed on orally and by way of routine practices but the popularity gained by "chemically" produced medicines in the sixteenth century among the general population,[653] and the rise of the "nerves" that started in the late seventeenth century[654] offer vivid proof that the premodern lay medical culture was fundamentally adaptable and open to innovation. Even the preeminent significance of uroscopy for early modern lay medical culture did not by all appearances arise from "folk medicine" but was crucially owed to the great appreciation uroscopy had enjoyed in the learned medicine of the Middle Ages.

My research into theories and explanatory models that guided everyday medical practice strongly suggests that learned Renaissance physicians, in turn, were prepared to move much closer towards the medical world of laypeople than their published polemics against the ignorance of the "vulgus" would make as believe. As Nancy Siraisi, Danielle Jacquart, Luke Demaitre, Chiara Crisciani, Joel Agrimi, and others have shown, the doctrine of "dyscrasia" or "intemperies" – that is, a disrupted balance of the four natural humors and the body's four primary qualities – still enjoyed a very prominent place in medieval medicine, not just in theory but also in practice.[655] Sources like consultation letters suggest that medieval physicians relied to a far greater extent on the traditional doctrine of humoral balance than physicians in the Renaissance. And as we have seen, this doctrine was still

---

653 Cf. Eamon, Science (1994).
654 Stolberg, Experiencing illness (2011), pp. 170–195.
655 E.g. Joel Agrimi and Chiara Crisciani, leading experts in the field of medieval medical theory and practice, have explicity characterized this concept as the dominant one (Agrimi/Crisciani, Malato (1980), p. 39).

playing a greater role in the university lectures of the sixteenth century, which were largely based on the canon of medical literature passed down from antiquity, than on the ground, in actual medical practice. In other words, the concept of an impure, foreign morbid matter whose mobilization and evacuation was considered decisive for a successful treatment may have been old, but its towering significance in the medical practice of the sixteenth century, which by that time far surpassed that of the doctrine of dyscrasia and *intemperies,* was by all appearances the result of a relatively new development within learned medicine.

The humanist (re)discovery of the works by Galen, Hippocrates, and other ancient authors cannot explain this pronounced shift towards an understanding of disease which focused on unclean, rotting, corrupted, and otherwise preternatural, morbid matter, which formed and accumulated in the body due to insufficient concoction, obstructions, or disrupted excretions. The only plausible explanation for this interpretive shift, it seems to me, is that these ideas had been prevalent among the lay populace for a considerable period of time and now, during the Renaissance, were increasingly taken up by learned medicine.

This immediately raises another question: what might have led the learned physicians to give more credit in their daily practice to the disease concepts that were prevalent among laypeople and thereby devalue the traditional doctrine of humoral balance, which was the basis of learned medical theory before and supported by the great classical authorities? Answering this question will necessarily involve some degree of speculation, but I would like to propose some hypotheses.

A central factor doubtlessly was the physicians' socialization. As Peter Burke stressed in a seminal article years ago, the educated upper classes of the seventeenth and eighteenth centuries began to set themselves off from the "folk culture" of the "common people". In the sixteenth century, this "folk culture" still largely shaped everyone's mental world and everyday behavior. A growing educated elite only had additional access to a second culture, a scholarly culture that was largely grounded in antiquity.[656] In our context this means that the physicians – and especially the growing number of physicians from a comparatively humble social background – belonged to both worlds. For their first two decades or so, in childhood and youth, they were socialized into the "folk culture" shared by their community. Like everyone else, they thus grew up with the ideas about the body and its diseases that prevailed among the lay population and learnt to accept them as unquestioned,

---

656 Burke, Popular culture (1978), pp. 23–28 and, on the long-term developments, pp. 244–286.

self-evident truths. Every day, they experienced how people in their community trusted traditional diagnostic and therapeutic practices and recovered after they took medicines or were bled, after they engaged in a sympathetic ritual or resorted to a healing charm. The critical attitude physicians expressed in their publications toward lay practices and lay healers was a result of their later academic studies and part of their professional identity. But it could hardly dislodge the physicians' ideas and images of the body and its diseases that inextricably bound them to the traditional lay medical culture – the culture they had grown up with and which had become second nature to them.[657]

Another reason for the physicians' openness for popular medical ideas and practices would have been the shifting constellations of power on the contemporary health market. Some time ago, in two oft-quoted contributions, the British sociologist Nicholas Jewson, drawing on British sources, formulated fundamental theses about the physician-patient relationship in the early modern period. According to Jewson, physicians treated only a small number of socially high-ranking patients, with whom they were involved in a relationship of patronage. Under these conditions, physicians had to accommodate most of their patients' wishes and preferences if they wanted to retain their favor and secure sufficient income for themselves.[658] Jewson's theses have been justly criticized in some points. In England as on the European continent, a "relationship of patronage" between patients and their learned physicians was in no way prevalent during the time he investigated. Only very few physicians depended on the favor of a handful of patients of high standing. Even imperial and royal court physicians commonly treated sick people in the respective residential city along with the ruler and his family. As becomes evident in Handsch's notebooks, in physicians' practice journals, and in published case histories, large parts of the population at least occasionally sought the advice of a physician. In the small town of Zwickau, Hiob Finzel treated about 6,000 different patients in a period of seventeen years.[659]

---

[657] Similarly, Helman, Culture (2007), p. 125, has pointed out for modern medicine that physicians remain "also part of the 'folk' world for most of their lives – both before and after graduating from medical school. Both as individuals and as members of a particular family, community, religion or social class, they bring with them a specific set of ideas, assumptions, experiences, prejudices and inherited folklore, and this can greatly influence their medical practice."
[658] Jewson, Medical knowledge (1974); idem, Disappearance (1976).
[659] Stolberg, A sixteenth-century physician (2019).

Nevertheless, Jewson's theses prove helpful for an understanding of physicians' motives in accommodating the ideas and practices of laypeople. While the relationship between physicians and patients may only exceptionally be characterized as patronage, it is true that patients were in a comparatively powerful position for a simple reason: they had a choice. In larger towns and cities, a number of different physicians commonly worked parallel to one another, and even in places that could only boast a single learned practitioner, patients could usually just as well consult a barber, barber-surgeon, or one of the many lay healers, or make do with home remedies. Moreover, the number of learned physicians rose steeply in the course of the sixteenth century, and they increasingly settled in places where no physician had practiced before. At the same time, medicine turned into a profession that physicians relied on entirely to earn their bread and butter. While many physicians in the Middle Ages still counted among a small elite and were quite often able to secure their livelihood through sinecures from the church, most sixteenth-century physicians largely depended on the income from their practice to make a living. Also, most physicians no longer lived in celibacy but started families. Many of them had several mouths to feed and had to prepare to pay for the dowry of their daughters and the education of their sons. In a situation in which physicians knew that their patients could turn their backs on them at any time if they disliked their diagnosis or treatment, the incentive was great to make diagnoses, give explanations, and offer treatment methods that would satisfy the expectations and wishes of patients and relatives, and thus fall in line with their medical worldview.

Yet, why were the physicians unable to establish the traditional model of humoral balance in the world of laypeople? What made the explanation of diseases as resulting from raw, unclean, or spoiled morbid matter that needed to be evacuated from the body so attractive, to the point that physicians had to adapt the patients' way of thinking in this regard? We might want to look for an answer in Mary Douglas's famous study *Purity and danger*.[660] Foreign or at least insufficiently concocted and assimilated morbid matter that could be found in the body and to which laypeople attributed most diseases, was "matter out of place" in the sense of Douglas's famous definition of "dirt", and therefore unclean. According to Douglas, the collective fear of dirt and uncleanliness for its part may as a rule be understood as something that expresses the fear of a border violation, of a threat to national, ethnic, or cultural identities. In this sense, Douglas Biow has interpreted the general appreciation of clean streets and squares and the measures Italian cities of the Renaissance adopted to fight the omnipresent dirt

---

660 Douglas, Purity and danger (1978).

as a response to the experience of diverse border violations: the warring between the city states, increasing social mobility, changes in family structure, and the inherently transgressive outbreaks of the plague.[661]

However, the perception of a threat to the boundaries of a community can be found in almost any place in the world at almost any time in history. The most satisfactory explanation for the particular attraction and tenacity of the notions and images of an impure, foreign morbid matter which needed to be evacuated seems to me to be another one. It is in a broader sense a phenomenological explanation, one that involves the subjective experience of the body. We will have to exercise caution here: even the seemingly natural subjective bodily experience is culturally shaped and framed. This is vividly demonstrated by the bodily sensations – commonly described by early modern patients but no longer comprehensible to us in this way – of a rising uterus, for example, or hot vapors that found a way to rise up.[662] But if we compare it to the interpretation of diseases as resulting from an imbalance of the humors and qualities the doctrine of unclean, unnatural morbid matter clearly had advantages. The *intemperies* of traditional humoral pathology was based on an understanding of illness as a gradual deviation from a state of balance that was construed as ideal for each individual. Disease here affected the whole body which was always at the risk of a shift away from an ideal balance and the individual constantly had to make sure to maintain and, if necessary reestablish, this balance. The explanation of illness as the result of unclean, insufficiently concocted, spoiled or otherwise exogenous substances by contrast fitted in seamlessly with an ontological conception of disease. Here, it was not the body as such that became pathologically altered but the disease was like an object, something the body "had" temporarily, something external that befell it, that possibly even literally entered it like a foreign creature.[663] This also meant that it would be possible to defeat the illness once and for all by mobilizing the morbid matter and evacuating it from the body.

Individuals who lived in this period believed that they could literally experience through their senses the purifying effect of such evacuations on their own body. They felt relieved, set free, which is a sensation to which many individuals today are likely still able to relate. The black, phlegmy blood from bloodletting;

---

661 Biow, Culture (2006).
662 Stolberg, Experiencing illness (2011); see also the classical study by Norbert Elias on the rise of the modern "homo clausus" (Elias, Prozeß (1979)).
663 In his analysis of contemporary ego-documents, Robert Jütte has likewise found that illness was experienced as something that came from the outside and indeed frequently as an "autonomous being" (Jütte, Ärzte (1991), p. 124).

the mucous, bilious matter that was evacuated through vomiting; the sometimes greenish or yellowish sputum; the unpleasant stench of sweat; the waste matter produced by the intestines; the unappetizing matter that drained from pustules and abscesses, all this underscored time and again the idea that the body by its own efforts or supported by human interventions freed itself from waste matter – and then recovered in the vast majority of cases.

I would argue that no other explanatory model in the history of Western medicine corresponded so precisely and directly with subjective human experience,[664] neither the ancient and medieval model of humoral balance nor the later iatrochemical and mechanistic theories, and least of all modern biomedicine. No other explanatory model appealed directly to the senses to the same degree or conveyed a sense of empowerment and control in a comparable way. Illness was something that happened to the body, an outside influence that occupied it and appeared in the form of a materially tangible agent. The body's natural, healthy core remained unaffected. If one succeeded in rendering the morbid matter harmless and evacuating it, the disease was removed and the patient was healed.

Witchcraft and Magic

We have seen, then, how physicians and laypeople shared basic assumptions about the causes and the treatment of diseases, and how physicians, by all appearances, even shifted their views towards those of laypeople. There is one important area, however, where we have to add nuance to this notion of a shared medical worldview, namely regarding magic and sympathetic healing. As we will see, even here no distinct line can be drawn between lay or "folk" medicine on the one hand and learned medicine on the other but academically trained physicians tended to take a much more skeptical attitude than laypeople.

The belief in inflicted diseases or diseases that were "laid on" somebody as a spell seems to have been very common among the population. Handsch and his colleagues encountered it time and again. Above all, diseases with rare, unusual and persistent manifestations and sexual dysfunctions raised suspicion. For example, Handsch and Mattioli saw an approximately fifty-year-old man

---

[664] Wear, Popularized ideas (1986), p. 238, has arrived at a very similar conclusion for the seventeenth century, namely that medicine "was very close to people's perceptions and sensations of illness". As he put it, purging and bloodletting, for example, "both allowed the patient to see for himself superfluous humours being removed. If one believed that there was a mass of impurity in the body, what better for the patient than actually to see it leaving?".

from the country who for years had been experiencing a strange fit that befell him almost every month: he would feel nauseous and have intense pain in his left thigh. He would not eat for days and stand leaning against a wall without moving a muscle or saying a word until he collapsed and fainted. During the fit, the man complained, it felt as if a wild animal was lying on top of him. He could not move but only kicked about with his feet, beset by great fear. The sick man suspected that the complaint had been inflicted on him, a *maleficium*, as Handsch conveyed this suspicion. His father's lover had once cast a *maleficium* upon his mother and he feared that it had transferred to him.[665]

This was not an isolated case. An impotent decan believed that a maid had cast a spell on him.[666] Even a noblewoman like the Baroness of Hungerkasten wondered whether perhaps her husband's lover had cast a spell, giving her severe headaches and other complaints.[667] Another noblewoman sought Willenbroch and Mattioli's help because she had been unable to sleep for eight days and was trembling. She, too, believed that the cause was a *maleficium*. Handsch learnt that she had had an impotent husband whom Mattioli had cured with a "remedy for *maleficia*" that he had found in Arnaldo de Villanova's writings.[668] When a strapping young man in the service of the court was gripped by madness, people believed that a certain woman had bewitched him.[669] According to Handsch's stepmother, St. John's wort (*hypericum perforatum*) helped women in childbed ward off diabolical *maleficia*.[670] Even an old man who suffered from nothing more than burning when he passed water believed that this was due to a *maleficium* a female neighbor had cast.[671]

Handsch and the physicians in his professional environment did not doubt that diseases could be inflicted or that spells could be cast. Handsch took pride in a remedy he had invented to counteract a love spell that caused newlyweds, like his brother-in-law Heinrich, to become impotent: St. John's wort, acting as a "fuga daemonum", had to be laid in the man's bed. St. John's wort also helped with Lehner's dog, which stopped barking for two weeks; now it was barking again. And it further helped with sheep who were under a spell.[672]

---

[665] Cod. 11183, foll. 288r-289v.
[666] Cod. 11205, fol. 256v.
[667] Ibid., fol. 502r.
[668] Cod. 11183, fol. 117r.
[669] Ibid., fol. 478v.
[670] Cod. 11205, fol. 417v.
[671] Ibid., fol. 572r.
[672] Ibid., fol. 406r-v and fol. 417v.

The existence of demons and witches was generally recognized among educated people, and philosophers and theologians at the time were involved in a highly complex and sophisticated scholarly debate on the topic.[673] This scholarly demonology borrowed elements from lay culture but ultimately built a complex theoretical edifice which served to justify torture and death sentences for alleged witches.[674] Physicians, however, increasingly raised doubts. As Martin von Drembach (1500–1571) stated in 1548, it had to be conceded that demons could attack the body, but it could not be denied that the raging of *atra bilis*, or black bile, could cause very similar changes in melancholics.[675] Johann Weyer and Thomas Erastus denied that alleged witches possessed any supernatural abilities at all, saying that they were unable by their own efforts to make people sick with a spell. Rather, the originator of these misdeeds was the devil. He was very skilled at deceiving people, making them believe that the illness in question was caused by people. Erastus nevertheless demanded punishment on the grounds that the women had after all entered a pact with the devil.[676]

Physicians introduced similarly subtle distinctions when it came to magical healing. The population was familiar with a broad spectrum of practices relating to sympathetic magic and folk piety.[677] Handsch noted down a great number of them. People said that if bitten by a rabid dog, one had to put the dog's hair in the wound.[678] From a captain he heard that wounds caused by a knife, a sword, or a nail did not fester if one thrust the weapon or the nail into a piece of bacon.[679] A patient showed him an amulet that had cured his impotence.[680] The town scribe of Leipa told him about a woman suffering from a fever who recovered the instant someone put an amulet with a curative slip of paper around her neck. It read: "I, Margaretha, have the cold. Thunder, lightning, and hellish fire come into me, so it will soon go away".[681] A schoolmaster working for the Count of Donin was familiar with the use of the wood of gallows, accompanied

---

673 Cf. the magisterial study by Clark, Thinking with demons (1997).
674 Institoris, Malleus (1511); Handsch knew this work (Cod. 9666, fol. 141r; Cod. 11200, fol. 241v).
675 Drembach, De atra bile ([1548]), conclusio XX.
676 Weyer, De praestigiis (1564); Erastus, De lamiis (1578); cf. Gunnoe, Debate (2002); on Weyer see Waardt, Johann Wier (2018), with further references.
677 For a rich regional study, focussing on the Saar area see Labouvie, Verbotene Künste (1992), esp. pp. 95–110.
678 Cod. 11183, fol. 218r.
679 Cod. 11205, fol. 151r.
680 Cod. 11183, fol. 87r.
681 Cod. 11205, fol. 700v: "Ich Margaretha habe das Kalde. Donner, Pliz und hellisch Fewer komme in mich, so vergehts mich bald."

by pious prayer, to cure diseases.⁶⁸² And Handsch even thought it worthwhile to note down the exact wording of various healing charms. With fever, for example, one was to take three pieces of bread and on the first piece write "pax pater", draw a cross and say the Lord's Prayer three times, as well as three Ave Marias. On the second, one was to write "Amor. Amor filius", add two crosses, and say five Lord's Prayers and five Ave Marias, because of the Five Holy Wounds. On the third piece, one was to write "virtus spiritus sancti", say seven Lord's Prayers and seven Ave Marias, because of the seven gifts of the Holy Spirit.⁶⁸³ "Black magic" as well had Handsch's attention, for example the belief that a man would became impotent if one sewed a needle into his clothing that had been used to sew a corpse into a shroud.⁶⁸⁴

Some physicians met such procedures with a certain skepticism and denounced them as "Aberglaube" or in Latin as "superstitio".⁶⁸⁵ Handsch occasionally used this term as well. For example, he wrote "superstitio" in the margin of an entry about the way some people treated fevers. He had learned that some peeled a hardboiled egg and put it in an anthill. When the egg was consumed, so too was the fever, they claimed.⁶⁸⁶ He also thought it was "superstitio" when people believed that the fever would end when you had the sick person drink from the hand of a hangman.⁶⁸⁷ He used the term "Affenglaube" (the faith of apes) – a common synonym for "Aberglaube" (superstition) at the time – when he commented on the treatment of a "Nabelverstürzung" in an infant, carried out with the help of a fire poker that was held to the navel, while the following words were spoken: "Arrange yourself, stomach and navel, like this handle and the poker, in the name of etc."⁶⁸⁸

Yet, there are also many entries in which Handsch described the successful use of magical, sympathetic procedures without taking a critical distance and without showing any doubt that patients recovered due to these procedures. He described, for example, how his four-year-old niece fell seriously ill with a fever. She coughed, vomited, and had a strong nosebleed. To stop the latter, a certain Martha – presumably a maid – tied long pieces of red yarn around the girl's knees, elbows, wrists, and several other joints. Apparently, the sympathetic effects of the color red and the "stanching" were supposed to stop the flow of

---

682 Cod. 11183, fol. 2r.
683 Cod. 11006, fol. 186r.
684 Cod. 11183, fol. 210r; on early modern love magic see Hacke, Wirkungsmächtigkeit (2001).
685 On the history of the concept see Grodzynski, Superstitio (1974).
686 Cod. 11183, fol. 472r.
687 Cod. 11205, fol. 469r.
688 Ibid., fol. 118r.

blood. The hope was fulfilled: the child felt better the very next day. The nosebleed came back intermittently, but then stopped completely.[689] A member of the high nobility like Sigismund von Berka was familiar with this practice as well. He sent a string of red yarn to a sick man, advising him to wrap it around his fingers and the joints of his arms.[690] Twice, in two separate entries, Handsch came back to the healing effects of pepper that supposedly grew on the grave of Jaroslaw von Bernstein. Everyone in the village who was suffering from a fever had been given some of the pepper and everyone had been rid of their fever.[691]

Physicians were not fundamentally opposed to amulets either. Handsch declared that the classic incantation "Abracadabra", written on a piece of paper and hung around the neck as an amulet, was an effective remedy for fevers, even if he did not think it advisable to reveal this to patients and their relatives. To avoid appearing "superstitiosus", the physician was to put the slip of paper in a fragrant apple without the patient's knowledge and put the apple around the patient's neck.[692] From Gallo, Handsch heard a story about a certain Dr. Herdwig, whose tenacious quartan fever the physicians had been unable to cure. When an old woman finally advised him to use an amulet, the physicians allegedly gave their explicit permission. The following day, the febrile attacks were so severe that the sick man was ready to throw away the amulet, but then the attacks did not happen again.[693] Attending to a young woman with a toothache, Gallo achieved good results when he applied another sympathetic healing procedure. Based on Gallo's notes, Handsch described the procedure in detail: the *tetragrammaton* was to be written on a piece of paper – this probably refers to the letters that make up the Hebrew word for "God" or to the letters I, N, R, and I – leaving a gap between each of the letters. Then one was to pound a horseshoe nail through one letter after the other until one came to the letter that made the pain subside. As long as the nail remained there, the pain would not come back.[694]

Confronted with such evidence that academic physicians were open to magical procedures medical historians of the past have often deplored such "backwardness". They found it difficult to understand why even famous sixteenth- and seventeenth-century authors adhered to "superstitious" ideas. In their eyes, this

---

689 Cod. 11183, fol. 208v.
690 Ibid.
691 Ibid., foll. 188v-189r and fol. 240r.
692 Cod. 11200, fol. 242v.
693 Cod. 11207, fol. 153v; elsewhere in his notes (Cod. 11205, fol. 1v) Handsch mentioned a doctor of law by the name of Andreas Herdwig in Breslau.
694 Cod. 11207, fol. 83v.

was in contradiction to the rational medicine that ultimately gave rise to modern, science-based medicine. Taking a closer look at the medical debates of that period, however, leads us to a very different assessment. By no means was it primarily the old-fashioned physicians, the *antiqui*, who believed in amulets and sympathetic magical healing. On the contrary: the belief in the efficacy of magical procedures was in some respects the more modern one. It was yet another expression of the increased appreciation of empirical knowledge. It was a fundamental principle of empirically-based natural philosophy that the multifarious hidden powers and actions that appertained to natural things could only be recognized by observing effects, an idea that was developed and harnessed in the concept of *magia naturalis*.[695] The magnet's attractive force that was as inexplicable as it was undeniable and the paralyzing power of the torpedo fish, which produces electric shocks – as we know today – were vivid and oft-quoted examples. They contradicted the Aristotelian dogma that things could only act on each other by immediate contact. So, why should one exclude the possibility that such occult forces played an important role in causing and curing diseases? A renowned seventeenth-century physician like Balthasar Timaeus von Güldenklee (1600–1667) still emphatically endorsed the numerous observations and reports by various authors on such matters, asserting that they could not be discounted as mere fiction and fables. Timaeus included examples from first-hand experience, even from his own family: his servants had quarreled with an old woman who was suspected of sorcery. Soon after, Timaeus's seven-year-old daughter developed strange symptoms; she had horrible nightmares and screamed at night. Only when the old woman was burnt as a witch did the girl's condition improve.[696]

With all of this in mind, it is not surprising that a leading proponent of orthodox Galenic medicine like Johannes Lange (1485–1565) also arrived at a carefully weighed judgment: amulets, "ligatures", and similar *periapta* – objects with healing powers that were put around the neck or attached to the body to prevent or treat sickness – could certainly be effective. This was because special hidden properties ("proprietates occultae") inhered in many substances and things due to their nature or the specific influence of the stars at the time of their creation. For example, leading authors confirmed that certain plants, like St. John's wort or the herb moly had a powerful effect on evil spirits ("malignos spiritus"), protecting the houses in which they were hung. Similarly, it was

---

695 On changing concepts of magic see Müller-Jahncke, Von Ficino zu Agrippa (1979); on magic and empirical evidence Dear, Meanings (2006), esp. p. 110.
696 Timaeus von Güldenklee, Casus (1691), p. 328.

claimed, wolf dung tied to the body cured colic, and black cumin seed cured catarrh.

Lange made one important qualification: the effects had to originate from the hidden, specific, material properties of these substances. Amulets were effective because and only if certain vapors flowed from them like "atoms" ("velut atomi") into the body where they acted upon the disease. While Alexander von Tralles, Gordonius, and other, older authors might have made claims to the contrary, mere words and written characters, quotes from the Bible or demon names did not possess a curative and protective effect, no matter whether they were spoken by a conjurer or written on a slip of paper and carried on the body. The same was true of rings and seals in which, supposedly, the curative powers of stars had been harnessed. Placing one's faith in such objects, according to Lange, was superstition.[697] In his disputation *De amuletis,* Thomas Erastus (1524–1583) arrived at a similar conclusion: to credit mere words, characters, and the like with real curative power was nothing but superstition, and contradicted reason. They lacked the principles of effect that could explain a physical change.[698]

Yet, under the influence of Renaissance Platonism and its appreciation of immaterial powers and influences, there were also scholarly voices who advocated against such "moderate" views. In his influential publication *De triplici vita,* Marsilio Ficino had ascribed a significant effect even to mere words.[699] Handsch considered it noteworthy, for example, that Girolamo Cardano, based on personal experience ("propria experientia"), found that bleeding could be stanched by saying, "Blood stay inside you. Like Christ in himself", three times.[700] In the sixteenth and early seventeenth centuries, physicians with a Paracelsian orientation were particularly open to these kinds of ideas.

Some physicians even saw a commercial potential. The Nuremberg physician and Paracelsian Heinrich Wolff (1520–1581) offered the physician and poet Johannes Posthius (1520–1581) and his wife two copies of a *sigillum in piscibus,* asking two talers apiece; this included instructions on how to use it and a de-

---

697 Lange, Epistolarum (1589) pp. 159–167 (= book 1, letter 34: "De physicis medicorum ligaturis & periaptis & anulis").
698 Published posthumously in Erastus, Disputationum (1595), foll. 95–109v, Disputatio XXII: De amuletis; on Erastus and his position on central issues in contemporary medicine see also Kühlmann/Telle (1985), pp. 265–271.
699 Ficino, De triplici vita (1498); see also Müller-Jahncke, Von Ficino zu Agrippa (1979), pp. 32–39.
700 Cod. 11200, fol. 242v: "Sanguis mane in te. Sicut Christus in se"

scription of the illnesses against which it helped. He said that he had the *sigillum* produced for several gentlemen and seven copies remained.[701]

The majority of orthodox Galenic physicians until far into the seventeenth century appear to have had a certain faith in amulets and other curative objects attached to the body only in so far as the effects could be explained through their intrinsic, material powers. Some expressed skepticism even in this regard. They would not even accept Galen's claim that he cured an epileptic boy by hanging a peony around his neck.[702] For others, amulets – in the sense of substances with proven curative powers that were hung around the neck or otherwise attached to the body – formed an important part of their therapeutic repertoire. Augustin Thoner (1567–1655) in Ulm, for example, recommended an amulet made of shiny red coral for a patient's insomnia and bad dreams.[703] Numerous authors confirmed the efficacy of arsenic and mercury amulets as preventatives against the plague.[704] Following in this vein, the Berlin physician Johann Georg Magnus offered the advice that one could protect oneself from the plague not only by putting incense powder on hot coals in the morning and the evening to cleanse the air and by smelling a scented sachet at noon, but also by wearing an amulet with mercury and bezoar over the heart.[705]

Incidentally, even critically-minded contemporaries like Weyer and Erastus conceded that magic spells and amulets containing allegedly curative words or letters sometimes seemed to produce spectacular effects. They merely explained them differently, calling them the work of the Devil, who knew how to skillfully manipulate natural things and deceive humans. The purported curative success was thus demonic and using such means was against the divine order.[706]

Weyer offered a further explanation, which may strike us as remarkably modern in hindsight: the healing power of amulets and charms was owed to the power of the human mind ("vis animi nostri"), that is to the sheer belief in the efficacy of these means. Faith, he claimed, could go a long way, especially with the uneducated. This was very apparent with toothaches, for which these procedures were often used. If a sick person had no faith in the treatment or even

---

[701] Fürstlich Oettingen-Wallersteinsches Archiv Harburg, Oe.B. VII.2° 6, pp. 371f, letter from Wolff to Posthius, 24 January 1572 (www.aerztebriefe.de/id/00004767, M. Huth).
[702] Letter from the Coburg physician Peter Hofmann to Sigismund Schnitzer, Coburg 13 November 1602, in: Hornung, Cista medica [1626], pp. 386f.
[703] Thoner, Observationum (1649), p. 351; on Thoner see Kutzer, Herrgott (2000).
[704] Letter from Sigismund Schnitzer (d. 1622) to an unnamed physician, in Hornung, Cista medica ([1626]), pp. 47–54, with numerous references.
[705] Staatsbibliothek Berlin, Ms. germ. qu. 34, foll. 24r-29r, undated letter from Magnus to Sigismund von Goetze (www.aerztebriefe.de/id/00015550, S. Schlegelmilch).
[706] Erastus, Disputationum (1595), foll. 95r-110v.

thought it laughable, or if bystanders scorned it, the soothsayer ("praecantans") could do nothing. He had witnessed this in the case of a girl from the nobility, Weyer added. At first, the magic spell had relieved her toothache, but when she was reproached about it on religious grounds, the pain came back.[707]

The great influence of faith on the therapeutic result – today we would speak of placebo effects – was demonstrated vividly in stories like the one told again by Weyer, about a woman who was suffering from an eye complaint. She improved considerably after an amulet was placed around her neck. In the end, she was so much better that she took the amulet off. Someone opened it and found a slip of paper that, as it turned out, did not have biblical quotations written on it but the words: "May the Devil scratch your eyes out and shit in the holes". In his sarcastic comment, Weyer added that if spells like this were truly effective, the woman would have lost her eyes.[708] Gallo – who, according to Handsch,[709] generally thought highly of amulets – offered a similar story about an amulet that, in the judgment of physicians, could hardly have produced the good results that were attributed to it.[710] The amulet seemed to have cured a girl of tertian fever. Then a man opened it, found a slip of paper with a verse from the psalms, threw it in the fire – and the fever came back. The man consoled the girl and pretended to write the verse on another piece of paper. In fact, however, he only wrote down nonsense words. The amulet with the piece of paper was put back around the girl's neck and the fever went away again. Handsch attributed what had happened to the girl to her belief in the amulet's efficacy.[711] It was not the amulet that helped but the belief in it, he noted in another entry, commenting on a similar story, or perhaps even the same.[712]

---

[707] Weyer, De praestigiis (1564), pp. 432–434.
[708] Ibid., p. 429: "Der Teuffel kratze dir die Augen auß, scheisse dir in die Löcher".
[709] Cod. 11200, fol. 241v.
[710] Cod. 11207, fol. 154r.
[711] Cod. 9671, foll. 122v-123r, "fixa fides est quae sanat interdum".
[712] Cod. 11207, fol. 154v: "Quod signum est, amuleta non conferre sed fidem."

Conclusion

Georg Handsch was not one of the great, famous protagonists of Renaissance medicine. As a witness of his time, however, he is unique thanks to the thousands of pages of personal notes he left to posterity. Based on Handsch's notebooks and numerous other manuscript and printed sources, the aim of this book has been to reconstruct the world and the practice of Renaissance physicians with a level of differentiation and an attention to everyday realities that has not yet been attained in historical research.

This is not the right place for a full summary of the many different subject areas and issues that Handsch's notebooks illuminate, ranging from the theoretical and practical study of medicine at university to the interpretation, diagnosis, and treatment of widespread diseases in quotidian medical practice to questions regarding the physician-patient relationship, and from the role of the town and court physicians to the physicians' learned habitus and their involvement in humanism all the way to questions of personal hygiene and sexuality.

Above and beyond the sheer inexhaustible variety of detailed information they offer, Handsch's notes serve to enrich and correct our understanding of the medicine of the Renaissance period in fundamental ways. Thanks to their concrete nature and their groundedness in everyday life as well as their relaying of the perspective and language of laypeople, and supplemented by sources penned by other physicians, they permit us to paint a much more precise and realistic picture of the medicine of the time than more theory-oriented medical printed writing on which historians of Renaissance medicine have mostly relied. Looking just at the study of medicine, these sources offer new insights, for example, on the clinical teaching in hospitals and private homes, on the acquisition of practical skills like uroscopy and the manual examination of the patient, which research had hitherto assumed was not practiced by physicians, and on the in-depth anatomical training which took place outside the large anatomical demonstrations and was connected to questions of medical and surgical practice. With regard to the medical doctrine of diseases, we saw how the traditional interpretation of diseases as a result of an upset balance of humors and qualities in the body, which has often been described as the prevailing theory of that time, was almost irrelevant to the practicing physicians' understanding and treatment of diseases in the Renaissance. The majority of diseases were attributed to spoiled, rotten, acrid, burnt, or otherwise harmful morbid matter. At most, the preternatural humors were occasionally said to originate in an *intemperies* of individual organs, above all the liver. What was much more powerful and decisive for the understanding and the treatment of most diseases than the notion of imbalance, was the idea that such morbid matter resulted from the insufficient concoction of food, from putrefactive processes inside the body, from a pathogenic, searing heat – as in the case of fevers – or from blocked natural excretion. The doctrine which foregrounded the role of mobile morbid matter that could accumulate anywhere in the body went hand in hand with a pronounced tendency toward localizing disease processes in the body. This tendency in turn gave rise to a new appreciation for autopsies on deceased patients. Post-mortems were widely carried out as early as the sixteenth century, and physicians valued them highly as a source of new knowledge. To name another important finding of the research that went into this book: reading Handsch's notes, we may be surprised how actively physicians and laypeople exchanged knowledge. Handsch and the physicians in his professional environment took seriously the medical knowledge, the experience, and practices of laypeople, and even of lay healers, whom they, in the printed medical literature, lambasted and contested, calling them ignorant bunglers. In an effort to explain presumed disease processes and recommend treatments to patients and their families using accessible language and imagery, physicians drew substantially on a very limited number of explanatory elements that were familiar to laypeople. And not only that, to some degree, they also adapted their disease concepts and therapies to the expectations and wishes of laypeople.

The medical world that emerges here is colorful and fascinating but also often foreign. One of the great challenges in writing this book was to find ways of doing justice to the foreign aspects as well as to the familiar ones. I have sought to strike a careful balance between relaying the fundamental otherness of the period's conceptions of the body and disease and its diagnostic and therapeutic practices on the one hand and highlighting some of the long-term developments that, from today's perspective, marked the path toward modern medicine on the other.

Many of the ideas about the body and its diseases that I have presented in this book may appear foreign if not outright absurd to the modern reader. Judged by today's medical standards, the copious bloodletting and the drastic purgatives that were a mainstay of therapy at the time were harmful rather than beneficial in most cases. Yet, like the medicine practiced by the physicians' less educated competitors and like the various forms of medicine that still exist in different parts of the world today, the medicine of the Renaissance undoubtedly fulfilled an important function: it offered refuge and orientation. It conveyed hope, the consoling belief that it was possible to control and eliminate diseases rather than finding oneself helplessly at their mercy. And as sick people and practitioners alike saw it, this trust proved to be justified time and again. After all, at the risk of repeating myself: most illnesses as we know them today sooner or later heal by themselves or improve temporarily at least, whether treated or not. It is their natural course. Across historical periods and across cultures, however, such favorable outcomes are inevitably attributed to whichever treatment was applied. They are perceived as proof of a correct diagnosis and of the efficacy of the chosen treatment, no matter whether a patient recovers after being treated with a drastic laxative, a healing charm, homeopathic pills, or an intravenous antibiotic. And any "successful" treatment, in turn, confirms the validity of the underlying theories and explanatory models that guide diagnosis and therapy. We ask the wrong question when we wonder why people adhered to ideas about the body and its diseases that often appear absurd today, why they willingly agreed to be assailed with harsh laxatives and emetics, with bloodletting, or even with cautering irons. The question is why they should have given up their faith in practices that had, in their perception, been tried and tested for centuries and so often proved effective in everyday experience. Patients at the time may sometimes have had reason to doubt the diagnostic and therapeutic abilities of individual medical practitioners when they did not get better. But in that case they could quite simply seek the help of a different healer, without doubting the well-established principles and the practices of medicine as such.

Side by side with much that may seem foreign and bewildering to us, this book has also traced phenomena and developments in academic medicine that show the Renaissance period as occupying an important place in the development of modern medicine. The image of academic medicine during the Renaissance as a dusty, book-based science that, apart from anatomy and botany, was characterized by blind obedience to authority proves to be a caricature. Certainly, an excellent knowledge of the important works of ancient medicine and of the more recent medical writings continued to be considered indispensable. It was central to the self-image of learned physicians and was a crucial aspect of physicians' efforts to set themselves off from their lesser educated competitors. Yet, during the Renaissance, the number of academic physicians rose quickly and most of them relied on their practice to make a living. In the process, practical knowledge and skills took on central importance. Even the printed medical writings from that time reflect a clear shift toward practically-oriented and practice-based genres, such as the *observationes* and *curationes*, and toward collections of proven medicines, on which physicians could draw for their own practice. At the leading Northern Italian universities, conventional lectures now had practical training as a counterpart, bedside teaching, as it is still today at the core of medical training. Students were schooled thoroughly in identifying internal pathological processes from the patient's medical history, subjective complaints and external symptoms, and in developing a therapy, on this basis, that would address the disease causes hidden inside the body. They also acquired many diagnostic and therapeutic skills, including a knowledge of numerous medicinal plants in their natural condition and as medical preparations. Even the philological activities of the physician-humanists – removed from medical practice as they may seem at first glance – ultimately aimed at giving access to the true, pure, and – such was the hope – superior medicine of Hippocrates, Galen, and other ancient authorities, and thus making better therapeutic outcomes possible.

The concerted effort of Renaissance physicians to provide more reliable diagnoses and more effective therapies in everyday practice was accompanied by a decided turn toward empirical knowledge. The frequently invoked "scientific revolution" of the seventeenth century that made empiricism and experimentation a central source of knowledge was set in motion in no small way by the learned physicians of the Renaissance. While an increased appreciation for empirical approaches has been documented and described by many authors in the context of anatomy and botany, research in these two fields was no end in itself. Furthered above all by physicians, botany was often concerned with the medicinal use of plants. Anatomy may have served well to demonstrate the miracle of divine creation,[713] but physicians also hoped to gain a better understanding of bodily processes and thereby of the development of diseases in order to improve treatment. This is the reason why they made great efforts to shed light on disease processes by performing autopsies on deceased patients. Historical research has severely underestimated these activities, only because the physicians of the time interpreted the alterations they observed through the lens of their very different conceptions of the body and disease, classifying them accordingly. For similar reasons, because the efforts bore little fruit from a modern perspective, historians have hitherto failed to give due regard to the efforts of Renaissance physicians' quest for new, more effective medicines. This search is reflected in practice journals and notebooks, and in extensive personal collections of recipes for tried and tested medications, which many physicians created at the time. Most notably, it culminated in tests with potential antidotes, that is in early comparative, and in a modern understanding, experimental studies with human subjects.

Enhancing the status of empiricism in this fundamental way, Renaissance medicine in certain respects paved the way for the epistemological principles on which modern medicine came to be built. Yet, it would be centuries before academic medicine developed therapies and medications that could be said, also from today's vantage point, to noticeably and reliably change the course of diseases for the better. There were also intervening crosscurrents in the seventeenth and early eighteenth centuries. Many physicians tried their luck with new explanatory systems based primarily in natural philosophical axioms, including iatrochemistry and Helmontianism, or in hydraulic, mechanistic concepts like

---

713 Nutton, Wittenberg anatomy (1993).

Cartesianism. Beginning in the late seventeenth century, vitalism as well as animism, established by Georg Ernst Stahl, became increasingly influential. These schools of thought gave central importance to the specific properties of the living organism or attributed a pre-eminent role to the soul in controlling all bodily processes. Alongside traditional concepts such as "obstruction", unprecedented importance was now given to the nerves, their sensitivity and irritability. When it came to treating illness, however, people continued to rely on the methods that had, in their perception, proven their worth for centuries. Purgatives, baths, and bloodletting continued to be of paramount importance. Many patients, still in the nineteenth century, demanded bloodletting and powerful laxatives and expressed their disappointment if a dramatic result failed to materialize.[714] In France, for a limited period of time, the application of leeches even became the most important therapeutic procedure of all. The treatment remained largely the same, only the effects were explained differently: bloodletting now counteracted "irritability" and hours-long baths softened and relaxed the hardened nerves, instead of cleansing the body.

It was only in the course of the nineteenth and early twentieth centuries, with the increasing monopolization of healthcare by academic physicians, the development of the hospital into a key medical institution, and a growing openness on the part of broad sections of the population toward new, scientific findings, that physicians could radically distance themselves from the old, established conceptions and practices, without having to fear that they might be rejected by patients and ultimately risk losing their livelihood. With the exception of surgery, it would be another several decades, however, before the medical treatment of illness would be able – from today's perspective – to show clearly superior results. Among the innumerable drugs thrown on the market by the up-and-coming pharmaceutical industry in the late nineteenth and early twentieth centuries, there were, according to current knowledge, only few preparations, like the (highly toxic) syphilis drug *Salvarsan*, that were actually effective medications. This only changed with the introduction of antibiotics following the Second World War. By that time, academic medicine had already largely supplanted those traditional ideas that it had largely espoused in previous centuries. Only some fragmentary elements are still alive in today's lay medical culture, for example in the widespread notion of a "detox" or "cleanse", in the disease concepts

---

[714] See my analysis of more than 200 handwritten medical topo- and ethnographies penned by Bavarian district physicians between 1828 and 1837 (Staatsarchiv Bamberg K3FIII 1481) and in the 1860s (Bayerische Staatsbibliothek München, Cgm 6874) in Stolberg, Heilkunde (1986).

and therapies of naturopathy and homeopathy,[715] and in the many still commonly used terms such as "one's spirits", "catarrh", "hypochondria", and "melancholy", whose original meanings have long since vanished from general linguistic consciousness.

Historians have become very reluctant to speak of "progress" and the shortcomings of modern biomedicine are well known. Yet, its superior therapeutic outcomes and indeed its unprecedented successes in the treatment of many disease can hardly be denied. In this sense, it would be difficult or indeed foolish to describe the eclipse of many of the notions and practices I have outlined in this book as a history of loss. But there is a price to pay. In the Renaissance, a thorough understanding of the explanatory models and images that governed the understanding and treatment of diseases was not the prerogative of a small elite of medical experts. The patients and their relatives could easily grasp them and they seemed to be confirmed by their subjective bodily experience. Today, physicians can at best resort to images and comparisons in an attempt to translate the complex theories about the physical and biochemical processes in the sick body to the ordinary patient, which, in fact, are often not even thoroughly understood by the average medical practitioner. The shared medical world of physicians and patients in the Renaissance, with its wealth of concepts that were closely oriented on the body and experience, is indeed irretrievably lost.

---

715 This goes, in particular, for the homeopathic concept of *psora*. It attributes virtually all chronic diseases to morbid matter retained in the body after previous disease episodes.

Sources

Visual sources – List of illustrations

Cover: Egbert van Panderen (1581–1637?), Physician (from: "The medical practitioner as Christ, angel, man and devil"), Wellcome Collection, London.

Fig. 1	Joris Hoefnagel, Innsbruck with the castle of Ambras (after Alexander Colin), in: Civitates Orbis Terrarum, part 5, Cologne 1598, n° 58.
Fig. 2	Page from one of Georg Handsch's notebooks (Österreichische Nationalbibliothek, Vienna, Cod. 11183, fol. 434r).
Fig. 3	Michiel Jansz van Mierevelt, Anatomy lesson of Dr Willem van der Meer, 1617, Museum Prinsenhof, Delft.
Fig. 4	Bernard van Orley, Portrait of the physician Joris van Zeile, Musées royaux des Beaux-Arts de Belgique, Brussels.
Fig. 5	Statue of St Cosmas, with urine glass, Wellcome Collection, London.
Fig. 6	Rheubabarum in: Pietro Andrea Mattioli, I discorsi nelli sei libri di Pedacio Dioscoride Anazarbeo, Venice 1568, Wellcome Collection, London.
Fig. 7	Painful surgical treatment, oil painting by Gerrit Lundens, 1649, Wellcome Collection, London.
Fig. 8	Lukas van Leiden, Dentist, 1523, Wellcome Collection, London.
Fig. 9	Unknown painter, after Frans van Mieris (orig. 1657), The doctor's visit, Wellcome Collection, London.
Fig. 10	Distilling oven (balneum Mariae) in: Pietro Andrea Mattioli, Kreutterbuch, 1611, Universitätsbibliothek Erfurt, Sign. 13 – MA 2° 23t.
Fig. 11	Unknown artist, Guy de Chauliac performing a dissection, gouache after a 15th-century illuminated manuscript, Wellcome Collection, London.
Fig. 12	Francesco Segala, relief portrait of Archduke Ferdinand II, around 1580, Kunsthistorisches Museum, Vienna, KK 3085.
Fig. 13 and 14	Egbert van Panderen (1581–1637?), The medical practitioner as Christ, angel, man and devil, Wellcome Collection, London.
Fig. 15	Frans van Mieris, The doctor's visit, 1667, Paul Getty Museum, Los Angeles.
Fig. 16	Bath chamber with clients in a tub, on a sweating bench and undergoing cupping, Herzog August-Bibliothek, Wolfenbüttel, Cod. Guelf. 8.7. Aug. 8°, fol. 139r.

Manuscript Sources

Avignon, Bibliothèque municipale
Ms. 1998, album amicorum of Isaac Perusset

Bamberg, Staatsbibliothek
Bamberger Sammlung, Msc. misc. 385, *Memoriale practicum* by Erasmus Reinhold

Bamberg, Staatsarchiv
K3FIII 1481, collection of medical topographies and ethnographies, 1828–1837

Berlin, Staatsbibliothek
Ms. bor. 680 und 682, correspondence of Leonhard Thurneisser
Ms. germ. fol. 99, 420a, 420b, 421a, 422b, 423a, 423b, 424, 425 und 426, correspondence of Leonhard Thurneisser
Ms. lat. qu. 41, loci communes, Salomon Alberti
Hdschr. 311, medical and anatomical notes, Italy, late 16th century
Hdschr. 442, recipe book, 16th century

Bethesda, National Library of Medicine
Ms. E 63, practice notes by Bartholomäus Carrichter
Ms. E 77, album amicorum of Conrad Gessner

Bologna, Biblioteca dell'Arciginnasio
Ms. A 46, notes by an unidentified student on a private lecture by Antonio Fracanzano in Padua 1555.

Cesena, Biblioteca comunale
Ms. 167–29 treatises by Elideo Padovani on the diseases of women, on the diseases of children, and on simples

Copenhagen, Det Kongelige Bibliotek
Ms. Gl. Kongl. 4 1691, *Farrago medica* by Isaac Habrecht (1606)
Ms. Gl. kongl. S. 4° 1694, collection of medical *observationes* by Caspar Weckerlin (1616)

Dresden, Sächsische Landes- und Universitätsbibliothek
Ms. C 337, collection of consilia by French physicians

Erlangen, Universitätsbibliothek
Ms. 909, student notes from Bologna and Padua by Johannes Brünsterer, around 1550
Ms. 910, collection of student notes on collegia in Padua, around 1550
Ms. 911, student notes by Johannes Brünsterer
Ms. 935, *Mnemoneutikon* by Joachim Camerarius II.
Ms. 981, lecture notes on Alessandro Massaria, *De morbis mulierum*, 1591
Ms. 1206, loci communes by Ambrosius Prechtl

Ferrara, Biblioteca Ariostea
Collezione Antonelli, Ms. 531, student notes on the *curationes* of Antonio Musa Brasavola and other physicians in Ferrara in the 1540s

Forlì, Biblioteca comunale Aurelio Saffi
Fondo antico, Ms. 94, collection of case histories by an unknown author, early 1540s

Freiburg, Universitätsbibliothek
HS 99, Practica medicinae

Göttingen, Staats- und Universitätsbibliothek
Ms Meibom 20, notes of an unidentified medical student in Padua, around 1550
Ms Meibom 146, collection of consilia by Jacob Horst

Halle, Marienbibliothek
Ms. 92, album amicorum by Joachim Oelhafen

Heidelberg, Universitätsbibliothek
Cpl 1895-1, practice journal of Johannes Magenbuch (copy of the original in the Biblioteca Vaticana, Rome)

Innsbruck, Tiroler Landesarchiv
Ferdinandea 164, Miscellanea, including documents on Georg Handsch's death

Kopialbuch "Geschäft vom Hof", 1572, 1575 and 1576

Jena, Thüringer Universitäts- und Landesbibliothek
Ms. Prov. fol. 26 (16), Johann Altenburger's account of the death of Anna of Saxony

Leipzig, Universitätsbibliothek
Ms. 2494, *Volumen locorum communium conscriptorum*, around 1600

London, British Library
Ms Sloane 727, notes on the courses of Giovanni Domenico Sala, Padua, for the preparation of medical exams, 1620

London, Wellcome Library
Western Manuscripts 330, recipe book

Montpellier, Bibliothèque de la Ville
Manuscrits Germain, Ms. 111, *Liber procuratoris* (copy)

Munich, Bayerische Staatsbibliothek
Cgm 3733, Tobias Geiger, *Discursus medicus und politicus* (1656)
Cgm 6874, collection of medical topographies and ethnographies by Bavarian district physicians, 1860s
Clm 25087, Michael Braun, *Formula loquendi vulgariter in iudicio urinali*, early 16th century

Münster, Stadtarchiv
A-RatsA_A II Nr. 20, minutes of the town magistrate, vol. 42 (1610)

New Haven, Medical Historical Library, Yale University, no shelf mark, medical manuscript, around 1552

Nürnberg, Stadtbibliothek
Ms. Cent. V, 10b, practice journal of Georg Palm

Nürnberg, Germanisches Nationalmuseum
Hs 100.822, practice journal of Georg Palm

Padua, Archivio antico dell'Università
n. 476 and n. 477, *Epistolario della nazione degli artisti*, 1565–1647

St. Gallen, Kantonsbibliothek Vadiana
Ms. 408, medical *loci communes* by an unidentified writer

Stockholm, Kungliga Biblioteket
X 101 *Receptur-Diarium* of Petrus Kirsten, 1612–1616

Stuttgart, Hauptstaatsarchiv
A 209, Bü 725, proceedings regarding unauthorized medical practice
A 228, Bü 68, includes various letters written by physicians
A 282, Bü. 1301, personnel file of Johann Schwartz

Ulm, Stadtarchiv
J1 Autographen, L 74–76, correspondence of the family Gockel

Utrecht, Universiteitsbiblioteek
ms. VII E 49, medical journal of Cornelis Booth

Valence, Archives départementales de la Drôme
Ms. D 17, list of doctoral degrees

Venice, Archivio di Stato
Riformatori allo Studio di Padova 419 and 449, correspondence

Venice, Biblioteca Marciana
Cod. lat. VII 66 (=9684), Girolamo Amalteo

Vienna, Österreichische Nationalbibliothek
NB: In this book, shelf marks that are limited to a „Cod." followed by a four- or five-digit number refer to the holdings of the Österreichische Nationalbibiothek
Cod. 9550, 9607, 9650 9666, 9671, 9821, 11006, 11130, 11141–3, 11153, 11183, 11200, 11204–11208, 11210, 11226, 11231, 11238–40 and 11251, manuscripts of Georg Handsch
Cod. 11083, consilium of an unidentified physician on the prevention of kidney stones, probably written for Archduke Ferdinand II
Cod. 11144, Paracelsian manuscript, by an unidentified writer
Cod. 11155, copies of two consilia for Archduke Ferdinand II, one by Renato Brasavola (wrongly dated 1554) and one written collectively by Giulio Alessandrini, Pietro Andrea Mattioli and Christoph Heuberger, around 1571
Cod. 11158, consilium by Andrea Gallo for Emperor Maximilian II, around 1555
Cod. 11182, medico-surgical miscellanea
Cod. 11228, *Annotationes in Nonum Rhasis ad Almansorem dictatae a doctore Augustino Schurphio in schola Vitebergensi Anno 1537*

Washington DC, Folger Library
Bd.w. 158-133q, album amicorum of Johann Ulrich Höcklin, 1564–1574

Weimar, Anna-Amalia-Bibliothek
Stb 134, album amicorum of David Wirsung

Weimar, Thüringisches Hauptstaatsarchiv
Ernestinisches Gesamtarchiv, Reg. Rr 1-316, 803, personnel file of Antonius Juncker.

Wrocław, Biblioteka Uniwersytecka
Library of the Church of Maria Magdalena, M. 1024, practice notes by Bartholomäus Carrichter

Zwickau, Ratschulbibliothek
Ms. QQQQ1, Ms. QQQQ1a und Ms QQQQ1b, *Ratiocinium* (practice journal and account book of Hiob Finzel)

Printed Works

Abe, Rudolf Horst: *Die Erfurter medizinische Fakultät in den Jahren 1392–1524*. Leipzig 1974.
Absmeier, Christine: *Das schlesische Schulwesen im Jahrhundert der Reformation. Ständische Bildungsreformen im Geiste Philipp Melanchthons*. Stuttgart 2011.
Achillini, Alessandro: *Opera omnia in unum collecta cum annotationibus excellentissimi doctoris Pamphilii Montii Bononiensis*. Venice 1545.
Adam, Melchior: *Vitae Germanorum medicorum, qui seculo superiori, et quod excurrit, claruerunt*. Heidelberg 1620.
Aëtius of Amida: *Libri XVI*. Vol. 3. Transl. by Giovanni Battista da Monte. Basel 1535.
Aewerdieck, Björn: *Register zu den Wunderzeichenbüchern Job Fincels*. Frankfurt am Main 2010.
Agasse, Jean-Michel: Introduction. In: idem and Concetta Pennuto (eds): *Une correspondance entre deux médecins humanistes. Girolamo Mercuriale – Johann Crato von Krafftheim*. Geneva 2016, pp. 9–133.
Agricola, Georgius: *De ortu et causis subterraneorum libri V. De natura eorum quae effluunt ex terra libri IV. De natura fossilium libri X. De veteribus et novis metallis libri II. Bermannus sive de re metallica dialogus*. Basel 1546.
Agrimi, Jole and Chiara Crisciani: *Consilia médicaux*. Turnhout 1994.
Aho, James: *Confession and bookkeeping. The religious, moral, and rhetorical roots of modern accounting*. Albany, NY 2005.
Albrecht, Stefan: Prag. In: Wolfgang Adam and Siegrid Westphal (eds): *Handbuch kultureller Zentren der Frühen Neuzeit. Städte und Residenzen im alten deutschen Sprachraum*. Berlin/Boston 2012, pp. 1649–1694.
Alciati, Andrea: *Emblematum liber*. Augsburg 1531.
Algazi, Gadi: Eine gelernte Lebensweise: Figurationen des Gelehrtenlebens zwischen Mittelalter und Früher Neuzeit. In: *Berichte zur Wissenschaftsgeschichte* 30 (2007), pp. 107–118.
Algazi, Gadi: Food for thought. Hieronymus Wolf grapples with the scholarly habitus. In: Rudolf Dekker (ed.): *Egodocuments and history. Autobiographical writing in its social context since the Middle Ages*. Hilversum 2002, pp. 21–44.
Algazi, Gadi: "Geistesabwesenheit". Gelehrte zuhause um 1500. In: Alf Lüdtke and Reiner Prass (eds): *Gelehrtenleben. Wissenschaftspraxis in der Neuzeit*. Köln/Weimar/Vienna 2007, pp. 215–234.
Algazi, Gadi: Habitus, familia und forma vitae. Die Lebensweise mittelalterlicher Gelehrter in muslimischen, jüdischen und christlichen Gemeinden – vergleichend betrachtet. In: Frank Rexroth (ed.): *Beiträge zur Kulturgeschichte der Gelehrten im späten Mittelalter*. Ostfildern 2010, pp. 185–217.
Algazi, Gadi: Scholars in households. Refiguring the learned habitus, 1480–1550. In: *Science in context* 16 (2003), pp. 9–42.
Algazi, Gadi, Valentin Groebner and Bernhard Jussen (eds): *Negotiating the gift. Pre-modern figurations of exchange*. Göttingen 2003.
Alkemeyer, Thomas, Gunilla Budde and Dagmar Freist (eds): *Selbst-Bildungen. Soziale und kulturelle Praktiken der Subjektivierung*. Bielefeld 2013.
Alkemeyer, Thomas: Subjektivierung in sozialen Praktiken. Umrisse einer praxeologischen Analytik. In: Alkemeyer, Budde and Freist, *Selbst-Bildungen* (2013), pp. 33–68.

Allen, Percy Stafford: Some letters of masters and scholars 1500–1530. In: *The English historical review* 22 (1907), pp. 740–754.
Alpinus, Prosper: *De praesagienda vita et morte aegrotantium libri septem*. Frankfurt 1601.
Amatus Lusitanus: *Curationum medicinalium centuria prima, multiplici variaque rerum cognitione referta*. Florence 1551.
Amatus Lusitanus: *Curationum medicinalium centuria prima, multiplici variaque rerum cognitione referta*. Paris 1552.
Amatus Lusitanus: Introitus ad aegrotantem. Simulque disgressio de crisi et diebus decretoribus. In: idem: *Curationum* (1552), pp. 1–61.
Alvarez, Antonio: *Epistolarum et consiliorum medicinalium pars prima*. Naples 1585.
Andreozzi, Alfonso: Le leggi penali degli antichi Chinesi: discorso proemiale sul diritto e sui limiti del punire e traduzioni originali dal cinese. Florence 1878.
Andreska, Jan: Losos labský v historických záznamech a v současnosti I. In: *Živa* (2010), pp. 178–182.
Andretta, Elisa and Marilyn Nicoud (eds): *Être médecin à la cour (Italie, France, Espagne, XIIIe -XVIIIe siècle)*. Florence 2013.
Andretta, Elisa: *Roma medica. Anatomie d'un système médical au XVIe siècle*. Rome 2011.
Arbenz, Emil and Hermann Wartmann (eds): *Die Vadianische Briefsammlung der Stadtbibliothek St. Gallen*. Part 6 and 7. St. Gallen 1906–1913.
Arber, Agnes: *Herbals. Their origin and evolution*. Cambridge 1986.
Arcaeus, Franciscus: *De recta curandorum vulnerum ratione libri II*. Antwerp 1574.
Argenterio, Giovanni: *De morbis libri XIIII*. Florence 1556.
Arrizabalaga, Jon, John Henderson and Roger French: *The great pox. The French disease in Renaissance Europe*. New Haven 1997.
Assion, Peter and Joachim Telle: Der Nürnberger Stadtarzt Johannes Magenbuch. Zu Leben und Werk eines Mediziners der Reformationszeit. In: *Sudhoffs Archiv* 56 (1972), pp. 353–421.
Augenio, Orazio: *Epistolarum et consultationum medicinalium prioris tomi libri XII*. Venice 1602.
Aumüller, Gerhard: Professor in Marburg und Leibarzt in Kassel? Lebensbilder hessischer Ärzte zur Zeit des Landgrafen Philipp (1504–1567) und die weitere Entwicklung der Medizin unter Landgraf Moritz (1572–1632). In: Irmtraut Sahmland and Kornelia Grundmann (eds): *Perspektiven der Medizingeschichte Marburgs. Neue Studien und Kontexte*. Darmstadt/ Marburg 2011, pp. 11–46.
Austrius, Sebastianus: *De infantium sive puerorum morborum et symptomatorum dignitione tum curatione liber*. Basel 1540.
Avicenna, *Canon medicinae*. Ed. and comm. by Giovanni Costeo. Venice 1595.
Baader, Gerhard: Medizinische Theorie und Praxis zwischen Arabismus und Renaissancehumanismus. In: Gundolf Keil, Bernd Moeller Bernd and Winfried Trusen (eds): *Der Humanismus und die oberen Fakultäten*. Weinheim 1987, pp. 185–213.
Bacchelli, Franco: Antonio Musa Brasavola archiatra di Ercole II duca di Ferrara. In: *Micrologus* 16 (2008), pp. 327–346.
Bachmann, Hans: Dr. Johann Peter Merenda. Aus dem Leben eines Innsbrucker Hofarztes, 1542 bis 1567. In: *Tiroler Heimatblätter* 28 (1953), pp. 5–10.
Bacon, Francis: *Twoo bookes [. . .] Of the proficience and advancement of learning, divine and humane*. London 1605.
Baillou, Guillaume: *Consiliorum medicinalium libri II*. 3 vols. Ed. by Jacques Thevart. Paris 1635.

Banzer, Marcus: *Fabrica receptarum. Id est: methodus brevis, perspicua ac facilis in qua quae sint remediorum compositorum formae, quae earundem differentiae, quae componendi & praescribendi ratio [. . .] planissime edocetur.* Augsburg 1622.
Barker-Benfield, G. J.: *The culture of sensibility. Sex and society in eighteenth-century Britain.* Chicago/London 1992.
Bartholinus, Thomas: *De libris legendis dissertationes.* Ed. by Joh. Gerh. Meuschen. Frankfurt 1711.
Bauch, Gustav: *Valentin Trozendorf und die Goldberger Schule.* Berlin 1921.
Bauer, Barbara: Die Rolle des Hofastrologen und Hofmathematikus als fürstlicher Berater. In: August Buck (ed.): *Höfischer Humanismus.* Weinheim 1989, pp. 93–117.
Bauhin, Caspar: *Gynaeciorum sive de mulierum affectibus commentarii.* Basel 1586.
Bayle, Ariane: Thériaque et triacleurs chez Pierre-André Mathiole. In: Sarah Voinier and Guillaume Winter (eds): *Poison et antidote dans l'Europe des XVIe et XVIIe siècles.* Paris 2011, pp. 33–47.
Bedini, Gianni: *L'orto botanico di Pisa. Piante, storia, personaggi, ruoli / The botanic garden of Pisa. Plants, history, people, roles.* Pisa 2007.
Beer, Karl: Philippine Welser als Freundin der Heilkunst. In: *Gesnerus* 7 (1950), pp. 80–86.
Beierlein, Paul Reinhard: Der kursächsische Leibarzt Sigismund Kohlreuter (1534–1599). In: *Sudhoffs Archiv* 38 (1954), pp. 70–83.
Belloni Speciale, Gabriella: Falloppia, Gabriele. In: *Dizionario biografico degli Italiani* 44 (1994) (http://www.treccani.it/enciclopedia/gabriele-falloppia_%28Dizionario-Biografico%29/)
Belmas, Elisabeth and Serenella Nonnis Vigilante (eds): *Les relations médecin-malade des temps modernes à l'époque contemporaine.* Villeneuve d'Ascq-France 2013.
Ben-Chaim, Michael: *Experimental philosophy and the birth of empirical science. Boyle, Locke, and Newton.* Aldershot 2004.
Benivieni, Antonio: *De abditis nonnullis ac mirandis morborum et sanationum causis.* Ed. by Giorgio Weber. Florence 1994.
Benzenhöfer, Udo and Wilhelm Kühlmann (eds): *Heilkunde und Krankheitserfahrung in der Frühen Neuzeit.* Tübingen 1992.
Bergdolt, Klaus: *Das Gewissen der Medizin. Ärztliche Moral von der Antike bis heute.* Munich 2004.
Berg, Alexander: *Der Krankheitskomplex der Kolik- u[nd] Gebärmutterleiden in Volksmedizin und Medizingeschichte unter besonderer Berücksichtigung der Volksmedizin in Ostpreußen. Ein Beitrag zur Erforschung volkstümlicher Krankheitsvorstellungen.* Berlin 1935.
Bergdolt, Klaus, Berndt Hamm and Andreas Tönnesmann (eds): *Das Kind in der Renaissance.* Wiesbaden 2008.
Bernardi, Francesco: *Prospetto storico-critico. Dell'origine, facoltà, diversi stati, progressi, e vicende del Collegio medico chirurgico, e dell'arte chirurgica in Venezia.* Venice 1797.
Berthold, Andreas: *Compendium breve de terrae sigillatae usu commodissimo & utilissimo.* Sine loco 1589.
Berthold, Andreas: *Nützlicher unnd nothwendiger Bericht von der Krafft, Würckung, Tugendt und Eigenschafften, der hülffreichen Terrae Sigillatae.* Frankfurt 1597.
Berthold, Andreas: *Terrae sigillatae nuper in Germania repertae vires atque virtutes admirandae eiusque administrandae ac usurpandae ratio.* Frankfurt 1583.

Berthold, Andreas: *The wonderfull and strange effect and vertues of a new Terra sigillata lately found out in Germanie, with the right order of the applying and administring of it: being oftentimes tried and experienced.* London 1587.
Bertolaso, Bartolo: La cattedra "De pulsibus et urinis" (1601–1748) nello studio padovano. In: *Castalia* 16 (1960), pp. 109–117.
Bertolaso, Bartolo: Richerche d'archivio su alcuni aspetti dell'insegnamento medico presso la Università di Padova nel cinque- e seicento. In: *Acta medicae historiae patavina* 6 (1958–59), pp. 17–37.
Beukers, Harm: Clinical teaching in Leiden from its beginning until the end of the eighteenth century. In: idem and J. Moll (eds): *Clinical teaching, past and present.* Amsterdam/Atlanta, GA, pp. 139–152.
Bianchi, Massimo Luigi: Il tema dell'esperienza in Paracelso. In: Marco Veneziani (ed.): Experientia. Florence 2002, pp. 199–216.
Bianchi, Massimo Luigi: Occulto e manifesto in Jean Fernel e Pietro Severino. In: *Atti e memorie dell'Accademia toscana di scienze e lettere "La Colombaria"* 47 (1982), pp. 185–248.
Bienert, Karl J.: Böhm[isch] Leipa, das Verkehrs-, Wirtschafts- und Kulturzentrum Böhmens. In: *Heimat-Buch.* Bodenbach a. Elbe [c. 1937], pp. 1–5.
Bigotti, Fabrizio: *Physiology of the soul. Mind, body and matter in the Galenic tradition of the late Renaissance (1550–1630).* Turnhout 2019.
Biow, Douglas: The culture of cleanliness in Renaissance Italy. Ithaca/London 2006.
Blair, Ann: Humanist methods in natural philosophy. The commonplace book. In: *Journal of the history of ideas* 53 (1992), pp. 541–551.
Blair, Ann: Reading strategies for coping with information overload, ca. 1550–1700. In: *Journal of the history of ideas* 64 (2003), pp. 11–28.
Blair, Ann M.: *Too much to know. Managing scholarly information before the modern age.* New Haven/London 2010.
Bloch, Iwan: *Der Ursprung der Syphilis. Eine medizinische und kulturgeschichtliche Untersuchung.* 2 vols. Jena 1901/1911.
Bodenstein, Adam von (ed.): *Metamorphosis.* Basel 1572.
Bodin, Jean: *Universae naturae theatrum: in quo rerum omnium effectrices causae et fines contemplantur et continuae series quinque libris discutiuntur.* Lyon 1596.
Boehm, Laetitia u.a. (ed.): *Biographisches Lexikon der Ludwig-Maximilians-Universität München.* Part 1: *Ingolstadt-Landshut 1472–1826.* Berlin 1998.
Boissier de Sauvages, François: *Nosologia methodica sistens morborum classes juxta Sydenhami mentem et botanicorum ordinem.* Vol. 1. Venice 1773.
Bonnet, Théophile: *Sepulchretum sive anatomia practica ex cadaveribus morbo denatis.* Geneva 1679.
Bösch, Alexander: *Liber familiarum personalium, das ist, Verzeichnus waß sich mit mir, und der meinigen in meiner haußhaltung, sonderliches begeben und zugetragen hatt. Lebensbericht und Familiengeschichte des Toggenburger Pfarrers Alexander Bösch (1618–1693).* Ed. by Lorenz Heiligensetzer. Basel 2001.
Boscius, Joannis Loneus: *De lapidibus qui nascuntur in corpore humano, et praecipue renibus ac vesica, et ipsorum curatione theses. Respondente Andrea Helepyro.* Ingolstadt 1580.
Botalli, Leonardo: *Commentarioli duo, alter de medici, alter de aegroti munere.* Lyon 1565.
Bottoni, Albertino: *De morbis muliebribus.* Padua 1585.

Boudewijns, Michael: *Ventilabrum medico-theologicum, quo omnes casus cum medicos tum aegros aliosque concernentes eventilantur, et quod SS. PP. conformius, scholasticis probabilius, & in conscientia tutius est, secernitur.* Antwerp 1666

Boudon-Miller, Véronique and Guy Cobolet: *Lire les médecins Grecs à la Renaissance.* Paris 2004.

Bourbon, Florence: Jean Liebault (1535–1596), médicin hippocratique. Vers la gynécologie moderne. In: *Renaissance and Reformation* 33 (2010), pp. 61–84.

Bourdieu, Pierre: *Esquisse d'une théorie de la pratique, précédé de trois études d'ethnologie kabyle.* Geneva 1972.

Bourdieu, Pierre: Les trois états du capital culturel. In: *Actes de la recherche en sciences sociales* 30 (1979), pp. 3–6.

Bourdieu, Pierre: The forms of capital. In: John G. Richardson (ed.): *Handbook of theory and research for the sociology of education.* New York 1986, pp. 241–60.

Braembussche, A. A. van den: Het biografisch element in de geschiedschrijving. Een geschiedstheoretische verkenning. In: *Tijdschrift voor sociale geschiedenis* 15 (1989), pp. 26–60.

Brambilla, Giovanni Alessandro: *Scuola Longobarda: Pavesi, Milanesi, Piemontesi, Genovesi, Piacentini, Parmigiani, Modenesi, Ferraresi, Bolognesi, Veronesi, Padovani ec.* Vol. 2, 1: *Secolo XVI.* Milan 1781.

Brasavola, Antonio Musa: *In octo libros aphorismorum Hippocratis et Galeni commentaria et annotationes.* Basel 1541.

Brendecke, Arndt (ed.): *Praktiken der Frühen Neuzeit. Akteure – Handlungen – Artefakte.* Cologne/Weimar/Vienna 2015.

Brendel, Johann Philipp (ed.): *Consilia medica celeberrimorum quorundam Germaniae medicorum.* Frankfurt 1615.

Brockliss, Laurence W.B.: Curricula. In: Ridder-Symoens, *History* (1996), pp. 565–620.

Brockliss, Laurence W.B.: *French higher education in the seventeenth and eighteenth centuries. A cultural history.* Oxford 1987.

Brockliss, Laurence W.B. and Colin Jones: *The medical world of early modern France.* Oxford 1997.

Bröer, Ralf: *Höfische Medizin. Strukturen der medizinischen Versorgung eines frühneuzeitlichen Fürstenhofes am Beispiel des Wiener Kaiserhofes (1650–1750).* Habilitationsschrift. Heidelberg 2006.

Brosseder, Claudia: *Im Bann der Sterne. Caspar Peucer, Philipp Melanchthon und andere Wittenberger Astrologen.* Berlin 2004.

Brugi, Biagio: *Gli scolari dello studio di Padova nel cinquecento. Discorso inaugurale.* Padua 1903.

Brunfels, Otto: *Theses seu communes loci totius rei medicae.* Strasbourg 1532.

Brunschwig, Hieronymus: *Buch der Cirurgia. Hantwirckung der Wund Artzney.* Augsburg 1497.

Brunschwig, Hieronymus: *Großes Destillierbuch.* Strasbourg 1512.

Brunschwig, Hieronymus: *Das Buch zu Destilliren die zusamen gethonen Ding.* Strasbourg 1519.

Brunschwig, Jacques and Geoffrey E. R. Lloyd (eds), in collaboration with Pierre Pellegrin: *Greek thought. A guide to classical knowledge.* Cambridge/London 2000.

Buchwald, Georg: Simon Wilde aus Zwickau. Ein Wittenberger Studentenleben zur Zeit der Reformation. In: *Mitteilungen der Deutschen Gesellschaft in Leipzig* 9 (1894), pp. 61–111.

Bünz, Enno: Leibärzte. In: Werner Paravicini (ed.): *Höfe und Residenzen im spätmittelalterlichen Reich. Bilder und Begriffe.* Vol. I: *Begriffe.* Ostfildern 2005, pp. 156–157.
Burckhardt, Jacob: *Die Cultur der Renaissance. Ein Versuch.* Basel 1860.
Burke, Peter: Images as evidence in seventeenth-century Europe. In: *Journal of the history of ideas* 64 (2003), pp. 273–296.
Burke, Peter: Individuality and biography in the Renaissance. In: Enno Rudolph (ed.): *Die Renaissance und die Entdeckung des Individuums in der Kunst. Die Renaissance als erste Aufklärung II.* Tübingen 1998, pp. 65–78.
Burke, Peter: *Popular culture in early modern Europe.* London 1978.
Buschmann, Nicolaus: Persönlichkeit und geschichtliche Welt. Zur praxeologischen Konzeptualisierung des Subjekts in der Geschichtswissenschaft. In: Alkemeyer, Budde and Dagmar Freist, *Selbst-Bildungen* (2013), pp. 125–149.
Bůžek, Václav: *Ferdinand von Tirol zwischen Prag und Innsbruck. Der Adel aus den böhmischen Ländern auf dem Weg zu den Höfen der ersten Habsburger.* Cologne/Weimar 2009.
Bylebyl, Jerome J.: *Cardiovascular physiology in the sixteenth and early seventeenth centuries.* PhD-thesis, Yale University. New Haven 1969.
Bylebyl, Jerome J.: Medicine, philosophy and humanism in Renaissance Italy. In: John W. Shirley and F. David Hoeniger (eds): *Science and the arts in the Renaissance.* Washington, D.C. 1985, pp. 27–49.
Bylebyl, Jerome J.: The school of Padua: humanistic medicine in the sixteenth century. In: Charles Webster (ed.): *Health, medicine and mortality in the sixteenth century.* Cambridge 1979, pp. 335–370.
Bylebyl, Jerome: The manifest and the hidden in the Renaissance clinic. In: William F. Bynum and Roy Porter (eds): *Medicine and the five senses.* Cambridge 2004, pp. 40–60.
Calabritto, Monica: Medicina practica, consilia and the illnesses of the head in Girolamo Mercuriale and Giulio Cesare Claudini. Similarities and differences of the sexes. In: *Medicina e storia* 11 (2006), pp. 63–83.
Calabritto, Monica: Curing melancholia in sixteenth-century medical *consilia* between theory and practice. In: *Medicina nei secoli* 24 (2012), pp. 627–664.
Camerarius, Joachim: *Arithmologia ethica, loci communes, et epigrammata.* Leipzig 1552.
Capivaccia, Girolamo: De modo interrogandi aegros. In: idem: *Opera omnia.* Ed. by Johann Hartmann Beyer. Frankfurt 1603, pp. 236–237.
Cappelletti, Elsa M.: Le piante coltivate nell'orto botanico di Padova ai tempi di Luigi Squalermo detto Anguillara. In: Minelli, *L'orto* (1995), pp. 162–171.
Cardano, Girolamo: *De malo recentiorum medicorum medendi usu libellus.* Venice 1536.
Cardano, Girolamo: *Opera quaedam lectu digna.* Basel 1562.
Carlino, Andrea: *Books of the body. Anatomical ritual and Renaissance learning.* Chicago 1999.
Carrichter, Bartholomaeus: *Kräutterbuch. Darinnen begriffen, under welchem Zeichen Zodiaci, auch in welchem Gradu ein jedes Kraut stehe, wie sie in Leib, und zu allen Schäden zu bereiten, und zu welcher Zeit sie zu colligieren sein.* Strasbourg 1609.
Castelli, Bartolommeo: *Lexicon medicum graecolatinum [. . .] ex Hippocrate, et Galeno desumptum.* Messana 1598
Castro, Roderigo da: *Medicus-politicus: sive de officiis medico-politicis tractatus.* Hamburg 1614.
Castro, Roderigo da: *Universa mulierum medicina.* Part 2. Hamburg 1662 (1st edn 1603).

Cavallo, Sandra and Tessa Storey: *Healthy living in late Renaissance Italy*. Oxford 2014.
Celsus, Aulus Cornelius: *De medicina libri octo*. Ed. by Johannes Antonides van der Linden, Leiden 1657.
Celtis, Konrad: *Quattuor libri amorum secundum quattuor latera Germaniae. Germania generalis. Accedunt carmina aliorum ad libros amorum pertinentia*. Ed. by Felicitas Pindter. Leipzig 1934.
Champier, Symphorien: *Claudii Galeni Pergameni historiales campi [. . .] in quatuor libros congesti et commentariis non poenitendis illustrati*. Basel 1532.
Chauliac, Guy de: *Chirurgia*. Leiden 1559.
Chauliac, Guy de: *Guigonis de Caulhiaco inventarium sive chirurgia magna*. Ed. by Michael R. McVaugh, vol. 1: *Text*. Leiden 1997.
Chifflet, Jean: *Singulares tam ex curationibus, quam cadaverum sectionibus observationes*. Paris 1612.
Ciancio, Luca: "Per questa via s'ascende a magior seggio". Pietro Andrea Mattioli e le scienze mediche e naturali alla corte di Bernardo Cles. In: *Studi Trentini. Storia* 94 (2015), pp. 159–184.
Ciancio, Luca: Many gardens – real, symbolic, visual – of Pietro Andrea Mattioli. In: Juliette Ferdinand (ed.): *From art to science. Experiencing nature in the European garden 1500–1700*. Treviso 2016, pp. 35–45
Cicero, Marcus Tullius: *Epistulae ad familiares*. Venice 1471.
Cipolla, Carlo M.: *Public health and the medical profession in the Renaissance*. Cambridge 1976.
Clark, Stuart: *Thinking with demons. The idea of witchcraft in early modern Europe*. Oxford 1997
Clauser, Christoph: *Das die Betrachtung des Menschenn Harns on anderen Bericht unnütz*. Sine loco [1543].
Clouse, Michele L.: *Medicine, government and public health in Philip II's Spain. Shared interests, competing authorities*. Farnham 2011.
Codronchi, Baptista: *De christiana ac tuta medendi ratione*. Ferrara 1591.
Coiter, Volcher: *Externarum et internarum principalium humani corporis partium tabulae, atque anatomicae exercitationes observationesque variae*. Nürnberg 1573.
Collinus, Matthaeus et alii: *Prima farrago sacri argumenti poematum ab aliquot studiosis poeticae bohemis scriptorum diversis temporibus ad nobilem et clarissimum virum D. Ioannem Seniorem Hoddeiovinum ad Hoddeiova*. Prague [1561].
Collinus, Matthaeus et alii: *Tertia farrago poematum*. Prague 1561.
Collinus, Matthaeus et alii: *Quarta farrago poematum*. Prague 1562.
Colombo, Realdo: *De re anatomica libri XV*. Venice 1559.
Comparetti, Andrea: *Saggio della Scuola Clinica nello Spedale di Padova*. Padua 1793.
Cook, Harold J.: Good advice and little medicine. The professional authority of early modern English physicians. In: *Journal of British studies* 33 (1994), pp. 1–31.
Cook, Harold J.: Medicine. In: Katharine Park and Lorraine Daston (eds): *Early modern science* (= The Cambridge History of Science, vol. 3). Cambridge 2006, pp. 407–434.
Cook, Harold J.: Physicians and natural history. In: Nicholas Jardine, James Secord and Emma Spary (eds): *Cultures of natural history*. Cambridge 1996, pp. 91–105.
Cook, Harold J.: *Trials of an ordinary doctor: Joannes Groenevelt in seventeenth-century London*. Baltimore 1994.

Cook, Harold J.: Victories for empiricism, failures for theory. Medicine and science in the seventeenth-century. In: Charles T. Wolfe and Ofer Gal (eds): *The body as object and instrument of knowledge. Embodied empiricism and early modern science*. Dordrecht 2010, pp. 9–32.
Cooper, Glen M.: Approaches to the critical days in late medieval and Renaissance thinkers. In: *Early science and medicine* 18 (2013), pp 536–565.
Cordus, Euricius: *De urinis. Das ist von rechter Besichtigunge des Harns und ihrem Mißbrauch*. Ed. by J. Dryander. Frankfurt 1543.
Cordus, Valerius: *Pharmacorum omnium, quae quidem in usu sunt, conficiendorum ratio: vulgo vocant dispensatorium pharmacopolarum*. Nürnberg 1546.
Cornarius, Janus: *Medicina, sive medicus, liber unus. Eiusdem orationes II: I. Hippocrates, sive doctor verus: II. de rectis medicinae studiis amplectendis*. Basel 1556.
Cornaro, Alvise: *Discorsi della vita sobria*. Milan 1627.
Crato, Johannes: *Consiliorum et epistolarum medicinalium liber*. Ed. by Lorenz Scholz. Frankfurt am Main 1591.
Crato, Johannes: *Consiliorum et epistolarum medicinalium liber quintus*. Hanau 1594.
Cunsolo, Elisabetta: Giulio Casserio e la pubblicazione del *De Vocis Auditusque Organis* tra Padova e Ferrara all'inizio del '600. In: *Mélanges de l'école française de Rome* 120–122 (2008), pp. 385–405.
Da Monte, Giovanni Battista: *Consilia medica omnia, quae ullibi extant, partim antea, partim nunc primum edita*. Ed. by Girolamo Donzellini. Nürnberg 1559.
Da Monte, Giovanni Battista: *Consultationum medicinalium centuria prima*. Ed. by Valentinus Lublinus. Venice 1554 (further edn 1556).
Da Monte, Giovanni Battista: *Consultationum medicinalium ad varia morborum genera, centuria tertia*. Venice 1558.
Da Monte, Giovanni Battista: *Consultationum medicinalium centuria secunda*. Venice 1559.
Da Monte, Giovanni Battista: *Consultationum medicarum opus absolutissimum*. Ed. by Johannes Crato. Basel 1565.
Da Monte, Giovanni Battista: De uterinis affectibus. In: idem: *Opuscula*. Ed. by Valentinus Lublinus. Venice 1554, foll. 63r-109v.
Da Monte, Giovanni Battista: *Lectiones de urinis*. Ed. by Franz Emmerich. Vienna 1552.
Da Monte, Giovanni Battista: *Methodus de elementis, cui accessit De syphillidos lue tractatus, unacum regulari cura huius morbi Benedicti faventini*. Vienna 1553.
Da Monte, Giovanni Battista: *Opuscula varia ac praeclara*. 2 vols. Basel 1558.
Darmon, Pierre: *Le tribunal de l'impuissance*. Paris 1979.
Daston, Lorraine: Perché i fatti sono brevi? In: *Quaderni storici* 108 (2001), pp. 745–770.
Daston, Lorraine: Taking note(s). In: *Isis* 95 (2004), pp. 443–448.
Daston, Lorraine and Katharine Park: *Wonders and the order of nature, 1150–1750*. New York 1998.
Davis, Dona Lee and Richard G. Whitten: Medical and popular traditions of nerves. In: *Social science and medicine* 26 (1988), pp. 1209–1222.
Davis, Dona Lee and Setha M. Low (eds): *Gender, health, and illness. The case of nerves*. New York 1989.
De Renzi, Salvatore (ed.): *Collectio salernitana*. 5 vols. Naples 1852–1859.
De Renzi, Silvia: A career in manuscripts: Genres and purposes of a physician's writing in Rome, 1600–1630. In: *Italian studies* 66 (2011), pp. 234–248.

Dear, Peter: The meanings of experience. In: Katharine Park and Lorraine Daston (eds): *Early modern science* (= The Cambridge History of Science, vol. 3). Cambridge 2006, pp. 106–131.
Debru, Armelle: Galen. In: Brunschwig/Lloyd,*Greek thought* (2000), pp. 618–630.
Debus, Allen G.: *The French Paracelsians. The chemical challenge to medical and scientific tradition in early modern France.* Cambridge 1991.
Delisle, Candice: The letter: Private of public place? The Mattioli–Gesner controversy about the *aconitum primum*. In: *Gesnerus* 61 (2004), pp. 161–176.
Dell'Acqua, Gioan Battista: Giovanni Manardo medico e clinico. In: *Atti del convegno internazionale per la celebrazione del V centenario della nascita di Giovanni Manardo 1462–1536*. Ferrara 1963, pp.8–42.
Demaitre, Luke: *Medieval medicine. The art of healing from head to toe.* Santa Barbara/Denver/Oxford 2013.
Demaitre, Luke: Medieval notions of cancer. Malignancy and metaphor. In: *Bulletin of the history of medicine* 72 (1998), pp. 609–637.
Demaitre, Luke: Straws in the wind. Latin writings on asthma between Galen and Cardano. In: *Allergy and asthma proceedings* 23 (2002), pp. 61–93.
Dinges, Martin, Kay Peter Jankrift, Sabine Schlegelmilch and Michael Stolberg (eds): *Medical practice, 1600–1900. Physicians and their patients.* Leiden 2016.
Donati, Marcello: *De medica historia mirabili libri sex.* Venice 1588.
Dodoens, Rembert: *Medicinalium observationum exempla rara, recognita et aucta.* Cologne 1581.
Dondi, Raffaele Flaminio: Elideo Padovani. Medico forlivese del secolo XVI. In: *Atti e memorie dell'Accademia di storia dell'arte sanitaria* 117 (1951), pp. 139–144.
Dondi, Raffaele Flaminio: Cenni sul medico forlivese Alessandro Padovani (?–1637) e sulla sua biblioteca. In: *Rivista di storia della medicina* 19 (1975), pp. 190–198.
Dotzauer, Winfried: Deutsches Studium und deutsche Studenten an europäischen Hochschulen (Frankreich, Italien) und die nachfolgende Tätigkeit in Staat, Kirche und Territorium in Deutschland. In: Erich Maschke and Jürgen Sydow (eds): *Stadt und Universität im Mittelalter und in der frühen Neuzeit*. Tübingen 1974, pp. 112–141.
Douglas, Mary: *Purity and danger. An analysis of concepts of pollution and taboo.* London 1978.
Drembach, Martin von: *De atra bile disputatio medica.* Resp. Blasius Thammüller. [Leipzig]: [1548].
Drexel, Jeremias: *Aurifodina artium et scientiarum omnium excerpendi solertia.* Munich 1638.
Duden, Barbara: *Geschichte unter der Haut. Ein Eisenacher Arzt und seine Patientinnen um 1730.* Stuttgart 1987.
Dulieu, Louis: Félix Platter, étudiant de l'École de médecine de Montpellier. In: Ulrich Tröhler (ed.): *Felix Platter (1536–1614) in seiner Zeit*. Basel 1991, pp.17–20.
Dulieu, Louis: Guillaume Rondelet. In: *Clio medica* 1 (1966), pp. 89–111.
Dulieu, Louis: *La médecine à Montpellier.* Vol. 2: *La Renaissance.* Avignon 1979.
Dunus, Thaddaeus: *Muliebrium morborum omnis generis remedia.* Strasbourg 1565.
Durling, Richard J.: A chronological census of Renaissance editions and translations of Galen In: *Journal of the Warburg and Courtauld Institutes* 24 (1961), pp. 230–305.
Durling, Richard J.: Conrad Gesner's "Liber amicorum" 1555–1565. In: *Gesnerus* 22 (1965), pp. 134–159.

Durling, Richard J.: Girolamo Mercuriale's *De modo studendi*. In: *Osiris* N. S. 6 (1991), pp. 181–195.
Dumaître, Paule: *Ambroise Paré. Chirurgien de quatre rois de France.* Paris 1986.
Eadie, Mervyn J. and Peter F. Bladin: *A disease once sacred. A history of the medical understanding of epilepsy.* Eastleigh 2001.
Eamon, William: How to read a book of secrets. In: Elaine Leong and Alisha Rankin (eds): *Secrets and knowledge in medicine and science, 1500–1800.* Farnham 2011, pp. 23–46.
Eamon, William: *Science and the secrets of nature. Books of secrets in medieval and early modern culture.* Princeton 1994.
Ebelová, Ivana (ed.): *Pamětní kniha města české Lípy.* Ústí nad Labem 2005.
Eckart, Wolfgang U.: Anmerkungen zur "Medicus politicus"- und "Machiavellus Medicus"- Literatur des 17. und 18. Jahrhunderts. In: Benzenhöfer/Kühlmann, *Heilkunde* (1992), pp. 114–129.
Eisenberg, Leon: The physician as interpreter. Ascribing meaning to the illness experience. In: *Comprehensive psychiatry* 22 (1981), pp. 239–248.
Elias, Norbert: *Über den Prozeß der Zivilisation. Soziogenetische und psychogenetische Untersuchungen.* 2 vols. 6th edn. Frankfurt 1979.
Elkeles, Barbara: Arzt und Patient in der medizinischen Standesliteratur der Frühen Neuzeit. In: Benzenhöfer/Kühlmann, *Heilkunde* (1992), pp. 131–143.
Elkeles, Barbara: Medicus und Medikaster: Zum Konflikt zwischen akademischer und "empirischer" Medizin im 17. und frühen 18. Jahrhundert. In: *Medizinhistorisches Journal* 22 (1987), pp. 197–211.
D'Elvert, Christian: *Zur Geschichte der Pflege der Naturwissenschaften in Mähren und Schlesien, insbesondere der Naturkunde dieser Länder, mit Rücksicht auf Böhmen und Österreich.* Brünn 1868.
Erastus, Thomas: *De lamiis seu strigibus.* Basel 1578.
Erastus, Thomas: *De medicina nova Philippi Paracelsi.* 4 parts. Basel 1572–1573.
Erastus, Thomas: *Disputationum et epistolarum medicinalium volumen doctissimum.* Ed. by Theophilus Maderus. Zürich 1595.
Elkeles, Barbara: Arzt und Patient in der medizinischen Standesliteratur der Frühen Neuzeit. In: Benzenhöfer/Kühlmann, *Heilkunde* (1992), pp. 131–143.
Ellenbog, Nikolaus: *Briefwechsel.* Ed. by Andreas Bigelmair and Friedrich Zoepfl. Münster 1938.
Enenkel, Karl A. E.: Die Grundlegung humanistischer Selbstpräsentation im Brief-Corpus: Francesco Petrarcas *Familiarium rerum libri XXIV.* In: van Houdt, *Self-presentation* (2002), pp. 367–384.
Enenkel, Karl A. E.: In search of fame. Self-representation in neo-Latin humanism. In: Stephen Gersh and Bert Roest (eds): *Medieval and Renaissance humanism: Rhetoric, representation and reform.* Leiden 2003, pp. 93–113.
Erasmus, Desiderius: *De conscribendis epistolis.* Cambridge 1521.
Erasmus, Desiderius: *De duplici copia verborum ac rerum commentarii duo.* Paris 1514.
Ettmüller, Michael: *Opera omnia theoretica et practica.* Part 2. Lyon 1685.
Evans, Jennifer and Sara Read: *Maladies and medicine. Exploring health and healing 1540–1740.* Barnsley 2017.
Fabiani, Giuseppe: *La vita di Pietro Andrea Mattioli.* Ed. by Luciano Bianchi. Siena 1872.
Fabricius, Wilhelm: *Opera omnia quae extant.* Frankfurt 1646.

Fabricius, Wilhelm: *Wund-Artzney. Gantzes Werck, und aller Bücher, so viel deren vorhanden.* Frankfurt 1652.
Facciolati, Jacobus: *Fasti Gymnasii Patavini [. . .] collecti ab anno MDXVII quo restitutae scholae sunt ad MDCCLVI.* Padua 1757.
Falloppia, Gabrielle: De cauteriis tractatus. Appended to idem: *Tractatus de compositione medicamentorum dilucidissimus.* Venice 1570, foll. 65r-72v.
Falloppia, Gabrielle: *De humani corporis anatome compendium.* Venice 1571.
Falloppia, Gabrielle: *De medicatis aquis atque de fossilibus.* Venice 1564.
Falloppia, Gabrielle: De tumoribus praeter naturam. In: idem: *Opera genuina omnia.* Vol 3. Venice 1606, foll. 1r-109v.
Falloppia, Gabrielle: *Expositio in librum Galeni de ossibus. Huic accesserunt observationes anatomicae eiusdem authoris.* Ed. by F. Michinus. Venice 1570.
Falloppia, Gabrielle: *Observationes anatomicae ad Petrum Mannam.* Venice 1561.
Falloppia, Gabrielle: Tractatus de decoratione. In: idem: *Opuscula. Part 2.* Padua 1566, foll. 34r-51v
Fantuzzi, Giovanni: *Notizie degli scrittori bolognesi.* Vol. 6. Bologna 1788.
Fausti, Daniela (ed.): *La complessa scienza dei semplici. Atti delle celebrazioni per il V centenario della nascita di Pietro Andrea Mattioli, Siena, 12 marzo-19 novembre.* Siena 2001.
Favaro, Antonio (ed.): *Atti della Nazione Germanica Artista nello Studio di Padova.* Vol. 1. Venice 1911.
Favaro, Giuseppe: Contributi alle biografia di Girolamo Fabrici d'Acquapendente. In: *Memorie e documenti per la storia della Università di Padova.* Vol. 1. Padua 1922, pp. 241–348.
Favaro, Giuseppe: *Gabrielle Falloppa modenese (MDXXII-MDLXII). Studio biografico.* Modena 1928.
Faventinus, Leonellus de Victoriis: *De aegritudinibus infantium tractatus admodum salutifer.* Venice 1557.
Fernel, Jean: Consiliorum liber. Cui accesserunt responsa quaedam clarorum medicorum Parisiensium. In: idem: *Universa medicina.* Geneva 1644, pp. 247–397 (appended to *De abditis rerum*).
Fernel, Jean: De abditis rerum causis libri duo. In: Fernel, *Universa medicina* (1644) (separate pagination).
Fernel, Jean: *Universa medicina.* Geneva 1542.
Fernel, Jean, *Universa medicina.* Geneva 1644.
Ferrarius, Omnibonus: *De arte medica infantium quorum duo priores de tuenda eorum sanitate, posteriores de curandis morbis agunt.* Brixen 1577.
Ferretto, Silvia: *Bassiano Lando e la "scienza" della medicina tra filosofia e teologia nel XVI secolo.* Tesi, Università degli Studi di Trento, ciclo XXII, 2006–2009.
Ferretto, Silvia: *Maestri per il metodo di trattar le cose Bassiano Lando, Giovan Battista da Monte e la scienza della medicina nel XVI secolo.* Padua 2012.
Ferri, Sara (ed.): *Pietro Andrea Mattioli, Siena 1501-Trento 1578. La vita, le opere.* Perugia 1997.
Ferri, Sara: Il "Dioscoride", i "Discorsi", i "Commentarii": Gli amici e i nemici. In: eadem, *Mattioli* (1997), pp. 15–48.
Feustel, Robert: *Grenzgänge. Kulturen des Rauschs seit der Renaissance.* Munich 2013.
Fichtner, Gerhard: Padova e Tübingen: La formazione medica nei secoli XVI e XVII. In: *Acta medicae historiae patavina* 19 (1972–73), pp. 43–62.
Ficino, Marsilio: *De triplici vita: libri tres.* Venice 1498 (repr. Hildesheim 1978).

Findlen, Paula and Pamela H. Smith (eds): *Merchants and marvels. Commerce and the representation of nature in early modern Europe*. New York 2002.
Findlen, Paula: *Possessing nature. Museums, collecting, and scientific culture in early modern Italy*. Berkeley/Los Angeles/London 1994.
Findlen, Paula: The formation of a scientific community. Natural history in sixteenth-century Italy. In: Anthony Grafton and Nancy Siraisi (eds): *Natural particulars. Nature and the disciplines in Renaissance Europe*. Cambridge, MA, 1999, pp. 369–400.
Findlen, Paula: The death of a naturalist: Knowledge and community in Renaissance Italy. In: Gideon Manning and Cynthia Klestinec (eds): *Professors, physicians and practices in the history of medicine: Essays honoring Nancy Siraisi*. New York 2017, pp. 127–167.
Finkler, Kaja: The universality of nerves. In: Davis/Low, Gender (1989), pp. 169–179.
Finucci, Valeria: *The prince's body. Vincenzo Gonzaga and Renaissance medicine*. Cambridge/London 2015.
Finzel, Hiob: *Wunderzeichen. Warhafftige Beschreybung und gründlich Verzeichnuß schröcklicher wunderzeichen und Geschichten, die von dem Jar an M. D. XVII bis auff yetziges Jar M.D.LVI geschehen und ergangen sindt nach der Jarzal*. Nürnberg 1556.
Fischer, Klaus: *Hartmann Schedel in Nördlingen. Das pharmazeutisch-soziale Profil eines spätmittelalterlichen Stadtarztes*. Würzburg 1996.
Fischer-Homberger, Esther: *Hypochondrie. Melancholie bis Neurose. Krankheiten und Zustandsbilder*. Bern 1970.
Fissell, Mary: *Vernacular bodies. The politics of reproduction in early modern England*. Oxford 2004.
Flamm, Heinz: Bader – Wundarzt – Medicus. In: idem and Karl Mazakarini (eds): *Bader – Wundarzt – Medicus. Heilkunst in Klosterneuburg. Begleitpublikation zur Ausstellung*. Klosterneuburg 1996, pp. 7–40.
Fonseca, Rodericus: *Opusculum, quo adolescentes ad medicinam facile capessendam instruuntur, casus omnium febrium methodice discutiuntur, & curantur*. Florence 1596.
Forcher, Michael: *Erzherzog Ferdinand II. Landesfürst von Tirol. Sein Leben. Seine Herrschaft. Sein Land*. Innsbruck/Vienna 2017.
Foreest, Pieter van: *Observationum et curationum medicinalium libri XXXII*. Leiden 1603–1606.
Foreest, Pieter van: *Observationum et curationum chirurgicarum libri quatuor posteriores, de vulneribus, ulceribus, fracturis, luxationibus*. Leiden 1601.
Foreest, Pieter van: *Uromanteia. Das ist warhafftiger und wolgegründter Bericht von den vielfaltigen Urtheilen unnd Weissagungen auß den Urinen oder Wassern*. Frankfurt 1620.
Foreest, Pieter van: *Observationum et curationum medicinalium ac chirurgicarum opera omnia*. Frankfurt 1634.
Fortuna, Stefania: The Latin editions of Galen's *Opera omnia* (1490–1625) and their prefaces. In: *Early science and medicine* 17 (2012), pp. 391–412.
Fossati, Pier Maria (ed.): *Girolamo Fabrizi da Acquapendente. Medico e anatomista. La vita e le opere. Note in margine alla mostra*. Acquapendente 1988.
Fracanzano, Antonio: *De morbo gallico fragmenta quaedam elegantissima, ex lectionibus anni MDLXII Bononiae*. Appended to Gabrielle Falloppi, *De morbo gallico liber*. Venice 1574, pp. 186–219.
Fracanzano, Antonio: *De morbo gallico liber*. Ed. by Camillo Cochio. Bologna 1564.
Fracastoro, Girolamo: *Syphilis sive morbus gallicus*. Verona 1536.
French, Roger: *Medicine before science. The rational and learned doctor from the Middle Ages to the Enlightenment*. Cambridge 2003.

Friedrich, Udo: *Naturgeschichte zwischen artes liberales und frühneuzeitlicher Wissenschaft. Conrad Gessners "Historia animalium" und ihre volkssprachige Rezeption.* Tübingen 1995.
Friedrich IV. von der Pfalz: Das Tagebuch und Ausgabenbuch des Churfürsten Friedrich IV. von der Pfalz. Ed. by J. Wille. In: *Zeitschrift für die Geschichte des Oberrheins* 33 (1880), pp. 201–295.
Frijhoff, Willem: Patterns. In: Ridder-Symoens, *History* (1996), pp. 43–105.
Fuchs, Leonhard: *De historia stirpium commentarij insignes.* Basel 1542.
Fučíková, Eliška et alii (eds): *Rudolf II and Prague. The court and the city.* London 1997.
Fürst, Susanne: *Das Arztporträt in der Frühen Neuzeit.* Diss. med. Regensburg 2009.
Galen: *De morborum & symptomatum differentijs & causis libri 6.* Transl. by Wilhelm Copus. Lyon 1547.
Galen: *Opera omnia.* 20 vols. Ed. by C. G. Kühn. Leipzig 1822 (repr. Hildesheim 1964).
Galen: Quod optimus medicus sit quoque philosophus. Transl. by Desiderius Erasmus. In: idem: *Protreptikos logos pros tas technas [. . .]. Ad artes exhortatio. De optima doctrina. Quod optimus medicus sit quoque philosophus.* Paris 1547, pp. 27–31.
Gallo, Andrea: *Fascis de peste, peripneumonia pestilentiali cum sputo sanguinis, febre pestilentiali, ac quibusdam symptomatibus, in quinque fasciculos digestus.* Brixen 1567.
Gasser, Achilles Pirmin: *Ainfeltiger und gegrünter Bericht, wie menigklich sich in pestilentzischem Übergang, mit Artznyen, und anderer Lybsnot, halten, beweren und genören soll.* Nürnberg 1544.
Gasser, Achilles Pirmin: *Catalogus regum omnium, quorum sub christiana professione per Europam adhuc regna florent.* Augsburg 1552.
Gasser, Achilles Pirmin: *De regibus Hierosolymitanis.* Basel 1555.
Gasser, Achilles Pirmin: *Historiarum et chronicorum mundi epitome velut index.* Basel 1532.
Gaudin, Léon (ed.): *Félix et Thomas Platter à Montpellier, 1552–1559, 1595–1599. Notes de voyage de deux étudiants balois.* Montpellier 1892.
Gentilcore, David: *Food and health in early modern Europe. Diet, medicine and society, 1450–1800.* London 2016.
Gentilcore, David: *Healers and healing in early modern Italy.* Manchester 1998.
Gentilcore, David: Was there a "popular medicine" in early modern Europe? In: *Folklore* 115 (2004), pp. 151–166.
Germain, Alexandre Charles: La médecine arabe et la médecine grecque à Montpellier. In: idem (ed.): *Mélanges académiques d'histoire et d'archéologie.* Vol. 5. Montpellier 1877 (separate pagination).
Germain, Alexandre Charles: *Les anciennes thèses de l'École de médecine de Montpellier. Collation des grades et concours professoraux.* Montpellier 1886.
Germain, Alexandre Charles: *Les étudiants de l'École de médecine de Montpellier au XVIe siècle. Étude historique sur le* Liber procuratoris studiosorum. Paris 1876.
Germain, Alexandre Charles: Les pèlerins de la science à Montpellier. In: *Bulletin de la Société Languedocienne de Géographie* 1 (1878), pp. 161–181.
Gersdorff, Hans von: *Feldtbuch der Wundartzney.* Strasbourg 1517.
Gessner, Conrad: *Historia animalium.* Zürich 1551–1558 and 1587.
Gessner, Conrad, *Pandectae sive partitionum universalium [. . .] libri XXI.* Zürich 1548.
Gessner, Conrad: *Sanitatis tuendae praecepta: cum aliis, tum literarum studiosis hominibus, & iis qui minus exercentur, cognitu necessaria; contra luxum conviviorum; contra notas astrologicas ephemeridum de secandis venis.* Zürich 1556.

Gillet, Johann Franz Albert: *Crato von Crafftheim und seine Freunde. Ein Beitrag zur Kirchengeschichte.* 2 parts. Frankfurt am Main 1860.

Glaubitz, Michael von: *Zwo Haußtaffeln und Underricht fur die Reichen und Armen zur Sommer und Winterzeit wider die fürstehende schrecklich und wegfressende Pestilentz.* Mainz 1584.

Glück, Helmut: *Deutsch als Fremdsprache in Europa vom Mittelalter bis zur Barockzeit.* Berlin/ New York 2002.

Good, Byron J.: *Medicine, rationality and experience. An anthropological perspective.* Cambridge 1994.

Gößwein, Elisabeth: *Mater puerorum. Das epileptische Kind im Fokus ärztlicher Fallberichte der Frühen Neuzeit.* Diss. med. Univ. Regensburg 2016.

Graf-Stuhlhofer, Franz: *Humanismus zwischen Hof und Universität. Georg Tannstetter (Collimitius) und sein wissenschaftliches Umfeld im Wien des frühen 16. Jahrhunderts.* Vienna 1996.

Grafton, Anthony: *Cardano's cosmos. The worlds and works of a Renaissance astrologer.* Cambridge, MA 1999.

Green, Monica: Women's medical practice and health care in medieval Europe. In: *Signs* 14 (1989), pp. 434–473.

Green, Monica: *Making women's medicine masculine: The rise of male authority in pre-modern gynecology.* Oxford 2008.

Greenblatt, Stephen: *Renaissance self-fashioning. From More to Shakespeare.* Chicago/ London 1980.

Greiner, J.: Dinkelsbühler Arzt-Instruktionen von 1556. In: *Sudhoffs Archiv* 28 (1935), pp. 123–125.

Grell, Ole Peter: Conflicting duties: Plague and the obligations of early modern physicians towards patients and commonwealth in England and the Netherlands. In: Andrew Wear, Johanna Geyer-Kordesch and Roger French (eds): *Doctors and ethics: The earlier historical setting of professional ethics.* Amsterdam 1993, pp. 131–152.

Grell, Ole Peter (ed.): *Paracelsus: The man and his reputation, his ideas and their transformation.* Leiden 1998.

Grendler, Paul F.: *The universities of the Italian Renaissance.* Baltimore 2002.

Grodzynski, Denise: Superstitio. In: *Revue des études anciennes* 76 (1974), pp. 36–60.

Groß, Dominik and Jan Steinmetzer: Strategien ärztlicher Selbstautorisierung in der frühneuzeitlichen Medizin. Das Beispiel Volcher Coiters (1534–1576). In: *Medizinhistorisches Journal* 40 (2005), pp. 275–320.

Größing, Sigrid-Maria: *Kaufmannstochter im Kaiserhaus. Philippine Welser und ihre Heilkunst.* [Vienna] 1992.

Größing, Sigrid-Maria: *Die Heilkunst der Philippine Welser, Außenseiterin im Hause Habsburg.* Augsburg 1998.

Gryll, Lorenz: *Oratio de peregrinatione studii medicinalis ergo suscepta.* [Ingolstadt] 1566.

Guarino, Mauro: Profilo storico degli ospedali di Bologna e Ferrara. In: Graziano Campanini, Mauro Guarino and G. Lippi (eds): *Le arti della salute. Il patrimonio culturale e scientifico della sanità pubblica in Emilia-Romagna.* Milan 2005, pp. 77–93.

Guidi, Guido: De curatione generatim, in: idem: *Opera omnia sive ars medicinalis.* Frankfurt 1626 (separate pagination).

Gunnoe, Charles: The debate between Johann Weyer and Thomas Erastus on the punishment of witches. In: James van Horn Melton (ed.): *Cultures of communication from Reformation*

to Enlightenment. Constructing publics in the early modern German lands. Aldershot 2002, pp. 257–285.
Gunnoe, Charles D.: Thomas Erastus and his circle of anti-Paracelsians. In: Joachim Telle (eds): *Analecta paracelsica. Studien zum Nachleben Theophrast von Hohenheims im deutschen Kulturgebiet der frühen Neuzeit*. Stuttgart 1994, pp.127–148.
Guth, Gustav: Das Idyll von den Teplitzer Heilquellen (Idyllion de thermis teplicensibus) des Thomas Mitis (1550). In: *Erzgebirgszeitung* 51, n° 9 (1930), pp. 125–129, 142–145 and 161–163.
Haag, Sabine and Sandbichler, Veronika (eds): *Ferdinand II. 450 Jahre Tiroler Landesfürst*. Innsbruck 2017.
Hacke, Daniela: Von der Wirkungsmächtigkeit des Heiligen: Magische Liebeszauberpraktiken und die religiöse Mentalität venezianischer Laien in der frühen Neuzeit. In: *Historische Anthropologie* 3 (2001), pp. 311–332.
Handsch, Georg: Ad lectorem. In: Petrus Sibyllenus: *De peste liber*. Prague 1564.
Handsch, Georg: Calendarium novum rythmicis sententiis apposite ad unumquodque tempus vel festum accomodatis concinnatum. In: Matthaeus Collinus: *Elementarius libellus in lingua latina & boiemica pro novellis scholasticis*. Prague 1550.
Handsch, Georg: *Die Elbefischerei in Böhmen und Meißen*. Ed. by Ottokar Schubert. Prague 1933.
Handsch, Georg: [Two letters to Simon Ennius and a letter to Matthaeus Collinus]. In: *Časopis Musea království českého* 87 (1913), pp. 167–169 and p. 179.
Handsch, Georg: In effigiem reginae Mariae. In: Thomas Mitis (ed.): *In felicem inaugurationem sereniss[imi] regis Maximiliani, & sereniss[imae] reginae Mariae, chorus davidicus*. Prague 1562.
Handsch, Georg: In icona R[egis] Maximiliani. In: Thomas Mitis (ed.): *In felicem inaugurationem sereniss[imi] regis Maximiliani, & sereniss[imae] reginae Mariae, chorus davidicus*. Prague 1562.
Handsch, Georg: Dedicatory poem. In: Wenzel Nicolaides (ed.): *Cantiones evangelicae ad usitatas harmonias, quae in ecclesiis boemicis per totius anni circulum canuntur, accomodatae, praecipua Christi beneficia breviter complectentes*. Wittenberg 1554.
Handsch, Georg: Zum Leser. In: Mattioli, *Kreutterbuch* (1563).
Handsch, Georg (ed.): *Secunda farrago elegiarum et idylliorum ab aliquot studiosis poeticae bohemis scriptorum diversis temporibus ad nobilem et clarissimum virum D. Ioannem Seniorem Hoddeiovinum ad Hoddeiova*. Prague 1561.
Hankinson, Robert J.: *The Cambridge companion to Galen*. Cambridge 2008.
Hantschel, Franz: *Heimatkunde des politischen Bezirkes B.-Leipa*. Böhmisch Leipa 1911.
Hart, James: *The arraignment of urines, wherein are set downe the manifold errors and abuses of ignorant urine-monging [sic!] empirickes, cozening quacksalvers, women-physitians and the like stuffe*. London 1623.
Harvey, William: *Exercitatio anatomica de motu cordis et sanguinis in animalibus*. Frankfurt 1628.
Hase, Eduard Friedrich: Dr. Thomas Reinesius, Stadtphysikus und Bürgermeister zu Altenburg. Ein Lebensbild aus dem 17. Jahrhundert. In: *Mitteilungen der Geschichts- und Altertumsforschenden Gesellschaft des Osterlandes* 4 (1858), pp. 309–348.
Hasse, Hans Peter and Günther Wartenberg (eds): *Caspar Peucer 1525–1602. Wissenschaft, Glaube und Politik im konfessionellen Zeitalter*. Leipzig 2004.

Havenreuter, Johann Ludwig: *Theses medicae de iis rebus quae in principio artis medicae Galeni traduntur.* Resp. Joh. Sebastian Frid. Strasbourg 1568.
Heide, Anton de: *Vertoog over de onzekerheit der piskijkerij en bedrieglijkheit der piskijkeren.* Amsterdam 1682.
Heigel, Karl Theodor von: Schrenck von Notzing. In: *Allgemeine Deutsche Biographie* 32 (1891), pp. 485–488.
Hechstetter, Philippus: *Rararum observationum medicinalium decades tres.* Augsburg 1624.
Heischkel, Edith: Die Welt des praktischen Arztes. In: Walter Artelt and Walter Rüegg (eds): *Der Arzt und der Kranke in der Gesellschaft des 19. Jahrhunderts.* Frankfurt 1967, pp. 1–16.
Hejnic, Josef: *Dva humanisté v roce 1547 (Jan Šentygar a Bohuslav Hodějovský).* Prague 1957.
Hejnová, Miroslava: *Pietro Andrea Mattioli 1501–1578. U příležitosti 500. výročí narození/In occasione del V. centenario della nascita.* Prague 2001.
Helm, Jürgen: Die Galenrezeption in Philipp Melanchthons De anima (1540/1552). In: *Medizinhistorisches Journal* 31 (1996), pp. 298–321.
Helm, Jürgen: Zwischen Aristotelismus, Protestantismus und zeitgenössischer Medizin. Philipp Melanchthons Lehrbuch "De anima" (1540/1552). In: Jürgen Leonhardt (ed.): *Melanchthon und das Lehrbuch des 16. Jahrhunderts.* Rostock 1997, pp. 175–191.
Helman, Cecil G.: *Culture, health and illness.* 5th edn. Boca Raton 2007.
Helman, Cecil G.: "Feed a cold, starve a fever". Folk models of infection in an English suburban community and their relation to medical treatment. In: *Culture, medicine and psychiatry* 2 (1978), pp. 107–137.
Helmich, Egon: *Die Briefe Konrad Gesners an Crato von Krafftheim nach der Briefsammlung von 1566.* Diss. med. Düsseldorf 1938.
Henderson, John: *The Renaissance hospital. Healing the body and healing the soul.* New Haven 2006.
Henkel, Arthur and Albrecht Schöne (eds): *Emblemata. Handbuch zur Sinnbildkunst des XVI. und XVII. Jahrhunderts.* Stuttgart/Weimar 1996.
Herbst, Klaus-Dieter: *Biobibliographisches Handbuch der Kalendermacher von 1550 bis 1750* (https://www.presseforschung.uni-bremen.de/dokuwiki/doku.php?id=startseite).
Herbst, Klaus-Dieter: Der Arzt als Autor von Jahreskalendern. In: Salatowsky/Stolberg, *Göttliche Kunst* (2019), pp. 80–93.
Herz, Josef (ed.): Das Tagebuch des Augsburger Arztes und Stadtphysicus Dr. Philipp Hoechstetter 1579–1635. In: *Zeitschrift des Historischen Vereins für Schwaben und Neuburg* 70 (1976), pp. 180–224.
Herzog, E.: Zwei alte Physikat-Bestallungen aus den Jahren 1523 und 1546. In: *Vereinte deutsche Zeitschrift für die Staats-Arzneikunde*, N.F. 3 (1848), n° 1, pp. 194–200.
Hess, Volker and Sabine Schlegelmilch: Cornucopia officinae medicae: Medical practice records and their origin. In: Dinges et alii, *Medical practice* (2016), pp. 11–38.
Hessus, Helius Eobanus: *Helii Eobani Hessi [. . .] et amicorum ipsius epistolarum familiarium libri XII.* Marburg 1543.
Heusinger, Tobias: *Das zitternde Herz des Monarchen. Kommentierte Edition eines ärztlichen Konsils von Andrea Gallo für Kaiser Maximilian II.* Diss. med. Würzburg [2021] (in preparation).
Hild, Heike: *Das Stammbuch des Medicus, Alchemisten und Poeten Daniel Stolcius als Manuskript des Emblembuches Viridarium Chymicum (1624) und als Zeugnis seiner Peregrinatio Academica.* Diss. TU Munich 1991.
Hindson, Betham: Attitudes towards menstruation and menstrual blood in Elizabethan England. In: *Journal of social history* 43 (2009), pp. 89–114.

Hippocrates: *Aphorismi cum Galeni commentariis*. Transl. by Niccolò Leoniceno. Venice 1538.
Hippocrates: *Œuvres complètes d'Hippocrate*. Ed. by Émile Littré. Paris 1839–1861 (repr. Amsterdam 1978).
Hippocrates: *De aere, aquis et locis libellus*. Transl. by Janus Cornarius. Basel 1529.
Hirai, Hiro: *Medical humanism and natural philosophy: renaissance debates on matter, life and the soul*. Boston/Leiden 2011.
Hirai, Hiro: The new astral medicine. In: Brendan Dooley (ed.): *A companion to astrology in the Renaissance*. Leiden/Boston 2014, S. 267–286.
Hirn, Josef: *Erzherzog Ferdinand II. von Tirol. Geschichte seiner Regierung und seiner Länder*. 2 vols. Innsbruck 1885/1887.
Hlaváčková, Ludmila and Petr Svobodný: *Dějiny lékařství v českých zemích*. Prague 2004.
Hlaváčková, Ludmila, Petr Svobodný and Josef Adamec: *Biografický slovník pražské lékařské fakulty 1348–1939*. 2 vols. Prague 1988 and 1993.
Hoffmann, Friedrich: *Medicus politicus sive regulae prudentiae secundum quas medicus juvenis studia sua & vitae rationem dirigere debet, si famam sibi felicemque praxin & cito acquirere & conservare cupit*. Leiden 1708.
Hoffmann-Axthelm, Walter: *Die Geschichte der Zahnheilkunde*. Berlin 1973.
Hoppe, Brigitte: Bildungseifrige Apotheker der Frühen Neuzeit. In: *Pharmazeutische Zeitung* 137 (1992), n. 44, pp. 38–44.
Horer, Ananius: *Artzney-Teuffel, oder kurtzer Discurs, darinn diesem Ertzmörder seine Larve abgezogen*. Sine loco 1634.
Hörnigk, Ludwig von: *Politia medica*. Frankfurt am Main 1636.
Hornung, Johannes: *De uroscopia fraudulenta discursus. Kurtzer Bericht von dem unvollkommenen und betrüglichen Urtheil des menschlichen Borns oder Harns*. Herborn 1611.
Hornung, Johannes (ed.): *Cista medica*. Nürnberg [1626].
Horský, Zdeněk: Die europäische Bedeutung der böhmischen Tradition der "neuen Wissenschaft" im 16. Jahrhundert. In: Hans-Bernd Harder (ed.): *Studien zum Humanismus in den böhmischen Ländern*. Cologne/Vienna 1988, pp.275–289.
Horst, Gregor: *Büchlein von dem Schorbock, gemynem Vatterlandt zum besten Teutsch beschrieben*. Gießen 1615.
Horst, Horst: *Observationum medicinalium singularium libri quatuor posteriores*. Ulm 1628.
Horst, Jakob: *Brevis et dilucida enarratio libri Hippocratis De corde (with other texts connected to Horst's doctoral exam)*. Frankfurt an der Oder 1563.
Horst, Jakob: Oratio de remoris discentium medicinam earumque remediis. In: idem: *Epistolae philosophicae et medicinales*. Leipzig 1596, pp. 530–593.
Houdt, Toon van et alii (eds): *Self-presentation and social identification. The rhetoric and pragmatics of letter-writing in early modern times*. Leuven 2002.
Houllier, Jacques: *De morborum internorum curatione liber I*. Paris 1567.
Huber, Katharina: *Felix Platters "Observationes". Studien zum frühneuzeitlichen Gesundheitswesen in Basel*. Basel 2003.
Hubmann, Astrid: *Der Zahnwurm. Die Geschichte eines volksheilkundlichen Glaubens*. Diss. med. Univ. Regensburg 2008.
Hutten, Ulrich von: *Von der wunderbarlichen Artzney des Holtz Guaiacum genant, und wie man die Frantzosen oder Blatteren heilen sol*. Transl. by Thomas Murner. Strasbourg 1519.
Ingegno, Alberto: Astrologia, magia e ordine del mondo. In: Pietro Rossi and Carlo A. Viano (eds): *Storia della filosofia. 3. Dal Quattrocento al Seicento*. Roma/Bari 1995, pp. 85–113.

Ijsewein, Jozef: *Companion to Neo-Latin studies*. Part 2: *Literary, linguistic, philological and editorial questions*. 2nd edn. Leuven 1998.
Institoris, Heinrich: *Malleus maleficarum*. Cologne 1511.
Jackson, Mark: *Asthma. The biography*. New York 2009.
Jackson, Stanley W.: *Melancholia and depression. From Hippocratic times to modern times*. New Haven/London 1986.
Jacquart, Danielle: Theory, everyday practice, and three fifteenth-century physicians. In: *Osiris* 6 (1990), pp. 140–160.
Jakubcová, Alena, Matthias Johannes Pernerstorfer and Hubert Reitterer: *Theater in Böhmen, Mähren und Schlesien. Von den Anfängen bis zum Ausgang des 18. Jahrhunderts. Ein Lexikon*. Vienna 2013.
Jaumann, Herbert: Iatrophilologia. "Medicus philologicus" und analoge Konzepte in der frühen Neuzeit. In: Ralph Häfner (ed.): *Philologie und Erkenntnis. Beiträge zu Begriff und Problem frühneuzeitlicher "Philologie"*. Tübingen 2001, pp.151–176.
Jenny, Beat Rudolf (ed.): *Die Amerbachkorrespondenz*. Vol. 6 and Vol. 9,1. Basel 1967 and 1982.
Jensen, Kristian: The humanist reform of Latin and Latin teaching. In: Jill Kraye (ed.): *The Cambridge companion to Renaissance humanism*. Cambridge/New York 1996, pp. 63–81.
Jewson, Nicholas D.: Medical knowledge and the patronage system in 18th century England. In: *Sociology* 8 (1974), pp. 369–385.
Jewson, Nicholas D.: The disappearance of the sick-man from medical cosmology, 1770–1870. In: *Sociology* 10 (1976), 225–244.
Jones, Colin: *The smile revolution in eighteenth century Paris*. Oxford 2014
Jouanna, Jacques: Die Entstehung der Heilkunst im Westen. In: Mirko Dražen Grmek (ed.): *Die Geschichte des medizinischen Denkens. Antike und Mittelalter*. Munich 1996, pp.28–80.
Jouanna, Jacques: Hippocrates. In: Brunschwig/Lloyd, *Greek thought* (2000), pp. 649–659.
Joubert, Laurent: *Le première et seconde parti des erreurs populaires, touchant la médecine et le regime de santé*. Rouen 1601.
Joubert, Laurent: *Oratio de praesidiis futuri excellentis medici*. Geneva 1580.
Joutsivuo, Timo: *Scholastic tradition and humanist innovation. The concept of neutrum in Renaissance medicine*. Helsinki 1999.
Junghans, Helmar: Zeitpunkt und Ort von Luthers Turmerlebnis angesichts neuer Ausgrabungen. In: Christopher Spehr (ed.): *Lutherjahrbuch* 84 (2017), pp. 11–50.
Jütte, Robert: *Ärzte, Heiler und Patienten. Medizinischer Alltag in der frühen Neuzeit*. Munich/Zürich 1991.
Jütte, Robert: "Wo kein Weib ist, da seufzet der Kranke". Familie und Krankheit in der Frühen Neuzeit. In: *Jahrbuch des Instituts für Geschichte der Medizin der Robert Bosch Stiftung* 7 (1989), pp. 7–24.
Kalina von Jätenstein, Matthias: *Nachrichten über böhmische Schriftsteller und Gelehrte*. 2 vols. Prague 1818/1819.
Karcher, Johannes: Thomas Erastus (1524–1583), der unversöhnliche Gegner des Theophrastus Paracelsus. In: *Gesnerus* 14 (1957), pp. 1–13.
Kaartinen, Marjo: "Pray, Dr, is there reason to fear a cancer?' Fear of breast cancer in early modern Britain." In: Jonas Liliequist (ed.): *A history of emotions, 1200–1800*. London 2012, pp. 153–166 and pp. 241–243 (notes).
Kassell, Lauren: Casebooks in early modern England. Medicine, astrology, and written records. In: *Bulletin of the history of medicine* 88 (2014), pp. 595–625.

Kassell, Lauren: *Medicine and magic in Elizabethan London: Simon Forman – astrologer, alchemist, and physician*. Oxford 2005.
Kegler, Caspar: *[Quaestiones de vacuationibus purgationibusque medicinae studiosis disputandae]*. Broadsheet. [Leipzig] c. 1500.
Kerger, Martin: *Methodus excerpendi, Drexeliana succinctior* (= appended to Drexel, *Aurifodina*). Breslau 1695.
Kijper, Albert: *Medicinam rite discendi et exercendi methodus*. Leiden 1643.
King, Helen: *Hippocrates' woman. Reading the female body in ancient Greece*. London/ New York 1998.
King, Helen: *Midwifery, obstetrics and the rise of gynaecology. The uses of a sixteenth-century compendium*. Aldershot 2007.
King, Helen: Once upon a text. Hysteria from Hippocrates. In: Sander I. Gilman et alii (eds): *Hysteria beyond Freud*. Berkeley 1993, pp. 3–90.
King, Helen: *The one-sex body on trial. The classical and early modern evidence*. Farnham 2013.
Kintzinger, Martin: Status medicorum. Mediziner in der städtischen Gesellschaft des 14. bis 16. Jahrhunderts. In: Peter Johanek (ed.): *Städtisches Gesundheits- und Fürsorgewesen vor 1800*. Cologne 2000, pp. 63–92.
Kinzelbach, Annemarie: *Gesundbleiben, Krankwerden, Armsein in der frühneuzeitlichen Gesellschaft 1500 –1700. Gesunde und Kranke in den Reichsstädten Ulm und Überlingen*. Stuttgart 1995.
Kinzelbach, Annemarie: Heilkundige Frauen im oberdeutschen Raum, 1450–1700. In: *Historische Anthropologie* 7 (1999), pp. 165–190.
Kinzelbach, Annemarie: Zur Sozial- und Alltagsgeschichte eines Handwerks in der frühen Neuzeit. "Wundärzte" und ihre Patienten in Ulm. In: *Ulm und Oberschwaben* 49 (1994), pp. 111–144.
Kinzelbach, Annemarie, Stephanie Neuner und Karen Nolte: Medicine in practice. Knowledge, diagnosis and therapy. In: Dinges et alii, *Medical practice* (2016), pp. 99–130.
Kirwan, Richard: Introduction: Scholarly self-fashioning and the cultural history of universities. In: idem (ed.): *Scholarly self-fashioning and community in the early modern university*. Farnham 2013, pp. 1–20.
Kistner, Nikolaus: *Opuscula historica et politico-philologa tributa in libros IV*. Ed. by Quirin Reuter. Frankfurt 1611.
Kitti, Jurina: *Vom Quacksalber zum Doctor medicinae. Die Heilkunde in der deutschen Graphik des 16. Jahrhunderts*. Cologne 1985.
Klaas, Philip, Hubert Steinke and Alois Unterkircher: Daily business. The organization and finances of doctors' practices. In: Dinges et alii, *Medical practice* (2016), pp. 71–98.
Klestinec, Cynthia: *Theaters of anatomy. Students, teachers, and traditions of dissection in Renaissance Venice*. Baltimore 2011.
Klibansky, Raymond, Erwin Panofsky and Fritz Saxl: *Saturn und Melancholie. Studien zur Geschichte der Naturphilosophie und Medizin, der Religion und der Kunst*. Frankfurt 1992.
Klose, Wolfgang: *Corpus alborum amicorum. Beschreibendes Verzeichnis der Stammbücher des 16. Jahrhunderts*. Stuttgart 1988.
Knoedler, Franz (ed.): *De egestionibus: Texte und Untersuchungen zur spätmittelalterlichen Koproskopie*. Pattensen 1979.

Koch, Hans Theodor: Anatomie als universitäres Lehrfach. In: Jürgen Helm and Karin Stukenbrock (eds): *Anatomie. Sektionen einer medizinischen Wissenschaft im 18. Jahrhundert.* Wiesbaden 2003, pp. 163–188.

Koch, Hans Theodor: Die Wittenberger Medizinische Fakultät (1502–1652). Ein biobibliographischer Überblick. In: Stefan Oehmig (ed.): *Medizin und Sozialwesen in Mitteldeutschland zur Reformationszeit.* Leipzig 2007, pp. 289–343.

König, Klaus G.: *Der Nürnberger Stadtarzt Dr. Georg Palma (1543–1591).* Stuttgart 1961.

Koning, Jan de: Lo sviluppo della botanica nel XVI secolo. In: Minelli, *L'orto* (1995), pp. 11–31.

Kostenzer, Otto: Die Leibärzte Kaiser Maximilians I. in Innsbruck. In: *Veröffentlichungen des Tiroler Landesmuseums Ferdinandeum* 50 (1970), pp. 73–111.

Kotthorst, Lotte: Gelehrte Mediziner am Niederrhein. Das Italienstudium der Ärzte am Hof Wilhelms V. von Jülich-Kleve-Berg (1539–1592). In: Kaspar Gubler and Rainer C. Schwinges (eds): *Gelehrte Lebenswelten im 15. und 16. Jahrhundert.* Zürich 2018, pp. 129–156.

Kraack, Gerhard: Die Anfänge der medizinischen Versorgung in Flensburg und die Gründung der Ratsapotheke im Jahr 1604. In: Broder Schwensen (ed.): *Flensburg um 1600.* Flensburg 2006, pp. 283–306

Kragius, Andreas: *Laurea apollinea monspelliensis.* Basel 1586.

Kramarczyk, Andrea: Der Arzt Johannes Naevius (1499–1574) – ein Freund des Joachim Camerarius. In: Rainer Kößling and Günther Wartenberg (eds): *Joachim Camerarius.* Tübingen 2017, pp. 337–348.

Kramarczyk, Andrea and Antonia Krüger (eds): *Im Dienste von Kaiser und Kurfürst. Die Leibärzte Johannes und Caspar Neefe und ihre Familie.* Chemnitz 2014.

Kühlmann, Wilhelm: Poet, Chymicus, Mathematicus. Das Stammbuch des böhmischen Paracelsisten Daniel Stoltzius. In: Joachim Telle (ed.): *Parerga Paracelsica. Paracelsus in Vergangenheit und Gegenwart.* Stuttgart 1991, pp. 275–300.

Kühlmann, Wilhelm and Joachim Telle (eds): *Der Frühparacelsismus.* Vol. 1. Tübingen 2001.

Kühlmann, Wilhelm and Joachim Telle: Humanismus und Medizin an der Universität Heidelberg im 16. Jahrhundert. In: Wilhelm Doerr (ed.): *Semper apertus. Sechshundert Jahre Ruprecht-Karls-Universität Heidelberg 1386–1986.* Vol. 1: *Mittelalter und Frühe Neuzeit 1386–1803.* Berlin 1985, pp. 255–289.

Kühnel, Harry: Pietro Andrea Matthioli. Leibarzt und Botaniker des 16. Jahrhunderts. In: *Mitteilungen des Österreichischen Staatsarchivs* 15 (1962), pp. 63–92.

Kuhn, Werner: *Die Studenten der Universität Tübingen zwischen 1477 und 1534. Ihr Studium und ihre spätere Lebensstellung.* Göppingen 1971.

Kusukawa, Sachiko: Aspectio divinorum operum: Melanchthon and astrology for Lutheran medics. In: Ole Peter Grell and Andrew Cunningham (eds): *Medicine and the Reformation.* London 1993, pp. 33–56.

Kutschmann, Werner: *Der Naturwissenschaftler und sein Körper. Die Rolle der "inneren Natur" in der experimentellen Naturwissenschaft der frühen Neuzeit.* Frankfurt am Main 1986.

Kutschmann, Werner: Der Naturwissenschaftler und sein Körper. Naturwissensschaftsgeschichte aus antrhopologischer Perspektive. In: *Berichte zur Wissenschaftsgeschichte* 14 (1991), pp. 137–146.

Kutzer, Michael: Herrgott, Heiler und Harnschau: Das Vermächtnis des Ulmer Stadtarztes Augustin Thoner (1567–1655). In: *Medizinhistorisches Journal* 35 (2000), pp. 149–173.

Labouvie, Eva: *Andere Umstände. Eine Kulturgeschichte der Geburt.* Cologne 1998.

Labouvie, Eva: *Verbotene Künste. Volksmagie und ländlicher Aberglaube in den Dorfgemeinden des Saarraumes (16.-19. Jahrhundert).* St. Ingbert 1992.

Lachmund, Jens and Gunnar Stollberg: *Patientenwelten. Krankheit und Medizin vom späten 18. bis zum frühen 20. Jahrhundert im Spiegel von Autobiographien.* Opladen 1995.
Lachmund, Jens and Gunnar Stollberg: The doctor, his audience, and the meaning of illness. The drama of medical practice in the late 18th and early 19th centuries. In: iidem (eds): *The social construction of illness. Illness and medical knowledge in past and present.* Stuttgart 1992, pp. 53–66.
Lahr, Beer: *Original-Denkwürdigkeiten eines Zeitgenossen am Hofe Johann Wilhelm's III. Herzogs von Jülich, Cleve, Berg. Nebst einem Anhange von Original-Briefen und Verhandlungen betreffend den Proceß der Herzogin Jakobe.* Ed. by E[rich] K[ühlwetter] und F[ranz Wilhelm] C[ustodis]. Düsseldorf 1834.
Laín Entralgo, Pedro: La historica clinica. Historia y teoria del relato patografico. Barcelona 1961.
Laín Entralgo, Pedro: *La relacion medico-enfermo. Historia y teoria.* Madrid 1964.
Lambeck, Peter: *Commentariorum de Augustissima Bibliotheca Caesarea Vindobonensi liber.* Ed. by Adam Frantisek Kollár. 2nd edn. Vienna 1769.
Lammel, Hans-Uwe: Hofmedizin als interdisziplinäre Forschungsaufgabe – eine Bilanz. In: *Medizinhistorisches Journal* 53 (2018), pp. 197–216.
Lane Furdell, Elizabeth: *The royal doctors 1485–1714. Medical personnel at the Tudor and Stuart courts.* New York 2001.
Lange, Johannes: *Epistolarum medicinalium volumen tripartitum.* Frankfurt 1589.
Lange, Johannes: *Medicinalium epistolarum miscellanea, varia ac rara.* Basel 1554.
Lange, Johannes: *Secunda medicinalium epistolarum miscellanea, varia ac rara.* Basel 1560.
Laqueur, Thomas W.: *Making sex. Body and gender from the Greeks to Freud.* Cambridge, MA/London 1990.
Laschinger, Johannes: Dr. Hartmann Schedel als Stadtarzt in Amberg (1477–1481). In: *Mitteilungen des Vereins für Geschichte der Stadt Nürnberg* 80 (1993), pp. 137–145.
Lawrence, Christopher (ed.): *Medical theory, surgical practice. Studies in the history of surgery.* London/New York 1992.
Lawrence, Christopher: Democratic, divine and heroic. The history and historiography of surgery. In: Lawrence, *Medical theory* (1992), pp. 1–47.
Lawrence, Christopher: Medical minds, surgical bodies. corporeality and the doctors. In: Lawrence/Shapin, *Science incarnate* (1998), pp. 156–201.
Lawrence, Christopher and Steven Shapin (eds): *Science incarnate. Historical embodiments of natural knowledge.* Chicago 1998.
Ledvinka, Václav and Jiří Pešek: The public and private lives of Prague's burghers. In: Fučíková, *Rudolf II* (1997), pp. 287–301.
Leinkauf, Thomas: *Die Philosophie des Humanismus und der Renaissance.* Munich 2020.
Leong, Elaine: Collecting knowledge for the family: Recipes, gender and practical knowledge in the early modern English household. In: *Centaurus* 55 (2013), pp. 81–103.
Leong, Elaine: *Recipes and everyday knowledge. Medicine, science and the household in early modern England.* Chicago/London 2018.
Lesser, Andreas: *Die albertinischen Leibärzte vor 1700 und ihre verwandtschaftlichen Beziehungen zu Ärzten und Apothekern.* Petersberg 2015.
Leven, Karl-Heinz: *Die Geschichte der Infektionskrankheiten. Von der Antike bis ins 20. Jahrhundert.* Landsberg 1997.
Leven, Karl-Heinz: Krankheiten – historische Deutung versus retrospektive Diagnose. In: Norbert Paul and Thomas Schlich (eds): *Medizingeschichte. Aufgaben, Probleme, Perspektiven.* Frankfurt 1998, pp. 153–185.

Liber decanorum fac[ultatis] phil[sophiae] ab anno 1367, usque ad annum 1585. Part 2. Prague 1832.

Liébault, Jean: *Trois livres appartenans aux infirmitez et maladies des femmes*. Paris 1582.

Lind, L. R.: *Pre-Vesalian anatomy. Biography, translations, documents*. Philadelphia 1975.

Lindeboom, G. A.: Medical education in the Netherlands 1575–1750. In: C. D. O'Malley (ed.): *The history of medical education*. Berkeley 1970, pp. 201–234.

Lindemann, Mary: *Medicine and society in early modern Europe*. 2nd edn. Cambridge 2010.

Lingo, Alison Klairmont: *The rise of medical practitioners in sixteenth-century France. The case of Lyon and Montpellier*. PhD-Dissertation. Berkeley 1980.

Lingo, Alison Klairmont: Empirics and charlatans in early modern France. In: *Journal of social history* 19 (1986), pp. 583–603.

Liphimeus, Sabalathrus: *Warnung wider den Harn-Teuffel*. Nürnberg 1626.

Lockwood, D. P.: *Ugo Benzi. Medical philosopher and physician, 1376–1439*. Chicago 1951.

Long, Pamela O.: *Artisan/practitioners and the rise of the new science, 1400–1600*. Corvallis, OR 2001.

Lonie, Iain M.: Fever pathology in the sixteenth century. Tradition and innovation. In: William F. Bynum and Vivian Nutton (eds): *Theories of fever from antiquity to the Enlightenment*. London 1981, pp. 19–44.

Lonie, Iain M.: The "Paris Hippocratics". Teaching and research in Paris in the second half of the sixteenth century. In: Wear, French and Lonie, *Medical Renaissance* (1985), pp. 169–174.

López Pinero, José María: *Ciencia y técnica en la sociedad espanola de los siglos XVI y XVII*. Barcelona 1979.

López Pinero, José María: The medical profession in 16th century Spain. In: Russell, *Town and state physician* (1981), pp. 85–98.

Löwenstein, Jakob Samuel: Biographien und Schriften der ordentlichen Professoren der Medicin an der Hochschule zu Frankfurth a.O. in den Jahren 1506 bis 1811. In: *Janus* (1848), pp. 283–315 and pp. 419–443.

Low, Setha M: Culturally interpreted symptoms or culture-bound syndromes. A cross-cultural review of nerves. In: *Social science and medicine* 21 (1985), pp. 187–196.

Low, Setha M: Embodied metaphors: nerves as lived experience. In: Thomas J. Csordas (ed.): *Embodiment and experience. The existential ground of culture and self*. Cambridge 1994, pp. 139–162.

Ludovicus, Laurentius (ed.): *Compendium etymologiae et syntaxis in usum gymnasii Gorlicensis. Addita sunt gnorismata regularum in syntaxi, usurpata a Valentino Trozedorfio, in schola Goldbergensi*. Görlitz 1572.

Ludwig, Walther: *Das Stammbuch als Bestandteil humanistischer Kultur. Das Album des Heinrich Carlhack Hermeling (1587–1592)*. Göttingen 2006.

Ludwig, Walther (ed.): *Vater und Sohn im 16. Jahrhundert. Der Briefwechsel des Wolfgang Reichart genannt Rychardus mit seinem Sohn Zeno (1520–1543)*. Hildesheim 1999.

Lunel, Alexandre: *La maison médicale du roi. XVIe-XVIIIe siècle. Le pouvoir royal et les professions de santé*. Seyssel 2008.

Luther, Martin: *Werke. Kritische Gesamtausgabe. Briefwechsel*. Vol. 5: *1529–1530*. Ed. by O. Clemen. Weimar 1934.

MacDonald, Michael: *Mystical Bedlam. Madness, anxiety, and healing in seventeenth-century England*. Cambridge 1981.

Mache, Ursula: *Anatomischer Unterricht in Padua im 16. Jahrhundert. Edition, Übersetzung und Kommentierung der Aufzeichnungen eines böhmischen Studenten*. Duisburg 2019 (= Diss. med. dent. Regensburg 2019).
MacKinney, Loren C.: Medical education in the Middle Ages. In: *Cahiers d'histoire mondiale* 2 (1955), pp. 835–861.
MacKinney, Loren C.: Medical ethics and etiquette in the early middle ages. The persistence of Hippocratic ideals. In: *Bulletin of the history of medicine* 26 (1952), pp. 1–31.
Maclean, Ian: *Logic, signs and nature in the Renaissance. The case of learned medicine*. Cambridge 2002.
Maclean, Ian: The medical republic of letters before the Thirty Years War. In: *Intellectual history review* 18 (2008), pp. 15–30.
Maclean, Ian: *The Renaissance notion of woman. A study in the fortunes of scholasticism and medical science in European intellectual life*. Cambridge 1987.
Maiwald, V[incenz]: *Geschichte der Botanik in Böhmen*. Vienna/Leipzig 1904.
Malatesta, Maria (ed.): *Doctors and patients. History, representation, communication from antiquity to the present*. Berkeley 2015.
Manardi, Giovanni: *Epistolae medicinales, in quibus multa recentiorum errata et antiquorum decreta reserantur*. Ferrara 1521.
Manardi, Giovanni: *Epistolarum medicinalium libri XX*. Venice 1557.
Mantese, Giovanni: *Per una storia dell'arte medica in Vicenza alla fine del sec. XVI*. Vicenza 1969.
Manzke, Walter: *Remedia pro infantibus. Arzneiliche Kindertherapie im 15. und 16. Jahrhundert, dargestellt anhand ausgewählter Krankheiten*. Diss. rer. nat. Marburg 2008.
Marinello, Giovanni: *Le medicine partenenti alle infermità delle donne*. Venice 1563.
Marland, Hilary: *Dangerous motherhood. Insanity and childbirth in Victorian Britain*. Basingstoke/New York 2004.
Martínek, Jan: *Jan Hodějovský a jeho literární okruh*. Ed. by Marta Vaculínová, together with Dana Martínková. Prague 2012.
Martínková, Dana: Beschreibungen böhmischer und mährischer Städte im Zeitalter des Humanismus. In: Hans-Bernd Harder (ed.): *Studien zum Humanismus in den böhmischen Ländern. Part III: Die Bedeutung der humanistischen Topographien und Reisebeschreibungen in der Kultur der böhmischen Länder bis zur Zeit Balbins*. Cologne 1993, pp.25–34.
Martínková, Dana: *Literární druh veršovaných popisů měst v naší latinské humanistické literatuře*. Posthumous edition by Marta Vaculínová (together with Martínek, *Jan Hodějovský*). Prague 2012.
Martínková, Dana: *Poselství ducha. Latinská próza českých humanistů*. Prague 1975.
Marzell, Heinrich: Die Haselwurz (Asarum europaeum L.) in der alten Medizin. In: *Sudhoffs Archiv für Geschichte der Medizin und der Naturwissenschaften* 42 (1958), pp. 319–325.
Massaria, Alessandro: *Praelectiones de morbis mulierum*. Ed. by Heinrich Osthausen. Leipzig 1600.
Mattioli, Pietro Andrea: *Commentarii in libros sex Pedacii Dioscoridis de materia medica*. Venice 1554.
Mattioli, Pietro Andrea: *Commentarii in P. Dioscoridis De materia medica*. Venice 1565.
Mattioli, Pietro Andrea: *Commentarii in sex libros Pedacii Dioscoridis Anazarbei de medica materia*. Venice 1570.
Mattioli, Pietro Andrea: *Epistolarum medicinalium libri quinque*. Prague 1561.
Mattioli, Pietro Andrea: *Epistolarum medicinalium libri quinque*. Lyon 1564.

Mattioli, Pietro Andrea: *Il Magno Palazzo del Cardinale di Trento*. Venice 1539.
Mattioli, Pietro Andrea: Morbi gallici novum ac utilissimum opusculum. In: Niccolò Leoniceno et alii: *Liber de morbo gallico*. Venice 1535 [no pagination].
Mattioli, Pietro Andrea: *New Kreutterbuch mit den allerschönsten und artlichsten Figuren aller Gewechsz, dergleichen vormals in keiner Sprach nie an Tag kommen.* Transl. and ed. by Georg Handsch. Venice 1563.
Mattioli, Pietro Andrea: *Kreutterbuch.* Ed. by Joachim Camerarius. Frankfurt am Main 1586.
Mauch, Adolf: *Libellus de aegritudinibus infantium. Ein Buch über Kinderkrankheiten von Paolo Bagellardi (Padua 1472), ins Deutsche übertragen.* Diss. med. Bottrop 1937.
Mauss, Marcel: *Die Gabe. Form und Funktion des Austauschs in archaischen Gesellschaften.* Frankfurt 1990.
Mayer, Maximilian: *Verständnis und Darstellung des Skorbuts im 17. Jahrhundert. Mit einer Edition und Übersetzung der Fallgeschichten zu 'Skorbut' bei Johannes Frank.* Diss. med. Würzburg 2012 (http://opus.bibliothek.uni-wuerzburg.de/frontdoor/index/index/docId/6241).
Mazzetti, Serafino: *Repertorio di tutti i professori antichi, e moderni della famosa Università, e del celebre Istituto delle Scienze di Bologna.* Bologna 1847.
Mazzuchelli, Giammaria: *Gli scrittori d'Italia cioè notizie storiche, e critiche intorno alle vite, e agli scritti dei letterati Italiani.* Vol. 1.1. Brescia 1758.
McClive, Cathy: *Menstruation and procreation in early modern France.* Farnham 2015.
McVaugh, Michael R.: *The rational surgery of the Middle Ages.* Tavarnuzze/Impruneta 2006.
Meibom, Johann Heinrich: *Hippocratis magni Orkos [graece] sive jusjurandum, recensitum, et libro commentario illustratum.* Leiden 1643.
Melanchthon, Philipp: *Commentarius de anima.* Wittenberg 1540.
Melanchthon, Philipp: *Liber de anima.* Wittenberg 1552.
Melanchthon, Philipp: *Loci communes rerum theologicarum seu hypotyposes theologicae.* Wittenberg 1521.
Melhofer, Philipp: *Lasstafel oder Almannach [. . .] Auff das MDXLIII Jare.* Augsburg 1543.
Menčik, Ferdinand (ed.): *Dopisy M. Matouše Kollína z Chotěřiny a jeho přátel ke Kašparovi z Nydbrucka, tajnému radovi krále Maximiliána II.* Prague 1914.
Menini, Cesare: "Curationes A. M. Brasavoli". Contributo alla conoscenza delle opere di Antonio Musa Brasavolo come medico pratico. In: *Rivista della storia delle scienze mediche e naturali* 43 (1952), pp. 255–261.
Mercado, Luìs: *De mulierum affectionibus.* Venice 1587.
Mercuriale, Girolamo: *De morbis cutaneis.* Transl. by Richard L. Sutton as: *Sixteenth century physician and his methods. Mercurialis on diseases of the skin.* Kansas City 1986.
Mercuriale, Girolamo: *De morbis muliebribus praelectiones.* 4th edn. Venice 1601.
Mercuriale, Girolamo: *De morbis puerorum tractatus.* Venice 1583.
Mercuriale, Girolamo: De ratione discendi medicinam epigraphe. In: Joachim Georg Schenck, (ed.): *De formandis medicinae studiis et schola medica constituenda enchiridion selectum.* Strasbourg 1607, pp. 18–35.
Merenda, Giovanni P.: *Evacuandi ratio tribus in libris luculenter perstricta.* Basel 1547.
Mertens, Dieter: Zur Sozialgeschichte und Funktion des *poeta laureatus* im Zeitalter Maximilians I. In: Rainer Christoph Schwinges (ed.): *Gelehrte im Reich. Zur Sozial- und Wirkungsgeschichte akademischer Eliten des 14. bis 16. Jahrhunderts.* Berlin 1996, pp. 327–348.
Merula, Gaudenzio: *Memorabilium opus.* Lyon 1556.
Metzger, Nadine: *Wolfsmenschen und nächtliche Heimsuchungen: Zur kulturhistorischen Verortung vormoderner Konzepte von Lykanthropie und Ephialtes.* Remscheid 2011.

Meyer, Stefanie: *Der "Discursus medicus et politicus" von Tobias Geiger (1656). Edition und Kommentar*. Diss. med. Würzburg 2021.
Micale, Mark S.: *Approaching hysteria. Disease and its interpretations*. Princeton 1995.
Mikkeli, Heikki: *An Aristotelian response to Renaissance humanism. Jacopo Zabarella on the nature of arts and sciences*. Helsinki 1992.
Mikkeli, Heikki: *Hygiene in the early modern medical tradition*. Helsinki 1999.
Miller, Genevieve: A seventeenth-century astrological diagnosis. In: Edgar Ashworth Underwood (ed.): *Science, medicine and history. Essays on the evolution of scientific thought and medical practice*. London 1953, pp. 27–33.
Milton, J. R.: Induction before Hume. In: *British journal for the philosophy of science* 38 (1987), pp. 49–74.
Moehsen, J. C. W.: *Leben Leonhard Thurneissers zum Thurn. Ein Beitrag zur Geschichte der Alchemie wie auch der Wissenschaften und Künste in der Mark Brandenburg gegen Ende des 16. Jahrhunderts*. Berlin/Leipzig 1783.
Minelli, Alessandro (ed.): *L'orto botanico di Padova, 1545–1995*. Venice 1998.
Mone, Franz Joseph: Ueber Krankenpflege, vom 13. bis 16. Jahrhundert. In: *Zeitschrift für die Geschichte des Oberrheins* 2 (1851), pp. 257–291.
Monnetus, Io[annis] Carolus: Ad lectorem. In: Giovanni Battista da Monte: *In tertium primi Epidemiorum sectionem explanationes*. Ed. by Valentinus Lublinus. Venice 1554.
Montagnana, Marco Antonio: *De herpete, phagedaena, gangraena, sphacelo et cancro, tam cognoscendis, tam curandis tractatio accuratissima*. Venice 1589.
Montaigne, Michel de: *Die Essais*. Selected and ed. by Arthur Franz. Leipzig 1953.
Moran, Bruce: *The alchemical world of the German court. Occult philosophy and chemical medicine in the circle of Moritz of Hessen (1572–1632)*. Stuttgart 1991.
Moss, Ann: Power and persuasion. Commonplace culture in early modern Europe. In: David Cowling and Mette B. Bruun (eds): *Commonplace culture in Western Europe in the early modern period*. Leuven 2011, pp. 1–17.
Moss, Ann: *Printed commonplace-books and the structuring of Renaissance thought*. Oxford 1996.
Muccillo, Maria: Da Monte (De Monte, Dei Monte), Giovanni Battista. In: *Dizionario biografico degli Italiani* 32 (1986) (http://www.treccani.it/enciclopedia/da-monte-giovanni-battista-detto-montano_%28Dizionario-Biografico%29/).
Müller, Harald: "Specimen eruditionis". Zum Habitus der Renaissance-Humanisten und seiner sozialen Bedeutung. In: Frank Rexroth (ed.): *Beiträge zur Kulturgeschichte der Gelehrten im späten Mittelalter*. Ostfildern 2010, pp. 117–151.
Müller, Nikolaus: *Philipp Melanchthons letzte Lebenstage, Heimgang und Bestattung nach den gleichzeitigen Berichten der Wittenberger Professoren. Zum 350. Todestage Melanchthons*. Leipzig 1910.
Müller-Jahncke, Wolf-Dieter: Von Ficino zu Agrippa. Der Magia-Begriff des Renaissance-Humanismus im Überblick. In: Antoine Faivre and Rolf Christian Zimmermann (eds): *Epochen der Naturmystik. Hermetische Traditionen im wissenschaftlichen Fortschritt*. Berlin 1979, pp. 24–51.
Mugnai Carrara, Daniela: Epistemological problems in Giovanni Mainardi's commentary on Galen's *Ars parva*. In: Anthony Grafton and Nancy Siriasi (eds): *Natural particulars. Nature and the disciplines in Renaissance Europe*. Cambridge, MA 1999, pp. 251–273.
Mugnai Carrara, Daniela: Profilo di Nicolò Leoniceno. In: *Interpres. Rivista di studi quattrocenteschi* (1979), pp. 169–212.

Mugnai Carrara, Daniela and Maria Conforti: L'insegnamento della medicina dall'istituzione delle università al 1550. In: Antonio Clericuzio and Germana Ernst (eds): *Il Rinascimento italiano e l'Europa*. Vol. 5: *Le scienze*. Treviso/Costabissara 2008, pp. 455–478.

Murphy, Hannah: *A new order of medicine. The rise of physicians in Reformation Nuremberg*. Pittsburgh 2019.

Nagy, Doreen Evenden: *Popular medicine in seventeenth-century England*. Bowling Green 1988.

Nance, Brian: *Turquet de Mayerne as Baroque physician. The art medical portraiture*. Amsterdam/New York 2001.

Neefe, Caspar: *De missione sanguinis, quam phlebotomiam appellant, disputatio*. Leipzig 1548.

Nelles, Paul: Reading and memory in the universal library: Conrad Gessner and the Renaissance book. In: Donald Beecher and Grant Williams (eds): *Ars reminiscendi. Mind and memory in Renaissance culture*. Toronto 2009, pp. 147–169.

Nettesheim, Agrippa von: *Die Eitelkeit und Unsicherheit der Wissenschaft und die Verteidigungsschrift*. Ed. by Fritz Mauthner. Vol. 2. Munich 1913.

Neuburger, Max: *Die Lehre von der Heilkraft der Natur im Wandel der Zeiten*. Stuttgart 1926.

Neumeister, Sebastian and Conrad Wiedemann (eds): *Res publica litteraria. Die Institutionen der Gelehrsamkeit in der frühen Neuzeit*. Wiesbaden 1987.

Neuser, Wilhelm H.: Das Stammbuch des Zacharias Ursinus (1553–1563 und 1581). In: *Blätter für pfälzische Kirchengeschichte und religiöse Volkskunde* 31 (1964), pp. 101–155.

Newton, Hannah: *The sick child in early modern England, 1580–1720*. Oxford 2012.

Nicoud, Marilyn: Medici, lettere e pazienti. Pratica medica e retorica nella corrispondenza della cancelleria sforzesca. In: Andretta/Nicoud, *Être médecin* (2013), pp. 213–233.

Nováková, Julie: Rytmické kalendarium Jiřího Handsche. In: *Listy filologické* 89 (1966), pp. 315–320.

Nutton, Vivian: Continuity or rediscovery? The city physician in classical antiquity and mediaeval Italy. In: Russell, *Town and state physician* (1981), pp. 9–46.

Nutton, Vivian.: Hippocrates in the Renaissance. In: Gerhard Baader and Rolf Winau (eds): *Die Hippokratischen Epidemien. Theorie – Praxis – Tradition*. Stuttgart 1989, pp. 420–439.

Nutton, Vivian: Humanist surgery. In: Wear, French and Lonie, *Medical Renaissance* (1985), pp. 75–99.

Nutton, Vivian: Introduction. In: idem, *Medicine* (1990), pp. 1–14.

Nutton, Vivian: John Caius und Johannes Lange. Medizinischer Humanismus zur Zeit Vesals. In: *NTM* 21 (1984), pp. 81–87.

Nutton, Vivian (ed.): *Medicine at the courts of Europe, 1500–1837*. London/New York 1989.

Nutton, Vivian: Medicine at the German Universities, 1348–1500. A Preliminary Sketch. In: *Würzburger medizinhistorische Mitteilungen* (1997), pp. 173–187.

Nutton, Vivian: Roman medicine, 250 BC to AD 200, and medicine in late antiquity and the early Middle Ages. In: Conrad Lawrence et alii: *The Western medical tradition, 800 BC to AD 1800*. Cambridge, 1995, pp. 39–70.

Nutton, Vivian: The diffusion of ancient medicine in the Renaissance. In: *Medicina nei secoli* N. S. 14 (2002), pp. 461–478.

Nutton, Vivian and Roy Porter (eds): *The history of medical education in Britain*. Amsterdam/Atlanta,GA 1995.

Nutton, Vivian: The reception of Fracastoro's theory of contagion. The seed that fell among thorns? In: *Osiris* 6 (1990), pp. 196–234.

Nutton, Vivian.: Wittenberg anatomy. In: Ole Peter Grell (ed.): *Medicine and the Reformation*. London 1993, pp. 11–32.
Oberrauch, Lukas: Medizin. In: Martin Korenjak (ed.): *Tyrolis latina. Geschichte der lateinischen Literatur in Tirol*. Vol. 1: *Von den Anfängen bis zur Gründung der Universität Innsbruck*. Vienna 2012, pp. 363–377.
Oetheus, Jakob: *Gründtlicher Bericht, Lehr unnd Instruction von rechtem und nutzlichem Brauch der Artzney*. Dillingen 1574.
Oetheus, Jakob: *Theses de methodo therapeutica, secundum dogmaticam, ac rationalem medicinam*. Resp. Philipp Menzel. Ingolstadt 1569.
Ofenhitzer, Franziska: *Praxisalltag in der Frühen Neuzeit. Das Rezeptdiarium (1612–1616) von Petrus Kirstenius aus Breslau*. Diss. med. Univ. Würzburg 2015.
Ogilvie, Brian W.: *The science of describing. Natural history in Renaissance Europe*. Chicago/London 2006.
Olmi, Giuseppe: Molti amici in vari luoghi. Studio della natura e rapporti epistolari nel XVI secolo. In: *Nuncius* 6 (1991), pp. 3–31.
O'Malley, Charles D.: *Andreas Vesalius of Brussels, 1514–1564*. Berkeley/Los Angeles 1965.
O'Malley, Charles D.: Medical education during the Renaissance. In: idem (ed.): *History of medical education*. Berkeley/Los Angeles 1970, pp. 89–102.
Ongaro, Giuseppe: La medicina nello Studio di Padova e nel Veneto. In: *Storia della cultura veneta. Dal primo Quattrocento al Consilio di Trento*. Vol III/III. Vicenza 1981, pp. 75–134.
Ongaro, Giuseppe: L'insegnamento clinico di Giovan Battista da Monte (1489–1551). Una revisione critica. In: *Physis* 31 (1994), pp. 357–369.
Ongaro, Giuseppe: Medicina. In: Piero del Negro (ed.): *L'Università di Padova. Otto secoli di storia*. Padua 2001, pp. 153–193.
Ongaro, Giuseppe: *Wirsung a Padova 1629–1643*. Treviso 2010.
Orsolato, Giuseppe: Sulla prima fondazione di una clinica in Padova e sul monumento a G. B. Da Monte nella casa che fu del professore G. A. Giacomini. In: *Rivista periodica dei lavori della Reale Accademia di scienze, lettere ed arti in Padova* 23 (1872–73), pp. 127–152.
Padovani, Elideo: *Processus, curationes et consilia in curandis in particularibus morbis quae prosperos habuerunt eventus*. Ed. by Johannes Wittich. Leipzig 1607.
Pagel, Walter: *Das medizinische Weltbild des Paracelsus. Seine Zusammenhänge mit Neuplatonismus und Gnosis*. Wiesbaden 1962.
Palmer, Richard: Physicians and the state in post-medieval Italy. In: Russell, *Town and state physician* (1981), pp. 47–61.
Panáček, Jaroslav: *Testament Georga Handsche z roku 1578*. Bezděz 2013.
Pancino, Claudia: Doctor and patient in the modern age: words, gazes and gestures. In: Maria Malatesta (ed.): *Doctors and patients. History, representation, communication from antiquity to the present*. San Francisco 2015, pp. 81–107.
Pánek, Jaroslav: The nobility in the Czech lands, 1550–1650. In: Fučíková, *Rudolf II* (1997), pp. 270–286.
Panke-Kochinke, Birgit: *Die Geschichte der Krankenpflege (1679–2000). Ein Quellenbuch*. Frankfurt 2003.
Paracelsus: *Grosse Wundartzney. Von allen Wunden, Stich, Schüsß Bränd, Bisß, Beynbrüch*. Ulm 1536.
Paracelsus: *Von der Bergsucht oder Bergkranckheiten drey Bücher*. Dillingen 1567.
Paracelsus: *Von der frantzösischen Kranckheit drey Bücher*. Nürnberg 1530.

Pardi, Giuseppe: *Titoli dottorali conferiti dallo studio di Ferrara nei sec. XV e XVI*. Lucca 1901 (repr. Bologna 1970).
Paré, Ambroise: *Les œuvres*. Paris 1575.
Paré, Ambroise: *Opera chirurgica*. Frankfurt 1594.
Paré, Ambroise: *Response [. . .] aux calomnies d'aucuns médecins, et chirurgiens, touchant ses œuvres*. [Paris 1575].
Park, Katherine: *Doctors and medicine in early Renaissance Florence*. Princeton/New York 1985.
Park, Katharine: Observations in the margins, 500–1500. In: Lorraine Daston and Elizabeth Lunbeck (eds): *Histories of scientific observation*. Chicago/London 2011, pp. 15–44.
Park, Katharine and Robert A. Nye: Destiny is anatomy. In: *The New Republic* 18 February 1991, pp. 53–57.
Paullini, Christian Franz: *Wie nemlich mit Koth und Urin fast alle, ja auch die schwerste, gifftige Kranckheiten, und bezauberte Schaden, vom Haupt biß zun Füssen inn- und äusserlich glücklich curirt worden*. Frankfurt 1696.
Paulos von Aegina: *Paulos' von Aegina, des besten Arztes sieben Bücher*. Transl. and ed. by Julius Berendes. Leiden 1914.
Pawlik, Christian: *Martin Stainpeis: Liber de modo studendi seu legendi in medicina. Bearbeitung und Erläuterung einer Studienanleitung für Mediziner im ausgehenden Mittelalter*. Diss. med. TU Munich 1980.
Pellegrin, Pierre: Medicine. In: Brunschwig/Lloyd, *Greek thought* (2000), pp. 414–432.
Pennuto, Concetta: The debate on critical days in Renaissance Italy. In: Anna Akasoy, Charles Burnett and Ronit Yoeli-Tlalim (eds): *Astro-medicine. Astrology and medicine, East an West*. 2008, pp. 75–98.
Pešek, Jiří: Prague between 1550 and 1650. In: Fučíková, *Rudolf II* (1997), pp. 252–269.
Pfeil, Brigitte and Tilmann Walter: Im Dienst der Reichsstadt. Der spätmittelalterliche Stadtarzt Amplonius von der Buchen (1403–1438) und seine Briefe an die Stadt Nördlingen. In: *Jahrbuch des Historischen Vereins für Nördlingen und das Ries* 35 (2017), pp. 57–91.
Phaer, Thomas: *The regiment of life [. . .] with the boke of children*. London 1545.
Piccinini, Gabriella: Tra scienza ed arti. Lo Studio di Siena e l'insegnamento della medicina (secoli XIII-XVI). In: *L'Università di Siena. 750 anni di storia*. Milan 1991, pp. 145–158.
Pictorius, Georg: *Von Zernichten Artzten*. Strasbourg 1557.
Pieters, Jürgen and Julie Rogiest: Self-fashioning in de vroegmoderne literatuur- en cultuurgeschiedenis: genese en ontwikkeling van een concept. In: *Frame* 22 (2009), pp. 43–59.
Placotomus, Johannes [alias Johannes Brettschneider]: *De ratione discendi ac praecipue medicinam*. Leipzig 1552.
Planer, Andreas: *Theses med[ico]-phys[icae] de concoctione, eiusque differentiis*. Resp. Israel Spach. Strasbourg 1577.
Planerio, Giovanni: Epistolae morales. In: idem: *Varia opuscula*. Venice 1584 (separate pagination).
Planerio, Giovanni: Brevis patriae suae descriptio. In: idem: *Varia opuscula*. Venice 1584 (separate pagination).
Platter, Felix: *Beschreibung der Stadt Basel 1610 und Pestbericht 1610/11*. Ed. by Valentin Lötscher. Basel/Stuttgart 1987.
Platter, Felix: *De corporis humani structura et usu libri III. Tabulis methodice explicati, iconibus accurate illustrati*. Basel 1583.

Platter, Felix: *Observationum in hominis affectibus plerisque corpori et animo [. . .] incommodantibus libri tres*. Basel 1614.
Platter, Felix: *Quaestionum medicarum paradoxarum & endoxarum, iuxta partes medicinae dispositarum centuria posthuma*. Ed. by Thomas Platter. Basel 1625.
Platter, Felix: *Tagebuch (Lebensbeschreibung) 1536–1567*. Ed. by Valentin Lötscher. Basel 1976.
Plinius: *Epistolarum libri X*. Lyon 1539.
Pomata, Gianna: A word of the empirics: The ancient concept of observation and its recovery in early modern medicine. In: *Annals of science* 65 (2011), pp. 1–25.
Pomata, Gianna: *La promessa di guarigione. Malati e curatori in antico regime. Bologna XVI-XVIII secolo*. Bari 1994.
Pomata, Gianna: Observation rising. Birth of an epistemic genre, 1500–1600. In: Lorraine Daston and Elizabeth Lunbeck (eds): *Histories of scientific observation*. Chicago/London 2011, pp. 45–80.
Pomata, Gianna: *Praxis historialis*. The uses of *historia* in early modern medicine. In: Pomata/Siraisi, Historia (2005), pp. 105–146.
Pomata, Gianna: Sharing cases: The *observationes* in early modern medicine. In: *Early science and medicine* 15 (2010), pp. 193–236.
Pomata, Gianna and Nancy G. Siraisi (eds): *Historia. Empiricism and erudition in early modern Europe*. Cambridge, MA 2005.
Pons, Jacobus: *Medicus seu ratio, ac via aptissima ad recte tum discendam, tum exercendam medicinam. Ad tyrones*. Lyon 1600.
Pormann, Peter E. and Emily Savage Smith: *Medieval Islamic medicine*. Cairo 2007.
Porter, Roy and George S. Rousseau: *Gout. The patrician malady*. New Haven/London 1998.
Porter, Roy: The rise of physical examination. In: W. F. Bynum and Roy Porter (eds): *Medicine and the five senses*. Cambridge 2004, pp. 179–197.
Poynter, F. N. L. and W. J. Bishop (eds): *A seventeenth-century doctor and his patients: John Symcotts, 1592?-1662*. Streatley 1951.
Premuda, Loris: Un discepolo di Leoniceno tra filologia ed empirismo. G. Manardo e il "libero esame" dei classici della medicina in funzione di più spreguidicati orientamenti metodologici. In: *Atti del convegno internazionale per la celebrazione del V centenario della nascita di Giovanni Manardo 1462–1536*. Ferrara 1963, pp. 43–56.
Prioreschi, Plinio: Did the Hippocratic physician treat hopeless cases? In: *Gesnerus* 49 (1992), pp. 341–350.
Procházka, Faustin: *De saecularibus liberalium artium in Bohemia et Moravia fatis commentarius*. Prague 1782.
Pulz, Waltraud: *Nüchternes Kalkül – verzehrende Leidenschaft. Nahrungsabstinenz im 16. Jahrhundert*. Cologne/Weimar/Vienna 2007.
Purš, Ivo: Die Bibliothek Erzherzog Ferdinands II. auf Schloss Ambras. In: Sabine Haag and Veronika Sandbichler (eds): *Ferdinand II. 450 Jahre Tiroler Landesfürst*. Innsbruck 2017, pp. 99–104.
Quaranta, Alessandra: Medici trentini e *Respublica medicorum* europea: scambi culturali e scientifici nella seconda metà del Cinquecento. In: *Studi Trentini. Storia* 97 (2018), pp. 83–120.
Questel, Caspar: *Dissertatio academica de pulvinari morientibus non subtrahendo, von Abziehung der Sterbenden Haupt=Küssen, ex moralibus, divinis, juris item ac artis medicae principis methodice proposita, et exemplis rarioribus illustrata*. Jena 1678.

Ragland, Evan R.: "Making trials" in sixteenth- and early seventeenth-century European academic medicine. In: *Isis* 108 (2017), pp. 503–528.
Raimondi, C.: Lettere di P.A. Mattioli ad Ulisse Aldrovandi. In: *Bullettino senese di Storia patria* 13 (1906), pp. 121–185.
Ramsey, Matthew: *Professional and popular medicine in France, 1770–1830. The social world of medical practice.* Cambridge 1988.
Rankin, Alisha: Becoming an expert practitioner: Court experimentalism and the medical skills of Anna of Saxony (1532–1585). In: *Isis* 98 (2007), pp. 23–53.
Rankin, Alisha: On anecdote and antidotes. Poison trials in early modern Europe. In: *Bulletin of the history of medicine* 91 (2017), pp. 274–302.
Rankin, Alisha: *Panaceia's daughters. Noblewomen as healers in early modern Germany.* Chicago/London 2013.
Rankin, Alisha: *The poison trials. Wonder drugs, experiment, and the battle for authority in Renaissance science.* Chicago 2021.
Raphael, Lutz: Habitus und sozialer Sinn. Der Ansatz der Praxistheorie bei Pierre Bourdieu. In: Friedrich Jäger and Jürgen Straub (eds): *Handbuch der Kulturwissenschaften.* Vol. 2. Stuttgart 2004, pp. 266–276.
Rasori, Giovanni: *Sul metodo degli studi medici prolusione.* Milan 1809.
Rath, Gernot: *Die Entwicklung des klinischen Unterrichts.* Göttingen 1965.
Rath, Gernot: Moderne Diagnosen historischer Seuchen. In: *Deutsche medizinische Wochenschrift* 81 (1956), pp. 2065–2069.
Rather, L. J.: *The genesis of cancer: A study in the history of ideas.* Baltimore 1978.
Reckwitz, Andreas: Grundelemente einer Theorie sozialer Praktiken. Eine sozialtheoretische Perspektive. In: *Zeitschrift für Soziologie* 32 (2003), pp. 282–301.
Read, Sara: *Menstruation and the female body in early modern England.* Basingstoke 2013.
Reeds, Karen Meier: *Botany in medieval and Renaissance universities.* New York/London 1991.
Reger, Brigitte: *Affectio hypochondriaca. Das Krankheitsbild der Hypochondrie in der Frühen Neuzeit.* Diss. med. Regensburg 2015.
Resende, Garcia de: *Crónica de D. João II e miscelânea.* Coimbra 1798 (facsimile reprint Lisbon 1991).
Renner, Franz: *Ein new wolgegründet nützlichs unnd haylsams Handtbüchlein gemeiner Praktik aller innerlicher und eusserlicher Erzney wider die Krankheit der Franzosen.* Nürnberg 1557.
Reusnerus, Nicolaus: *Icones sive imagines virorum literis illustrium.* Strasbourg 1590.
Rhazes (Al-Rāzī): *Al-Rāzī, on the treatment of small children (De curis puerorum). The Latin and Hebrew translations.* Ed. by Michael McVaugh. Leiden 2015.
Richards, Jennifer: Useful books: Reading vernacular regimens in sixteenth-century England. In: *Journal of the history of ideas* 73 (2012), pp. 247–271.
Richardson, Linda Deer: The generation of disease. Occult causes and diseases of the total substance. In: Wear, French und Lonie, *Medical Renaissance* (1985), pp. 175–194.
Richter, David: *Genealogia Lutherorum.* Berlin/Leipzig 1733.
Ridder-Symoens, Hilde de (ed.): *A history of the university in Europe.* Vol. II: *Universities in early modern Europe (1500–1800).* Cambridge 1996.
Riddle, J. M.: Three previously unknown sixteenth-century contributors to pharmacy, medicine and botany. Ioannes Manardus, Franciscus Frigimelica and Melchior Guilandinus. In: *Pharmacy in history* 21 (1979), pp. 143–155.

Ritzmann, Iris: *Sorgenkinder. Kranke und behinderte Mädchen und Jungen im 18. Jahrhundert.* Cologne/Weimar/Vienna 2008.
Roeck, Bernd: *Der Morgen der Welt. Geschichte der Renaissance.* Munich 2017.
Roger, Jacques: *Jean Fernel et les problèmes de la médecine de la Renaissance.* Paris 1960.
Rondelet, Guillaume: *Libri de piscibus marinis in quibus verae piscium effigies expressae sunt.* Lyon 1554.
Ronsseus, Balduinus: *Miscellanea seu epistolae medicinales.* Leiden 1590.
Rosenberg, Daniel: Early modern information overload. In: *Journal of the history of ideas* 64 (2003), pp. 1–9.
Rosenheim, Max: *The album amicorum. Communicated to the Society of Antiquaries.* Oxford 1910.
Rudel, Otto: *Beiträge zur Geschichte der Medizin in Tirol. Gesammelt für das Etschländer Ärzteblatt.* Bozen 1925.
Ründal, Erik O.: "daß seine Mannschaft ganz unvollkommen sey". Impotenz in der Frühen Neuzeit. Diskurse und Praktiken in Deutschland. In: *Österreichische Zeitschrift für Geschichtswissenschaft* 22, N. 2 (2011), pp. 50–74.
Ruland, Martin: *Curationum empiricarum et historicarum, in certis locis et notis personis optime expertarum et rite probatarum centuria prima.* Basel 1578.
Russell, Andrew W. (ed.): *The town and state physician in Europe from the Middle Ages to the Enlightenment.* Wolfenbüttel 1981.
Sacchini, Franciscus: *De ratione libros cum profectu legendi.* Ingolstadt 1614.
Salatowsky, Sascha and Michael Stolberg (eds): *Eine göttliche Kunst. Medizin und Krankheit in der Frühen Neuzeit* (exhibition catalogue, Forschungsbibiothek Gotha). Gotha 2019.
Sander, Sabine: *Handwerkschirurgen. Sozialgeschichte einer verdrängten Berufsgruppe.* Göttingen 1989.
Santa Maria, Angiolgabriello di: *Biblioteca, e storia di quei scrittori cosi della città come del territorio di Vicenza che pervennero fin' ad ora a notizia.* Vol. 3 and Vol. 4. Vicenza 1772.
Santing, Catrien: *Geneeskunde en humanisme. Een intellectuele biografie van Theodericus Ulsenius (c. 1460–1508).* Rotterdam 1992.
Santoro, Marco: *Uso e abuso delle dediche. A proposito del "Della dedicatione de' libri" di Giovanni Fratta.* Rome 2006.
Sassonia, Ercole: *Pantheum medicinae selectum: sive medicinae practicae templum, omnibus omnium fere morborum insultibus commune, libris undecim distinctum.* Frankfurt 1603.
Savoia, Paolo: The book of the sick of Santa Maria della Morte in Bologna and the medical organization of a hospital in the sixteenth-century. In: *Nuncius* 31 (2016), pp. 163–235
Savonarola, Michele: *Practica.* Venice 1502.
Sawyer, Ronald C.: Friends or foes? Doctors and their patients in early modern England. In: Yosio Kawakita, Shizu Sakai and Yasuo Otsuka (eds.): *History of the doctor-patient relationship.* Tokyo/Brentwood 1995, pp. 31–53.
Sawyer, Ronald C.: Patients, healers, and disease in the Southeast Midlands, 1587–1634. Unpublished PhD-thesis, University of Wisconsin 1986.
Schäfer, Daniel: Regimina infantium. Die Sorge um die Gesundheit der Kinder in der Renaissance. In: Bergdolt, Hamm and Tönnesmann, *Kind* (2008), pp. 71–100.
Schaffrath, Ulrich: Läuse, Muscheln und Tabak. Das Herbar Ratzenberger. In: *Philippia* 15 (2012), pp. 191–214.
Schattner, Angela: *Zwischen Familie, Heilern und Fürsorge. Das Bewältigungsverhalten von Epileptikern in deutschsprachigen Gebieten des 16.-18. Jahrhunderts.* Stuttgart 2012.

Schatzki, Theodore R., Karin Knorr Cetina and Eike von Savigny (eds): *The practice turn in contemporary theory*. London/New York 2001.

Schenck, Johann von Grafenberg: *Observationum medicarum, rararum, novarum, admirabilium, et monstrosarum libri*. 2 vols. Freiburg 1597/1599.

Schiebinger, Londa: Skeletons in the closet. The first illustrations of the female skeleton in eighteenth-century anatomy. In: *Representations* 14 (1986), pp. 42–82.

Schieß, Traugott: *Briefe aus der Fremde von einem Zürcher Studenten der Medizin (Dr. Georg Keller) 1550–1558* (= Neujahrblatt Nr. 262). Zürich 1906.

Schild, Wolfgang: Das Blut des Hingerichteten. In: Christina von Braun and Christoph Wulf (eds): *Mythen des Bluts*. Frankfurt 2007, pp. 126–154.

Schilling, Ruth, Sabine Schlegelmilch and Susan Splinter: Stadtarzt oder Arzt in der Stadt? Drei Ärzte der Frühen Neuzeit und ihr Verständnis des städtischen Amtes. In: *Medizinhistorisches Journal* 46 (2011), pp. 99–133.

Schirrmeister, Albert: *Triumph des Dichters. Gekrönte Intellektuelle im 16. Jahrhundert.* Cologne/Weimar/Vienna 2003.

Schlegelmilch, Sabine: *Ärztliche Praxis und sozialer Raum im 17. Jahrhundert. Johannes Magirus (1615–1697)*. Cologne 2018.

Schlegelmilch, Sabine: Das Selbstbewußtsein der Chirurgen. Tobias Geigers Traktat *Discursus Medicus et Politicus* (1656). In: Mariacarla Gadebusch Bondio, Christian Kaiser and Manuel Förg (eds): *Menschennatur in Zeiten des Umbruchs. Das Ideal des "politischen" Arztes in der Frühen Neuzeit*. Oldenburg 2020, pp. 141–176.

Schlegelmilch, Sabine: Promoting a good physician a town physician. Letters of application to German town authorities (1500–1700). In: Andrew Mendelsohn, Annemarie Kinzelbach and Ruth Schilling (eds): *Civic medicine. Physician, polity, and pen in early modern Europe*. Abingdon 2019, pp. 88–109.

Schlegelmilch, Sabine: "What a magnificent work a good physician is". The medical practice of Johannes Magirus (1615–1697). In: Dinges et alii, *Medical practice* (2016), pp. 151–168.

Schlegelmilch, Ulrich: Surgical disputations in Basel at around 1600. In: Meelis Friedenthal, Hanspeter Marti and Robert Seidel (eds): *Early modern disputations and dissertations in an interdisciplinary and European context*. Leiden 2021, pp. 255–287.

Schmid, Alois: "Poeta et orator a Caesare laureatus". Die Dichterkrönungen Kaiser Maximilians I. In: *Historisches Jahrbuch* 109 (1989), pp. 56–108.

Schmidt, Erich Ludwig: *Deutsche Volkskunde im Zeitalter des Humanismus und der Reformation*. Berlin 1904.

Schmidt, Paul Gerhard: Mediziner oder Poet? Soziale Lage und Lebenspläne hessischer Humanisten. In: August Buck and Tibor Klaniczay (eds): *Sozialgeschichtliche Fragestellungen in der Renaissanceforschung*. Wiesbaden 1992, pp.107–117.

Schmidt-Biggemann, Wilhelm: *Topica universalis. Eine Modellgeschichte humanistischer und barocker Wissenschaft*. Hamburg 1983.

Schmitt, Charles B.: Aristotle among the physicians. In: Wear, French and Lonie, *Medical Renaissance* (1985), pp. 1–15 and notes pp. 271–279.

Schmitt, Charles B.: *Aristotle and the Renaissance*. Cambridge 1983.

Schnell, Bernhard: Arzt und Literat. Zum Anteil der Ärzte am spätmittelalterlichen Literaturbetrieb. In: *Sudhoffs Archiv* 75 (1991), pp. 44–57.

Schober, Karl and Emil Neder: *Sechshunderjahrfeier der Stadt Böhmisch Leipa, 1337–1937*. Böhmisch-Leipa 1929.

Scholz, Lorenz: *Catalogus arborum, fruticum et plantarum, tam indigenarum quam exoticarum, horti medici Laurentii Scholzii medici Vratisl.* Breslau 1594.
Scholz, Lorenz (ed.): *Consiliorum et epistolarum medicinalium [. . .] liber secundus.* Frankfurt 1592.
Scholz, Lorenz (Hrg.): *Consiliorum et epistolarum medicinalium Ioannis Cratonis à Kraftheim liber septimus.* Hannover 1611.
Scholz, Lorenz (ed.): *Consiliorum medicinalium conscriptorum a praestantiss[imis] atque exercitatiss[imis] nostrorum temporum medicis liber singularis.* Frankfurt 1598.
Scholz, Lorenz (ed.): *Epistolarum philosophicarum, medicinalium ac chymicarum a summis nostrae aetatis philosophis ac medicis exaratum volumen.* Frankfurt 1598.
Schrauf, Karl and Wenzel Hartl: *Fünf Wiener Ärzte und Naturforscher aus dem XVI. Jahrhundert. Johann Aicholz, Diomedes Cornarius, Mathias Cornax, Wilhelm Coturnossius, Andreas Dadius.* Vienna 1894.
Schrick, Michael: *Von den ausgebrannten Wassern.* Augsburg 1481.
Schuster, Daniel: *"Die Festung des Lebens zu stürmen". Körper- und Krankheitsmetaphern in der medizinischen Ratgeberliteratur des 16. und 17. Jahrhunderts.* Diss. med. Würzburg 2021.
Schütte, Jana Madlen: *Medizin im Konflikt: Fakultäten, Märkte und Experten in deutschen Universitätsstädten des 14. bis 16. Jahrhunderts.* Leiden 2017.
Schwarz, Christiane: *Studien zur Stammbuchpraxis der Frühen Neuzeit. Gestaltung und Nutzung des Album amicorum am Beispiel eines Hofbeamten und Dichters, eines Politikers und eines Goldschmieds (etwa 1550–1650).* Frankfurt 2002 (= Diss. phil. Munich 1999).
Scipio, Rosario (ed.): *Girolamo Fabrici l'Acquapendente.* Viterbo 1978.
Seidl, Katharina: " . . . how to assuage all outer and inner malady . . . ". Medicine at the court of Archduke Ferdinand II. In: Sabine Haag and Veronika Sandbichler (eds): *Ferdinand II. 450 years sovereign ruler of Tyrol.* Exhibition catalogue. Innsbruck/Vienna 2017, pp. 67–71.
Senfelder, Leopold: Georg Handsch von Limus. Lebensbild eines Arztes aus dem XVI. Jahrhundert. In: *Wiener klinische Rundschau* (1901), pp. 495–499, pp. 514–516 and pp. 533–535.
Sennert, Daniel: *Opera omnia.* Lyon 1656.
Sennert, Daniel: *Institutionum medicinae libri V.* Wittenberg 1620.
Sevilla, Isidor of: *Praeclarissimum opus [. . .] quod ethimologiarum intitulat[ur].* Paris 1509.
Sharpe, Kevin: *The politics of reading in early modern England.* New Haven 2000.
Sherman, W. H.: *Used books. Marking readers in Renaissance England.* Philadelphia 2008.
Sherrington, Charles: *The endeavour of Jean Fernel.* Cambridge 1946.
Simons, Madelon: *"Een Theatrum van Representatie?" Aartshertog Ferdinand van Oostenrijk stadhouder in Praag tussen 1547 en 1567.* Diss. phil. Amsterdam 2009.
Simons, Ronald C. and Charles C. Hughes (eds): *The culture-bound syndromes. Folk illnesses of psychiatric and anthopological interest.* Dordrecht 1985.
Siraisi, Nancy G.: Anatomizing the past. Physicians and history in Renaissance culture. In: *Renaissance quarterly* 53 (2000), pp. 1–30.
Siraisi, Nancy G.: *Avicenna in Renaissance Italy. The "Canon" and medical teaching in Italian universities after 1500.* Princeton 1987.
Siraisi, Nancy G.: Baudouin Ronsse as writer of medical letters. In: Ann Blair and Anja-Silvia Going (eds): *For the sake of learning. Essays in honor of Anthony Grafton.* Leiden/Boston 2016, pp. 123–139.

Siraisi, Nancy G.: *Communities of learned experience. Epistolary medicine in the Renaissance.* Baltimore 2013.
Siraisi, Nancy G.: Die medizinische Fakultät. In: Walter Rüegg (ed.): *Geschichte der Universität in Europa.* Vol. I: *Von der Reformation zur Französischen Revolution (1500–1800).* Munich 1996, pp. 321–342.
Siraisi, Nancy G.: Disease and symptom as problematic concepts in Renaissance medicine. In: Eckhard Kessler and Ian Maclean (eds): *Res et verba in der Renaissance.* Wiesbaden 2002, pp. 217–240.
Siraisi, Nancy G.: *History, medicine and the traditions of Renaissance learning.* Ann Arbor 2007.
Siraisi, Nancy G.: L'individuale nella medicina tra medioevo e umanesimo: i 'casi clinici'. In: Roberto Cardini and Mariangela Regoliosi (eds): *Umanesimo e medicina. Il problema dell'individuale.* Rome 1996, pp. 33–62.
Siraisi, Nancy G.: Medicina practica. Girolamo Mercuriale as teacher and textbook author. In: Emidio Campi, Simone De Angelis, Anja-Silvia Goeing and Anthony T. Grafton (eds): *Scholarly knowledge. Textbooks in early modern Europe.* Geneva 2008, pp. 287–305.
Siraisi, Nancy G.: *Medicine and the Italian universities 1250–1600.* Leiden 2001.
Siraisi, Nancy G.: Medicine, 1450–1620, and the history of science. In: *Isis* 103 (2012), pp. 491–514.
Siraisi, Nancy G.: *Medieval & early Renaisance medicine.* Chicago/London 1990.
Siraisi, Nancy G.: Oratory and rhetoric in Renaissance medicine. In: *Journal of the history of ideas* 65 (2004), pp. 191–211.
Siraisi, Nancy G.: Segni evidenti, teoria e testimonianza nelle narrazioni di autopsie del Rinascimento. In: *Quaderni storici* 36 (2001), pp. 719–744.
Siraisi, Nancy G.: *Taddeo Alderotti and his pupils. Two generations of Italian medical learning.* Princeton 1981.
Siraisi, Nancy G.: *The clock and the mirror. Girolamo Cardano and Renaissance medicine.* Princeton 1997.
Siraisi, Nancy G.: The faculty of medicine. In: Ridder-Symoens, *History* (1992), pp. 360–387.
Slater, John, and Maria Luz López Terrada: Scenes of mediation: Staging medicine in the Spanish interludes. In: *Social history of medicine* 24 (2011), pp. 226–243.
Smith, Pamela: *The body of the artisan. Art and experience in the scientific revolution.* Chicago/London 2004.
Smolka, Josef and Marta Vaculínová: Renesanční lékař Georg Handsch (1529–1578). In: *DVT – Dějiny věd a techniky* 43 (2010), pp. 1–26.
Sole, Brunoroa and Jacob Schultes: *Loci communes juris caesarei, pontificii et saxonici. Opus legentibus, consulentibus, judicibus, advocatis utile, facile, necessarium.* Leipzig 1607.
Solenander, Rainer: *Consiliorum medicinalium Reineri Soleandri [. . .] sectiones quinque [. . .] cum consiliis celeberrimi medici Ioannis Montani.* 2nd edn. Hannover 1609.
Spach, Israel (ed.): *Gynaeciorum sive de mulierum tum communibus, tum gravidarum, parientium, et puerperarum affectibus et morbis libri.* Strasbourg 1597.
Spach, Israel: *Nomenclator scriptorum medicorum. Hoc est: Elenchus eorum, qui artem medicam suis scriptis illustrarunt, secundum locos communes ipsius medicinae.* Strasbourg 1591.
Span, Lorenz: *Epicedion nobili ac excellentissimo domino D. Andreæ de Gallis tridentino.* Prague 1560.
Spitzer, Gabriele: *Leonhard Thurneysser zum Thurn und die von ihm gegründete Berliner Druckerei (1574–1591).* 3 vols. Diss. phil. Berlin 1987.

Spitzner, Hermann Rudolf: *Die Salernitanische Gynäkologie und Geburtshilfe unter dem Namen der "Trotula"*. Diss. Leipzig 1921.
Staden, Heinrich von: Incurability and hopelessness. The Hippocratic corpus. In: Paul Potter (ed.): *La maladie et les maladies dans la collection hippocratique. Actes du VIe Colloque International Hippocratique.* Québec 1990, pp. 75–112.
Starn, Randolph: A postmodern Renaissance? In: *Renaissance quarterly* 60 (2007), pp. 1–24.
Statuta Dominorum Artistarum Achademiae [sic] Patavina [Padua [?] c. 1600]
Stainpeiss, Martin: *Liber de modo studendi seu legendi in medicina*. Vienna 1520.
Starck, Andreas: *Krancken Spiegel*. Mülhausen 1598.
Steiger, Anselm Johann: *Melancholie, Diätetik und Trost. Konzepte der Melancholie-Therapie im 16. und 17. Jahrhundert*. Heidelberg 1996.
Stein, Claudia: *Negotiating the French pox in early modern Germany*. Farnham 2009.
Stengel, Johann: *Theses de venae sectione*. Würzburg 1602.
Sterzi, Giuseppe: *Giulio Casseri anatomico e chirurgo (1552c.-1616)*. Venice 1909.
Stocker, Johannes: *Empirica: sive medicamenta varia, experientia diuturna comprobata et stabilita, contra plerosque omnes corporis humani morbos tam internos quam externos.* Ed. by Tobias Dornkrell ab Eberhertz. Frankfurt 1601.
Stöhsel, Robert: *Die Fieberlehre an den Universitäten Montpellier und Pavia im 14. und 15. Jahrhundert. Mitteilung eines handschriftlichen "Sermo utilis de febribus" von Antonius Guaynerius*. Diss. med. Würzburg 1923.
Stolberg, Michael: "Abhorreas pinguedinem": Fat and obesity in early modern medicine (c. 1500–1750) In: *Studies in the history and philosophy of biology and biomedical sciences* 43 (2012), pp. 370–378.
Stolberg, Michael, Accounting, religion, and the economics of medical care in 16th-century Germany. Hiob Finzel's *Rationarium praxeos medicae*, 1565–1589. In: Axel Hüntelmann and Oliver Falk (eds): *Accounting for health. Calculation, paperwork, and medicine, 1500–2000*. Manchester 2021, pp. 35–55.
Stolberg, Michael: Active euthanasia in early modern society. Learned debates and popular practices. In: *Social history of medicine* 20 (2007), pp. 205–221.
Stolberg, Michael: A sixteenth-century physician and his patients: The practice journal of Hiob Finzel, 1565–1589. In: *Social history of medicine* 32 (2019), pp. 221–240.
Stolberg, Michael: A woman down to her bones. The anatomy of sexual difference in the sixteenth and early seventeenth centuries. In: *Isis* 94 (2003), pp. 274–299.
Stolberg, Michael: A woman's hell? Medical perceptions of menopause in preindustrial Europe. In: *Bulletin of the history of medicine* 73 (1999), pp. 408–428.
Stolberg, Michael: Bedside teaching and the acquisition of practical skills in mid-sixteenth-century Padua. In: *Journal of the history of medicine and allied sciences* 69 (2014), pp. 633–661.
Stolberg, Michael: "Cura palliativa". Begriff und Diskussion der palliativen Krankheitsbehandlung in der vormodernen Medizin (ca. 1500–1850). In: *Medizinhistorisches Journal* 42 (2007), pp. 7–29.
Stolberg, Michael: Der gesunde Leib. Zur Geschichtlichkeit frühneuzeitlicher Körpererfahrung. In: Paul Münch (ed.): *"Erfahrung" als Kategorie der Frühneuzeitgeschichte* (= Historische Zeitschrift, Beiheft 31 (2001)), pp. 37–57.
Stolberg, Michael: *Die Geschichte der Palliativmedizin. Medizinische Sterbebegleitung von 1500 bis heute*. Frankfurt 2011.

Stolberg, Michael: Die Homöopathie auf dem Prüfstand. Der erste Doppelblindversuch der Medizingeschichte im Jahr 1835. In: *Münchener Medizinische Wochenschrift* 138 (1996), pp. 364–366.
Stolberg, Michael: Emotions and the body in early modern medicine. In: *Emotion review* 11 (2019), pp. 113–122.
Stolberg, Michael: Empiricism in sixteenth-century medical practice. The notebooks of Georg Handsch. In: *Early science and medicine* 18 (2013), pp. 487–516.
Stolberg, Michael: Enthüllungen. Die uroskopische Schwangerschaftsdiagnose und ihre Darstellung in der frühneuzeitlichen Kunst. In: Daniel Hornuff and Heiner Fangerau (eds): *Visualisierung des Ungeborenen*. Paderborn 2020, pp. 51–68.
Stolberg, Michael: Erfahrungen und Deutungen der weiblichen Monatsblutung in der Frühen Neuzeit. In: Barbara Mahlmann-Bauer (ed.): *Scientiae et artes. Die Vermittlung alten und neuen Wissens in Literatur, Kunst und Musik*. Wolfenbüttel 2004, pp. 913–931.
Stolberg, Michael: Examining the body (c. 1500–1750) In: Sarah Toulalan and Kate Fisher (eds): *The Routledge history of sex and the body, 1500 to the present*. Oxford 2013, pp. 91–105.
Stolberg, Michael: *Experiencing illness and the sick body in early modern Europe*. London 2011.
Stolberg, Michael: Formen und Funktionen ärztlicher Fallberichte in der Frühen Neuzeit (1500–1800). In: Johannes Süßmann, Susanne Scholz and Gisela Engel (eds): *Fallstudien: Theorie – Geschichte – Methode*. Berlin 2007, pp. 81–95.
Stolberg, Michael: *Heilkunde zwischen Staat und Bevölkerung. Angebot und Annahme medizinischer Versorgung in Oberfranken im frühen 19. Jahrhundert*. Diss. med. TU Munich 1986.
Stolberg, Michael: Metaphors and images of cancer in early modern Europe. In: *Bulletin of the history of medicine* 88 (2014), pp. 48–74.
Stolberg, Michael: Keeping the body open. Impurity, excretions, and healthy living in the early modern period. In: James Kennaway and Rina Knoeff (eds): *Lifestyle and medicine in the Enlightenment. The six non-naturals in the long eighteenth century*. New York/London 2020, pp. 205–222.
Stolberg, Michael: Kommunikative Praktiken. Ärztliche Wissensvermittlung am Krankenbett im 16. Jahrhundert. In: Arndt Brendecke (ed.): *Praktiken der Frühen Neuzeit. Akteure – Handlungen – Artefakte*. Cologne/Weimar/Vienna 2015, pp. 111–121.
Stolberg, Michael: Konservierte Pflanzen für die Wissenschaft. In: Salatowsky/Stolberg, *Göttliche Kunst* (2019), pp. 122–124.
Stolberg, Michael: Krankheitsgeschehen und leibärztliche Praxis am Hof von Erzherzog Ferdinand II. Die Aufzeichnungen des Georg Handsch (1529–1578). In: Elena Taddei and Marina Hilber (eds): *In fürstlicher Nähe. Ärzte bei Hof (1450–1800)*. Innsbruck 2021, pp. 91–110.
Stolberg, Michael: Learning anatomy in late sixteenth-century Padua. In: *History of science* 56 (2018), pp. 381–402.
Stolberg, Michael: Learning from the common folks. Academic physicians and medical lay culture in the sixteenth century. In: *Social history of medicine* 27 (2014), pp. 649–667.
Stolberg, Michael: Lykanthropie. In: Manfred Landfester (ed.): *Der Neue Pauly*. Vol. 15/1: *Wissenschafts- und Rezeptionsgeschichte La–Ot*. Stuttgart/Weimar 2001, pp. 243–246.
Stolberg, Michael: Medical note-taking in the sixteenth and seventeenth centuries. In: Alberto Cevolini (ed.): *Forgetting machines: Knowledge management evolution in early modern Europe*. Leiden/Boston 2016, pp. 243–264.

Stolberg, Michael: Medizinische Loci communes. Formen und Funktionen einer ärztlichen Aufzeichnungspraxis im 16. und 17. Jahrhundert. In: *NTM – Zeitschrift für Geschichte der Wissenschaften, Technik und Medizin* 21 (2013), pp. 37–60.

Stolberg, Michael: "Mein askulapisches Orakel!": Patientenbriefe als Quelle einer Kulturgeschichte der Krankheitserfahrung im 18. Jahrhundert. In: *Österreichische Zeitschrift für Geschichtswissenschaft* 7 (1996), pp. 385–404.

Stolberg, Michael: Menstruation and sexual difference in early modern medicine. In: Andrew Shail and Gillian Howie (eds): *Menstruation. A cultural history*. Basingstoke 2005, pp. 90–101.

Stolberg, Michael: Metaphors and images of cancer in early modern Europe. In: *Bulletin of the history of medicine* 88 (2014), pp. 48–74.

Stolberg, Michael: Möglichkeiten und Grenzen einer retrospektiven Diagnose. In: Waltraud Pulz (ed.): *Zwischen Himmel und Erde. Körperliche Zeichen der Heiligkeit*. Stuttgart 2012, pp. 209–227.

Stolberg, Michael: Negotiating the meanings of illness. Medical popularization and the patient in the 18th century. In: Wilhelm de Blécourt and Cornelie Usborne (eds): *Cultural approaches to the history of medicine. Mediating medicine in early modern and modern Europe*. Basingstoke/New York 2004, pp.89–107.

Stolberg, Michael: Post-mortems, anatomical dissections and humoural pathology in the sixteenth and early seventeenth centuries. In: Silvia De Renzi, Marco Bresadola and Maria Conforti (eds): *Pathology in practice. Diseases and dissections in early modern Europe*. New York/London 2017, pp. 79–95.

Stolberg, Michael: Probleme und Perspektiven einer Geschichte der Volksmedizin. In: Thomas Schnalke and Claudia Wiesemann (eds): *Die Grenzen des Anderen. Medizingeschichte aus postmoderner Perspektive*. Vienna 1998, pp. 49–73.

Stolberg, Michael: Studying medicine in 16th-century Padua and Montpellier. A comparative analysis from the perspectives of medical students. In: Delia Gavrus and Susan Lamb (eds): *History of medical education*. Montreal 2022 [in preparation].

Stolberg, Michael: Sweat. Learned concepts and popular perceptions, 1500–1800. In: Manfred Horstmannshoff, Helen King and Claus Zittel (eds): *Blood, sweat and tears. The changing concepts of physiology from antiquity to early modern Europe*. Leiden/Boston 2012, pp. 503–522.

Stolberg, Michael: Teaching anatomy in post-Vesalian Padua. An analysis of student notes. In: *Journal of medieval and early modern studies* 48 (2018), pp. 61–78.

Stolberg, Michael: The decline of uroscopy in early modern learned medicine, 1500–1650. In: *Early science and medicine* 12 (2007), pp. 313–336.

Stolberg, Michael: The doctor-patient relationship in the Renaissance. In: *European journal for the history of medicine and health* 1 (2021), pp. 1–29, open access: https://doi.org/10.1163/26667711-bja10001

Stolberg, Michael: The many uses of writing. A humanist physician in sixteenth-century Prague. In: Andrew Mendelsohn, Annemarie Kinzelbach and Ruth Schilling (eds): *Civic medicine. Physician, polity, and pen in early modern Europe*. London 2019, pp. 67–87.

Stolberg, Michael: The monthly malady: A history of premenstrual suffering. In: *Medical history* 44 (2000), pp. 301–322.

Stolberg, Michael: Tödliche Menschenversuche im 16. Jahrhundert. In: *Deutsches Ärzteblatt*, Ausgabe A 111 (2014), pp. 2060–2062.

Stolberg, Michael: *Uroscopy in early modern Europe*. Farnham/ Burlington, VT, 2015.

Stolberg, Michael: "You have no good blood in your body". Oral communication in sixteenth-century physicians' medical practice. In: *Medical history* 59 (2015), pp. 63–82.
Stolberg, Michael: "Zorn, Wein und Weiber verderben unsere Leiber." Krankheit und Affekt in der frühneuzeitlichen Medizin. In: Johann Anselm Steiger and Ralf Georg Bogner (eds): *Passion, Affekt und Leidenschaft in der Frühen Neuzeit.* Wiesbaden 2005, pp. 1033–1059.
Stolberg, Michael: Zwischen Identitätsbildung und Selbstinszenierung. Ärztliches Self-Fashioning in der Frühen Neuzeit. In: Dagmar Freist (ed.): *Diskurse – Körper – Artefakte. Historische Praxeologie in der Frühneuzeitforschung.* Bielefeld 2015, pp. 33–55.
Stolberg, Michael and Tilmann Walter: Martin Luthers viele Krankheiten. Ein unbekanntes Konsil von Matthäus Ratzenberger und die Problematik der retrospektiven Diagnose. In: *Archiv für Reformationsgeschichte* 109 (2018), pp. 126–151.
Stolz, Michael: *Artes-liberales-Zyklen: Formationen des Wissens im Mittelalter.* Vol. 1. Tübingen/Basel 2004.
Storchová, Lucie: *Bohemian school humanism and its editorial practices (ca. 1550–1610).* Turnhout 2014.
Storchová, Lucie: Collinus, Matthaeus. In: eadem (ed.): *Companion to Central and Eastern European humanism. Vol. 2: Czech lands, part 1: A-L.* Berlin 2020, pp. 298–316.
Storchová, Lucie: Handsch, Georg. In: eadem (ed.): *Companion to Central and Eastern European humanism. Vol. 2: Czech lands, part 1: A-L.* Berlin 2020, pp. 512–522.
Storchová, Lucie: Humanist occasional poetry and strategies for acquiring patronage. The case of Georg Handsch. In: Sylva Dobalová and Jaroslava Hausenblasová: *Archduke Ferdinand II of Austria: A second-born son in Renaissance Europe* [in preparation].
Storchová, Lucie: *Paupertate styloque connecti. Utváření humanistické učenecké komunity v českých zemích.* Prague 2011.
Storchová, Lucie: "The tempting girl, I know so well": Representations of gout and the self-fashioning of Bohemian humanist scholars. In: *Early science and medicine* 21 (2016), pp. 511–530.
Strobelberger, Johann Stefan: *Laureationum medicarum apud exteros promeritarum adversum obtrectatores breves vindiciae, in honorem Scholae medicae Monspeliensis propositae.* Nürnberg 1628.
Stroh, Walter: *Aerztliche Bewerbungen, Berufungen, Bestallungen des 15. und des 16. Jahrhunderts, aus Esslingen, sowie Verwandtes zum ärztlichen Standeswesen jener Zeit.* Diss. med. Leipzig 1920.
Stromer, Heinrich: *Algorithmus linealis numerationem, additionem, subtractionem, duplationem, mediationem, multiplicationem, divisionem et progressionem una cum regula de tri perstringens.* Vienna 1520.
Stübler, Eberhard: *Geschichte der medizinischen Fakultät der Universität Heidelberg 1386–1925.* Heidelberg 1926.
Stupanus, Johann Niklaus: *De praefocatione matricis.* Exhibet Rudolph Heinrich Groshaus. Basel 1612.
Sudhoff, Karl: *Erstlinge der pädiatrischen Literatur. Drei Wiegendrucke über Heilung und Pflege des Kindes.* Munich 1925.
Sudhoff, Karl: *Iatromathematiker vornehmlich im 15. und 16. Jahrhundert.* Breslau 1902.
Sudhoff, Karl: Kurpfuscher, Ärzte und Stadtbehörden am Ende des 15. Jahrhunderts. Handschriften- und Aktenstudie. In: *Archiv für Geschichte der Medizin* 8 (1915), pp. 98–124.

Sudhoff, Karl: *Versuch einer Kritik der Echtheit der Paracelsischen Schriften.* 2 vols. Berlin 1898/99.
Sudhoff, Karl: Zur Geschichte der Lehre von den kritischen Tagen im Krankheitsverlaufe. In: *Sudhoffs Archiv* 21 (1929), pp. 1–22.
Sullivan, Erin: *Beyond melancholy. Sadness and selfhood in Renaissance England.* Oxford 2016.
Svobodný, Petr: The medical faculty. In: Ivana Čornejová and Michal Svatoš (eds): *A history of Prague University, 1348–1802.* Prague 2001, pp. 171–185.
Sylvius, Jacobus: *Ordo et ordinis ratio in legendis Hippocratis et Galeni libris.* Paris 1548.
Talbot, Charles: *Medical education in the Middle Ages.* In: O'Malley, *History* (1970), pp. 73–87.
Tanfani, Gustavo: "I consilia medica" di Vittore Trincavella. In: *Rivista di storia delle scienze mediche e naturali* 43 (1952), pp. 248–254.
Tanner, Jakob: *Historische Anthropologie zur Einführung.* Hamburg 2004.
Tannstetter, Georg: *Artificium de applicatione astrologiae ad medicinam, deque conviventia earundem.* Ed. and comm. by Rosemarie Eichinger. Vienna/Münster 2006 (orig.: Strasbourg 1531).
Telle, Joachim: Arzneikunst und der "gemeine Mann". Zum deutsch-lateinischen Sprachenstreit in der frühneuzeitlichen Medizin. In: Herzog August Bibliothek Wolfenbüttel, (ed.): *Pharmazie und der gemeine Mann. Hausarznei und Apotheke in deutschen Schriften der frühen Neuzeit.* Wolfenbüttel 1982, pp. 43–48.
Telle, Joachim: Bartholomäus Carrichter. Zu Leben und Werk eines deutschen Fachschriftstellers des 16. Jahrhunderts. Mit einem Werkverzeichnis von Julian Paulus. In: *Daphnis, Zeitschrift für mittlere deutsche Literatur* 26 (1997), pp. 715–751.
Temkin, Owsei: An historical analysis of the concept of infection. In: idem: *Studies in intellectual history.* Baltimore 1968, pp. 123–147.
Temkin, Owsei: Fernel, Joubert, and Erastus on the specificity of cathartic drugs. In: Allen G. Debus (ed.): *Science, medicine and society in the Renaissance.* Vol. 1. New York 1972, pp. 61–68.
Temkin, Owsei: *Galenism: Rise and decline of a medical philosophy.* Ithaca, N.Y. 1973.
Temkin, Owsei: Studien zum "Sinn"-Begriff in der Medizin. In: *Kyklos* 2 (1929), pp. 21–105.
Temkin, Owsei: *The falling sickness. A history of epilepsy from the Greeks to the beginnings of modern neurology.* 2nd edn. Baltimore/London 1971.
Theodosius, Ioannes Baptista: *Medicinales epistolae LXVIIII.* Basel 1553.
Thoner, Augustinus: *Observationum medicinalium haud trivialium libri quatuor.* Ulm 1649.
Thurn, Nikolaus: Deutsche neulateinische Städtelobgedichte. Ein Vergleich ausgewählter Beispiele des 16. Jahrhunderts. In: *Neulateinisches Jahrbuch* 4 (2002), pp. 253–269.
Thurneisser zum Thurn, Leonhard: *Pison. Das erst Theil. Von kalten, warmen minerischen und metallischen Wassern, sampt der Vergleichunge der Plantarum und Erdgewechsen 10. Bücher.* Frankfurt an der Oder 1572.
Timaeus von Güldenklee, Balthasar: *Casus medicinales praxi triginta sex annorum observati.* Leipzig 1667.
Timaeus von Güldenklee, Balthasar: *Casus et observationes practicae triginta sex annorum.* Leipzig 1691.
Timaeus von Güldenklee, Balthasar: *Responsa medica et diaeteticon opus posthumum.* Leipzig 1668.
Tiraboschi, Girolamo: *Biblioteca modenese.* Vol. II. Modena 1782.

Touwaide, Alain: Galien et la toxicologie. In: Wolfgang Haase (ed.): *Aufstieg und Niedergang der römischen Welt*. Part II: *Principat*. Vol. 37,2. Berlin/New York 1994, pp. 1887–1986.
Tovazzi, Giangrisostomo: *Familiarium tridentinum*. Trento 2006 (http://www.db.ofmtn.pcn.net/ofmtn/files/biblioteca/TOVAZZI%20FAMILIARIUM%20TRIDENTINUM.pdf).
Toxites, Michael: *Spongia stibii adversus Lucae Stenglini medicinae doctoris et physici augustani aspergines*. Strasbourg 1567.
Traister, Barbara Howard: *The notorious astrological physician of London. Works and days of Simon Forman*. Chicago/London 2001.
Trevor-Roper, Hugh: The court physician and Paracelsism. In: Nutton, *Medicine* (1990), pp. 79–94.
Triebs, Michaela: *Die Medizinische Fakultät der Universität Helmstedt (1576–1810). Eine Studie zu ihrer Geschichte unter besonderer Berücksichtigung der Promotions- und Übungsdisputation*. Wiesbaden 1995.
Trincavella, Vettore: *Consilia medica post editionem venetam et lugdunensem, accessione CXXVIII consiliorum locupletata, et per locos communes digesta*. Basel 1587.
Trincavella, Vettore: *Consiliorum medicinalium libri III. Epistolarum medicinalium libri III*. Venice 1586.
Trincavella, Vettore: *De ratione curandi particulares humani corporis affectus praelectiones*. Venice 1575.
Truc, Miroslav: Die gesellschaftliche Aufgabe der Prager Karls-Universität in der zweiten Hälfte des 16. und am Anfang des 17. Jahrhunderts. In: Hans-Bernd Harder (ed.): *Später Humanismus in der Krone* Böhmens *1570–1620*. Dresden 1998, pp. 203–210.
Tulpius, Nicolaus: *Observationum medicarum libri tres*. Amsterdam 1641.
Uhlig, Paul: Auf der Suche nach Stadtärzten: Zwickauer Ratsprotokolle berichten. In: *Sudhoffs Archiv für Geschichte der Medizin und der Naturwissenschaften* 31 (1938), pp. 330–336.
Ullmann, Manfred: *Die Medizin im Islam*. Leiden/Cologne 1970.
Valleriola, François: *Loci medicinae communes, tribus libris digesti*. Lyon 1562.
Valleriola, François: *Loci medicinae communes, tribus libris digesti*. Venice 1563.
Valleriola, François: *Loci medicinae communes, tribus libris digesti, quibus accessit appendix, universa complectens ea, quae ad totius operis integritatem deesse videbantur*. Lyon 1589.
Valleriola, François: *Observationum medicinalium libri sex*. Lyon 1573.
Vanzan-Marchini, Nelli-Elena: *I mali e i rimedi della serenissima*. Venice 1995.
Varanda, Jean: *De morbis mulierum libri III*. Montpellier 1620.
Vekerdy, Lilla: Paracelsus's *Great Wound Surgery*. In: Elizabeth Lane Furdell (ed.): *Textual healing. Essays on medieval and early modern medicine*. Leiden/Boston 2005, pp. 77–99.
Vesal, Andreas: *De humani corporis fabrica*. Basel 1543.
Vieler, Ingrid: *Die deutsche Arztpraxis im 19. Jahrhundert*. Diss. med. Mainz 1958.
Vietor, Peter: *Theses medicae de praefocatione uteri*. Basel 1610.
Vigo, Giovanni da: *The most excellent workes of chirurgerye*. [London] 1543.
Vinař, Josef: *Obrazy z minulosti českého lékařství*. Prague 1959.
Vischer, Christoph: Die Stammbücher der Universitätsbibliothek Basel: ein beschreibendes Verz[eichnis]. In: *Festschrift Karl Schwarber*. Basel 1949, pp.247–264.
Vittore, Benedetto: Medicatio empirica singulorum morborum. Paris 1551.
Vittori, Leonello: *De aegritudinibus infantium tractatus admodum salutifer*. Venice 1557.
Vives, Juan Luís: *De conscribendis epistolis*. Basel 1536.

Vives, Juan Luís: *The passions of the soul* (1543). Ed. by Carlos G. Noreña. Lewiston/Queenston 1990.
Voigtlaender, Heinz: *Löhne und Preise in vier Jahrtausenden*. Speyer 1994.
Waardt, Hans de: Johann Wier. Hofarzt von Herzog Wilhelm und Vorkämpfer für Toleranz. In: Guido von Büren, Ralf-Peter Fuchs and Georg Mölich (eds): *Herrschaft, Hof und Humanismus. Wilhelm V. von Jülich-Kleve-Berg und seine Zeit*. Bielefeld 2018, pp. 573–590.
Wackerbauer, Anton: Dr. Reiner Solenander (Reinhard Gathmann) ein niederrheinischer Arzt, Leibarzt am Düsseldorfer Hofe (1524–1601). In: *Düsseldorfer Jahrbuch. Beiträge zur Geschichte des Niederrheins* 37 (1932/33), pp. 95–140.
Wagner, Wolfgang Eric: Doctores – Practicantes – Empirici. Die Durchsetzung der Medizinischen Fakultäten gegenüber anderen Heilergruppen in Paris und Wien im späten Mittelalter. In: Rainer C. Schwinges (ed.): *Universität im öffentlichen Raum*. Basel 2008, pp. 15–43.
Wallis, Patrick: Competition and cooperation in the early modern medical economy. In: Mark S. R. Jenner and Patrick Wallis (eds): *Medicine and the market in England and its colonies, c. 1450–c. 1850*. London 2007, pp. 47–68.
Walter, Tilmann: Ärztliche Selbstdarstellung im Zeitalter der Fugger und Welser. Epistolarische Strategien und Repräsentationspraktiken bei Felix Platter (1536–1614). In: Angelika Westermann and Stefanie von Welser (eds): *Personen und Milieu. Individualbewusstsein? Persönliches Profil und soziales Umfeld*. Husum 2013, pp. 285–314.
Walter, Tilmann: Ärztehaushalte im 16. Jahrhundert. Einkünfte, Status und Praktiken der Repräsentation. In: *Medizin, Geschichte und Gesellschaft* 27 (2008), pp. 31–73.
Walter, Tilmann: New light on Antiparacelsianism (c. 1570–1610). The medical republic of letters and the idea of progress in science. In: *Sixteenth century journal* 43 (2012), pp. 701–725.
Wear, Andrew: Explorations in Renaissance writings on the practice of medicine. In: Wear, French and Lonie, *Medical Renaissance* (1985), pp. 118–145.
Wear, Andrew: *Knowledge & practice in English medicine, 1550–1680*. Cambridge 2000.
Wear, Andrew: Medical practice in late seventeenth- and early eighteenth-century England: Continuity and union. In: idem, R. K. French and I. M. Lonie (eds): *The medical revolution of the seventeenth century*. Cambridge 1989, pp. 294–320.
Wear, Andrew: Medicine in early modern Europe 1500–1700. In: Conrad Lawrence, Michael Neve, Vivian Nutton, Roy Porter and Andrew Wear: *The Western medical tradition, 800 BC to AD 1800*. Cambridge, 1995, pp. 215–361.
Wear, Andrew: Popularized ideas of health and illness in seventeenth-century France. In: *Seventeenth century French studies* 8 (1986), pp. 229–242.
Wear, Andrew: The spleen in Renaissance anatomy. In: *Medical history* 21 (1977), pp. 43–60.
Wear, Andrea, Roger French and Iain Lonie (eds): *The medical Renaissance of the sixteenth century*. Cambridge 1985.
Webster, Charles: *Paracelsus: Medicine, magic and mission at the end of time*. New Haven/London 2008.
Wehrli, Gustav A.: *Die Bader, Barbiere und Wundärzte im alten Zürich*. Zürich 1927.
Wehrli, Gustav: *Der Zürcher Stadtarzt Dr. Christoph Clauser und seine Stellung zur Reformation der Heilkunde im 16. Jahrhundert. Nebst Faksimileausgabe seiner Harnschrift und seiner Kalender*. Zürich 1924.

Weisser, Olivia: *Ill composed. Sickness, gender, and belief in early modern England.* New Haven/London 2015.
Wellner, Axel: Bergmedicus Christian August Mithoff (1615–1657). Ein Beitrag zur Medizingeschichte des Harzes. In: *Allgemeiner Harz-Berg-Kalender für das Jahr 1984* (1984), pp. 36–38.
Welsch, Georg Hieronymus: *Curationum exotericarum chiliades II.* Ulm 1676.
Welsch, Georg Hieronymus: *Consiliorum medicinalium centuriae IV.* Ulm 1676.
Weston, Robert: *Medical consulting by letter in France, 1665–1789.* Farnham 2013.
Weyer, Johannes: *De praestigiis daemonum libri V.* Basel 1564.
Widmann, Martin and Christoph Mörgeli: *Bader und Wundarzt. Medizinisches Handwerk in vergangenen Tagen.* Zürich 1998.
Wiedemann, Theodor: *Geschichte der Reformation und Gegenreformation im Lande unter der Enns.* Vol. 3: *Die reformatorische Bewegung im Bisthume Passau.* Prague 1882.
Wiegand, Hermann: Volkskunde und Ethnographie bei Konrad Celtis. In: Franz Fuchs (ed.): *Konrad Celtis in Nürnberg.* Wiesbaden 2004, pp. 51–73.
Wightman, William P.D.: Quid sit methodus? "Method" in the sixteenth century medical teaching and "discovery". In: *Journal of the history of medicine* 19 (1964), pp. 360–376.
Williams, Katherine E.: Hysteria in seventeenth-century case records and unpublished manuscripts. In: *History of psychiatry* 1 (1990), pp. 383–401.
Wilson, Adrian: On the history of disease concepts. The case of pleurisy. In: *History of science* 38 (2000), pp. 271–319.
Wittern, Wittern: Die Unterlassung ärztlicher Hilfeleistung in der griechischen Medizin der klassischen Zeit. In: *Münchener medizinische Wochenschrift* 121 (1979), pp. 731–734.
Wittich, Johannes: *Praeservator sanitatis. Ein nützlicher Bericht von den sechs unvormeidlichen [sic] Dingen, zur Gesundheit gantz ersprießlichen, wie man sich in denselben beydes zu Hause und auch über Land verhalten sol.* Leipzig 1590.
Wittstock, Antje: *Melancholia translata: Marsilio Ficinos Melancholie-Begriff im deutschsprachigen Raum des 16. Jahrhunderts.* Göttingen 2011.
Wolf, Kaspar (ed.): *Gynaeciorum, hoc est, de mulierum tum communibus, tum aliis, tum gravidarum, parientium, et puerperarum affectibus et morbis libri.* Basel 1566.
Wolff, Eberhard: "Volksmedizin": Abschied auf Raten. Vom definitorischen zum heuristischen Begriffsverständnis. In: *Zeitschrift für Volkskunde* 94 (1998), pp. 233–257.
Wolff, Fritz: *Kartographen – Autographen* (exhibition catalogue, Hessisches Staatsarchiv in Marburg). Marburg 1990.
Wolff, Jacob: *Die Lehre von der Krebskrankheit von den ältesten Zeiten bis zur Gegenwart.* Vol. 1, 2nd edn. Jena 1929.
Wolfangel, Doris: *Dr. Melchior Ayrer (1520–1579).* Diss. med. Würzburg 1957.
Wolkan, Rudolf: *Geschichte der deutschen Litteratur in Boehmen bis zum Ausgange des XVI. Jahrhunderts.* Prague 1894.
Wolkan, Rudolf: *Geschichte der deutschen Literatur in Böhmen und in den Sudentenländern.* Augsburg 1925.
Wolkan, Rudolf: Handsch, Georg. In: *Allgemeine Deutsche Biographie.* Vol. 49 (1904), pp. 749–751.
Wondrák, Eduard: Der Arzt und Dichter Laurentius Span (1530–1575). In: *Medizinhistorisches Journal* 18 (1983), pp. 238–249.
Worstbrock, Franz Josef (ed.): *Der Brief im Zeitalter der Renaissance.* Weinheim 1983.

Wotschke, Theodor: Johann Theobald Blasius, ein Lissaer Rektor des 16. Jahrhunderts. In: *Deutsche Wissenschaftliche Zeitschrift für Polen* 6 (1925), pp. 1–30.
Wustmann, Gustav: *Der Wirt von Auerbachs Keller. Dr. Heinrich Stromer von Auerbach (1482–1542). Mit sieben Briefen Stromers an Spalatin*. Berlin 1902.
Yeo, Richard: *Notebooks, English virtuosi, and early modern* science. Chicago/London 2014.
Zacchia, Paolo: *Quaestiones medico-legales*. 3rd edn. Amsterdam 1651.
Zahn, G.: Das Herbar des Dr. Caspar Ratzenberger (1598) in der Herzoglichen Bibliothek zu Gotha. In: *Mitteilungen des Thüringischen Botanischen Vereins*. N.F. 16 (1901), pp. 50–121.
Zaunick, Rudolph: Beiträge zur Geschichte der Leipziger chirurgisch-anatomischen Professur vor 1580. In: *Archiv für Geschichte der Medizin* 16 (1924/25), pp. 189–208.
Zedelmaier, Helmut: Navigieren im Text-Universum. Theodor Zwingers *Theatrum vitae humanae*. In: *metaphorik.de* 14 (2008), pp. 113–135.
Zerbi, Gabriele: *Opus perutile de cautelis medicorum*. [Venice, after 1494].
Zinn, Johann Conrad: *Disputatio de vulneribus capitis*. Basel 1595.
Zitter, Miriam: *Die Leibärzte der württembergischen Grafen im 15. Jahrhundert (1397–1496). Zur Medizin an den Höfen von Eberhard dem Milden bis Eberhard im Bart*. Leinfelden/Echterdingen 2000.
Zwinger, Theodor: *Theatrum vitae humanae*. Basel 1586.

Index

absinth 69, 339, 476, 509, 512, 525
acrimonies 133, 144, 189, 244, 265, 268, 276, 283–285, 308, 350, 372, 511
air 33, 35, 39, 100, 135, 146, 154, 197, 205, 233, 237, 245, 302–303, 319, 349, 352, 430, 499, 504, 524
alba amicorum 89–91, 111, 217
Alessandrini, Giulio (1506-1590) 177, 237
Amatus Lusitanus (1511-1568) 155, 272, 297, 311, 350, 389
amulets 277, 368
anatomy X, XIIXXI, XXIV, 8–10, 14, 25, 29, 4460, 67, 74–77, 79, 97, 105, 122, 180, 188, 214, 242, 269, 272, 279, 308, 323–327, 338, 340, 357–358, 360, 385, 392–394, 396–398, 400–401, 404, 411, 444, 517, 529
ancient medicine X, 4–5, 19, 27, 32–34, 36, 69, 76, 85, 90–91, 95, 97, 102, 105, 108, 117, 121, 150, 201, 205, 238, 248, 297, 323, 337, 357–358, 370, 401–403, 528, 531
animal spirits 275
antidotes 299, 360, 379–383, 385
antimony 272, 277, 286, 307, 366, 372–374, 462, 478, 502, 504, 527–528
apoplexy 121, 206, 221, 224–225, 275, 278–281, 431, 456, 458, 499, 515
apostemes 42, 179–180, 193, 266, 395–397
apothecaries 12, 14, 67, 70–73, 97, 125, 198, 247, 294, 320, 322, 354, 362, 373, 383–384, 414, 416–418, 435, 443–444, 466, 475–476, 484, 490, 505–506, 509, 511, 523, 526
Arabic medicine 27–28, 76, 288, 358
Argenterio, Giovanni (1513-1572) 41
aristocracy 7, 20, 84, 97, 239, 278, 295, 306, 310, 353, 362, 379, 383–384, 413, 424–425, 431, 433, 435, 457, 482, 497, 509, 512, 519
Aristotelianism 6–8, 26, 34, 282, 388, 529
Aristotle (384-322) 6, 8, 10, 351
arthritis 30, 192, 202, 248
ascites *see also* dropsy 76, 269, 400

asthma 49, 202, 221, 246, 361, 391, 496, 499
astrology 9, 150–154, 226, 286, 364, 430, 446
Avicenna / Ibn Sīnā (980-1037) 5–6, 26, 28, 30–31, 40, 42, 61, 99, 108, 133, 142, 193, 199, 209, 211, 227, 299, 357, 364, 367

Bacon, Francis (1561-1626) 402, 404
barber-surgeons XII, XXIII, 3, 13, 75, 80, 111, 192, 196, 214–219, 267, 299, 313, 349, 352, 411, 414, 421, 445, 466, 507, 513, 515–517, 533
Basel 12, 16–17, 24–25, 66, 81, 90, 100, 106, 384, 387, 411, 443
baths XXIII, 203, 254, 263, 287, 319–320, 353, 356, 431, 513, 515–517, 524–525
bath-masters 513, 515–517, 524
Bauhin, Caspar (1560-1624) 90, 108, 326
Bellocati, Alvise 29, 38, 44, 51, 56, 58, 160, 196, 210, 244, 272, 395
bezoars 299, 382–383
black bile XVIII, 4, 34, 36, 117, 123, 133, 170, 231, 265, 282, 284, 376
bladder- and kidney stones 133, 144, 214, 224, 252, 256, 258–262, 264, 390, 395, 398, 426, 495
blood XII, XVIII, XXIV, 4, 34–35, 36, 40–41, 49, 52, 64–65, 79, 103, 117, 123, 125–126, 128–131, 133–134, 136–137, 141–144, 147–149, 154, 156, 160–161, 164, 168, 170–173, 184, 190–200, 209–211, 215, 219–220, 230, 232, 234, 236–237, 240, 242, 244, 246–247, 252, 258, 264–265, 267–268, 270, 275, 278, 281, 283–284, 287, 289, 297–299, 325, 328–333, 336, 339–340, 346–347, 350–351, 353, 356, 374–376, 391, 397–400, 431, 470, 480, 483, 500–501, 505, 510, 524, 527, 529
blood letting 171, 173, 192–196, 199, 331, 478, 480

 Open Access. © 2022 Michael Stolberg, published by De Gruyter. This work is licensed under the Creative Commons Attribution-NonCommercial-NoDeratives 4.0 International License.
https://doi.org/10.1515/9783110733549-026

Bologna XXIII, 6, 9, 24, 43, 49, 51, 59–60, 66, 71, 74, 79–80, 136, 158, 177, 188, 198, 201, 208, 220, 262, 357, 389, 451
bones 35, 42, 61, 63–64, 76, 113, 229, 277, 290, 292, 304, 310, 325, 379, 395, 501
Bourdieu, Pierre (1930-2002) 11, 412
botanical gardens 69–73, 96
botany 18, 67, 69–74, 96, 99, 222, 357–358, 402, 404
brain 4, 35–36, 122, 139, 141, 206, 250, 275–276, 279–281, 283, 288, 339–340, 397, 430, 474, 508, 530
breast cancer 267–268, 396
breastfeeding 36, 318, 330, 471, 510
breasts 177, 267–268, 298, 318, 325, 330, 332, 347, 355–356, 396, 471, 527
Brettschneider (aka Placotomus), Johannes (1514-1577) 30–31, 43

calendars 9, 151
Camenicenus, Jacobus († 1565) 73, 172, 454, 477
Camerarius, Joachim II. (1534-1598) IX, 107, 364, 373
camphor 339, 355, 482, 512
Camuzio, Andrea (1512-1587) 432
cancer 55, 133, 221–222, 224, 265–269, 283, 285, 325, 329, 332, 396, 402, 466, 496–497, 509
Capivaccia, Girolamo (1523-1589) 44, 249, 326
Cardano, Girolamo (1501-1576) 151, 391, 405, 497
Carrichter, Bartholomäus († 1567) 375, 391
case histories 80, 96, 117, 119, 121, 151, 223–224, 241, 266, 290, 297, 316, 341, 359, 376, 386–389, 393–394, 404, 438, 485, 517, 532
catarrhs 38, 40, 52, 127, 139, 143, 155, 162, 229, 244, 250, 287, 309–310, 376, 391, 395, 459, 471, 515, 525, 529
catheters 257, 261, 263, 374, 486
Cellarius, Daniel 82, 89, 339
Celsus (fl. 2nd cent.) 76, 397, 498
Celtis, Konrad (1459-1508) 85, 102
childbed 192, 230, 286, 327, 355–356
children 20, 29, 35, 50, 199, 233, 240, 243, 245, 257, 262, 273, 283, 286, 297, 305, 316–321, 330, 333, 347, 352, 441, 447, 474, 489, 508, 524
chyme 123–124, 270
coctio 36, 123–129, 132–133, 138–139, 142, 147–148, 160–164, 170, 184, 201, 206–207, 238, 240, 249, 251, 259, 261, 300, 327, 331, 458, 478, 529, 531, 533
colics 132, 161, 188, 210, 239, 255–257, 259, 263, 277, 397, 434, 480–481, 502, 523
collegia 25, 45, 47, 54, 117, 121, 224, 317, 389, 520
Collinus, Matthaeus (1516-1566) IX, 20–21, 68, 73, 87, 178, 192, 250, 252, 291, 317, 329, 336, 344, 412–413, 462, 477–479, 504
Comes de Monte (aka Panfilio Pigatti) († 1587) 54, 59, 168, 171, 328, 331, 389, 457
complexio 34, 42, 55, 205, 284
consilia XXIII, 45, 48–49, 98, 119, 121, 209, 223, 317, 346, 374, 376, 412
consumption 39, 41, 48, 52, 57, 129, 136–137, 147, 165, 170, 221, 224, 229–230, 233, 241–247, 250, 262, 266, 268, 334, 380, 496–497, 499–500, 502, 523
contagion 39, 135–137, 233, 243, 245, 265, 295–298, 529
contagious diseases 14, 135–137, 209, 233, 243, 245–246, 295–297, 305, 418, 471, 529
contraception 345
convulsions 41, 187, 225, 273–275, 319, 322, 334, 397, 501, 509
coproscopy (examination of the stools) 167–169, 172
Cornarius, Janus (1500-1558) 111, 420
correspondence XI, XIV, XX, 8–9, 16, 25, 45, 83–84, 86–88, 91–99, 105, 111, 120, 134, 152, 206, 255, 394, 401, 410, 415, 420, 424, 433, 443–446, 457, 461, 468, 510
coughing 42, 52, 139, 144, 164, 192, 211, 215, 229, 242, 247, 270, 321, 391, 397, 477, 500–501, 506, 508, 523, 525
court physicians IX, XXIII, 22, 39, 84, 89, 92, 99, 153, 166, 169, 172, 271, 273, 372, 376, 384, 423–428, 430–435, 437, 439–440, 456, 468, 527, 532

Crato, Johannes von Krafftheim (1519-1585) 92, 94, 310, 372, 428, 435
critical days 238
culture-bound syndromes 222
cupping 13, 151, 197–199, 214, 251, 307, 310, 339, 355–356, 430, 490, 514–516, 524
Curaeus, Joachim (1532-1573) 26, 44, 62
curationes 49, 119, 181, 223, 297, 387, 389, 503
curative treatment 33, 181, 202, 247, 359, 362, 378, 432, 483, 497, 516, 522, 526
Curio, Georg (Georg Kleinschmidt) (1498-1556) 53

Da Monte, Giovanni Battista (1489-1551) 10, 29, 37–38, 47, 54–55, 245, 259, 275, 343, 358, 389, 498
death IX, XIII, XIX, 17, 20, 39, 48, 58, 86, 92, 100, 120, 174–176, 211, 226, 233, 240, 243, 274, 278, 280–281, 283, 286, 289, 318, 337, 354, 380–385, 394, 396, 404, 412, 427–428, 432, 440, 461–462, 479–480, 484, 492, 494–495, 497–498, 501–506
decubitus (pressure sores) 217
diagnosis XVIII, 3, 10, 14, 33, 37, 42–43, 53, 55–59, 107, 121, 142–143, 155, 157–158, 163–164, 166, 169, 172–173, 176, 180, 184, 221–222, 226, 228–229, 235, 241–242, 244, 246, 255, 268–269, 271, 281, 289, 306, 337, 340–341, 347–348, 367, 380, 386, 390, 395, 400, 423, 443, 445–446, 457–458, 461, 469–470, 472–474, 494–495, 533
dietetics 33, 146, 148, 204–205, 207–209, 430–431, 445, 482
disputation 82, 107
distillation 364, 370–371, 445, 528
dizziness 134, 278, 337, 340, 342–343, 391, 481
doctorate IX, 8–9, 12, 15–16, 44, 50, 52, 74, 81–83, 87, 220, 410, 413–414
domestic medicine 424, 508–509, 511
Douglas, Mary (1921-2007) 533
dreams XII, 157, 211, 214, 279
dropsy 48–49, 55, 57, 76, 126, 150, 171, 178, 180, 193, 202, 221, 224, 255, 266, 268–273, 368, 379, 389, 395–396, 400, 402, 457, 496, 499–502, 509, 527, 529
dyscrasia 42, 117, 530
dysentery 121, 136–137, 209, 236, 317, 480, 502, 512, 527

Ellenbog, Ulrich (ca 1435-1499) 8, 16
emaciation 126, 193, 203, 229, 243, 245–246, 268, 395, 495, 500–501, 523
emetics 236, 381, 470, 478
emotions 34, 103, 146, 148–150, 205, 230, 276, 280, 288, 290, 343, 351, 434, 460, 484
empiricism XIII, XXI, XXIII, XXIV45–110, 153, 240357, 359, 361, 367–368, 380, 385–386, 388, 392, 401–404, 524, 526, 529
empyema 48, 57, 59, 170, 216, 244, 500
enemas 68, 136, 188, 197, 214, 219, 263, 286, 479–480, 487, 490, 493, 502, 511, 519
England 24, 151, 236, 423, 532
ephemera (one-day-fever) 228–229
epilepsy 4, 39, 108, 144, 153–154, 158, 224, 255, 273–277, 280, 295, 317–319, 321, 336, 360, 368, 381, 490, 494–495
epistolary medical practice 46, 203, 205, 207, 251, 276, 430, 445–446, 469, 530
Erasmus of Rotterdam (1466-1536) 7, 104, 256
Erastus, Thomas (1524-1583) 90, 99, 309–310, 364, 366
errors, medical XII, XIV, 68, 120, 164, 217, 253, 379, 460, 462, 464
ethics, medical XIX, 385
ethnography 99, 101
excrements 52, 168, 185, 187, 203, 253, 284, 328, 378, 481, 483, 494, 510
expectoration 169, 215, 242–245, 247, 267, 332, 473
experimenta (proven remedies) 170, 181, 277, 311–312, 361–362, 368, 457
eye diseases 447

Fabrizi d'Acquapendente, Girolamo (1533-1619) 62, 75

faculties 5, 10, 13, 24, 33–35, 37, 41, 148, 183, 227, 282, 358–360, 368, 370, 378, 404, 520
fainting 76, 131, 165, 197, 221, 274, 332, 336, 340–342
Falloppia, Gabrielle (1522/23-1562) 51, 58, 61–65, 71, 75–78, 188, 196, 200–201, 203, 214, 240, 248, 269, 271–272, 279, 282, 295, 324–325, 371, 380, 385, 395, 526
Ferdinand II, Archduke (1529-1595) IX, XIII, XIV, 134, 203, 233, 288, 289, 292, 311, 370, 381, 426–427, 436, 446, 504
Fernel, Jean (1497-1558) 28, 32, 41, 108, 190, 227, 249–250, 275, 369, 393
Ferrara IX, 9, 44, 52, 59, 66, 74, 79–80, 82, 99, 170, 172, 176, 248, 317, 360, 380, 383, 389, 410, 460
fevers 29, 38, 42, 44, 48, 52, 55, 57–58, 59, 124, 133, 135, 143, 147, 153, 155–156, 160–161, 165, 171, 176–177, 189–191, 195, 201, 207–208, 221–222, 224, 226–240, 243, 246, 266, 268, 270, 274, 286, 317, 319, 321, 328, 332, 355, 362, 370, 376, 389–391, 395, 402, 455, 458, 461–462, 471, 477, 479, 484, 490, 493, 496, 504, 508, 510, 512, 518, 521, 525–526, 529
filth pharmacy (Dreckapotheke) 254, 273
Finzel, Hiob (Jobus Fincelius) (ca 1529-1589) XIX, XXIV, 120, 143, 145, 155, 194, 221, 225, 228–229, 266, 316, 337, 341, 352, 354–355, 421, 425, 440–444, 448, 451–452, 454–455, 532, 463–465
fluxes 38, 40, 52, 78, 121, 125, 127–128, 134, 143, 155, 162, 165, 209, 229, 244, 249–251, 259, 268, 280, 287, 291–292, 299, 308, 310, 376, 391, 395, 430, 458–459, 473, 515, 525–526, 528–529
foetor 244
fomentations 511
Foreest, Pieter van (1521-1597) 50, 80, 164, 387, 393
Fracanzano, Antonio († ca 1567) 26, 29, 38–39, 48, 51, 55, 57–59, 61–62, 67, 70–72, 156, 187, 228, 232, 235, 239, 245, 252, 293, 295–296, 298, 324, 326–327, 330, 333, 338, 350–353, 355, 389
French disease 29, 38, 48, 51, 111, 136–137, 156, 166, 185, 193–194, 221, 224, 251, 285, 289–290, 292–299, 303–307, 363, 366, 368, 370, 418, 456, 466, 471, 482, 487, 516–517, 528
Frigimelica, Francesco (1491/92-1558) 58
Fuchs, Leonhard (1501-1566) 32, 41, 68, 108, 194, 263

Galen 5–6, 7, 26–28, 31–33, 38, 40–43, 52, 61, 63, 65, 67, 69, 76, 78, 82, 108, 113, 122, 141–142, 157, 169, 187, 193–194, 212, 219, 227, 266, 270, 311, 323–324, 330, 340, 359, 364, 367, 371, 377, 400, 496, 502, 531
Galilei, Galileo (1564-1641/42) 8
Gallo, Andrea († 1560) 22–23, 73, 125, 134, 152–154, 166, 169, 176–180, 183–184, 186–187, 190, 193, 199, 201, 209, 211–212, 226, 229, 232, 234, 236–237, 241, 252–253, 257, 261, 263, 265, 270, 272, 276, 281, 284, 289, 292–293, 297, 299, 304, 306–307, 317, 320–321, 331, 338–339, 350, 353–354, 361–362, 370, 384, 390, 396, 412–413, 426, 428, 434, 439–441, 446, 456, 476–478, 480, 500–503, 505, 521
Gasser, Achilles Pirmin (1505-1577) 90, 100–101
genital discharge 156, 162, 209, 327, 333, 456, 486
genitals 139, 141, 210, 290, 323, 325, 327, 487
Gessner, Conrad (1516-1565) 75, 80, 89–91, 106, 326, 373, 436
gonorrhea *see also* genital discharge 156, 291–292, 296
gout *see also* podagra 39, 144, 187, 192, 203, 221, 224–225, 248–256, 261–262, 311, 368, 399, 475, 496, 512, 523
guaiacum 72, 299–300, 304–307, 398, 456, 488
gynecology 29, 50, 64, 224, 318, 323, 325–326, 345

habitus, learned XVII, XXI, 83, 110–111, 403
Habrecht, Isaac (1589-1633) 32, 108
Hagecius of Hajek, Thaddeus (1525-1600) 254, 504
hair 34, 55, 65, 75, 139, 156, 169, 202, 242–243, 277, 282, 290, 294, 303, 306, 320, 327, 382, 430, 508, 515–516
headaches 38, 127, 131, 133, 156, 189, 224, 233, 286, 290, 294, 300, 310, 329, 340, 376, 508, 515, 525
healing baths 263
healing charms 277, 359, 368, 532
healing contract 466
healing springs *see also* thermal springs 379, 488
heart 31, 35–36, 64, 69, 102–103, 128, 131, 133–134, 145, 149, 153, 155, 174–177, 183, 222, 225, 227, 229, 232, 234, 236, 260, 270, 280–281, 288, 319, 332, 336–340, 343, 351, 381, 397, 412, 430, 446, 467, 474, 481, 484, 511, 520, 530
heart tremble (tremor cordis) 153
hectic fevers 42, 228–229, 243, 246, 266, 395, 496
hellebore 67, 277, 373, 481
hematoscopy 171–173, 234
hemiplegia 279
hemoptysis (coughing up blood) 244
hemorrhoids 79, 139, 198, 203, 328, 332, 391
herbal remedies 71, 96, 188, 202, 252, 254, 262–263, 277, 307, 331, 351, 359, 371–373, 376, 475, 482, 489–490, 495, 500, 513, 526
hereditary diseases 39, 243, 250, 262, 279
hernias 77, 214, 218, 265, 488, 517
Hildebrand, archducal court surgeon 178, 216, 244, 267, 276, 286, 297, 303, 311–312, 320, 397–398, 518
Hippocratic medicine 4–5, 8, 26–27, 31, 43, 108, 113, 152, 169, 205–207, 209, 323–324, 364, 367, 459, 498, 531
Hoddeiovinus (Hodiejowsky of Hodiejowa), Johannes (1496-1566) 21, 87–88, 301, 304, 436
homeopathy 264, 378

hospitals 47–49, 50, 51, 53, 55, 66, 79, 117, 137, 158, 170, 186, 283, 379, 387, 397, 411, 414, 418, 439, 491
humanism IX, XXI, XXIII, XXIV27–3183, 85, 87, 89–90, 92–93, 95, 99, 101, 104, 107, 110–111, 249, 255, 289, 358, 388, 401, 403, 405, 437, 498, 531
humoral balance XVIII, XXIII, 42, 68, 117–118, 140–142, 144, 184, 223, 282, 530–531, 533
humors XVIII, XXIII, 4–5, 33, 40, 42, 64, 67, 107, 117–118, 123–125, 130, 132–134, 140–141, 144, 154, 157, 160, 165, 184–185, 187, 189–191, 200–202, 209, 221, 228, 230–233, 249, 252, 259, 265, 279, 282, 285, 298, 310, 341, 350, 359, 367, 370, 376, 390, 399–400, 471, 529–531, 533
hypochondria 179–180, 283, 288, 341, 376, 391
hysteria *see also* suffocation of the womb 334, 337, 341, 344, 402

impotence 210, 488
impurity XIX, XXIII, 7, 111, 122, 126–127, 130–132, 136, 138–139, 143, 160, 164, 169, 184, 191, 254, 267–268, 296, 305, 327, 329–330, 332–333, 470–471, 486, 515, 531
incurable patients 39, 246, 268, 457, 496–501, 503, 505
indurations 126, 130, 177, 179–180, 203, 267, 270–271, 284, 293–294, 329, 395–397, 399, 497
infants 225, 266, 274, 276–277, 316–317, 319–321, 356, 441, 471, 508
infection 135–136, 194, 209, 243, 265, 295–297, 471
infertility 77, 327, 329, 332, 345–346, 488
innate heat 5, 35–36, 55, 57–58, 123–124, 147–149, 160–161, 163, 185, 210, 227, 241, 262, 321, 323, 325, 327, 331, 351
intestines 36, 77, 132, 139, 156, 184–188, 194, 204, 206, 218, 259, 265, 317, 351, 383, 391, 397, 431, 483, 486, 502, 511, 527

jaundice 169, 172, 179, 190, 205–206, 221, 362, 522, 526
Jewish healers 298, 301
joints 40, 46, 127, 209, 248–254, 261, 294, 304, 309, 376
Joubert, Laurent (1529-1582) 347, 498

Keller, Georg († 1603) 8, 15, 17, 24–25, 75, 79
kidneys 36, 82, 123, 133, 139, 144, 156, 163, 209, 224, 234, 252, 255–256, 259–261, 263, 270–271, 395–396, 398–399, 496

Landi, Bassiano († 1562) 17, 32, 48, 141
Lange, Johannes (1485-1565) 80, 99, 216, 517
Latin schools 12, 19, 83, 85, 93, 421
lawyers 463
lay practitioners XII, XVIII, 39, 111, 121, 124, 129, 131, 165, 249, 252, 262–263, 273, 302, 309, 311, 329, 341, 349, 400, 411–412, 466, 507, 517–523, 525–528, 532–533
leeches 198, 524
Lehner, Ulrich (fl. 1550) 15, 20–21, 22, 73, 120, 134, 157, 161, 175–176, 186, 188, 191–192, 210, 215, 236, 238, 250, 252–253, 261, 278, 287–288, 293, 316, 321, 333, 339, 350, 361–362, 379, 413, 439, 441, 458, 486, 499, 502–503, 505, 521
Leiden 47, 314
Leipa (Česka Lipa) IX, XIII, 19, 22, 124, 131, 233, 262, 277, 356, 372, 412, 521–522, 525, 527–528
Leoniceno, Niccolo (1428-1524) 99, 295, 460
leprosy 39, 136, 139, 221, 255, 293–294, 306, 368, 418, 502
liberal arts 3, 5–6, 8–14, 16, 19–20, 23–24, 83, 403, 405, 436, 509–510, 516–517, 527
liver 36, 40, 52, 58–59, 66, 103, 122, 124–129, 131, 133, 139, 141–144, 146, 160, 163, 172, 177, 179–180, 189, 191, 193, 203, 206, 210, 221–222, 260, 265–268, 270–271, 283–284, 298, 375, 390–391, 395–397, 399–400, 431, 456, 458–459, 473, 520, 529
loci communes XXI, 104–111, 152, 401–404

Loxan, Katharina von († 1580) 171, 197, 269, 493
lunatics see also melancholia 288
lungs 36, 128, 170, 173, 189, 193, 229, 242, 244, 246–247, 267, 270, 288, 319, 376, 395, 397–400, 431, 459, 473, 500–501

madness 284–285
Magenbuch, Johannes (1487-1546) 438
magic 254, 277, 312, 353, 359, 363, 519, 532
Manardi, Giovanni (1462-1534) 99, 152, 255, 300, 460, 498
manual examination XVIII, 52, 55, 58–59, 130, 176–180, 271, 399, 487
manus Christi (sugary medicine) 183, 262, 476, 525
masturbation 209–210, 212, 262, 390
mathematics 8, 151
Mattioli, Pietro Andrea (1501-1577) IX, 67–68, 73, 89, 96, 99–101, 152–154, 168, 177–180, 187–188, 192–194, 197, 215, 229, 236, 238, 245, 247, 250–251, 257, 263, 269, 272, 285, 287, 289, 294, 299, 301, 304–308, 312, 318, 320, 340, 354, 361–363, 367, 369–370, 372–374, 376, 381, 383–384, 390, 396, 412–413, 426, 428, 432, 439–441, 456, 460–461, 469, 476–477, 480, 484, 488–489, 502, 504
measles 178, 317, 458, 493
medieval medicine 271, 530
melancholia (disease) 45, 133, 171, 274, 282–288, 341, 376
Melanchthon, Philipp (1497-1560) 10, 91, 106, 256, 371, 430, 506
menopause 268, 331–333
menstruation 40, 45, 49, 65, 130–131, 139, 144, 148, 186, 192–194, 197–198, 209, 211, 224, 230, 250, 260, 265, 268, 275, 287, 327–333, 339–340, 345–347, 349, 355–356, 372, 457, 471–473, 478, 485–486, 527
merchants 311, 438, 440, 455, 463
Mercuriale, Girolamo (1530-1606) 8, 31, 44, 108, 326

mercury 48, 147, 299–303, 305–307, 312, 315, 367, 375, 379–380, 383–384, 482–483, 487–488
midwives 14, 199, 316, 346, 351–354, 418, 486
milk 35, 254, 262, 273, 286, 297, 317, 321, 325, 334, 356, 430, 471
Mitis, Thomas (1523-1591) 21, 87–88, 95, 101, 157, 202
Montpellier 6, 8, 15, 17, 24–25, 43–44, 47, 53–54, 60, 66, 70, 72–73, 79, 82, 84, 177, 326, 357, 498, 519
morbid matter XIX, 39, 56, 122, 127, 135, 138–139, 142, 144, 146, 154–156, 160–162, 169–170, 172, 177, 179, 183–184, 186–193, 200–201, 215, 217, 221, 223, 228, 230–232, 234–238, 240–241, 244, 246, 249–254, 258–259, 263, 265, 279–280, 282–283, 290, 295, 297–300, 304, 310, 331, 339, 359, 395, 399, 471, 478, 482–484, 493, 510, 515, 529, 531, 533
Musa Brasavola, Antonio (1500-1555) 9, 44, 52, 59, 79, 82, 170, 317, 327, 360, 380, 389, 459
music 7, 13, 21, 205, 285

natural history 9, 84, 90, 95–96, 110, 150, 358, 387, 401
natural philosophy 4–5, 6, 11, 26, 33–34, 38, 402, 435
Neefe, Johann (1499-1574) 18, 74, 192, 203, 264, 283, 299, 339, 341, 361, 422, 426, 428, 486, 511, 521
nerves 35, 202, 209, 217, 250–251, 253, 276, 311, 334, 343, 398, 431, 530
non-naturals *see* dietetics
nosebleed 170, 198, 522
nursing 136, 164, 177, 321, 330–331, 339, 351, 356, 462, 470, 489–491, 493–494, 504–505

observationes XII, XIII, 10–97, 110, 119, 121, 181, 223, 241, 258, 316, 319, 328386, 387, 389–390, 394–395, 402–404, 436, 485, 494, 503

obstetrics 14, 199, 316, 346, 351–354, 418, 486
obstructions 58, 124, 129–130, 138–139, 143–144, 148, 155, 157, 163, 177, 180, 184, 189, 191, 193, 209, 221, 230, 236, 239, 250, 257, 263, 265, 268, 270–271, 275, 279–280, 283, 328, 330–331, 333, 347, 349, 376, 390, 431, 457–459, 472–473, 500, 502, 529, 531
one-sex model 323–325
opiates 39, 240, 252, 286, 311, 321, 385, 451, 476, 482, 502

Padovani, Elideo († 1575) 49, 52, 59, 79, 136, 389
Padua IX, XII, XXI, XXIV, 6, 8–9, 10, 14–17, 22–26, 28–29, 32, 37, 39, 41–45, 47–48, 50–51, 54, 59–64, 66, 68–72, 74–75, 78, 80–82, 84, 96, 101, 117, 121, 137, 141–142, 147, 149, 158, 168, 176, 189–190, 201, 203, 210, 224, 226, 232–233, 235–236, 238, 244–245, 252, 269–270, 272, 284, 291, 294–295, 317, 324, 326, 333, 336, 350–352, 357, 360, 363, 371, 383, 389, 395, 410, 412, 487, 515, 522, 526
pain 14, 38, 59, 76, 79, 111, 127–128, 131–133, 156, 161, 165–166, 178–180, 189, 194, 197–198, 200–201, 204, 211, 216, 218, 221, 224, 230, 233, 248–250, 252, 255–257, 259, 262, 264–265, 268, 286, 290, 292–294, 300, 304, 307–313, 315, 317, 320–321, 329, 332, 334, 337–338, 340, 343, 352, 356, 363, 374–376, 383, 391, 396–397, 422, 434, 461, 466, 477, 480, 482–484, 492, 495–497, 499, 502, 508, 511–512, 515, 525
palliative treatment 39, 181, 482, 496–497, 502
Palm, Georg (1543-1591) 438, 441
Paracelsianim 91, 129, 141, 167, 364–369, 371, 374–375, 377–378, 400, 445
Paracelsus (Theophrastus Bombastus von Hohenheim (1493-1541) 74, 80, 216, 363–364, 366–367, 370, 372, 374–375, 517, 524

paracentesis 76, 272
paralysis 202, 206, 221, 263, 279, 281, 306, 317, 361, 374, 382, 398, 431, 496, 509, 521
Paris 6, 15, 18, 24–25, 53, 66, 383
pathognomonic symptoms 42, 273
patient visits XXIII, 44, 47–48, 50–58, 78, 117, 158, 360, 386, 412, 424–425, 454, 502
pestilential fever 137, 191, 201, 228, 232, 236, 471
pharmacies 72, 254, 273, 417, 444
philonium 262, 502
philosophy 4–5, 6, 7, 8, 9, 10, 33, 405, 529
phlegm XVIII, 4, 34, 117, 123–126, 128, 131–133, 135, 138, 142, 144, 160, 162, 168, 170, 184, 189, 208, 230, 232, 259–261, 263, 275–276, 280, 303, 346, 376, 431, 470, 473–474, 489
physician-patient relationship 447–448, 451, 463, 469, 532
placebo 378
plague 14, 25, 39, 100, 137, 189, 199, 205, 232, 243, 289, 361–363, 368, 374, 380, 384, 413, 417, 503, 524
Planerio, Giovanni (1509-1600) 100–101
Platter, Felix (1536-1614) 17, 66, 70, 72, 82, 92, 100, 185, 332, 387, 411, 443, 519
plethora 144, 190, 281, 330
Pliny (61/62-ca 114) 67, 69, 93
podagra see also gout 39, 144, 187, 192, 203, 221, 224–225, 248–256, 261–262, 512, 523
poetry XXI, 11, 19, 21–22, 31–32, 84–90, 92–93, 101–102, 105, 111, 152, 373, 401, 403, 412, 430, 436, 463, 485
Posthius, Johannes (1537-1597) 85
post-mortems XXI, 43, 81, 141, 242, 259, 266, 270, 392–400, 404
practice journals XI, XIX, XXXXIV, 83–120, 143, 155, 194, 221, 223, 225, 229, 266, 316, 337, 341, 354, 376, 386, 425438, 442, 444, 448, 451, 454–455, 463–464, 532
pregnancy 60, 63, 108, 124, 152, 157, 165–166, 286–287, 318–319, 327, 330, 344–345, 347–350, 355–356, 447, 525

pregnancy diagnosis 349
prognosis XXII, 27, 41, 56, 58, 158, 164, 175, 268, 357, 386, 390, 445, 459–460, 462, 472, 479, 494–495, 499–500, 503, 505
proverbs 102
pulse diagnosis 53, 55–58, 107, 112, 149, 173–176, 195, 212, 235, 340, 382, 390, 454, 506
purgatives 154, 156, 183–189, 193–194, 203, 236, 238, 251, 253, 263, 300, 328, 359, 376–377, 471, 477, 483, 490, 498, 519, 525, 528
putrid fevers 56, 176, 228–229, 233, 236

quartan fevers 155, 221, 231–232, 234, 239–240, 268, 376, 496
quintessences 236, 368, 370, 509

radical moisture 227
rashes 111, 186, 193, 204, 214, 235, 286, 292, 306, 317, 320, 458–459, 462, 493
Ratzenberger, Caspar (1533-1603) 71, 96, 312
recipe books 363, 510
regimen see also dietetics 209, 430
Reichart, Zeno 14, 296
Reinesius, Thomas (1587-1667) 12
Reinhold, Erasmus (1511-1553) 107–108, 110
religion 11, 24, 88, 90, 94, 105, 138, 150, 166, 218, 278, 285, 316, 332, 343, 346, 410, 428, 456–457, 459, 463, 468, 493, 496, 505–506
republic of letters XXIII, 83–84, 90, 92–93, 96, 98, 224
retrospective diagnosis 242, 255, 343
Rhazes (854-925) 28, 30, 37, 42, 45, 235, 281, 289, 316
rhubarb 169, 184, 188, 273, 276, 370, 479, 483
Rondelet, Guillaume (1507-1566) 44, 326
rural population 5, 43, 451, 517, 521

scabies 48, 136–137, 233, 243, 292, 297, 299, 320, 374
Schedel, Hartmann (1440-1514) 74, 100, 414, 438

Schentigar, Johannes († 1554) 20, 87, 100–101, 521
scholastic medicine 7, 360
Schurff, Augustin (1495-1548) 30, 38, 67
Schwartz, Johann (fl. ca 1550) 15, 17–18, 66, 410, 427
scirrhus (hardened tumor) 58–59, 78
scurvy 136, 221, 283, 285, 402, 431
secret remedies 64, 311, 339, 361–363, 368, 375, 457
semen (male and female) 132, 139, 144, 209–212, 291, 344–346, 348, 390, 489
seminal flux (gonorrhoea) 156, 291–292, 296, 390
senna 187, 525
Sennert, Daniel (1572-1637) 17
sensibility 448
sexuality *see also* masturbation XII, 64, 178, 205, 209–212, 214, 276, 290–292, 295–297, 305, 344–348, 351, 390, 487, 489, 516
shame 351, 485–487
simples 50, 67–68, 71–73
skin 36, 39, 41, 55, 58, 77, 111, 133–134, 139, 148–149, 172, 177, 180, 186, 188, 193, 197–198, 200–202, 214, 217, 228, 233, 235, 237, 245, 248, 254, 257, 265–268, 282–284, 290, 292–293, 299–300, 303–305, 307, 310, 319–320, 324, 340, 356, 396, 399, 423, 430, 456, 480, 493, 495, 497, 501, 511, 513, 515–517, 525
sleep 146, 148, 205–207, 230, 270, 286, 296, 303, 321, 391, 459, 511
smallpox 295, 317
Solenander, Reiner (1524-1601) 425, 433
soul 7, 10, 34, 37, 94, 147–148, 183, 275, 368, 505
Spach, Israel (1560-1610) 326
Span, Laurentius (1530-1575) 85, 101, 435
specifics 61, 181, 223, 247, 263, 277
spleen 36, 49, 58–59, 122, 129, 131, 136, 143, 165, 179–180, 191, 203, 260, 271, 273, 282–284, 321, 376, 390, 399, 458, 473, 500, 527
sputum 169, 215, 242–245, 247, 267, 332, 473
St. Benedict's thistle 526
St. Gallen 18

stench 13, 100, 104, 184, 244–245, 265–267, 337, 397, 501, 524
stertian fever 171, 191, 221–222, 231, 236, 391, 402, 508, 518, 521
stomach 29, 31, 36, 38, 40, 59, 99, 122–129, 131–132, 134, 136, 139–144, 147, 162, 164–166, 168, 179, 183–185, 188, 194, 203–204, 206–208, 210, 232, 236, 251, 259–261, 266–267, 276, 332, 362, 367, 378, 391, 396–397, 399, 431, 458–459, 470, 472–474, 476–477, 481, 511, 529
stone disease 133, 144, 156, 214, 224, 252, 256–264, 390, 395, 398–399, 426, 495, 517, 525
stools 14, 139, 167–169, 185, 187–188, 203–204, 232, 238, 245, 253, 267, 284, 321, 329, 378, 470, 481, 483, 489, 494, 501, 510
Strobelberger, Johann Stefan (1593-1630) 53, 70, 72
Stromer, Heinrich (1482-1542) 12
studia humanitatis *see also* liberal arts 9, 19, 21
suffocation of the womb 40, 132, 143, 155, 224, 252, 281, 327, 329, 334, 336–343, 345, 355, 490, 529
surgeons *see also* barber-surgeons 3, 64, 74–76, 77, 79–81, 121, 138, 178, 180, 214–216, 218, 220, 244, 257, 264–265, 267–268, 276, 286, 297, 303, 308, 311–313, 320, 383, 397–398, 411, 423, 455, 466–467 507–508, 513, 516–517, 524
surgery 42, 76, 78–81, 154–155, 178, 193, 199, 203, 214, 216–218, 275, 320, 362–363, 396, 423, 495, 516–517
sweat 36, 41, 123, 139, 186, 191, 201, 204, 218, 221, 228, 230, 237–238, 251, 256, 299, 301, 303–304, 382–383, 489, 493, 514–516
Sylvius, Jacobus (1478-1555) 6, 27
symptom (concept) 40

tartaric diseases 129, 367, 400
teeth 61, 136, 189, 216, 233, 244, 264, 275, 303, 307–313, 315, 430, 478, 494, 516

temperament 34, 47, 54–55, 137, 140, 161, 199, 207, 282, 284, 327, 376, 380
terebinth 251, 263
terminal patients 501
terra sigillata 288, 383–384
tertian fevers 48, 155, 221, 231
theology 13–14, 24, 106, 367, 384
therapeutic outcomes 43, 241, 245, 265, 378, 380, 446, 489, 497, 503–504, 519
therapeutic success 16, 56, 77, 161, 187, 193, 196, 217–218, 252–253, 264, 298, 311, 323, 351, 353, 356, 358, 380, 405, 435, 506, 523
thermal springs 101, 202–203, 249, 263, 299, 379, 398–399, 488
Thurneisser, Leonhard (1531-1596) 376, 430, 433, 435, 445, 468
tinnitus 290, 294
tongue 83, 138, 169, 178, 186, 192, 235, 275, 294, 303, 363, 383, 462, 502
toothaches 308–312, 315
tophi 248–249, 252, 399
town physicians XIX, 6, 9, 13, 80, 84, 143, 220, 315, 387, 394, 409–410, 414–425, 435, 440, 443–444, 464, 520
Toxites, Michael (1514-1581) 364, 373, 375
Tremenus, Ludovicus (fl. 1560) 194, 215, 237, 292, 362
Trento 23, 95–96, 101, 196, 211, 219, 241, 263, 278, 284, 397, 410, 523
Trincavella, Vettore (1498-1563) 26, 29, 37, 44–46, 51, 55–56, 58, 78, 171, 210, 224, 228, 230, 232, 238, 270, 284, 295, 298, 328, 389, 526
Tübingen 53, 410
tumors 55, 58, 111, 130, 198, 211, 214, 216, 265–268, 290, 294, 320, 329, 397, 497, 501, 529

ulcers 42, 52, 55, 78, 111, 133, 139, 160, 169, 173, 200, 203, 209–210, 214–217, 244, 252, 259, 265–268, 283–285, 290, 292, 298, 304, 307, 320, 325, 398, 423, 466, 473, 487–488, 497, 508–509, 516–517
unicorn 379, 509, 512

uroscopy XVIII, 49, 53, 55, 107, 129, 158, 160–164, 166–167, 169, 172–173, 176, 234, 237, 258, 262, 348–349, 390, 411, 416, 445, 472–474, 530
uterus 40, 60, 63–64, 78, 128, 130–131, 134, 143, 145, 155, 157, 164, 180, 192–193, 196, 203, 211, 224, 230, 260, 267–268, 275, 318, 323–332, 334, 336–343, 345–347, 350–352, 354–355, 376, 396, 430, 458, 471, 473, 486, 490, 529

Vadian, Joachim (1494-1551) 85
Valleriola, François (1504-1580) 109
vapors 40, 128, 131–134, 139, 144, 160, 162, 164–165, 202, 250, 260, 275–276, 279, 283, 288, 319, 325, 329, 333, 337, 339–341, 373, 376, 459, 474, 516, 529
Venice 25, 39, 51, 54, 137, 187, 520
vertigo see also dizziness 295
Villanova, Arnaldo de (c. 1235-1311) 198, 253
vital heat 5, 35–36, 55, 57–58, 123–124, 133, 147–149, 160–161, 163, 185, 210, 227, 241, 262, 321, 323, 325, 327, 331, 351
vital spirits 57–58, 64, 147–149, 170, 175, 227–228, 340, 351, 353–354, 431

Weckerlin, Caspar (1580-1616) 391
Welser, Anna (1507-1571) 124, 154, 168, 216, 266, 306, 322, 509
Welser, Philippine (1527-1580) 185, 197, 203, 273, 289, 321, 336, 370, 493, 509
Weyer, Johannes (1515-1588) 426
whites (fluor albus) 139, 333
widows 165, 211
Willenbroch, Johannes 39, 125, 129, 153, 166, 169, 175, 177, 179, 194, 196, 219, 243, 247, 249, 272, 276, 286, 355, 360, 363, 367–368, 398, 400, 434, 441, 456, 478, 483, 501
winds 56, 131–132, 208, 259, 317, 367, 488
wine 20, 102–103, 129, 147, 183, 185, 197, 207–208, 218–219, 237, 240, 250, 261, 277, 291, 307, 311–312, 339, 351, 353–355, 357, 371, 375, 382, 391, 421, 425, 434, 465, 472, 476–477, 481, 486–487, 520

witchcraft *see also* magic 49, 212
Wittenberg 17, 25, 30, 38, 53, 66, 68, 91, 105, 144
worms 30, 157, 168, 232, 276–277, 317–319, 371, 458, 470, 509, 511

yellow bile 34, 36, 103, 123, 133, 139, 141, 161, 171, 191, 230–231, 283, 374

Zabarella, Jacopo (1533-1589) 8, 10
Zwinger, Theodor (1533-1588) 17, 90, 106, 109, 224, 434

www.ingramcontent.com/pod-product-compliance
Lightning Source LLC
Chambersburg PA
CBHW070253240426
43661CB00057B/2549